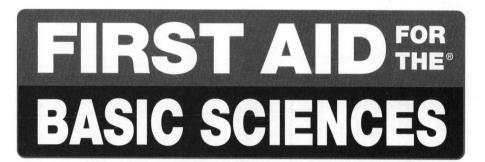

# General Principles

## Third Edition

**SENIOR EDITORS**

**TAO LE, MD, MHS**
Associate Clinical Professor
Chief, Section of Allergy and Immunology
Department of Medicine
University of Louisville

**WILLIAM L. HWANG, MD, PhD**
Resident, Harvard Radiation Oncology Program
Massachusetts General Hospital
Brigham & Women's Hospital

**EDITORS**

**LUKE R.G. PIKE, MD, DPhil**
Resident, Harvard Radiation Oncology Program
Massachusetts General Hospital
Brigham & Women's Hospital

**M. SCOTT MOORE, DO**
Clinical Research Fellow
Affiliated Laboratories, Scottsdale

Mc
Graw
Hill
Education

New York / Chicago / San Francisco / Athens / London / Madrid / Mexico City
Milan / New Delhi / Singapore / Sydney / Toronto

2 3 4 5 6 7 8 9   LMN   21 20 19 18

ISBN 978-1-25-958701-6
MHID 1-25-958701-0

Photo and line art credits for this book begin on page 469 and are considered an extension of this copyright page.
Portions of this book identified with the symbol ℞ are copyright © USMLE-Rx.com (MedIQ Learning, LLC).
Portions of this book identified with the symbol ℞ᵁ are copyright © Dr. Richard Usatine.
Portions of this book identified with the symbol ✳ are under license from other third parties. Please refer to page 469 for a complete list of those image source attribution notices.

---

### NOTICE

Medicine is an ever-changing science. As new research and clinical experience broaden our knowledge, changes in treatment and drug therapy are required. The authors and the publisher of this work have checked with sources believed to be reliable in their efforts to provide information that is complete and generally in accord with the standards accepted at the time of publication. However, in view of the possibility of human error or changes in medical sciences, neither the authors nor the publisher nor any other party who has been involved in the preparation or publication of this work warrants that the information contained herein is in every respect accurate or complete, and they disclaim all responsibility for any errors or omissions or for the results obtained from use of the information contained in this work. Readers are encouraged to confirm the information contained herein with other sources. For example and in particular, readers are advised to check the product information sheet included in the package of each drug they plan to administer to be certain that the information contained in this work is accurate and that changes have not been made in the recommended  dose or in the contraindications for administration. This recommendation is of particular importance in connection with new or infrequently used drugs.

---

The editor was Christina M. Thomas.
The production supervisor was Jeffrey Herzich.
Project management was provided by Rainbow Graphics.

**Library of Congress Cataloging-in-Publication Data**
Le, Tao.
 First aid for the basic sciences. General principles / Tao Le.
    p. ; cm.
 General principles
 Third edition. | New York : McGraw-Hill Education, [2017] | Includes bibliographical references and index.
 LCCN 2016018156 | ISBN 9781259587016 (pbk.) | ISBN 1259587010
 (pbk.)
 1.  MESH: Biological Science Disciplines | Medicine | Behavioral Sciences | Outlines.
 LCC R834.5 | NLM WB 18.2 | DDC 616.02/52–dc23 LC record available at https://lccn.loc.gov/2016018156
 R834.5.F57 2012
 616.02′52 — dc23

International Edition ISBN 978-1-25-992162-9; MHID 1-25-992162-X.

McGraw-Hill Education books are available at special quantity discounts to use as premiums and sales promotions, or for use in corporate training programs. To contact a representative please visit the Contact Us pages at www.mhprofessional.com.

## DEDICATION

To the contributors to this and future editions, who took time to share their knowledge, insight, and humor for the benefit of students and physicians everywhere.

*and*

To our families, friends, and loved ones, who supported us
in the task of assembling this guide.

# Contents

## CONTRIBUTING AUTHORS

**Ezra Baraban, MD**
Yale School of Medicine
Class of 2016

**Nashid H. Chaudhury**
Medical Scientist Training Program
Yale School of Medicine
Class of 2020

**Richard Giovane, MD**
Resident, Department of Family Medicine
University of Alabama

**Jessica F. Johnston, MSc**
Medical Scientist Training Program
Yale School of Medicine
Class of 2020

**Young H. Lim**
Medical Scientist Training Program
Yale School of Medicine
Class of 2020

**Margaret MacGibeny, MS**
Rutgers Robert Wood Johnson Medical School and
    Princeton University MD/PhD program
Class of 2020

**Benjamin B. Massenburg**
Icahn School of Medicine at Mount Sinai
Class of 2017

**Jake Prigoff, MD**
Resident, Department of Surgery
New York Presbyterian Hospital

**Ritchell van Dams, MD, MHS**
Intern, Department of Medicine
Norwalk Hospital

**Zachary Schwam, MD**
Yale School of Medicine
Class of 2016

## FACULTY REVIEWERS

**Susan Baserga, MD, PhD**
Professor, Molecular Biophysics & Biochemistry Genetics and
   Therapeutic Radiology
Yale School of Medicine

**Sheldon Campbell, MD, PhD**
Associate Professor of Laboratory Medicine
Co-director, Attacks and Defenses Master Course
Director, Laboratories at VA CT Healthcare System
Director, Microbiology Fellowship
Yale School of Medicine

**Conrad Fischer, MD**
Residency Program Director, Brookdale University Hospital
   Brooklyn, New York
Associate Professor, Medicine, Physiology, and Pharmacology
Touro College of Medicine

**Matthew Grant, MD**
Assistant Professor of Medicine (Infectious Disease)
Director, Yale Health Travel Medicine
Yale School of Medicine

**Marcel Green, MD**
Resident Physician, Department of Psychiatry
Mount Sinai Health System, St. Luke's–Roosevelt Hospital

**Peter Heeger, MD**
Irene and Arthur Fishberg Professor of Medicine
Translational Transplant Research Center
Department of Medicine
Icahn School of Medicine at Mount Sinai

**Jeffrey W. Hofmann, MD, PhD**
Resident, Department of Pathology
University of California, San Francisco

**Gerald Lee, MD**
Assistant Professor, Department of Pediatrics
University of Louisville School of Medicine

**Alexandros D. Polydorides, MD, PhD**
Associate Professor of Pathology and Medicine (Gastroenterology)
Icahn School of Medicine at Mount Sinai

**Sylvia Wassertheil-Smoller, PhD**
Distinguished University Professor and
   Molly Rosen and Maneoloff Chair in Social Medicine, Emerita
Department of Epidemiology and Population Health
Albert Einstein College of Medicine

**Howard M. Steinman, PhD**
Professor, Department of Biochemistry
Assistant Dean for Biomedical Science Education
Albert Einstein College of Medicine

**Peter Takizawa, PhD**
Assistant Professor, Department of Cell Biology
Director, Medical Studies
Yale School of Medicine

**George J. Trachte, PhD**
Professor, Department of Biomedical Sciences
University of Minnesota

**Prashant Vaishnava, MD**
Assistant Professor, Department of Medicine
Mount Sinai Hospital and Icahn School of Medicine at Mount
   Sinai

**Ana A. Weil, MD**
Instructor in Medicine
Massachusetts General Hospital

# Preface

With this third edition of *First Aid for the Basic Sciences: General Principles,* we continue our commitment to providing students with the most useful and up-to-date preparation guides for the USMLE Step 1. For the past year, a team of authors and editors have worked to update and further improve this third edition. This edition represents a major revision in many ways.

- Brand new Public Health and Patient Safety sections have been added.
- Every page has been carefully reviewed and updated to reflect the most high-yield material for the Step 1 exam.
- New high-yield figures, tables, and mnemonics have been incorporated.
- Margin elements, including flash cards, have been added to assist in optimizing the studying process.
- Hundreds of user comments and suggestions have been incorporated
- Emphasis on integration and linkage of concepts was increased.

This book would not have been possible without the help of the hundreds of students and faculty members who contributed their feedback and suggestions. We invite students and faculty to please share their thoughts and ideas to help us improve *First Aid for the Basic Sciences: General Principles.* (See How to Contribute, p. xiii.)

*Louisville*   Tao Le
*Boston*   William Hwang

# How to Use This Book

Both this text and its companion, *First Aid for the Basic Sciences: Organ Systems*, are designed to fill the need for a high-quality, in-depth, conceptually driven study guide for the USMLE Step 1. They can be used alone or in conjunction with the original *First Aid for the USMLE Step 1*. In this way, students can tailor their own studying experience, calling on either series, according to their mastery of each subject.

Medical students who have used the previous editions of this guide have given us feedback on how best to make use of the book.

- **It is recommended that you begin using this book as early as possible** when learning the basic medical sciences. We advise that you use this book as a companion to your preclinical medical school courses to provide a guide for the concepts that are most important for the USMLE Step 1.
- As you study each discipline, **use the corresponding section in *First Aid for the Basic Sciences: General Principles*** to consolidate the material, deepen your understanding, or clarify concepts.
- As you approach the test, use both *First Aid for the Basic Sciences: General Principles* and *First Aid for the Basic Sciences: Organ Systems* to review challenging concepts.
- Use the margin elements (ie, Flash Forward, Flash Back, Key Fact, Clinical Correlation, Mnemonic, Flash Cards) to test yourself throughout your studies.

To **broaden** your learning strategy, you can **integrate** your *First Aid for the Basic Sciences: General Principles* study with *First Aid for the USMLE Step 1*, *First Aid Cases for the USMLE Step 1*, and *First Aid Q&A for the USMLE Step 1* on a chapter-by-chapter basis.

# Acknowledgments

This has been a collaborative project from the start. We gratefully acknowledge the thoughtful comments and advice of the residents, international medical graduates, medical students, and faculty who have supported the editors and authors in the development of *First Aid for the Basic Sciences: General Principles*.

For support and encouragement throughout the process, we are grateful to Thao Pham and Louise Petersen.

Furthermore, we wish to give credit to our amazing editors and authors, who worked tirelessly on the manuscript. We never cease to be amazed by their dedication, thoughtfulness, and creativity.

Thanks to our publisher, McGraw-Hill Education, for their assistance and guidance. For outstanding editorial work, we thank Allison Battista, Christine Diedrich, Ruth Kaufman, Isabel Nogueira, Emma Underdown, Catherine Johnson, and Hannah Warnshuis. A special thanks to Rainbow Graphics, especially David Hommel, for remarkable production work.

We are also very grateful to the faculty at Uniformed Services University of the Health Sciences (USUHS) for use of their images and Dr. Richard Usatine for his outstanding dermatologic and clinical image contributions.

For contributions and corrections, we thank Abraham Abdul-Hak, Mohamed Abdulla, Zachary Aberman, Andranik Agazaryan, Zain Ahmed, Anas Alabkaa, Allen Avedian, Syed Ayaz, Andrew Beck, Michael Bellew, Konstantinos Belogiannis, Candace Benoit, Brandon Bodie, Aaron Bush, Robert Case, Jr., Anup Chalise, Rajdeep Chana, Sheng-chieh Chang, Yu Chiu, Renee Cholyway, Alice Chuang, Diana Dean, Douglas Dembinski, Kathryn Demitruk, Regina DePietro, Nolan Derr, Vikram Eddy, Alejandra Ellison-Barnes, Leonel Estofan, Tim Evans, Matt Fishman, Emerson Franke, Margaret Funk, Alejandro Garcia, William Gentry, Richard Godby, Shawn Gogia, Marisol Gonzalez, William Graves, Jessie Hanna, Clare Herickhoff, Joyce Ho, Jeff Hodges, David Huang, Andrew Iskandar, Anicia Ivey, Jeffrey James, Angela Jiang, Bradford Jones, Caroline Jones, Charissa Kahue, Sophie Kerszberg, Michael Kertzner, Mani Khorsand Askari, Peeraphol La-orkanchanakun, Juhye Lee, Jessica Liu, Jinyu Lu, James McClurg, Gregory McWhir, Rahul Mehta, Kristen Mengwasser, Aleksandra Miucin, Morgan Moon, Jan Neander, Michael Nguyen, Jay Patel, Nehal Patel, Iqra Patoli, Matthew Peters, Yelyzaveta Plechysta, Qiong Qui, Peter Francis Raguindin, Kenny Rivera, Luis Rivera, Benjamin Robbins, Jorge Roman, Julietta Rubin, Kaivan Salehpour, Abdullah Sarkar, Hoda Shabpiray, Neal Shah, Chris Shoff, Rachael Snow, Gregory Steinberg, Ryan Town, Michael Turgeon, Hunter Upton, Zack Vanderlaan, Christopher Vetter, Liliana Villamil Nunez, Sukanthi Viruthagiri, David Marcus Wang, and Andy Zureick.

*Louisville*   Tao Le
*Boston*   William Hwang

# How to Contribute

To continue to produce a high-yield review source for the USMLE Step 1, you are invited to submit any suggestions or corrections. We also offer paid internships in medical education and publishing ranging from three months to one year (see below for details). Please send us your suggestions for:

- New facts, mnemonics, diagrams, and illustrations
- High-yield topics that may reappear on future Step 1 examinations
- Corrections and other suggestions

For each new entry incorporated into the next edition, you will receive an **Amazon gift card** with a value of up to $20, as well as personal acknowledgment in the next edition. Significant contributions will be compensated at the discretion of the authors. Also let us know about material in this edition that you feel is low yield and should be deleted.

All submissions including potential errata should ideally be supported with hyperlinks to a dynamically updated Web resource such as UpToDate, AccessMedicine, and ClinicalKey.

We welcome potential errata on grammar and style if the change improves readability. Please note that *First Aid* style is somewhat unique; for example, we have fully adopted the *AMA Manual of Style* recommendations on eponyms ("We recommend that the possessive form be omitted in eponymous terms") and on abbreviations (no periods with eg, ie, etc).

The preferred way to submit new entries, clarifications, mnemonics, or potential corrections with a valid, authoritative reference is via our website: **www.firstaidteam.com.**

Alternatively, you can email us at: **firstaidteam@yahoo.com.**

## NOTE TO CONTRIBUTORS

All contributions become property of the authors and are subject to editing and reviewing. Please verify all data and spellings carefully. Contributions should be supported by at least two high-quality references. In the event that similar or duplicate entries are received, only the first complete entry received with valid, authoritative references will be credited. Please follow the style, punctuation, and format of this edition as much as possible.

## AUTHOR OPPORTUNITIES

The *First Aid* author team is pleased to offer part-time and full-time paid internships in medical education and publishing to motivated medical students and physicians. Internships range from a few months (eg, a summer) up to a full year. Participants will have an opportunity to author, edit, and earn academic credit on a wide variety of projects, including the popular *First Aid* series.

English writing/editing experience, familiarity with Microsoft Word, and Internet access are required. For more information, email us at **firstaidteam@yahoo.com** with a résumé and summary of your interest or samples of your work.

# CHAPTER 1

# Anatomy and Histology

## Cellular Anatomy and Histology

### THE CELL

The cell is the most basic structural and functional unit of life. Living organisms are composed of cells, which may exist as independent units or form more complex organisms. Each cell is a collection of integral, diverse components, required for the biochemical processes that sustain the life of the organism. The most important eukaryotic cellular components will be covered in the following sections.

### Plasma Membrane

Every eukaryotic cell is enveloped by an asymmetric lipid bilayer membrane. This membrane consists primarily of two sheets of **phospholipids,** each one-molecule thick (Figure 1-1B). Phospholipids are amphipathic molecules, containing both a water-soluble hydrophilic region and a fat-soluble hydrophobic region (Figure 1-1).

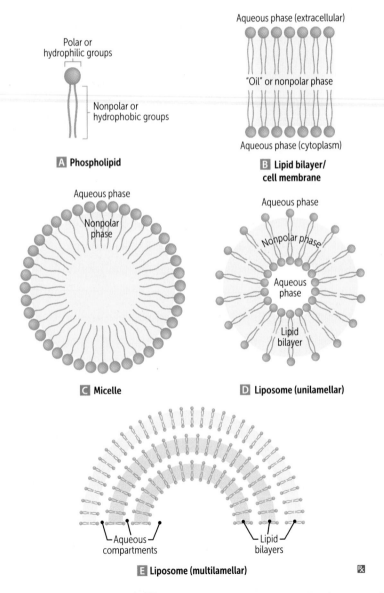

**FIGURE 1-1.** **Amphipathic lipids.** **A** Phospholipid, with a phosphate head group and a lipid tail; **B** lipid bilayer with both aqueous and nonpolar phases; **C** micelle in aqueous solution surrounding a nonpolar core; **D** unilamellar; and **E** multilamellar liposomes.

- The **hydrophilic** portions (ie, phosphate groups) of each phospholipid layer face both the aqueous extracellular environment as well as the aqueous cytoplasm.
- The **hydrophobic** portions of each phospholipid layer (ie, fatty acid chains) make up the fat-soluble center of the phospholipid membrane.

This bilayer membrane also contains **steroid** molecules (derived from **cholesterol**), glycolipids (fatty acids with sugar moieties), sphingolipids, proteins, and glycoproteins (proteins with sugar moieties). The cholesterol and glycolipid molecules alter the physical properties of the membrane (eg, increase the melting point) in relative proportion to their quantity. The proteins serve important and specific roles in the transport and trafficking of nutrients across the membrane, signal transduction, and interactions between the cell and its environment.

The cell membrane performs the following functions:

- Enhances cellular structural stability.
- Protects internal organelles from the external environment.
- Regulates the internal environment (chemical and electrical potential).
- Enables interactions with the external environment (eg, signal transduction and cellular adhesion).

### Nucleus and Nucleolus

The nucleus is the control center of the cell. The nucleus contains genetically encoded information in the form of DNA, which directs the life processes of the cell. It is surrounded by the nuclear membrane, which is composed of two lipid bilayers: The inner membrane defines the boundaries of the nucleus, and the outer membrane is continuous with the **rough endoplasmic reticulum (RER)** (Figure 1-2). In addition to DNA, the nucleus houses a number of important proteins that enable the maintenance (protection, repair, and replication), expression (transcription), and transportation of genetic material (capping, transport).

Most of the cell's **ribosomal RNA (rRNA)** is produced within the nucleus by the **nucleolus.** The rRNA then passes through the **nuclear pores** (transmembrane protein complexes that regulate trafficking across the nuclear membrane) to the cytosol, where it associates with the RER.

### Rough Endoplasmic Reticulum and Ribosomes

As previously described, the RER is home to the majority of the cell's ribosomes. The *rough* in rough endoplasmic reticulum comes from the many ribosomes that stud the membrane of the RER. Ribosomes associate with **transfer RNA (tRNA)** to translate **messenger RNA (mRNA)** into amino acid sequences and, eventually, into proteins (Figure 1-3). The RER functions primarily as the location for membrane and secretory protein production as well as protein modification (Figure 1-2). The RER is highly developed in cell types that produce secretory proteins (eg, pancreatic acinar cells or plasma cells).

### Smooth Endoplasmic Reticulum

The smooth endoplasmic reticulum (SER) is the site of fatty acid and phospholipid production and therefore is highly developed in cells of the adrenal cortex and steroid-secreting cells of the ovaries and testes. Hepatocytes also have a highly developed SER, as they are constantly detoxifying hydrophobic compounds through conjugation and excretion.

### Golgi Apparatus

Shortly after being synthesized, proteins from the RER are packaged into transport vesicles and secreted from the RER. These vesicles travel to and fuse with the **Golgi apparatus.** Within the lumen of the Golgi apparatus, secretory and membrane-bound

**KEY FACT**

Biologically important proteins include transmembrane transporters, ligand-receptor complexes, and ion channels. Protein dysfunction underlies many diseases.

 **FLASH FORWARD**

Genetic mutations may cause dysfunction of regulatory proteins, often leading to debilitating diseases. For example, xeroderma pigmentosum is an autosomal recessive disorder of nucleotide excision repair that leads to increased sensitivity to UV light and increased rates of skin cancer.

**KEY FACT**

The RER in neurons is referred to as Nissl body when viewed under a microscope.

 **FLASH FORWARD**

The cytochrome P-450 system is a family of enzymes located in the SER or mitochondria that metabolize millions of endogenous and exogenous compounds.

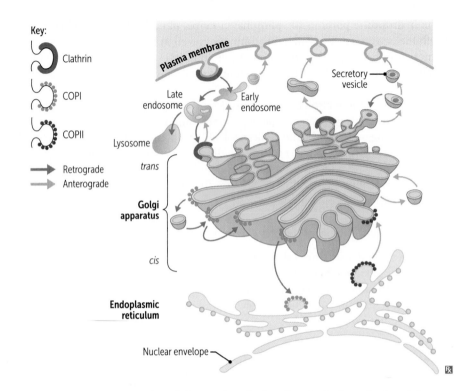

**Key:**

- Clathrin
- COPI
- COPII
- → Retrograde
- → Anterograde

FIGURE 1-2.     **Representation of the rough endoplasmic reticular branch of protein sorting.** Newly synthesized proteins are inserted into the endoplasmic reticulum membrane, or enter the lumen from membrane-bound polyribosomes, depicted as light blue spheres studding the endoplasmic reticulum. Those proteins are then transported out of the endoplasmic reticulum to the Golgi apparatus. Transport to the Golgi apparatus (anterograde transport) is mediated by COPII membrane proteins. Transport from the Golgi apparatus back to the endoplasmic reticulum (retrograde transport) is mediated by COPI membrane proteins. The proteins can be modified in the various subcompartments of the Golgi apparatus and are then segregated and sorted in the trans-Golgi network. Secretory proteins accumulate in secretory storage granules, from which they may be expelled. Proteins destined for the plasma membrane, or those that are secreted in a constitutive manner, are carried out to the cell surface in transport vesicles. This transport is mediated by clathrin membrane proteins. Some proteins enter prelysosomes (late endosomes) and fuse with endosomes to form lysosomes.

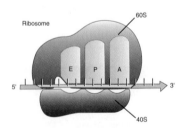

FIGURE 1-3.     **Schematic representation of translation.** Here, the 40S and 60S subunits of rRNA are shown, translating a portion of mRNA in the 5′ to 3′ direction. Many of these ribosomes are located within the membrane of the RER so that their initial protein product ends up within the lumen of the RER, where it undergoes further modification. **E** site, holds **E**mpty tRNA as it **E**xits; **P** site, accommodates growing **P**eptide; **A** site, **A**rriving **A**minoacyl tRNA.

proteins undergo modification. Depending on their final destination, these proteins may be modified in one of the three major regions of Golgi networks: **cis (CGN)**, **medial (MGN)**, or **trans (TGN)**. These proteins are then packaged in a second set of transport vesicles, which bud from the trans side and are delivered to their target locations (eg, organelle membranes, plasma membrane, and lysosomes; Figure 1-2).

### Functions of the Golgi Apparatus

- Distributes proteins and lipids from the endoplasmic reticulum to the plasma membrane, lysosomes, and secretory vesicles.
- Modifies *N*-oligosaccharides on asparagines.
- Adds O-oligosaccharides to serine and threonine residues.
- Assembles proteoglycans from core proteins.
- Adds sulfate to sugars in proteoglycans and tyrosine residues on proteins.
- Adds mannose-6-phosphate to specific proteins (targets the proteins to the lysosome).

### Lysosomes

The lysosome is the **trash collector** of the cell. Bound by a single lipid bilayer, the lysosome is responsible for hydrolytic degradation of obsolete cellular components. Extracellular materials, ingested via endocytosis or phagocytosis, are enveloped in an endo-some (temporary vesicle), which fuses with the lysosome, leading to enzymatic degradation of endosomal contents. Lysosomal enzymes (nucleases, proteases, and phosphatases) are activated at a pH below 4.8. To maintain this pH, the membrane of the lysosome contains a hydrogen ion pump, which uses adenosine triphosphate (ATP) to pump protons into the lysosome, against the concentration gradient.

## Mitochondria

The mitochondria are the primary site of **ATP** production in aerobic respiration. The proteins of the **outer membrane** enable the transport of large molecules (molecular weight ~10,000 daltons) for oxidative respiration. The **inner membrane** is separated from the outer by the intermembranous space and is more selectively permeable (Figure 1-4). The inner membrane has a large surface area due to its numerous folds, known as **cristae**, and it maintains its selectivity with transmembrane proteins. These transmembrane proteins constitute the electron transport chain, and maintain a proton gradient between the intermembranous space and the lumen of the inner membrane. The role of the electron transport chain is to generate energy for storage in the bonds of ATP.

## Microtubules and Cilia

Microtubules are aggregate intracellular protein structures important for cellular **support, rigidity,** and **locomotion**. They consist of α- and β-**tubulin** dimers, each bound to two guanosine triphosphate (GTP) molecules, giving them a positive and negative polarity. They combine to form cylindrical polymers of of 24 nm in diameter and variable lengths (Figure 1-5A). Polymerization occurs slowly at the positive end of the microtubule, but depolymerization occurs rapidly unless a GTP cap is in place.

Microtubules are incorporated into both flagella and **cilia**. Within cilia, the microtubules occur in pairs, known as **doublets**. A single cilium contains nine doublets around its circumference, each linked by an ATPase, **dynein** (Figure 1-5B). Dynein, anchored to one doublet, moves toward the negative end of the microtubule along the length of a neighboring doublet in a coordinated fashion, resulting in ciliary motion. Kinesin is another intracellular transport ATPase that moves toward the positive end of a microtubule, opposite of dynein.

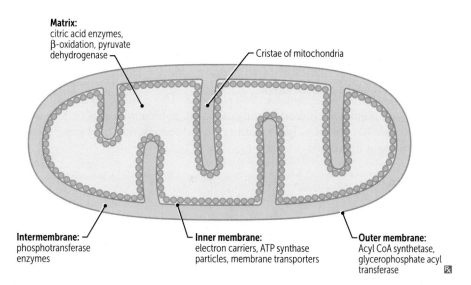

**Matrix:**
citric acid enzymes, β-oxidation, pyruvate dehydrogenase

— Cristae of mitochondria

**Intermembrane:**
phosphotransferase enzymes

**Inner membrane:**
electron carriers, ATP synthase particles, membrane transporters

**Outer membrane:**
Acyl CoA synthetase, glycerophosphate acyl transferase

**FIGURE 1-4.** **Structure of the mitochondrial membranes.** The inner membrane contains many folds, or cristae, and the enzymes for the electron transport chain, used in aerobic cellular respiration, are located here.

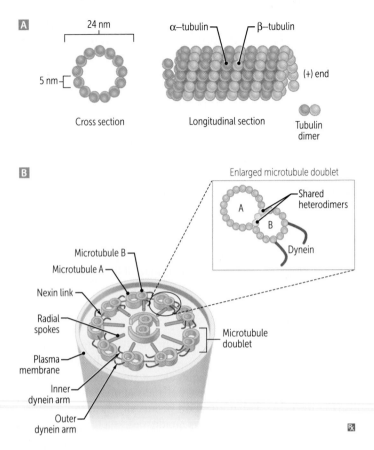

**FIGURE 1-5.** **Microtubules.** **A** Structure. The cylindrical structure of a microtubule is depicted as a circumferential array of 13 dimers of α- and β-tubulin. The tubulin dimers are being added to the positive end of the microtubule. **B** Ciliary structure. Nine microtubule doublets, circumferentially arranged, create motion via coordinated dynein ATP cleavage.

### Epithelial Cell Junctions

Transmembrane proteins mediate intercellular interaction by providing cellular adhesion and cell signaling. Cellular adhesion and communication are vitally important to both the integrity and the function of an organ.

Organs and tissues exposed to the external environment are the most resilient. These tissues are referred to as **epithelial,** primarily due to their embryologic origin. The epithelial cells of these external tissues contain an array of **cell junctions** that mediate cellular adhesion and communication processes. There are five principal types of cell junctions: **zonula occludens (tight junctions), zonula adherens (intermediate junctions), macula adherens (desmosomes), hemidesmosomes,** and **gap junctions (communicating junctions)** (Figure 1-6).

### Zonula Occludens

**Tight junctions,** also referred to as occluding junctions, have the following two primary functions:

- Determine epithelial cell polarity, separating the apical pole from the basolateral pole.
- Regulate passage of substances across the epithelial barrier (**paracellular transport**).

In a typical epithelial tissue, the membranes of adjacent cells meet at regular intervals to seal the paracellular space, preventing the paracellular movement of solutes. These connections occur during the interaction of the junctional protein complex with neighboring cells, composed of **claudins** and **occludins.**

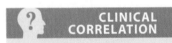

**CLINICAL CORRELATION**

Malignant epithelial cells contained by the basal membrane are termed **carcinoma in situ.** Loss of cell junctions allows penetration through the basement membrane as **invasive carcinoma.** When cells enter the bloodstream or lymphatics and establish new tumors at distant sites, they are considered **metastatic.**

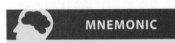

**MNEMONIC**

**CADHE**rins are **C**alcium-dependent **ADHE**sion proteins.

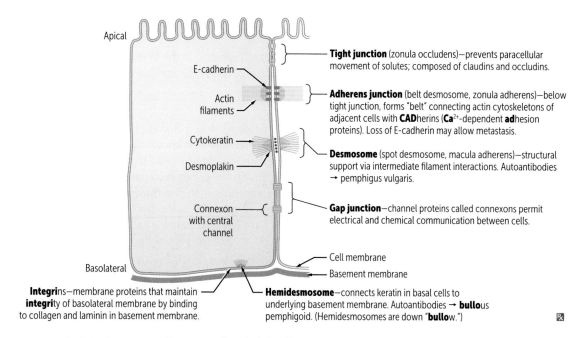

Apical

E-cadherin

Actin filaments

Cytokeratin

Desmoplakin

Connexon with central channel

Basolateral

**Tight junction** (zonula occludens)—prevents paracellular movement of solutes; composed of claudins and occludins.

**Adherens junction** (belt desmosome, zonula adherens)—below tight junction, forms "belt" connecting actin cytoskeletons of adjacent cells with **CAD**herins (**Ca**²⁺-dependent **ad**hesion proteins). Loss of E-cadherin may allow metastasis.

**Desmosome** (spot desmosome, macula adherens)—structural support via intermediate filament interactions. Autoantibodies → pemphigus vulgaris.

**Gap junction**—channel proteins called connexons permit electrical and chemical communication between cells.

Cell membrane

Basement membrane

**Integri**ns—membrane proteins that maintain **integri**ty of basolateral membrane by binding to collagen and laminin in basement membrane.

**Hemidesmosome**—connects keratin in basal cells to underlying basement membrane. Autoantibodies → **bullo**us pemphigoid. (Hemidesmosomes are down "**bullo**w.")

℞

**FIGURE 1-6.** **Epithelial cell junctions.** Five types of epithelial cell junctions are depicted along with their supporting and component proteins.

## Zonula Adherens

Intermediate junctions are located just below tight junctions, near the apical surface of an epithelial layer. Like the zonula occludens, the zonula adherens are located in a beltlike distribution. Inside the cell, these transmembrane protein complexes are associated with actin microfilaments. Outside the cell, **cadherins** from adjacent cells use a calcium-dependent mechanism to span wider intercellular spaces than can the zona occludens. Loss of E-cadherin may allow cancer cells to metastasize.

## Macula Adherens

As opposed to the beltlike distribution of the zonula occludens and adherens, desmosomes resemble spot welds—single rivets erratically spaced below the apical surface of the epithelium. Intracellularly, they are associated with keratin intermediate filaments, providing strength and rigidity to the epithelial surface. Like the zonula adherens, macula adherens are also mediated by calcium-dependent cadherin interactions.

## Hemidesmosomes

These asymmetrical anchors provide epithelial adhesion to the underlying connective tissue layer, the **basement membrane.** The hemidesmosomes contain **integrin** (instead of cadherins), an anchoring protein filament that binds the cell to the basement membrane. Although the intracellular portion structurally resembles that of the desmosome, none of the protein components are conserved, except for the cytoplasmic association with intermediate filaments.

## Gap Junctions

These intercellular junctions allow for rapid transmission of electrical or chemical information from one cell to the next. A connexon is formed from a complex of six **connexin** proteins. Each single **connexon** exists as a hollow cylindrical structure spanning the plasma membrane. When a connexon of one cell is bound to a connexon of an adjacent cell, a gap junction is formed, creating an open channel for fluid and electrolyte transport across cell membranes.

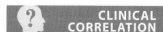

**CLINICAL CORRELATION**

**Pemphigus vulgaris:** An autoimmune disease of the skin due to anti-desmosome antibodies. This disrupts the cohesion between keratinocytes, leading to fragile blisters. The antibodies are distributed in a reticular or "net-like" pattern. Nikolsky sign is positive.

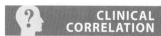

**CLINICAL CORRELATION**

**Bullous pemphigoid:** An autoimmune disease of the skin due to anti-hemidesmosome antibodies. These disrupt the dermal-epidermal junction resulting in separation of the layers in the form of tense bullae. The antibodies are distributed linearly along the basement membrane. Nikolsky sign is negative.

**FLASH FORWARD**

Gap junctions allow for "coupling" of cardiac myocytes, enabling the rapid transmission of electrical depolarization and coordinating contraction during the cardiac cycle.

## HEMATOPOIESIS

Hematopoietic cells are stem cells residing in the bone marrow that can give rise to all mature components of circulating blood cells and immune systems.

### Blood

Blood is composed of cells suspended in a liquid phase. This liquid phase, which consists of water, proteins, and electrolytes is known as **plasma**. $O_2$-carrying red blood cells, known as **erythrocytes**, make up about 45% of blood by volume. This percentage is known as the **hematocrit**. Erythrocytes can be separated from white blood cells, or **leukocytes**, and **platelets** by centrifugation. Erythrocytes form the lowest layer, and leukocytes form the next layer, also known as the **buffy coat**. Plasma from which the platelets and clotting factors have been extracted is called blood **serum**.

### The Pluripotent Stem Cell

The hematopoietic stem cell is the grandfather of all major blood cells. These cells reside within the bone marrow, where **hematopoiesis** (blood cell production) occurs. They are capable of asymmetrical reproduction: simultaneous self-renewal and differentiation.

- **Self-renewal,** integral to the maintenance of future hematopoietic potential, preserves the pool of stem cells.
- **Differentiation** leads to the production of specialized mature cells, necessary for carrying out the major functions of blood.

Two differentiated cell lines derive from the pluripotent stem cell: **myeloid** and **lymphoid** (Figure 1-7). These cells are considered committed, meaning that they have begun the process of differentiation and have lost some of their potential to become cells in an alternate lineage. The myeloid lineage produces six different types of colony-forming units (CFUs), each ending in a distinct mature cell: erythroid (producing erythrocytes), megakaryocyte (producing platelets), basophil, eosinophil, neutrophil, and monocyte (differentiates into macrophage). The lymphoid lineage produces two cell lines: T cells and B cells.

### Erythrocytes

Erythrocytes are nonnucleated, biconcave disks designed for gas exchange. These cells measure approximately 8 μm in diameter, and their biconcave shape increases their surface area for gas exchange, and allows them to squeeze through narrow capillaries. These cells lack organelles, which are extruded shortly after they enter the bloodstream. Instead, they contain only a plasma membrane, a cytoskeleton, hemoglobin, and glycolytic enzymes that help them survive via **anaerobic respiration** (90%) and the hexose monophosphate shunt (10%). This limits the red blood cell life span to approximately 120 days, after which they are mainly removed via macrophages in the spleen, and to a lesser extent, via the liver. Mature erythrocytes are replaced by immature **reticulocytes** produced in the bone marrow. Reticulocytes are distinguished from mature erythrocytes by their slightly larger diameter and reticular (mesh-like) network of ribosomal RNA. Erythropoietin is the hormone that stimulates erythroid progenitor cells to mature by binding to JAK2, a nonreceptor tyrosine kinase.

RBCs are highly dependent on glucose as their energy source, and glucose is transported across the RBC membrane via the glucose transporter (GLUT-1). They are susceptible to free radical damage, but can synthesize glutathione, an important antioxidant. Hemoglobin's ability to transport oxygen is closely associated with the production of 2,3-bisphosphoglycerate (2,3-BPG); 2,3-BPG decreases the affinity of hemoglobin for oxygen, thus improving oxygen delivery to tissues. The iron in hemoglobin is maintained in the ferrous state; ferric iron ($Fe^{3+}$) is reduced to the ferrous ($Fe^{2+}$) state via an NADH-dependent methemoglobin reductase system. Finally, RBCs contain certain enzymes

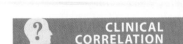

**CLINICAL CORRELATION**

RBC cytoskeletal abnormalities (eg, hereditary spherocytosis, elliptocytosis) and hemoglobinopathies (eg, thalassemias, sickle cell anemia) cause significant morbidity and mortality.

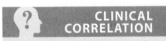

**CLINICAL CORRELATION**

The reticulocyte count increases when the bone marrow increases production to replenish red cell levels in the blood in response to anemia.

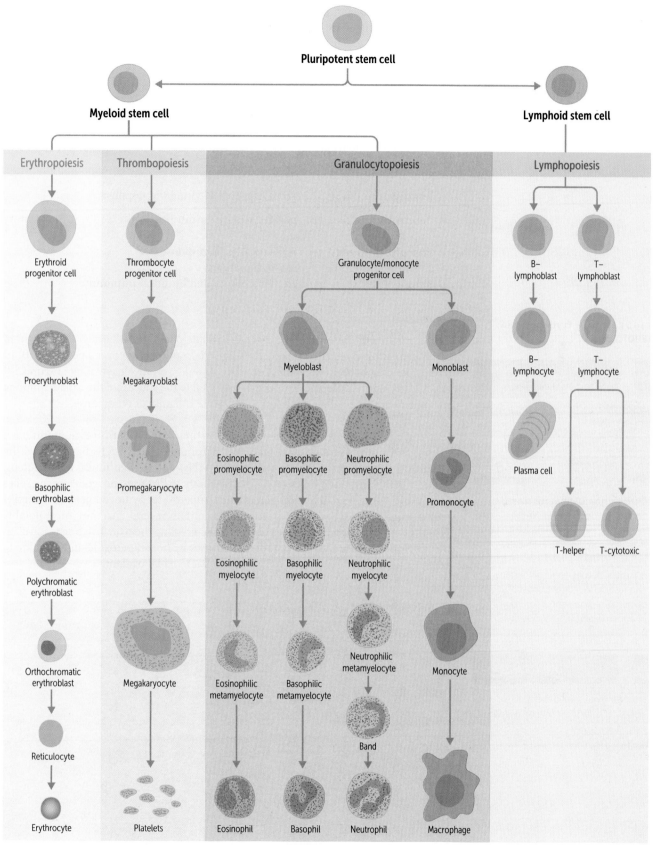

**FIGURE 1-7.    Blood cell differentiation.** A chart of the pluripotent hematopoietic stem cell's differentiation potential.

of nucleotide metabolism, and a deficiency in these enzymes (eg, adenosine deaminase, pyrimidine nucleotidase, and adenylate kinase) is involved in some of the hemolytic anemias.

## Leukocytes

Leukopoiesis is the process of white blood cell production from hematopoietic stem cells. **Neutrophils, basophils, mast cells,** and **eosinophils** develop through a common promyelocyte lineage. **Monocytes** develop from a monoblast. Lymphocytes, although separate from myeloid cells, are also considered leukocytes and arise from the lymphoid stem cell.

All leukocytes are involved in some aspect of the immune response:

- **Neutrophils** affect **nonspecific innate immunity** in the acute inflammatory response.
- **Basophils and mast cells** mediate **allergic responses.**
- **Eosinophils** help fight **parasitic infections.**
- **Lymphocytes** are integral to both **cellular** and **humoral immunity.**

## Neutrophils

These products of the myeloid lineage act as acute-phase granulocytes. They begin in the bone marrow as myeloid stem cells (Figure 1-7) and mature over a period of 10–14 days, producing both primary and secondary granules (promyelocyte stage; Figures 1-9 and 1-10). Once mature, these leukocytes are vital to the success of the innate immune system and are especially prominent in the acute inflammatory response.

Histologically, these cells are distinguished by their large spherical size, multilobed nuclei, and **azurophilic** primary granules **(lysosomes).** These cells have earned the alternative name **polymorphonucleocytes (PMNs)** due to their multilobed nucleus. The key to their immune function lies in the ability of PMNs to phagocytose microbes and destroy them via **reactive oxygen species** (superoxide, hydrogen peroxide, peroxyl radicals, and hydroxyl radicals). Neutrophils contain several enzymes, most notably **NADPH oxidase,** which produces $O_2^-$ radicals, directing the oxidative burst, as well as the **myeloperoxidase (MPO) system,** which uses hydrogen peroxide and chloride to generate hypochlorous acid (HOCl), a potent bactericidal oxidant.

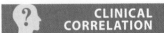
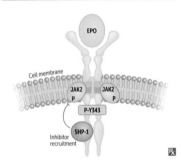

**FIGURE 1-8.** **Erythropoietin (EPO) receptor.**

### KEY FACT

*Leukos* = Greek for white.
*Cytos* = Greek for cell.

### CLINICAL CORRELATION

**Chronic granulomatous disease:** Congenital deficiency of NADPH oxidase impedes the oxidative burst in neutrophils, causing a difficulty in forming the reactive oxygen compounds used to kill pathogens. This results in recurrent bouts of bacterial infection, most commonly pneumonia and skin abscesses.

### KEY FACT

Important neutrophil chemotactic agents: C5a, IL-8, leukotriene B4 (LTB$_4$), kallikrein, platelet-activating factor.

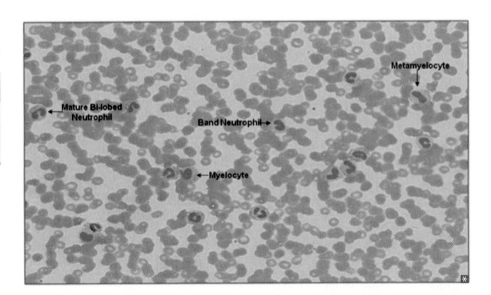

**FIGURE 1-9.** **Peripheral blood smear with neutrophilia.** This peripheral blood smear displays an extreme leukemoid reaction (neutrophilia). Most cells are band and segmented neutrophils.

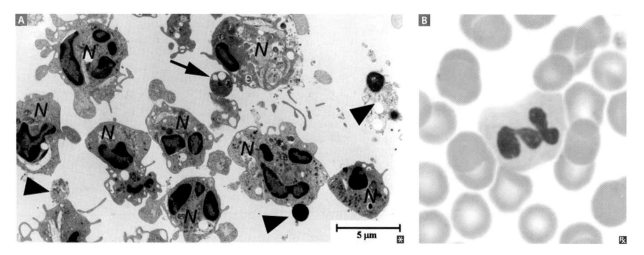

**FIGURE 1-10.    Electron microscopy of neutrophils.** **A** Highly activated neutrophils (N) with apoptotic neutrophils (black arrow) and cell debris (black arrowhead). **B** Neutrophil.

## Eosinophils

Eosinophils follow the same pattern of maturation as neutrophils, beginning in the bone marrow as eosinophilic CFUs. Eosinophils also contain granules with eosinophil peroxidase. However, they differ in that they are slightly larger than neutrophils with cationic proteins, such as **major basic protein** (antiparasitic) and **eosinophilic cationic protein** (antiparasitic) within **acidophilic** (ie, **eosinophilic**) granules. Once fully mature, eosinophils possess a large, bilobed nucleus (not multi-segmented like neutrophils) and sparse endoplasmic reticulum and Golgi vesicles (Figure 1-11).

## Basophils and Mast Cells

Distinguished by large, coarse, darkly staining granules, basophils produce peroxidase, **heparin,** and **histamine** (Figure 1-12). Basophils also release **kallikrein,** which acts as an eosinophil chemoattractant during hypersensitivity reactions, such as contact allergies and skin allograft rejection. Because they share a great deal of structural similarities, basophils can be considered the blood-borne counterpart of the **mast cell,** which resides within tissues, near blood vessels. Both mast cells and basophils produce histamine and

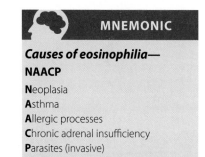

**MNEMONIC**

*Causes of eosinophilia—*
**NAACP**
**N**eoplasia
**A**sthma
**A**llergic processes
**C**hronic adrenal insufficiency
**P**arasites (invasive)

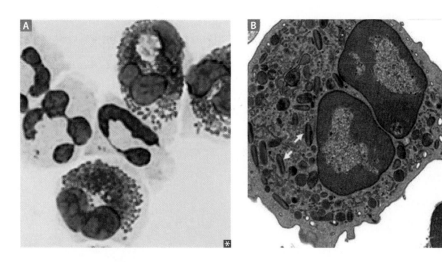

**FIGURE 1-11.    Eosinophil microscopy.** **A** Mature eosinophil with bright red granules. **B** Electron microscopy of eosinophils with bilobed nuclei and specific granules in the shape of a football with a crystalline core made from major basic protein.

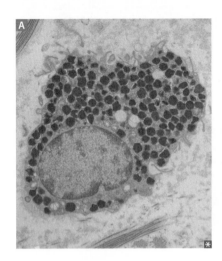
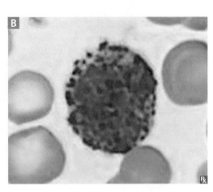

**FIGURE 1-12.** **Basophil microscopy.** A Electron micrograph of a normal intact mast cell with homogenous electron-dense granules. B Basophil.

heparin, but mast cells also contain serotonin (5-HT), which basophils lack. Mast cells degranulate during the acute phase of inflammation, acting, via their released granule contents, on the nearby vasculature. This leads to vasodilation, fluid transudation, and swelling of interstitial tissues.

## Monocyte Lineage

### Monocytes

Monocytes are the myeloid precursor to the mononuclear phagocyte, the tissue macrophage. Morphologically, they appear as spherical cells with scattered small granules, akin to lysosomes. The blood monocyte is a large (10–18 μm), motile cell that marginates along the vessel wall in response to the expression of specific cell adhesion proteins. During an inflammatory response, these cell adhesion proteins (namely, platelet endothelial cell adhesion molecule, or **PECAM-1**) facilitate monocyte **diapedesis** (transmigration) across vessel walls into surrounding tissues. Once in close proximity to the inflammatory foci, the monocyte differentiates into a macrophage with increased phagocytic and lysosomal activity (Figure 1-13).

### Macrophages

During differentiation, monocyte cell volume and lysosome numbers increase. These lysosomes fuse with phagosomes to degrade ingested cellular and noncellular material.

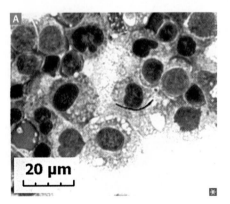
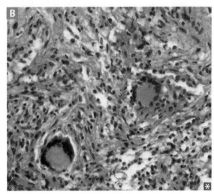

20 μm

**FIGURE 1-13.** **Macrophage microscopy.** A Active macrophage and B multinucleated giant cell.

Macrophages (20–80 µm) also contain a large number of cell surface receptors. These differ, depending on the tissue in which the macrophage matures, contributing to the diversity of macrophage functions (Table 1-1).

As described in Table 1-1, monocyte-derived cells are distributed among several organs and tissues (including connective tissue and bone) where they reside (termed tissue-resident macrophages). Alternatively, monocytes can migrate into tissues during an acute inflammatory response and, there, transform into reactive macrophages to aid the innate immune system. Once out of the circulation, monocytes have a half-life of up to 70 hours. Their numbers within inflamed tissues begin to overcome those of neutrophils after approximately 12 hours.

### Multinucleated Giant Cells

At sites of chronic inflammation, such as tuberculous lung tissue, macrophages sometimes fuse to produce multinucleated phagocytes (Figure 1-13). These microbicidal cells can be produced in vitro via interferon-γ (IFN-γ) or interleukin-3 (IL-3) stimulation.

### Antigen-Presenting Cells

Antigen-presenting cells (**APCs**) are essential to the adaptive immune system. These monocyte-derived phagocytic cells take up antigens (primarily protein particles), process them, display them bound to the **major histocompatibility complex (MHC) II** cell surface marker, and travel to lymph nodes, where they recruit other cells of the immune system into action. Dendritic cells are especially important in the initial exposure to a new antigen. Successful differentiation from monocytes depends on an endothelial cell signal that is secondary to foreign antigen exposure. In the absence of this second signal, these sensitized monocytes transform into macrophages.

### Lymphocytes

Lymphocytes are easily distinguished from other leukocytes by their shared morphology (Figures 1-14 and 1-15). After differentiating from lymphoblasts within the marrow, they migrate to the blood as spherical cells, 6–15 µm in diameter. Typically, the nucleus contains tightly packed chromatin, which stains a deep blue or purple and occupies approximately 90% of the cell cytoplasm.

As the primary actors in the adaptive immune response, lymphocytes undergo biochemical transformation into active immune cells via coordinated stimulatory signals. These activated lymphocytes then enter the cell cycle, producing a number of identical daughter cells. They eventually settle into $G_0$ as a memory cell while they await the

### CLINICAL CORRELATION

Lipid A from bacterial lipopolysaccharide (LPS) binds CD14 on macrophages to induce cytokine release. Toxic shock syndrome is caused by preformed *Staphylococcus aureus* toxic shock syndrome toxin (TSST-1), which acts as a superantigen and causes massive cytokine release.

### KEY FACT

Macrophages are activated by IFN-γ. They can function as antigen-presenting cells via MHC II.

### FLASH FORWARD

Dendritic cells are the most important APCs in the body and they are responsible for initiation of adaptive immunity.

**TABLE 1-1.** **Distribution of Mononuclear Phagocytes**

| | |
|---|---|
| Marrow | Monoblasts, promonocytes, monocytes, macrophages |
| Blood | Monocytes |
| Body cavities | Pleural macrophages, peritoneal macrophages |
| Inflammatory tissues | Epithelioid cells, exudate macrophages, multinucleated giant cells |
| Tissues | Liver (Kupffer cells), lung (alveolar macrophages), connective tissue (histiocytes), spleen (red pulp macrophages), lymph nodes, thymus, bone (osteoclasts), synovium (type A cells), mucosa-associated lymphoid tissue, gastrointestinal tract, genitourinary tract, endocrine organs, central nervous system (microglia), skin (dendritic cells) |

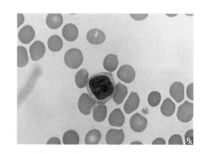

**FIGURE 1-14.** **Light microscopy of a lymphocyte from a blood smear.** Medium-sized agranular lymphocyte (stained purple) with a high nuclear to cytoplasmic ratio and a condensed chromatin pattern.

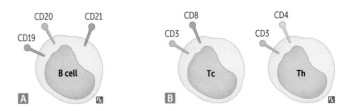

**FIGURE 1-15.** **Lymphocytes.** A B cell and B T cell.

next stimulation event. Alternatively, following replication, daughter cells can become terminally differentiated lymphocytes, primed for effector and secretory roles in immunologic defense of the host organism.

### B Cells and Plasma Cells

B cells are the "long-range artillery" in the adaptive immune response. After the lymphoblast stage, the lymphocyte lineage diverges into B cells and T cells, each performing separate roles in the adaptive, or **humoral, immune response.** Once committed, **B cells develop in the B**one marrow and then migrate to other lymphoid organs. As they develop, B cells express immunoglobulins (IgM and IgD) on their surface, in association with costimulatory proteins. These **B-cell antigen receptor complexes** allow for the recognition of foreign antigens and subsequent activation of the B cell. Downstream cell signaling leads to the expression of necessary genes for terminal differentiation to **plasma cells** that produce and secrete antibodies to aid the specific immune response. B cells that recognize self-antigens are triggered to undergo programmed cell death, or **apoptosis,** to reduce the chance of autoimmunity.

### T Cells

T cells are the "infantry" of the adaptive immune response. During maturation in the **T**hymus, early T cells begin expressing several surface receptors simultaneously, including the T-cell receptor (**TCR**), **CD4,** and **CD8.** If one of these CD receptors recognizes **receptors** of thymic APCs, either **MHC II** or **I,** respectively, then this T cell is **positively selected,** proliferates, and matures. If a T cell recognizes self-antigen, then it is **negatively selected,** and undergoes apoptosis. All T cells express CD3, and either CD4 (helper T cells), or CD8 (cytotoxic T cells).

### Helper T Cells

Two subtypes of T helper cells are derived from the CD4+ progenitor: Th1 and Th2. Th1 responses occur in the presence of intracellular pathogens. Helminthic or **parasitic infections,** on the other hand, drive Th2-mediated immune responses.

Helper T cells spring into action when they recognize foreign antigens bound to MHC II. Once activated, they secrete **cytokines,** chemical messengers that recruit and activate other immune effector cells. These cytokines, also called **interleukins,** specifically attract B cells, which, in turn, divide and differentiate into plasma cells. After the immune response is complete, some helper T cells become **memory cells**—quiescent immune cells that retain their specificity in case of a rechallenge with the same antigen in the future. The presence of memory cells increases the speed and efficiency of future immune responses.

### Cytotoxic T Cells

CD8+ T cells also proliferate in response to cytokines; however, they only recognize antigens in association with class I MHC. These cells are actively involved in immune surveillance of intracellular pathogens.

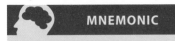

**MNEMONIC**

MHC × CD = 8 (eg, MHC II × CD4 = 8, and MHC I × CD8 = 8).

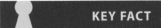

**KEY FACT**

Helper T cells "help" by mediating the specificity of the adaptive immune response. They act as a messenger between APCs and B cells, triggering humoral immunity.

**Every human cell contains MHC I, but only APCs contain MHC II.**

- A cell infected by an intracellular pathogen (ie, a virus) processes viral proteins and presents them on the surface via MHC I.
- A roving CD8+ T cell recognizes this signal and attaches to the infected cell via cell adhesion molecules.
- The activated cytotoxic T cell releases **perforins,** which are proteins that form holes in the plasma membrane of targeted cells.

# Gross Anatomy and Histology

## ABDOMINAL WALL ANATOMY

### Layers of the Abdominal Wall

The order of the layers of the anterior abdominal wall differs depending on location. They are depicted in Figure 1-16.

The abdominal muscle aponeuroses comprising the rectus sheath differ above and below the arcuate line. The arcuate line is a horizontal line at the level where the inferior epigastric vessels perforate the rectus abdominis (Figure 1-16). Above the umbilicus, the rectus abdominis muscle is enveloped in the aponeurosis of the internal oblique muscle, with the aponeurosis of the external oblique anterior to the rectus sheath. Below the arcuate line, the anterior rectus sheath is composed of all three abdominal muscle aponeuroses (external oblique, internal oblique, and transversus abdominis). Deep to the muscle layer is the extraperitoneal tissue and transversalis fascia. The parietal peritoneum is deep to that fascia.

### Inguinal Canal

The inguinal canal is an oblique, inferomedially directed channel through which the testes and its vessels and nerves traverse the abdominal wall to reach the scrotum (Figure 1-17). As the testis descends, it carries a sheath of peritoneal sac (tunica vaginalis) into which it invaginates acquiring a partial covering. The inguinal canal lies superior and parallel to the **inguinal ligament,** allows the passage of the **round ligament** of the uterus in women and the **spermatic cord** (ductus deferens and testicular vessels) in men. The canal has two openings: the **internal** (or **deep**) and **external** (or **superficial**) **inguinal rings.** The transversalis fascia evaginates through the abdominal wall and continues as a covering of structures passing through the abdominal wall. The superficial ring is actually an opening through the external oblique aponeurosis. If the protrusion occurs at the site of the deep inguinal ring, the hernia is indirect (Figure 1-18). If the weakness occurs medial to the inferior epigastric vessels, the hernia is direct (Figure 1-18).

### Retroperitoneum

The posterior abdominal cavity contains several important structures situated between the parietal peritoneum and the posterior abdominal wall. This region, the retroperitoneum, contains portions of the gastrointestinal, genitourinary, endocrine, and vascular systems (Figure 1-19).

### The Pectinate Line

The pectinate (dentate) line is the mucocutaneous junction where the endoderm meets the ectoderm in the anal canal. In the developing embryo, the endodermally derived hindgut fuses with the ectodermally derived external anal sphincter (Figure 1-20). Tissues on each side of this boundary are fed by separate neurovascular sources (Table 1-2).

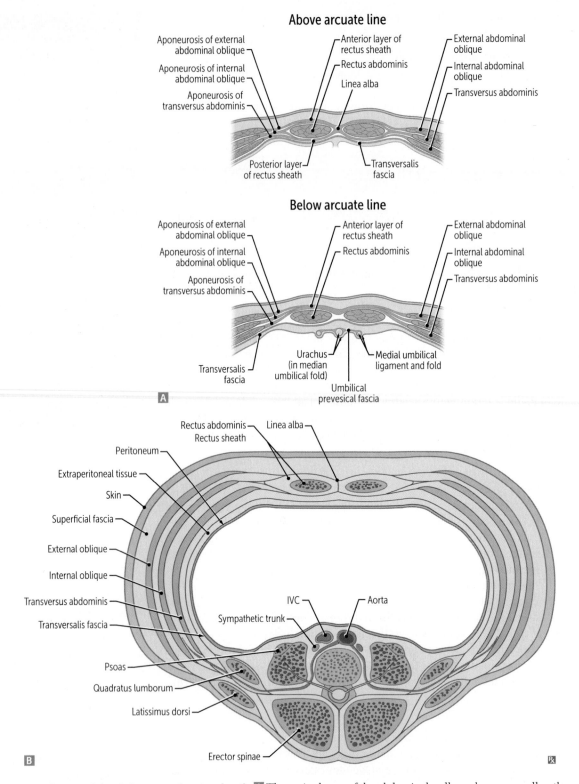

**Above arcuate line**

Aponeurosis of external abdominal oblique

Aponeurosis of internal abdominal oblique

Aponeurosis of transversus abdominis

Anterior layer of rectus sheath

Rectus abdominis

Linea alba

External abdominal oblique

Internal abdominal oblique

Transversus abdominis

Posterior layer of rectus sheath

Transversalis fascia

**Below arcuate line**

Aponeurosis of external abdominal oblique

Aponeurosis of internal abdominal oblique

Aponeurosis of transversus abdominis

Anterior layer of rectus sheath

Rectus abdominis

External abdominal oblique

Internal abdominal oblique

Transversus abdominis

Transversalis fascia

Urachus (in median umbilical fold)

Medial umbilical ligament and fold

Umbilical prevesical fascia

**A**

Rectus abdominis

Rectus sheath

Linea alba

Peritoneum

Extraperitoneal tissue

Skin

Superficial fascia

External oblique

Internal oblique

Transversus abdominis

Transversalis fascia

Psoas

Quadratus lumborum

Latissimus dorsi

IVC

Aorta

Sympathetic trunk

Erector spinae

**B**

**FIGURE 1-16.** **Layers of the abdomen and rectus sheath. A** The major layers of the abdominal wall are shown, as well as the relation of several retroperitoneal structures. IVC, inferior vena cava. **B** Superior to the arcuate line, the rectus abdominis muscle is wrapped by the aponeurosis of the internal oblique muscle. Inferior to the arcuate line, the rectus abdominis muscle lies posterior to the aponeuroses of both the internal oblique and transversus abdominis muscles; the posterior wall of the rectus sheath is only formed by the transversalis fascia.

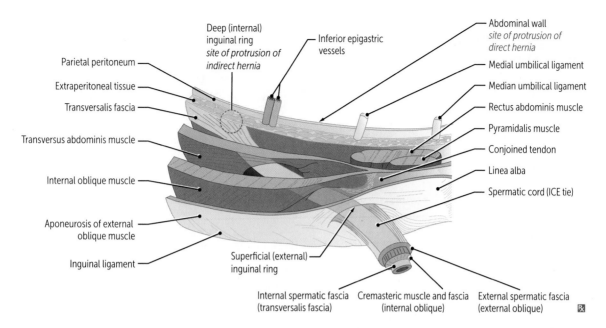

**FIGURE 1-17.** **Inguinal canal.** The location and contents of the male inguinal canal, as well as the abdominal wall layers it traverses, are shown. Other important anatomic relations are also highlighted, including umbilical ligaments and inferior epigastric vessels. The locations of direct and indirect hernias are also labeled.

## THE GASTROINTESTINAL SYSTEM

### Small Intestinal Layers

The small intestine, the major organ of nutrient absorption from the gut, is composed of several layers, each contributing to the coordination of digestion and transport (Figure 1-21).

- **Mucosa:** Absorption.
- **Submucosa:** Vascular and lymphatic supply.
- **Muscularis externa:** Mechanical mixing, dissociation, and propulsion.
- **Serosa:** Protection.

### Mucosa

The intestinal mucosa, the absorption barrier of the alimentary canal, is composed of polarized epithelial cells specialized in transport and uses several molecular and structural adaptations that allow it to efficiently extract nutrients from food.

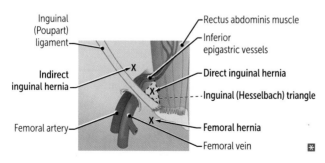
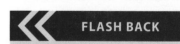

**FIGURE 1-18.** **Inguinal area.** Locations where indirect and direct inguinal hernias, and femoral hernias, may occur.

---

**MNEMONIC**

***Retroperitoneal structures—*
SAD PUCKER**

**S**uprarenal (adrenal) glands [not shown]
**A**orta and IVC
**D**uodenum (2nd through 4th parts)
**P**ancreas (except tail)
**U**reters [not shown]
**C**olon (descending and ascending)
**K**idneys
**E**sophagus (thoracic portion) [not shown]
**R**ectum (upper segment) [not shown]

---

**CLINICAL CORRELATION**

**Ulcers** can extend into the submucosa, inner, or outer muscular layer. **Erosions** are in the mucosa only.

---

**FLASH BACK**

Molecularly, the intestinal epithelium employs cell adhesion molecules to determine polarity and maintain the physical barrier between the body and the intestinal lumen (external environment).

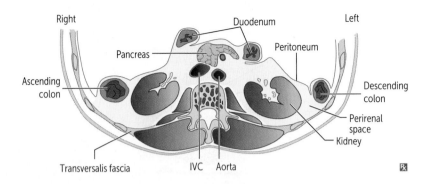

**FIGURE 1-19.** **Retroperitoneal structures.** The anatomic relations of important retroperitoneal structures are shown.

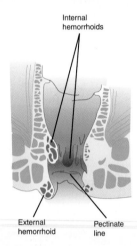

**FIGURE 1-20.** **Pectinate line.** A comparison of internal hemorrhoids (internal rectal vessels) and external hemorrhoids (external rectal vessels) is shown, highlighting their separation by the pectinate line. The endodermal and ectodermal origins of these structures underlie the anatomic distinction between them.

Structurally, the mucosa has four adaptations that increase the absorptive surface area:

- **Plicae circulares** (circular folds, or **valves of Kerckring**): Permanent folding of the mucosa and submucosa into the lumen of the small intestine. They begin in the duodenum, peak in distribution in the duodenojejunal junction, and end in the mid ileum.
- **Intestinal villi:** Finger-like projections of the mucosa into the lumen that extend deep into the mucosa to the muscularis mucosa. At the bottom of intestinal villi are intestinal glands.
- **Intestinal glands (or crypts of Lieberkühn):** Nonsecretory glands that enhance absorption.
- **Microvilli (brush border):** On the apical border of each enterocyte, or intestinal epithelial cell, the surface area is approximately 30-fold. Contains a core of parallel, cross-linked actin filaments bound to cytoskeletal proteins. The brush border is coated in a glycocalyx, a surface coat of glycoproteins excreted by columnar secretory goblet cells.

The luminal membrane of intestinal epithelial cells contains several intramembranous enzymes (eg, maltase, lactase, enterokinase) integral to digestion and small-molecule absorption. Intracytoplasmic enzymes break down absorbed di- and tripeptides.

## Submucosa

The submucosa is the site of vascular and lymphatic supply to the intestine. This layer, composed of loose connective tissue, contains a vascular plexus that extends capillaries into the surrounding layers. The lymphatic drainage of the submucosa begins as blind-ended channels, known as **lacteals,** within the core of the intestinal villi. These lacteals empty into a submucosal lymphatic plexus that shuttles antigens to nearby lymphatic nodules and emulsified fat-soluble nutrients to the liver.

**TABLE 1-2.** **Pectinate Line**

| CHARACTERISTICS | ABOVE | BELOW |
| --- | --- | --- |
| Cell types | Glandular epithelium | Squamous epithelium |
| Cancer type | Adenocarcinoma | Squamous cell carcinoma |
| Innervation | Visceral | Somatic |
| Hemorrhoids | Internal (painless) | External (painful) |
| Arterial supply | Superior rectal artery (branch of inferior mesenteric artery) | Inferior rectal artery (branch of internal pudendal artery) |
| Venous drainage | Superior rectal vein → inferior mesenteric vein → portal system | Inferior rectal vein → internal pudendal vein → internal iliac vein → common iliac vein → IVC |

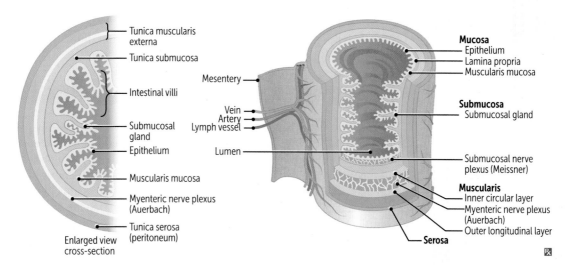

Tunica muscularis externa
Tunica submucosa
Intestinal villi
Submucosal gland
Epithelium
Muscularis mucosa
Myenteric nerve plexus (Auerbach)
Tunica serosa (peritoneum)
Enlarged view cross-section

Mesentery
Vein
Artery
Lymph vessel
Lumen

**Mucosa**
Epithelium
Lamina propria
Muscularis mucosa
**Submucosa**
Submucosal gland
Submucosal nerve plexus (Meissner)
**Muscularis**
Inner circular layer
Myenteric nerve plexus (Auerbach)
Outer longitudinal layer
**Serosa**

**FIGURE 1-21.    Anatomy of the small intestines, depicting the various tissue layers and nerve plexuses.**

Within the **duodenum,** the submucosa contains **Brunner glands,** tubuloacinar mucous glands that produce an alkaline (pH ~ 9) secretion to neutralize acidified chyme from the stomach. Within the **ileum** reside the lymphatic nodules that provide immunologic surveillance to the intestines. These nodules, also known as **Peyer patches** (Figure 1-22), or **mucosa-associated lymphoid tissue (MALT),** contain a germinal center of B cells surrounded by specialized APCs: **M cells** and dendritic cells. Antigens enter the Peyer patch through antigen presentation via M cells and dendritic cells. The B cells of the MALT germinal center are specialized; they produce a specific immunoglobulin, **IgA,** which can be secreted into the intestinal lumen to neutralize pathogens before they invade the epithelium.

The submucosa also houses one of the two neural plexuses located within the small intestine. The other (myenteric) plexus is located between the two layers of the muscularis externa. Considered part of the autonomic system, these neural networks receive a great deal of intrinsic input from the intestinal parenchyma. This allows the gut to operate nearly independently from the central nervous system, although its action can be modulated via extensive extrinsic neural input. Two networks control the activity of the small intestine: the **submucosal plexus of Meissner** and the **myenteric plexus of Auerbach**. They are extensively interconnected and probably equally modulate mucosal and muscular activity, coordinating action to maximize digestion.

## Muscularis Externa (Propria)

Intestinal motility is controlled by two layers of smooth muscle. One circular layer is surrounded by a second longitudinal layer (Auerbach's plexus resides between these two layers). Coordinated muscular contraction produces two types of mechanical results: **propulsion** and **segmentation.**

- **Propulsion** occurs when proximal contraction is coordinated with distal relaxation. This leads to increased upstream pressure, which slowly propels food through the digestive system. Contraction of proximal sphincters ensures that the food bolus only moves distally.
- **Segmentation** occurs when a bolus of food is mechanically compressed and split into portions as the lumen constricts near the bolus center, not merely proximal to it. If this contraction is not coordinated with distal relaxation, the bolus cannot be propelled forward. Instead, its contents are mixed by the muscular contractions.

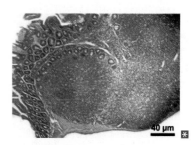

40 μm

**FIGURE 1-22.    Histology of Peyer patches in small intestine.**

### Serosa

The serosa is the visceral peritoneum covering the small intestine. It is lined by a single layer of mesothelium-derived cells.

## SPLENIC ANATOMY

The largest secondary lymphatic organ, the spleen, is located in the upper left quadrant of the abdominal cavity. It is completely surrounded by peritoneum, except at its hilum, where the vasculature enters and exits. It is bordered laterally and posteriorly by ribs 9–11, superiorly by the diaphragm, anteriorly by the stomach, inferiorly by the left colic flexure (splenic flexure), and medially by the left kidney. It is attached to the greater curvature of the stomach by the **gastrosplenic ligament** and to the posterior abdominal wall by the **splenorenal ligament.** The parenchyma of the spleen is composed of **red pulp** and **white pulp.**

### Red Pulp

The **splenic sinusoids** of the red pulp make up an interconnected network of vascular channels that aid the hematopoietic system by removing senescent and damaged erythrocytes from the circulation. These are lined by elongated endothelial cells and a discontinuous basement membrane made of reticular fibers (Figure 1-23). The walls separating the sinusoids are called **splenic cords** (cords of Billroth). The splenic cords contain plasma cells, macrophages, and blood cells supported by a connective tissue matrix. Macrophages adjacent to the sinusoids recognize opsonized bacteria, adherent antibodies, foreign antigens, and senescent red cells as they filter through the spleen.

### White Pulp

The white pulp is a site of immunologic reinforcements and is composed of nodules (Malpighian corpuscles) that contain B cells arranged in follicles and T cells arranged in sheaths. Arranged around a **central arteriole,** the white pulp contains immune cells in a specific orientation that facilitates hematogenous activation of the humoral immune system. As an antigen enters the central arteriole, the vasculature branches into radial arterioles (emanating from the central arteriole like spokes of a wheel), and the antigen passes through a surrounding sheath of T cells. This region, known as the periarterial lymphatic sheath (PALS), allows for sampling of the arteriolar contents.

The radial arterioles then empty their contents into the marginal zone, between the red and white pulp. This area contains specialized B cells and APCs that capture the blood-borne antigens for recognition by lymphocytes (Figure 1-23).

Activated T cells then travel to the adjacent lymphatic nodule for B-cell activation. This process produces active germinal centers within the white pulp where B cells mature. Mature B cells, or plasma cells, defend the host via soluble immunoglobulins secreted into the circulation.

## THE LYMPHATIC SYSTEM

### The Lymph Node

Like **little spleens** dispersed along the lymphatic system, these small secondary lymphatic organs aid regional adaptive immune responses by housing APCs, T cells, and B cells (Table 1-3). Each node possesses multiple afferent lymphatic channels that enter through the capsule of the lymph node near the cortex. The efferent lymphatics exit at the hilum, along with an artery and vein (Figure 1-24). From the afferent lymphatics, antigens and APCs in the lymph enter the **medullary sinus.** There, free antigens meet macrophages for phagocytosis and presentation in association with MHC II for T-cell

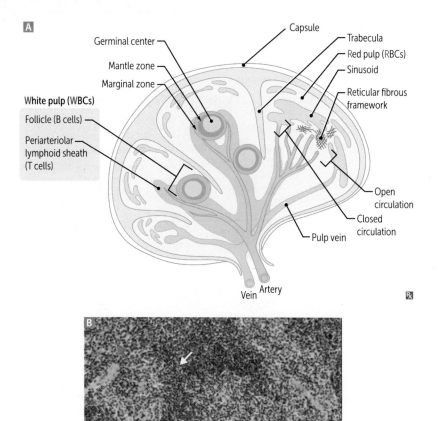

**FIGURE 1-23.** **Diagram of the functional units of the spleen and histologic section of splenic sinusoid.** **A** The important functional units of the spleen are delineated here, where a central arteriole enters and supplies blood first to the periarteriolar lymphoid sheath (PALS) T-cells, which is surrounded by the follicle of B cells. The marginal zone between the white pulp and red pulp contains antigen-presenting cells (APCs) and macrophages to capture blood-borne antigens for recognition by lymphocytes. **B** Histologic section of the splenic sinusoid showing vascular channels through the red pulp (red arrow), and T cells in the PALS (white arrow).

activation. Activated APCs bypass the adjacent **medullary cords** to reach the **paracortex,** where T cells await stimulation. Activated T cells move to the adjacent **cortical follicle,** where B cells await costimulatory signals. Once activated, mature B cells travel back to the medullary cords, where they develop into plasma cells and secrete immunoglobulins into the adjacent vascular supply.

**TABLE 1-3.** **Lymph Node Organization**

| REGION | DIVISIONS | CONTENTS AND FUNCTION |
|---|---|---|
| Cortex | Follicle (outer cortex) | ▪ Site of B-cell localization and proliferation<br>▪ 1° follicles are dense and contain dormant B cells<br>▪ 2° follicles have pale central active germinal centers |
| | Paracortex | ▪ Helper T cells reside between follicles and the splenic medulla<br>▪ High endothelial venules allow lymphocytes to enter circulation |
| Medulla | Sinus | ▪ Reticular cells and macrophages communicate with efferent lymphatics |
| | Cords | ▪ Closely packed lymphocytes and plasma cells |

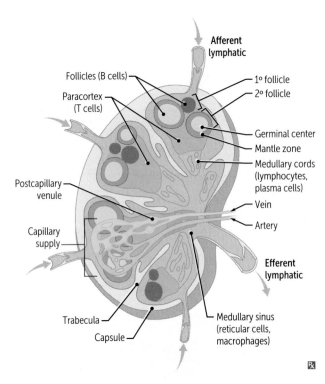

**FIGURE 1-24.** **Lymph node.** Schematic representation of the lymph node structure shows the major divisions of the node. The medulla consists of cords of plasma cells and sinuses of macrophages. The cortex consists of dormant and activated B-cell follicles, as well as a T-cell paracortex.

## Lymphatics

As part of the cardiovascular system, the lymphatic vessels **drain interstitial fluid from surrounding tissues** (Tables 1-4 and 1-5, and Figure 1-25). They are also integral to the process of transporting fats and fat-soluble nutrients and facilitating the humoral immune response. Their role in immunity involves carrying foreign antigens and APCs to lymph nodes for T- and B-cell activation.

The lymph vessels are analogous to veins in their structure and organization. The walls of the lymphatic capillary are made up of a layer of loosely bound endothelial cells, lacking tight junctions and bound to an incomplete basal lamina. This allows fluid to enter the lumen via hydrostatic pressure. As distal lymphatic capillaries merge, they produce larger vessels containing valves, just like veins, that maintain the direction of flow. In addition to interstitial hydrostatic pressure, muscular contractions aid the flow of lymph.

During its course back to the systemic circulation, lymphatic fluid is filtered through lymph nodes for immune surveillance. The remaining lymph reaches the bloodstream via one of two major routes: the larger **thoracic duct** or the smaller **right lymphatic duct**.

**TABLE 1-4.    Primary Lymph Drainage Routes**

| DRAINAGE ROUTE | ANATOMIC REGIONS DRAINED |
|---|---|
| Right lymphatic duct | Right arm, right half of head and right thorax |
| Thoracic duct | All other regions |

**TABLE 1-5.    Drainage Routes for the Major Lymph Nodes**

| LYMPH NODE CLUSTER | AREA OF BODY DRAINED |
|---|---|
| Cervical | Head and neck |
| Hilar | Lungs |
| Mediastinal | Trachea and esophagus |
| Axillary | Upper limb, breast, skin above umbilicus |
| Celiac | Liver, stomach, spleen, pancreas, upper duodenum |
| Superior mesenteric | Lower duodenum, jejunum, ileum, colon to splenic flexure |
| Inferior mesenteric | Colon from splenic flexure to upper rectum |
| Internal iliac | Lower rectum to anal canal (above pectinate line), bladder, vagina (middle third), prostate |
| Para-aortic | Testes, ovaries, kidneys, uterus |
| Superficial inguinal | Anal canal (below pectinate line), skin below umbilicus (except popliteal territory), scrotum |
| Popliteal | Dorsolateral foot, posterior calf |

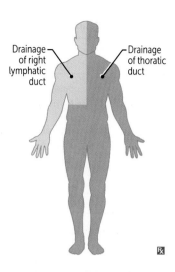

**FIGURE 1-25.    Areas of lymphatic drainage of the thoracic and right lymphatic ducts.** Note that the thoracic duct drains the lymphatic fluid from the entire body, except for the right half of the body superior to the diaphragm.

## PERIPHERAL NERVOUS SYSTEM

### Nerve Cells

During embryonic development, **neural crest cells** migrate into the peripheral tissues, where they differentiate into **neurons** of the following tissues:

- Sensory neurons of the dorsal root ganglia.
- Neurons of the cranial nerve ganglia.
- Neurons of the autonomic system (eg, vagus nerve or sympathetic ganglia).
- Neurons of the myenteric (Auerbach) and submucosal (Meissner) plexus.

Neuronal cells contain three major parts: the cell body (soma), **dendrites**, and **axons**.

- The soma houses the organelles (including the prominent nucleus and the well-developed RER, referred to as the **Nissl body**).
- **Dendrites** are afferent cytoplasmic processes arising from the soma that provide increased surface area for axonal synaptic connections, thus facilitating the reception and integration of information. Each neuron has many dendrites (Figure 1-26).
- An **axon** is the efferent cytoplasmic process sprouting from the soma at the **axon hillock** and ending in many **synaptic terminals**, or **boutons**. Each neuron has one axon.

Because neurons are specialized cells for signal transduction, they can secrete several different **neurotransmitters** (Table 1-6). These peptide molecules are produced in the RER, stored in secretory vesicles, transported through the axon along microtubules via molecular motors, and eventually released from the axon into the **synaptic cleft**. The synaptic cleft is the junction between the synaptic terminal and an adjacent cell. This vesicular secretion, which is triggered by a transmitted action potential, is the primary method of neural control.

### Schwann Cells

The Schwann cells (Figure 1-27) are descendents of neural crest cells and envelops only one peripheral nervous system (PNS) axon with myelin. This is in contrast to the

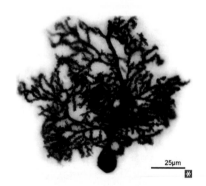

25µm

**FIGURE 1-26.    Histology of the Purkinje cell of the cerebellum, demonstrating characteristic extensive dendritic branching.**

**Q    QUESTION**

An 18-year-old man presents to his doctor complaining of fatigue and sore throat. On exam he has a fever, hepatosplenomegaly, and symmetrical lymphadenopathy of the posterior cervical chain of lymph nodes. He also has petechiae on his palate with enlarged tonsils. What is the most likely diagnosis?

**TABLE 1-6. Neurotransmitters**

| NEUROTRANSMITTER | LOCATION OF SYNTHESIS | ANXIETY | DEPRESSION | SCHIZOPHRENIA | ALZHEIMER DISEASE | HUNTINGTON DISEASE | PARKINSON DISEASE |
|---|---|---|---|---|---|---|---|
| Acetylcholine | Basal nucleus of Meynert | | | | ↓ | ↓ | ↑ |
| Dopamine | Ventral tegmentum, SNpc | | ↓ | ↑ | | ↑ | ↓ |
| GABA | Nucleus accumbens | ↓ | | | | ↓ | |
| Norepinephrine | Locus ceruleus | ↑ | ↓ | | | | |
| Serotonin | Raphe nucleus | ↓ | ↓ | | | | ↓ |

SNpc, substantia nigra pars compacta

Reproduced with permission from Le T, et al. *First Aid for the USMLE Step 1 2016*. New York, NY: McGraw-Hill Education; 2016: 455.

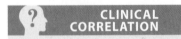

**CLINICAL CORRELATION**

The endoneurium is the target of the autoimmune inflammatory infiltrate in Guillain-Barré syndrome.

oligodendroglia of the central nervous system (CNS), which can myelinate multiple axons (Figure 1-27). Myelin increases conduction velocity due to saltatory conduction. Between myelinated segments are the nodes of Ranvier (Figure 1-28), and the myelinated segments are referred to as internodes.

### Peripheral Nerve

The peripheral nerve consists of a bundle of neuronal axons, Schwann cells, and protective connective tissues. It carries impulses from the CNS to the entire body. Although individual neurons are surrounded by Schwann cells, a nerve fiber is more complex (Figure 1-29). Each individual neuron, along with its associated Schwann cells, is encapsulated in endoneurium. Bundles of these nerves are called a nerve fascicle, which is encapsulated in perineurium. The perineurium acts as a permeability barrier that regulates nutrient transport from capillaries to the nerve fibers beneath. Nerve fascicles, and their vascular supply, are covered by epineurium (dense connective tissue), forming the peripheral nerve trunk.

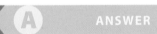

**ANSWER**

Infectious mononucleosis caused by Epstein-Barr virus. The diagnosis is confirmed by the presence of atypical lymphocytes and heterophile antibodies (Monospot).

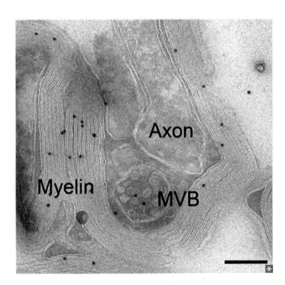

**FIGURE 1-27.** **Electron micrograph of myelinated axons in the optic nerve.** MVB, multivesicular bodies.

## Brachial Plexus

The motor portions of spinal nerves are organized differently from the sensory neurons. Instead of clear divisions organized by spinal level that serve successively distal regions of the body, a great deal of mixing of neurons from each spinal level produces a single nerve supplying a specific muscle group. The upper extremity's **brachial plexus** is a prime example. As motor neurons exit the spinal column between C5 and T1, the ventral rami begin to exchange individual fibers. These rami are considered the **roots** of the brachial plexus (Figure 1-30). As the five roots reach the inferior portion of the neck, C5 and C6 unite to form the **superior trunk**, as C8 and T1 unite to form the **inferior trunk**, leaving C7 as the **middle trunk**. These three trunks pass beneath the clavicle, where they each split into **anterior** and **posterior divisions**. The anterior divisions of the superior and middle trunks merge to form the **lateral cord** of the brachial plexus, and the anterior division of the inferior trunk becomes the **medial cord**. Both of these cords eventually supply the muscles of the anterior compartments of the upper limb. All three posterior divisions merge to form the **posterior cord,** which supplies the posterior compartments of the upper limb. From cords, the plexus divides further into its terminal infraclavicular **branches.** Common injuries associated with the brachial plexus are listed in Table 1-7, and shown in Figure 1-31.

## Dermatomes

Usually, successive spinal levels innervate successive caudal regions. The dermatomal organization of the body is displayed in Figure 1-32A and dermatomes of the hand are displayed in Figure 1-32B, as projected onto the skin.

## THE INTEGUMENTARY SYSTEM

### Skin

The skin has several functions:

- Mechanical protection
- Moisture retention
- Body temperature regulation
- Nonspecific immune defense
- Salt excretion
- Vitamin D synthesis
- Tactile sensation

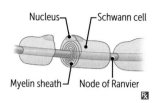

**FIGURE 1-28.** **Schwann cells.**

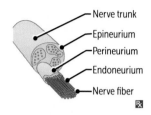

**FIGURE 1-29.** **Peripheral nerve layers.**

---

**KEY FACT**

Following trauma, the perineurium must be repaired via microsurgery to ensure proper nerve regeneration and functional restoration.

---

**MNEMONIC**

***Organization of the brachial plexus—***

**Randy Travis Drinks Cold Beer:**

**R**oots
**T**runks
**D**ivisions
**C**ords
**B**ranches

---

**MNEMONIC**

***Dermatomes—***

T**10** at the belly but-**10**
L**1** at I**L** (Inguinal **L**igament)
**L4**, down on **L-4**'s "all fours" (at the knees)

---

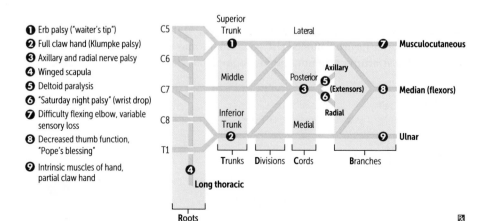

❶ Erb palsy ("waiter's tip")
❷ Full claw hand (Klumpke palsy)
❸ Axillary and radial nerve palsy
❹ Winged scapula
❺ Deltoid paralysis
❻ "Saturday night palsy" (wrist drop)
❼ Difficulty flexing elbow, variable sensory loss
❽ Decreased thumb function, "Pope's blessing"
❾ Intrinsic muscles of hand, partial claw hand

**FIGURE 1-30.** **Brachial plexus.** Schematic representation of the brachial plexus on the right. To the left are clinical correlations to some common brachial plexus injuries and the location of nerve lesions that create them.

**TABLE 1-7.    Common Brachial Plexus Injuries**

| LESION LOCATION | SYNDROME | DEFICITS |
|---|---|---|
| Superior trunk C5/C6 | Erb-Duchenne palsy ("waiter's tip") | ▪ Abduction (deltoid)<br>▪ Lateral rotation (infraspinatus, teres minor)<br>▪ Supination (biceps) and supinator muscle |
| Inferior trunk C8/T1 | Interphalangeal joint flexion and metacarpophalangeal joint extension paralysis (full "claw hand") | Intrinsic muscles of hand, forearm flexors of hand |
| Posterior cord C5/C6/C7/C8 | Axillary and radial nerve paralyses | Same as for axillary and radial nerves |
| Long thoracic nerve T1 | Winged scapula | Serratus anterior paralysis |
| Axillary nerve | Deltoid paralysis | Abduction |
| Radial nerve | "Saturday night palsy" | Wrist drop (supinator, brachioradialis, triceps, extensors of wrist/fingers) |
| Musculocutaneous nerve | Biceps paralysis | Elbow flexion, sensation on radial/lateral side of the forearm |
| Median nerve | "Pope's blessing" on making a fist | Thumb abduction, thumb opposition, fourth/fifth digit extension |
| Ulnar nerve | Fourth/fifth digit paralysis (partial "claw hand") | Grip strength, fourth/fifth digit flexion, intrinsic muscles of the hand |

**MNEMONIC**

**Layers of the epidermis—**

**Californians Like Girls in String Bikinis:**

Stratum **C**orneum
Stratum **L**ucidum
Stratum **G**ranulosum
Stratum **S**pinosum
Stratum **B**asalis

**KEY FACT**

The stratum lucidum is found only in areas of thick skin (eg, palms and soles).

**CLINICAL CORRELATION**

**Albinism:** Normal melanocyte number with **reduced melanin production** due to a decrease in **tyrosinase** activity or defective tyrosine transport. Can also be caused by failure of neural crest cell migration during development. Increased risk of skin cancer.

The skin is composed of three layers: the **epidermis** (ectodermally derived), the **deep dermis,** and the **hypodermis,** or subcutaneous tissues (the latter two of which are mesenchymally derived).

### Epidermis

The epidermis is predominantly made of **keratinocytes,** or epithelial cells named for the intermediate filament protein **keratin.** The epidermis is organized into five layers (Figure 1-33).

The **stratum basale** is composed of columnar keratinocytes bound to a basement membrane via hemidesmosomes. Cellular proliferation occurring at this level maintains the population of epidermal stem cells, replenishes sloughed skin cells, and contributes to epidermal wound healing. These columnar keratinocytes undergo a process of differentiation, as they move upwards toward the surface. At the level of the **stratum spinosum,** keratinocytes have a flattened polygonal shape and an ovoid nucleus. By the time they reach the **stratum corneum,** they are completely flattened and lack nuclei.

Erb-Duchenne palsy
("waiter's tip")

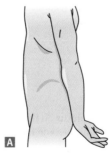

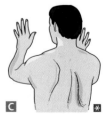

FIGURE 1-31.    **A** Erb palsy, **B** claw hand, and **C** winged scapula.

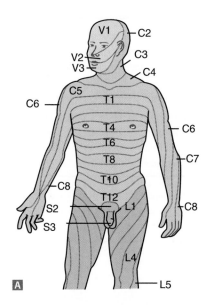

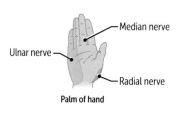

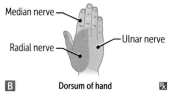

| Important Dermatomes | |
|---|---|
| Forehead | V1 |
| Thumb | C6 |
| Nipples | T4 |
| Umbilicus | T10 |
| Knee | L3/4 |
| Great toe | L5 |
| Anus | S5 |

**FIGURE 1-32.**    **Landmark dermatomes A, and dermatomes of the hand B.**

The epidermis also contains other cell types: **melanocytes, Langerhans cells,** and **Merkel cells.**

■ Melanocytes, derived from the neural crest, produce **melanin,** a tyrosine derivative responsible for skin pigmentation (Figure 1-34).
■ Langerhans cells are bone marrow–derived dendritic cells residing in the skin. Once activated, they migrate to secondary lymph organs to present antigens to T cells.
■ Merkel cells, found in the stratum basale, contribute to the function of the numerous **mechanoreceptors** present in the epidermis. A myelinated sensory axon actually ends in an unmyelinated portion, called the **nerve plate,** which synapses on the Merkel cell. This synapse allows the Merkel cell to signal tactile sensation.

In addition to Merkel cells, two other specialized sensory structures exist within the body: **Meissner corpuscles** in the dermis and **Pacinian corpuscles** in the deep tissues (Figure 1-36).

### Dermis

The epidermis is anchored to its basement membrane by hemidesmosomes. Two indistinct layers of the dermis, the **papillary layer** and the **reticular layer,** reside just below. The uppermost papillary layer (primarily loose connective tissue) consists of fibroblasts, collagen, and fine elastic fibers; the lower reticular layer contains mostly irregularly and densely packed collagen and elastic fibers.

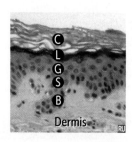

**FIGURE 1-33.    Epidermis layers.** C = stratum corneum; L = stratum lucidum; G = stratum granulosum; S = stratum spinosum; B = stratum basale.

**CLINICAL CORRELATION**

**Vitiligo:** Irregular areas of complete depigmentation. Caused by autoimmune destruction of melanocytes (Figure 1-35).

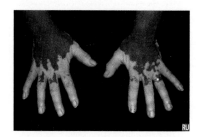

**FIGURE 1-35.    Clinical findings on a patient with vitiligo.**

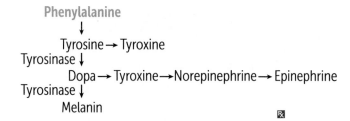

**FIGURE 1-34.    Albinism results from a complete deficiency of the tyrosinase.** Thus, the pigments eumelanin and phaeomelanin are not produced in the albinism tyrosine metabolic pathway.

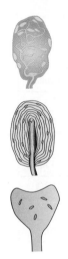

**Meissner** - Small, encapsulated nerve endings found in the dermis of palms, soles, and digits of skin. Involved in light discriminatory touch of glabrous (hairless) skin.

**Pacinian** - Large, encapsulated nerve endings found in deeper layers of skin at ligaments, joint capsules, serous membranes, and mesenteries. Involved in pressure, coarse touch, vibration, and tension.

**Merkel** - Cup-shaped nerve endings (tactile disks) in the stratum basale of the epidermis of fingertips, hair follicles, hard palate. Involved in light, and crude touch.

**FIGURE 1-36.** **Sensory corpuscles.**

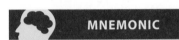

**MNEMONIC**

*Relation of the pulmonary artery to the bronchus at each lung hilum—*

**RALS**

**R**ight **A**nterior
**L**eft **S**uperior

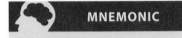

**MNEMONIC**

**E**ccrine glands: **E**verywhere

## Skin Appendages

Skin appendages (**hair follicles, sweat glands,** and **sebaceous glands**) are present in the dermis, as is the blood supply to the skin (Figure 1-37). Hair shafts are made of hardened keratin, and the follicular bulb where the hair originates contains stem cells capable of repopulating the follicular shaft, or even the epidermis following injury. Sebaceous glands are oil-producing glands that actually empty their contents into the hair follicle, the tubular invagination that the hair shaft follows as it grows to the surface. Sweat glands occur in two forms: (1) The **eccrine** sweat gland is a ubiquitous coiled gland innervated by sympathetic cholinergic nerves and used in temperature regulation. (2) The **apocrine** glands, regulated by adrenergic stimuli, only become active following puberty. These coiled glands are found in the axilla, mons pubis, and perianal regions.

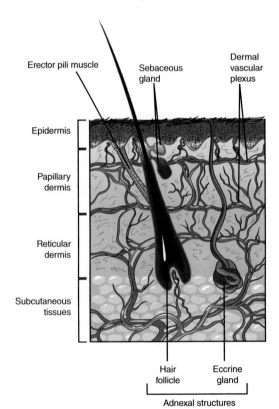

**FIGURE 1-37.** **Skin appendages.** The histologic schematic representation of skin demonstrates a complex organization of cells, connective tissue, blood vessels, and adnexal structures.

## THE RESPIRATORY SYSTEM

### Respiratory Histology

Once air has traveled through the **conducting zone** (nasal cavities, nasopharynx, oropharynx, larynx, trachea, bronchi, and bronchioles), it enters the **respiratory zone** (respiratory bronchioles, alveolar ducts, alveolar sacs, and alveoli [Figure 1-38]). Air exchange occurs in the respiratory zone.

### Bronchi and Bronchioles

Except for their smallest divisions, these airways are involved in conducting inhaled air to the lung, rather than gas exchange. Primarily, the walls of the conducting airways contain a **pseudostratified ciliated columnar epithelium,** composed of three cell types:

- **Ciliated epithelial cells:** Coordinated ciliary motion clears mucus (with trapped pathogens and debris) from the lungs. These cells extend distally to the beginning of the terminal bronchioles before transitioning to the cuboidal cells.
- **Goblet cells:** Produce mucus and protect the airway and lung tissue from inspired particles. Goblet cells extend to the end of the bronchi.
- **Basal cells:** Provide structural support to the airway and can differentiate into other epithelial cell types after injury.

### Alveolus

The alveolus is the basic functional unit of the lung. The lungs contain about 300 million alveoli, which increase the surface area for gas exchange to approximately 75 m$^2$. Each alveolar wall consists of two cell types, **type I** and **type II alveolar cells (pneumocytes),** serving separate physiologic functions (Figure 1-39).

The primary function of the type I pneumocytes is to form the first layer of the air-blood barrier. They are continuous with the low cuboidal epithelium of the adjacent respiratory bronchiole, and cover 97% of the alveolar surface, allowing deoxygenated blood to come into close proximity with inhaled environmental $O_2$. Below the type I cells is a fused (double) layer of basement membranes (from type I cells and endothelial cells) completing a semipermeable barrier that allows $O_2$ and $CO_2$ diffusion.

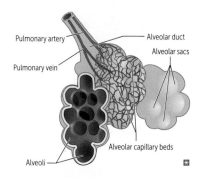

**FIGURE 1-38. Lung alveolus.** The respiratory unit of the lung is the alveolus.

> **KEY FACT**
>
> **Type I pneumocytes** are squamous and thin for optimal gas diffusion. They make up 97% of alveolar surfaces.

> **KEY FACT**
>
> **Type II pneumocytes** are cuboidal and clustered cells that secrete pulmonary surfactant to decrease alveolar surface tension and prevent alveolar collapse (atelectasis). Also serve as precursors to type I cells and other type II cells. Type II cells proliferate during lung damage.

> **FLASH FORWARD**
>
> Pulmonary surfactant reduces the surface tension at the air-fluid interface, thus decreasing the tendency for alveolar collapse.

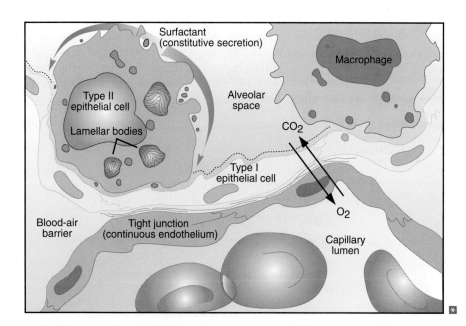

**FIGURE 1-39. Gas exchange barrier.** The thickness of the gas exchange barrier is highlighted, as well as the anatomic relations of important cell types: type I and type II epithelial cells, endothelial cells, macrophages, and red blood cells.

### FLASH FORWARD

Amniotic fluid surfactant levels can be used as a surrogate measure of fetal lung maturity. Steroids are given to premature infants to increase pneumocyte surfactant production.

### KEY FACT

Aspirated foreign bodies end up in the right main bronchus more often than in the left, because the right is wider and its course is more vertical than that of the left.

### KEY FACT

**Divisions of the bronchial tree:**
Trachea
Right and left main bronchi
Lobar bronchi
Segmental bronchi
Bronchioles
Terminal bronchioles
Respiratory bronchioles
Alveolar ducts
Alveoli

### MNEMONIC

**RALS**
**R**ight **A**nterior
**L**eft **S**uperior

---

The type II alveolar cell's primary function is the production of pulmonary surfactant. Type II alveolar cells also retain the ability to differentiate into type I alveolar cells if there is an injury to the lung. Clara cells, also known as C cells, also help produce surfactant in the lungs. C cells act as stem cells, which means they can differentiate and replace other damaged lung cells. Finally, C cells contain enzymes that can detoxify noxious substances in the lungs.

### Lung Anatomy

The lungs are enveloped in a serosal membrane, known as **pleura,** which has two layers. Apposed directly to the lung is the **visceral pleura.** The **parietal pleura** is adherent to the chest wall. Small amounts of fluid within the potential space between the visceral and parietal pleura, the pleural space or cavity, allows respiratory tissues to slide effortlessly as the lung expands.

Each lung is divided into **lobes,** which are further divided into **bronchopulmonary segments.** Each bronchopulmonary segment corresponds to a branch of the **bronchial tree** that delivers $O_2$ to the lung. The right lung is composed of three lobes, and the left lung, two (Figure 1-40). However, the superior lobe of the left lung contains a region, the **lingula,** which is analogous to the right lung's middle lobe. The **cardiac notch,** into which the apex of the heart protrudes, replaces the middle lobe on the left side. The bronchial tree begins at the trachea, which branches into right and left **main-stem bronchi.** The left bronchus is slightly longer, and the right bronchus makes a shallower angle (runs more vertically), with the trachea at its bifurcation. The intersection of the two mainstem bronchi with the trachea is called the **carina.**

The major vascular supply to each lung begins as a single branch of the **pulmonary artery** (carrying deoxygenated blood) and ends as two **pulmonary veins** (carrying oxygenated blood to the left atrium). Between these large vessels, the vasculature branches into intrasegmental pulmonary arteries, which travel with branching airways. The pulmonary veins are along the boundaries of the bronchopulmonary segment. Both end in a capillary network, within the alveolar septae, which facilitates gas exchange. The bronchial circulation delivers oxygenated blood from the thoracic aorta to supply the lung tissue.

### Anatomic Relations

The lungs reside within the rib cage, under the protection of the bony skeleton. The apices are at the level of the first rib, and the bases rest in the left and right costodiaphragmatic recesses. Posteriorly, the lungs extend more distally, deep into the costodiaphragmatic recess, at the 11th or 12th rib. Within the chest, each of the three lung

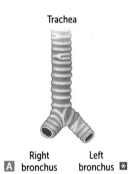

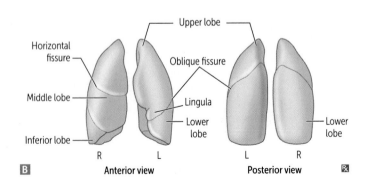

**FIGURE 1-40.**    **Lungs and bronchi.** ▣ Right bronchus is more vertical and wider in diameter than the left bronchus. ▣ Right lung has three lobes: superior lobe, middle lobe, and inferior lobe. In the left lung, there are two lobes and the lingula. The lingula is a small projection of the left lung homologous to the middle lobe.

surfaces (**mediastinal**, **costal**, and **diaphragmatic**) are in close proximity to important structures.

- **Mediastinal surface:** Marks the lateral extent of the **mediastinum**, which houses the heart, great vessels, esophagus, trachea, thoracic duct, bronchial hilum, and hilar lymph nodes, as well as the vagus and phrenic nerves.
- **Costal surface:** Primarily contacts the inside of the chest wall. As mentioned previously, two layers of pleura exist between the functional lung tissue and chest wall.
- **Diaphragmatic surface:** The diaphragm resides just below each lung.

The diaphragm, a thin sheet of muscle separating the thorax and abdomen, and the main muscle for respiration, is innervated by the **phrenic nerves**, which originate from cervical roots C3, C4, and C5. A number of vital structures cross the diaphragm to pass from the thoracic to the abdominal cavity. In particular, the **aorta, esophagus,** and **inferior vena cava** (IVC) each pierce the diaphragm at different thoracic vertebral levels. The IVC, the most anterior of the three structures, crosses at the level of T8. The esophagus crosses at T10, and the aorta crosses at T12 (Figure 1-41).

## THE ADRENAL GLANDS

### Adrenal Gland

Situated atop the kidney, the adrenal gland has an outer **cortex** surrounding an inner **medulla**. The mesodermally derived cortex produces **steroid hormones**, and the neuroectodermally derived medulla produces **catecholamines**.

### Cortex

The cortex is a three-story steroid hormone factory. Each of the three layers of the cortex (Figure 1-42) expresses specific enzymes for producing steroid hormones built from a cholesterol precursor.

- **Zona glomerulosa:** The outermost layer, which produces salt-regulating **aldosterone**.
- **Zona fasciculata:** The middle layer, which produces the stress hormone **cortisol**.
- **Zona reticularis:** The innermost layer, which produces sex hormones (**androgens**).

The zona glomerulosa is a region of concentrically arranged secretory epithelial cells, surrounded by a vascularized stroma. Residing just below the protective fibrous capsule of the gland, these cells are marked by a well-developed SER producing the mineralocorticoid aldosterone. **Angiotensin II**, produced from the conversion of angiotensin I by **angiotensin-converting enzyme** (ACE) in the lung, can trigger both release of aldosterone and hypertrophy of the zona glomerulosa.

The functional distinctions between the zona fasciculata and zona reticularis are less well developed, as are their morphologic boundaries. These regions are often treated as a functional unit. The columns of polygonal cells in the zona fasciculata occupy the majority of the cortex. Fenestrated capillaries intersperse these fascicles, delivering **adrenocorticotropic hormone (ACTH)** to regulate cortisol secretion back into the capillaries for systemic delivery. The zona reticularis, rather than forming columns or concentric circles, forms a network of cells, also surrounded by fenestrated capillaries for regulation by plasma ACTH.

### Medulla

The adrenal medulla oversees the systemic stress response. **Epinephrine** and **norepinephrine** (NE), two tyrosine-derived chemical messengers of the systemic stress response, are produced here. Although NE is also released within the synaptic cleft of adrenergic neurons, these catecholamines are released in bulk into the venous sinusoids of the

**MNEMONIC**

Phrenic nerve: **C3, 4, 5** keep the diaphragm alive!

**MNEMONIC**

**Structures that cross the diaphragm—**

**I 8 10 EGGs AT 12**

**I** = **I**VC
**8** = T**8**
**10** = T**10**
**EG** = **E**sopha**G**us
**G** = va**G**us nerve
**A** = **A**orta and **A**zygos vein
**T** = **T**horacic duct
**12** = T**12**

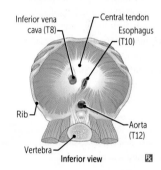

**FIGURE 1-41.** **Diaphragm structures.** Inferior view.

**CLINICAL CORRELATION**

Visceral diaphragmatic pain is conferred by nerves from C3–C5. Because these nerves also supply the shoulder, pain can be referred to the shoulder from the viscera (eg, from myocardial infarction or pleuritic pain).

**MNEMONIC**

**The deeper you go, the sweeter it gets:**

Zona glomerulosa: **Salt** hormones (aldosterone)
Zona fasciculata: **Sugar** hormones (glucocorticoids)
Zona reticularis: **Sex** hormones (androgens)
Or think of kidney **GFR** (**G**lomerular **F**iltration **R**ate), which adrenal gland sits above: **G**lomerulosa, **F**asciculata, **R**eticularis.

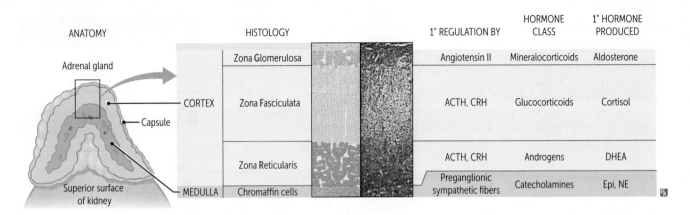

| ANATOMY | | HISTOLOGY | | 1° REGULATION BY | HORMONE CLASS | 1° HORMONE PRODUCED |
|---|---|---|---|---|---|---|
| | | Zona Glomerulosa | | Angiotensin II | Mineralocorticoids | Aldosterone |
| | CORTEX | Zona Fasciculata | | ACTH, CRH | Glucocorticoids | Cortisol |
| | | Zona Reticularis | | ACTH, CRH | Androgens | DHEA |
| | MEDULLA | Chromaffin cells | | Preganglionic sympathetic fibers | Catecholamines | Epi, NE |

**FIGURE 1-42.** **Schematic depiction of the cortex of the adrenal gland.** ACTH, adrenocorticotropic hormone; CRH, corticotropin-releasing hormone; DHEA, dehydroepiandrosterone; Epi, epinephrine; NE, norepinephrine.

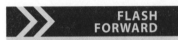

**FLASH FORWARD**

The catecholamine metabolites vanillylmandelic acid (VMA) and metanephrine can be measured in the urine. They are elevated in patients with **pheochromocytoma,** the most common tumor of the adrenal medulla in adults.

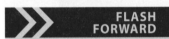

**FLASH FORWARD**

The most common tumors of the adrenal gland are adenomas from the cortex, neuroblastomas (in children) from medullary neural crest cells, and pheochromocytomas (in adults) arising from medullary chromaffin cells.

medulla. In fact, the adrenal medulla, like the autonomic nervous system, is derived from the neuroectoderm. They also receive innervation from sympathetic presynaptic neurons, thus acting as a modified sympathetic postganglionic neuron.

The medullary secretory cells, **chromaffin cells,** synthesize either epinephrine (80%) or NE (20%), but not both. These secretory products are produced from tyrosine (rather than cholesterol, as in the cortex).

# CHAPTER 2

# Biochemistry

# Molecular Biology

## NUCLEOTIDES

### General Structure

**Nucleotides** are composed of three subunits (Figure 2-1):

1. Pentose sugar
   - Ribose
   - Deoxyribose
2. Nitrogenous base
   - Purine
   - Pyrimidine
3. Phosphate group: Forms the linkages between nucleotides.

In contrast, a **nucleoside** is composed of only two units: a pentose sugar and a nitrogenous base. Nucleotides are linked by a **3′–5′ phosphodiester bond** (Figure 2-2). By convention, DNA sequences are written from the 5′ end to the 3′ end.

### Pentose Sugar

Can be either **ribose,** which is found in RNA, or **2-deoxyribose,** which is found in DNA (Figure 2-1). 2-Deoxyribose lacks a hydroxyl (–OH) group at the 2′ carbon (C2). **Ribose** can either retain its 2′ hydroxyl, in which case the subsequent nucleotide will be an RNA monomer, or the 2′ hydroxyl can be removed (reduced) by the key enzyme ribonucleotide reductase, creating **2-deoxyribose,** the five-carbon (pentose) sugar found in DNA (Figure 2-1).

### Nitrogenous Base

The two types differ by the number of rings comprising the base.

## PURINES VERSUS PYRIMIDINES

Each **purine** (adenine [A], guanine [G], xanthine, hypoxanthine, uric acid) is composed of two rings, whereas each **pyrimidine** (cytosine [C], uracil [U], thymine [T]) is composed of one ring (Figure 2-3). Note that **uracil** is found only in RNA, whereas

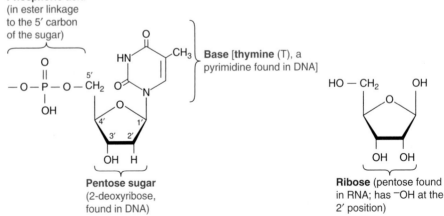

**FIGURE 2-1.** **The general structure of nucleotides.** Ribose and deoxyribose pentose sugars only differ at the 2′-carbon, in which deoxyribose lacks a hydroxyl (–OH) group.

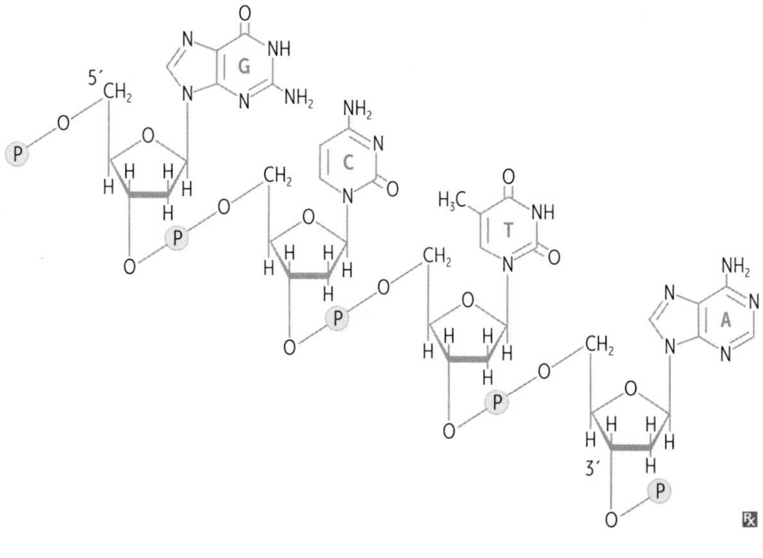

**FIGURE 2-2.** **Phosphodiester bond.** The phosphodiester bond links the 3′ end of a ribose sugar to the preceding sugar's 5′ carbon.

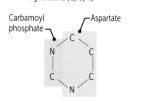

**FIGURE 2-3.** **Base structures of pyrimidines and purines.**

**thymine** is found only in DNA. All other bases are found in both RNA and DNA (Table 2-1). The pyrimidines may be derived from one another: deaminating cytosine results in uracil. Adding a methyl group to uracil produces thymine.

- Substrates for DNA synthesis include: dATP, dGTP, dTTP, dCTP (d = deoxy).
- Substrates for RNA synthesis include: ATP, GTP, UTP, CTP.

## BASE PAIRING

G-C bonds (3 H-bonds) are stronger than A-T bonds (2 H-bonds) (Figure 2-4). Increased G-C content increases the **melting temperature** ($T_m$), which is the temperature at which half of the DNA base-pair hydrogen bonds are broken. Chargaff's rule also dictates that the G content equals the C content, and the A content equals the T content.

# Nucleotide Synthesis

## PURINE NUCLEOTIDE SYNTHESIS

Occurs through either the de novo ("from scratch") or the salvage pathway. De novo synthesis utilizes elemental precursors and is used primarily for rapidly dividing cells. The salvage pathway recycles the nucleosides and nitrogenous bases that are released from degraded nucleic acids; it is considered the major route for synthesis in adults.

**TABLE 2-1.** **Purines Versus Pyrimidines**

| PURINES | PYRIMIDINES |
|---|---|
| Two rings | One ring |
| Adenine | Cytosine |
| Guanine | Thymine (found only in DNA) |
| Xanthine, hypoxanthine, uric acid | Uracil (found only in RNA) |

---

> **KEY FACT**
>
> Chargaff's rule: %A = %T and %G = %C. This is a simple consequence of the fact that A pairs with T, and C pairs with G. Another key principle of base pairing: purine bases (A and G) always base pair with pyrimidines (C and T), and vice versa. All base pairs (C**G** and T**A**) consist of one pyrimidine paired with one **purine.**

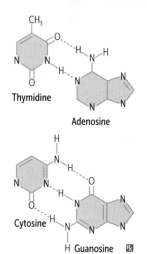

**FIGURE 2-4.** **Hydrogen bonding between base pairs.** Base pair "rules" arise from the fact that purine bases (containing two rings) are physically larger than pyrimidines. Therefore, a purine-purine base pair would be too large to fit into the double helix, whereas a pyrimidine-pyrimidine pair would not be able to reach across the double helix for hydrogen bonding.

**FLASH FORWARD**

Allopurinol and 6-mercaptopurine are purine analogs that inhibit PRPP amidotransferase.

**CLINICAL CORRELATION**

Nucleotide = phosphorylated nucleoside. Nucleoside kinases, the enzymes that convert nucleosides to nucleotides, are essential for converting nucleoside analog prodrugs like acyclovir into active drugs by phosphorylation. Herpesviruses such as varicella-zoster virus (VZV) and herpes simplex virus (HSV) express thymidine kinase, an enzyme that activates acyclovir to the active nucleotide, selectively within virally infected cells. Hence, acyclovir is commonly used to treat infections with these viruses. However, cytomegalovirus (CMV) is a herpesvirus that does not express thymidine kinase, and is therefore inherently resistant to acyclovir. Other antivirals, like ganciclovir and foscarnet, must be used instead.

### De Novo Synthesis

- Rate-limiting step by **glutamine PRPP (5-phosphoribosyl-1-pyrophosphate) amidotransferase.**
- PRPP amidotransferase is inhibited by downstream products (inosine monophosphate [IMP], guanosine monophosphate [GMP], adenosine monophosphate [AMP]) and purine analogs (allopurinol and 6-mercaptopurine).
- Required cofactors: tetrahydrofolate (THF), glutamine, glycine, aspartate.
- **Reciprocal substrate effect:** GTP and ATP are substrates in AMP and GMP synthesis, respectively. For example, $\downarrow$ GTP $\rightarrow$ $\downarrow$ AMP $\rightarrow$ $\downarrow$ ATP. This allows for balanced synthesis of adenine and guanine nucleotides.

### Purine Salvage Pathway

- Recycles ~90% of the preformed purines that are released when cells' nucleases degrade endogenous DNA and RNA and make new purine nucleotides (Figure 2-5).
- Catalyzed by hypoxanthine-guanine phosphoribosyltransferase (HGPRT), which is inhibited by IMP and GMP. HGPRT therefore "salvages" the free purine bases hypoxanthine and guanine to IMP and GMP, respectively. This rescues them from degradation to uric acid by xanthine oxidase.
- Nitrogenous base (guanine, hypoxanthine) + PRPP $\rightarrow$ GMP/IMP + inorganic pyrophosphate (PP$_i$).

## PURINE SALVAGE DEFICIENCIES

### Lesch-Nyhan Syndrome

X-linked recessive disorder of failed purine salvage due to the **absence of HGPRT.** HGPRT converts hypoxanthine $\rightarrow$ IMP and guanine $\rightarrow$ GMP. The inability to salvage purines leads to excess purine synthesis and consequent excess uric acid production.

### Presentation

Retardation, cerebral palsy, self-mutilation, aggression, gout, choreoathetosis, arthritis, nephropathy.

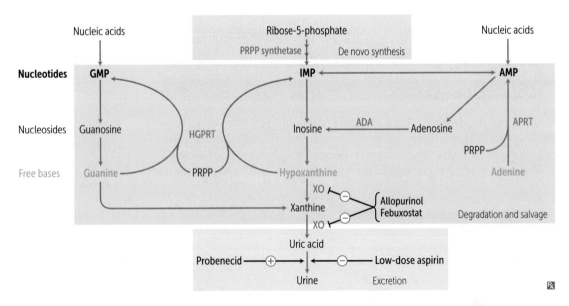

**FIGURE 2-5. Purine salvage pathway and deficiencies.** ADA, adenosine deaminase; AMP, adenosine monophosphate; APRT, adenine phosphoribosyltransferase; GMP, guanosine monophosphate; HGPRT, hypoxanthine guanine phosphoribosyltransferase; IMP, inosine monophosphate; PRPP, phosphoribosylpyrophosphate; XO, xanthine oxidase.

### Diagnosis

Orange crystals in diaper, difficulty with movement, self-injury, **hyperuricemia.**

### Treatment

**Allopurinol** inhibits xanthine oxidase, thereby **decreasing uric acid production.** Therefore, allopurinol can only be used to prevent gout attacks, not to treat them.

### Prognosis

Urate nephropathy, death in the first decade, usually as a result of renal failure.

## Gout

Disorder associated with **hyperuricemia,** due to either overproduction (90%) or underexcretion (10%) of uric acid. Uric acid is less soluble than hypoxanthine and xanthine, and, therefore, **sodium urate crystals** are deposited in joints and soft tissues, leading to arthritis.

- **Primary gout:** Due to hyperuricemia without evident cause. Affected individuals may have a familial disposition. May occur in association with PRPP synthetase hyperactivity or HGPRT deficiency of Lesch-Nyhan syndrome; most common form.
- **Secondary (acquired) gout:** Uric acid overproduction can be caused by leukemia, myeloproliferative syndrome, multiple myeloma, hemolysis, neoplasia, psoriasis, and alcoholism and is more common in men. Secondary gout due to urate underexcretion can be caused by kidney disease and drugs such as aspirin, diuretics, and alcohol.

### Presentation

Monoarticular arthritis of distal joints (eg, **podagra**—gout of the great toe), often with history of hyperuricemia for > 20–30 years, precipitated by a sudden change in urate levels (eg, due to large meals, alcohol), eventually leads to nodular **tophi** (urate crystals surrounded by fibrous connective tissue) located around the joints and Achilles tendon.

### Diagnosis

Arthritis, hyperuricemia, detection of **negatively bifringent** crystals from articular tap. Negatively birefringent crystals will be **yeLLow** when **paraLLel** to polarized light, blue when perpendicular. Note: **positively birefringent** crystals are characteristically found in **pseudogout.**

### Treatment

Normalize uric acid levels (allopurinol, probenecid for chronic gout), decrease pain and inflammation (colchicines, nonsteroidal anti-inflammatory drugs [NSAIDs] for acute gout), avoid large meals and alcohol.

## Severe Combined (T and B) Immunodeficiency

Autosomal recessive disorder caused by a deficiency in **adenosine deaminase (ADA).** Excess ATP and dATP cause an imbalance in the nucleotide pool via inhibition of **ribonucleotide reductase** (catalyzes ribose → deoxyribose). This prevents DNA synthesis and decreases the lymphocyte count. It is not understood why the enzyme deficiency devastates lymphocytes in particular.

Many genetic mutations can lead to the clinical syndrome of severe combined immunodeficiency disease (SCID). An important example is X-linked recessive SCID, which is due to a mutation in the common gamma chain—an important component of many interleukin (IL) receptors, most notably the IL-2 receptor, a key molecule for activation of T cells. It is such an important regulator of T-cell activation that monoclonal antibodies that block the IL-2 receptor, namely **daclizumab** and **basiliximab,** are clinically used to induce immunosuppression in transplant patients. This reduces the chances that the immune system will reject the graft.

**CLINICAL CORRELATION**

A feared complication of advanced cancer (especially leukemia and lymphoma) is **tumor lysis syndrome** (TLS)—massive release of intracellular contents from cancer cells, that can be seen after initiating chemotherapy. Released uric acid can crystallize in the nephrons and cause acute renal failure. **Rasburicase** is an enzyme that degrades urate into a harmless metabolite called allantoin, is used to treat and prevent TLS.

**MNEMONIC**

**Lesch-Nyhan Syndrome**

**L**acks
**N**ucleotide
**S**alvage (purine)

**FLASH FORWARD**

The same trio of drugs used to treat acute gout is used to treat acute pericarditis: NSAIDs, colchicine, and glucocorticoids. Note that allopurinol is used for gout prevention not treatment.

**FLASH FORWARD**

Far more common than SCID are **acquired** immunodeficiency states, such as HIV/AIDS and chronic corticosteroid use. All patients who lack functional T cells are vulnerable to opportunistic pathogens, such as **Pneumocystis carinii.** For this reason, HIV patients with CD4 counts below 200 require prophylactic trimethoprim-sulfamethoxazole. This regimen conveniently also controls **latent Toxoplasma infections.**

### Presentation

Children recurrently infected with bacterial, protozoan, and viral pathogens, especially *Candida* and *Pneumocystis jiroveci.*

### Diagnosis

No plasma cells or B or T lymphocytes on complete blood count (CBC), no thymus.

### Treatment

Gene therapy, bone marrow transplantation.

### Prognosis

Poor.

## PYRIMIDINE NUCLEOTIDE SYNTHESIS

Like purine bases, pyrimidine bases can be either synthesized from scratch ("de novo") or recycled through the salvage pathway. The salvage pathway relies on pyrimidine phosphoribosyl transferase enzyme, which is responsible for recycling orotic acid, uracil, and thymine, but not cytosine. De novo synthesis relies on a different set of enzymes.

### Hereditary Orotic Aciduria

Deficiency in orotate phosphoribosyl transferase and/or OMP decarboxylase (pyrimidine metabolism).

### Presentation

Retarded growth, severe anemia.

### Diagnosis

Low serum iron, leukopenia, megaloblastosis, white precipitate in urine.

### Treatment

Synthetic cytidine or uridine given to maintain pyrimidine nucleotide levels for DNA and RNA synthesis.

### Nucleotide Degradation

Products of purine degradation include **uric acid**, which is excreted in urine. Pyrimidine degradation yields **β-amino acids, $CO_2$,** and **$NH_4^+$.** For example, thymine is degraded into β-aminoisobutyrate, $CO_2$, and $NH_4^+$. Since thymine degradation is the only source of β-aminoisobutyrate in urine, **urinary β-aminoisobutyrate levels** are often used as an **indicator of DNA turnover** (↑ in chemotherapy, radiation therapy).

## DNA

### DNA Synthesis

- Building blocks: Deoxyribonucleotides.
- **dADP, dGDP, dCDP, dUDP synthesis:** Depends on **ribonucleotide reductase** enzyme, which converts ADP, GDP, CDP, and UDP into dADP, dGDP, dCDP, and dUDP, respectively. **dATP,** an allosteric inhibitor, strictly regulates ribonucleotide reductase in order to control the overall supply of dNDPs.
- **dTDP synthesis: Thymidylate synthase** catalyzes the transfer of one carbon from $N^5,N^{10}$-methylene tetrahydrofolate ($FH_4$) to dUDP, yielding dTDP. The $N^5,N^{10}$-$FH_4$ coenzyme then must be regenerated by **dihydrofolate reductase,** which uses reduced nicotinamide adenine dinucleotide phosphate (NADPH).

**FLASH FORWARD**

Chemotherapeutics exploit the following pathways: Hydroxyurea inhibits ribonucleotide reductase; 5-fluorouracil (5-FU) inhibits thymidylate synthase; methotrexate and pyrimethamine inhibit dihydrofolate reductase.

**FLASH FORWARD**

Bacterial dihydrofolate reductase is inhibited by the antimetabolite trimethoprim. It is often used in combination with sulfonamides (eg, sulfamethoxazole) to sequentially block folate synthesis. TRImethoprim structurally resembles the diuretic TRIamterene and can therefore cause **hyperkalemia.** Recall that diuretics that act by inhibiting the epithelial sodium channel (ENaC) are called K-sparing diuretics, because unlike loop and thiazide diuretics (which cause increased urinary K excretion, ie, K "wasting"), these drugs can increase plasma potassium.

## DNA Structure

The structure of DNA is characterized by its **polarity**, with a **5′ phosphate** end and a **3′ hydroxyl** end (Figure 2-6). It is composed of two polynucleotide strands that run **antiparallel** to each other (ie, in opposite directions). The two strands coil around a common axis to form a right-handed double helix (also called B-DNA). Nitrogenous bases sit inside the helix, whereas the phosphate and deoxyribose units sit outside. Each turn of the helix consists of 10 base pairs.

## Organization of Eukaryotic DNA Supercoiling

DNA helices can be tightly or loosely wound, and the physical strain on the helix depends on the action of topoisomerases. Topoisomerases nick the helix at its sugar-phosphate backbone, rendering it either loosely wound (negatively supercoiled DNA) or overwound (positively supercoiled DNA).

**Nucleosome** DNA is found associated with nucleoproteins as a protein-DNA complex (Figure 2-7). Negatively charged DNA is looped twice around positively charged histones composed of H2A, H2B, H3, and H4 proteins. The DNA-covered octamer of histone proteins (**beads on a string**) forms a unit called a **nucleosome** (also called 10-nm fibers). H1 histone and linker DNA tie one nucleosome to the next; the nucleosomes, in aggregate, condense further to form the 30-nm fiber. The 30-nm fibers associate and loop around scaffolding proteins. During mitosis, DNA condenses to form chromosomes.

## Heterochromatin

- Condensed.
- Transcriptionally inactive.
- Found in mitosis as well as interphase.

## Euchromatin

- Less condensed.
- Transcriptionally active.
- Includes the 10-nm and 30-nm fibers.

**FLASH FORWARD**

Fluoroquinolone antibiotics (eg, ciprofloxacin) antibiotics inhibit bacterial topoisomerase IV.

**KEY FACT**

Levels of DNA-protein organization: DNA → histones (H2A, H2B, H3, H4) → nucleosome (10-nm fiber) → 30-nm fiber

**QUESTION**

Why does histone acetylation cause increased gene transcription? How is the acetylation state of histones manipulated clinically to fight cancer?

**KEY FACT**

DNA + histones = beads (histones) on a string (DNA)

**KEY FACT**

DNA wraps around histones owing to electrostatic attractions between the negatively charged phosphodiester backbone of DNA and the positively charged side chains of abundant lysine and arginine residues within the histones.

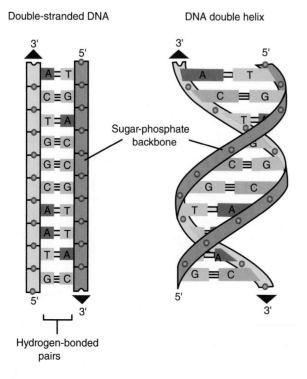

**FIGURE 2-6.** **Schematic representation of two complementary DNA sequences.**

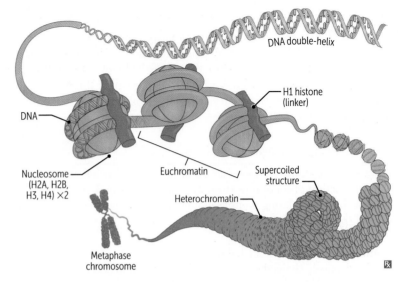

**FIGURE 2-7.    Chromatin structure and related proteins.**

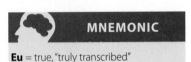

## Chromatin Structure

Influenced by both **DNA methylation** and **histone acetylation.** Usually, inactive genes have increased amounts of methylated DNA. Acetylation of histone loosens the chromatin structure. Loosened DNA is more accessible, and more genes can be transcribed.

## DNA Replication in Prokaryotes

### Semiconservative Replication

Each parent DNA strand serves as a template for the synthesis of one new daughter DNA strand. The resulting DNA molecule has one original parent strand and one newly synthesized strand (Figure 2-8).

### Separation of Two Complementary DNA Strands

Replication begins at a single, unique nucleotide sequence known as the **origin of replication**. A replication fork forms and marks a region of active synthesis. Replication is bidirectional with a leading and a discontinuous/lagging strand.

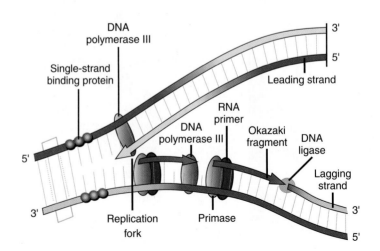

**FIGURE 2-8.    Prokaryotic DNA replication and DNA polymerases.** DNA replication with the leading and lagging strands.

- Leading strand is replicated **in the direction** in which the replication fork is moving. Synthesized continuously.
- Lagging strand is copied **in the opposite direction** of the moving replication fork. Synthesized discontinuously. The short, discontinuous fragments are known as **Okazaki fragments.**
- Involves several other proteins (Table 2-2).

## RNA Primer

The RNA primer is made by **primase;** necessary for DNA polymerase III to initiate replication.

## Chain Elongation

Chain elongation is catalyzed by **DNA polymerase III,** which has both polymerase and proofreading functions.

- Elongates the DNA chain by adding deoxynucleotides to the 3'-hydroxyl end of the RNA primer. Continues to add deoxynucleotides from the $5' \rightarrow 3'$ **direction** until it reaches the primer of the preceding fragment.
- Proofreads each newly added nucleotide. Has $3' \rightarrow 5'$ **exonuclease activity.**

## DNA Polymerase I

DNA polymerase I degrades RNA primer. Has $5' \rightarrow 3'$ exonuclease activity.

## DNA Ligase

DNA ligase seals the remaining nick by creating a phosphodiester linkage.

Overall, eukaryotic DNA replication is similar to that of prokaryotic DNA synthesis, with several notable exceptions (Table 2-3). Namely, replication begins at **consensus sequences** that are rich in A-T base pairs. Eukaryotic genome has multiple origins of replication. Eukaryotes have separate polymerases ($\alpha$, $\beta$, $\gamma$, $\delta$, $\varepsilon$) for synthesizing RNA primers, leading-strand DNA, lagging-strand DNA, mitochondrial DNA, and DNA repair (mutations and DNA repair are discussed later in the chapter).

## RNA

Building blocks are ribonucleotides connected by phosphodiester bonds.

**TABLE 2-2. Other Important Proteins Involved with Prokaryotic DNA Replication**

| PROTEIN | FUNCTION |
|---|---|
| DnaA protein | Binds to origin of replication and causes dsDNA to melt into a local region of ssDNA |
| DNA helicase | Unwinds double helix. Requires energy (ATP) |
| Single-stranded DNA-binding (SS-B) protein | Binds and stabilizes ssDNA to prevent reannealing |
| RNA primase | Synthesizes 10 nucleotide primer |
| DNA topoisomerase | Creates a nick in the helix to relieve the supercoils/strain imposed by DNA unwinding |

dsDNA, double-stranded DNA; ssDNA, single-stranded DNA.

## CLINICAL CORRELATION

Antihistone antibodies are found in patients with drug-induced lupus but not in patients with classic systemic lupus erythematosus (SLE). Medications commonly associated with this condition include **H**ydralazine, **I**soniazid, **P**rocainamide, and **P**henytoin. (It's not **HIPP** to have lupus).

## KEY FACT

DNA polymerase III has $5' \rightarrow 3'$ polymerase activity and $3' \rightarrow 5'$ exonuclease activity. The $3' \rightarrow 5'$ exonuclease activity of DNA polymerase simply means the enzyme can remove the nucleotide it just incorporated if it was incorrect. This is an important proofreading mechanism during DNA replication.

## KEY FACT

DNA polymerase I excises RNA primer with $5' \rightarrow 3'$ exonuclease.

## KEY FACT

Messenger RNA (mRNA) = largest type of RNA (massive = mRNA)
Ribosomal RNA (rRNA) = most abundant type of RNA (rampant = rRNA)
Transfer RNA (tRNA) = smallest type of RNA (tiny = tRNA)

## KEY FACT

**Origins** of replication always feature **AT-rich sequences.** Because AT base pairs are only held together by two hydrogen bonds, they are easier to melt apart, thereby making it easier for DNA replication to begin.

**TABLE 2-3.    Prokaryotic Versus Eukaryotic DNA Replication**

|  | PROKARYOTES | EUKARYOTES |
|---|---|---|
| DNA | Circular, small | Linear, long |
| Sites of replication | Only one (origin of replication, rich in AT base pairs), bound by DnaA proteins | Multiple sites that include a short sequence that is rich in AT base pairs (**consensus sequence**) |
| Primer synthesis | RNA primase | DNA polymerase α—primase activity, initiates DNA synthesis |
| Leading strand synthesis | DNA polymerase III (chain elongation, proofreading) | DNA polymerase α, δ—DNA elongation |
| Lagging strand synthesis | DNA polymerase I (degrades RNA primer) DNA polymerase III | DNA polymerase α, δ |
| DNA repair |  | DNA polymerase β, ε |
| Proofreading | DNA polymerase III | ?DNA polymerase α |
| Mitochondrial DNA | N/A | DNA polymerase γ—replicates mitochondrial DNA |
| RNA primer removal | DNA polymerase I | RNase H |

### RNA Versus DNA

RNA differs from DNA in the following ways:

- Smaller than DNA.
- Contains ribose sugar (deoxyribose in DNA).
- Contains uracil (thymine in DNA).
- Usually exists in single-strand form.

### Types of RNA

There are three types of RNA involved in protein synthesis, each with a specific function and location in the cell (Table 2-4).

### tRNA Structure

Transfer RNA has 75–90 nucleotides in a cloverleaf form. Anticodon end is opposite the 3′ aminoacyl end. All tRNAs, both eukaryotic and prokaryotic, have CCA at the 3′ end, in addition to a high percentage of chemically modified bases. The amino acid is covalently bound to the 3′ end of the tRNA. The anticodon of the tRNA is the same sequence as the DNA template strand (Figure 2-9).

**TABLE 2-4.    Comparison of the Three Types of RNA**

| RNA TYPE | FUNCTION | ABUNDANCE IN CELL (% OF TOTAL RNA) | NOTES |
|---|---|---|---|
| mRNA | Messenger—carries genetic information from nucleus to cytosol | 5 | Largest type |
| rRNA | Ribosomal—enzymatic function in protein translation | 80 | Most abundant type |
| tRNA | Transfer—serves as an adapter molecule that recognizes genetic code (the **codon**) that is carried by mRNA. A codon comprises three adjacent nucleotides and encodes one and only one amino acid. Carries and matches a specific amino acid that corresponds to the codon | 15 | Smallest type |

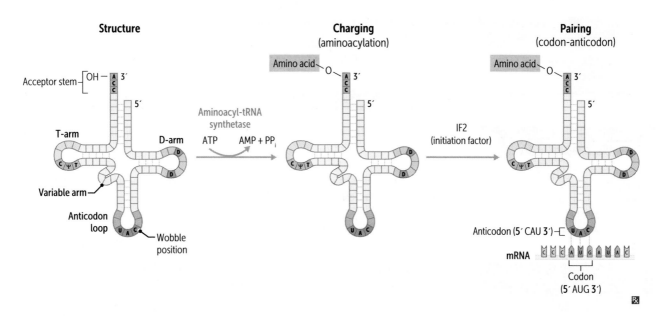

**FIGURE 2-9.** **tRNA structure.**

## FEATURES OF THE GENETIC CODE

### Central Dogma

The central dogma states that RNA is synthesized from a DNA template and protein is synthesized from an RNA template (Figure 2-10).

DNA and RNA sequences are read in triplets (a **codon**), in which each codon encodes either an amino acid (61 possible codons) or a "stop" signal (UGA, UAA, UAG). The **start codon** AUG (or rarely GUG) is the mRNA initiation codon. It fixes the reading frame and encodes slightly different amino acids in prokaryotes versus eukaryotes (Table 2-5). For both prokaryotes and eukaryotes, the genetic code is **unambiguous, redundant, and (almost) universal.**

### Unambiguous

1 codon → 1 amino acid.

### Degenerate/Redundant

More than 1 codon may code for the same amino acid (eg, three codons encode for the same stop signal).

### Universal

Used by almost all known organisms with some exceptions (eg, mitochondria, Archaebacteria, mycoplasma, and some yeasts).

**TABLE 2-5.** **Start Codon in Prokaryotes Versus Eukaryotes**

| Prokaryotes | AUG → *formyl*-methionine (f-met) |
|---|---|
| Eukaryotes | AUG → methionine (may be removed before translation is completed) |

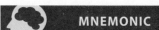

**MNEMONIC**

**Stop codons—**

**UGA** = **U** **G**o **A**way
**UAA** = **U** **A**re **A**way
**UAG** = **U** **A**re **G**one

**KEY FACT**

DNA and RNA are synthesized 5′ to 3′.
Protein is synthesized from N- to C-terminus.

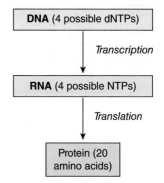

**FIGURE 2-10.** **The central dogma.** RNA is made from DNA, and protein is made from RNA.

### Direction of DNA, RNA, and Protein Synthesis

During DNA/RNA and protein synthesis, nucleotides and amino acids are always added in a set direction (Table 2-6).

## TRANSCRIPTION

The DNA template is transcribed into RNA by RNA polymerase in a process similar to that of DNA replication/synthesis.

RNA is composed of uracil (U) instead of thymine (T) bases. Therefore, in RNA, adenine (A) pairs with a uracil (U) instead of thymine (T).

The RNA immediately produced by RNA polymerase (before it undergoes modification) is known as the **primary transcript** or heterogeneous nuclear RNA (hnRNA).

■ Eukaryotes modify hnRNA, but prokaryotes do not (Table 2-7).
■ Eukaryotes and prokaryotes possess different RNA polymerases.

Whereas prokaryotes have only one RNA polymerase that synthesizes all RNA types, eukaryotes have several, each of which is responsible for making mRNA, rRNA, and tRNA.

### Transcription in Prokaryotes

In contrast to eukaryotes, prokaryotic RNA polymerase synthesizes all three types of RNA. It does not require a primer, and cannot proofread or correct mistakes. Structurally, it has two forms:

■ **Core enzyme** composed of four subunits ($\alpha_2\beta\beta'$).
■ **Holoenzyme,** a core enzyme with a sigma subunit that allows the enzyme to recognize promoter sequences.

Transcription occurs in three steps—initiation, elongation, and termination.

### Initiation

Sigma subunit of RNA polymerase recognizes promoter region of the sense strand of DNA, binds to DNA, and unwinds double helix. Upstream consensus sequences help the RNA polymerase find the promoter.

### Elongation

RNA grows as a polynucleotide chain from the 5′ end to the 3′ end. Meanwhile, RNA polymerase moves along the DNA template from the 3′ end to the 5′ end (Figure 2-11).

### Termination

RNA polymerase and/or specific termination factors (eg, rho factor in *Escherichia coli*) recognize special DNA sequences that cause their dissociation from the DNA template.

**TABLE 2-6.   Direction of DNA, RNA, and Protein Synthesis**

| MOLECULE TYPE | DIRECTION OF SYNTHESIS | NOTES |
|---|---|---|
| DNA | 5′ End of nucleotide added to | 5′ Triphosphate group is the energy source for the phosphodiester bond |
| RNA | 3′-OH group of growing DNA/RNA (**5′ → 3′**) | |
| Protein | Amino acids link N-terminus to C-terminus (**N → C**) | |

**TABLE 2-7.** **Factors That Affect Modification of the Primary Transcript**[a]

| RNA TYPE | POST-TRANSCRIPTIONAL MODIFICATION | |
| --- | --- | --- |
| | PROKARYOTES | EUKARYOTES |
| mRNA | No—identical with primary transcript | Yes |
| tRNA | Yes | Yes |
| rRNA | Yes | Yes |

[a]Whether the primary transcript is modified depends on the RNA type (mRNA, tRNA, rRNA) and the organism (eukaryotes versus prokaryotes).

- Termination can be rho dependent or independent.
- Rho-dependent termination requires participation of a protein factor.

Rho-independent termination requires a specific secondary structure (a hairpin loop followed by a string of Us) in the newly synthesized RNA (Figure 2-12).

### Transcription in Eukaryotes

Transcription in eukaryotes involves both RNA polymerase and additional transcription factors that bind to DNA. Different RNA polymerases are required to synthesize different types of eukaryotic RNA (Table 2-8).

### Regulation of Gene Expression at the Level of Transcription

Regulation is based on DNA sequences that may be located distant from, near, or within (eg, in an intron, which is not expressed) the gene being regulated (Figure 2-14). These DNA sequences include:

- **Promoters:** In eukaryotes, includes a TATA sequence (the **TATA box**) and/or a CAAT sequence 25 and 70 base pairs, respectively, upstream of ATG start codon (Figure 2-13). Critical for initiation of transcription. Mutations may decrease the quantity of gene transcribed.
- **Enhancer:** Stretch of DNA that increases the rate of transcription when bound by transcription factors (Figure 2-13).
- **Silencer:** Stretch of DNA that decreases the rate of transcription when bound.

### Transcription

Transcription follows the same steps as prokaryotes (initiation, elongation, and termination), but requires different RNA polymerase machinery.

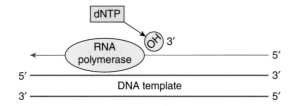

**FIGURE 2-11.** **Elongation step in transcription.** As new RNA is synthesized, it base pairs in an anti-parallel fashion with the template strand of DNA. After transcription is complete, the RNA will therefore have the same sequence as the nontemplate strand of DNA, except with U where the DNA contains T. The strand of DNA physically base pairing with the RNA as it is transcribed is called the *template*, or *anti-sense*, strand. The strand of DNA that shares a sequence with the nascent RNA (except has T instead of U) is therefore called the *sense*, or *coding*, strand.

**KEY FACT**

Prokaryotes have one RNA polymerase that makes *all* types of RNA. Eukaryotes have several RNA polymerases for each RNA type.

**KEY FACT**

The flow of genetic information: DNA → (replication) → DNA → (transcription) → mRNA, tRNA, rRNA → (translation) → protein.

**KEY FACT**

In **eukaryotes,** RNA processing occurs in the nucleus. In **prokaryotes,** RNA is not processed. The primary transcript is translated as soon as it is made.

**MNEMONIC**

**IN**trons stay **IN** the nucleus, whereas **EX**ons **EX**it and are **EX**pressed.

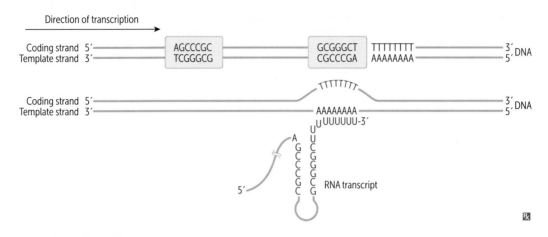

**FIGURE 2-12.** **Typical prokaryotic termination sequence.**

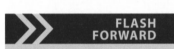
## RNA Processing

Unlike in prokaryotic mRNA, the primary transcript (hnRNA) is both spliced and modified with a 5′-cap and a 3′-tail before leaving the nucleus (Table 2-9). The cap contains 7-methylguanine, which protects it from nuclear digestion and helps ensure correct alignment of the RNA and ribosome for translation. The 3′ poly-A tail protects the mRNA from exonucleases, allows it to be exported from the nucleus, and is important for translation. Splicing prevents translation of introns. Once modified, the RNA is known as mRNA (Figure 2-15).

## Summary of Key Principles of DNA Replication and RNA Transcription

Double-stranded DNA and the RNA/DNA duplex that forms during transcription always base pair such that the two strands are anti-parallel, with the 5′ end of each strand physically far away from each other.

New monomers of DNA (dNTPs) and RNA (NTPs) always are added onto the 3′ OH group of the most recently incorporated nucleotide at the 3′ end of the nascent polymer.

To be eligible for incorporation into the growing chain of DNA or RNA, nucleotides must contain three phosphates (ie, ATP rather than ADP or AMP), because the reaction relies on the release of diphosphate for favorable energetics. The remaining phosphate becomes part of the phosphodiester backbone of the strand of DNA or RNA.

**TABLE 2-8.** **Eukaryotic RNA Polymerases and Their Function**

| RNA POLYMERASE | RNA TYPE MADE | NOTES |
|---|---|---|
| RNA polymerase I | rRNA | rRNA (28S, 18S, and 5.8S) |
| RNA polymerase II | mRNA | Cannot initiate transcription by itself, requires transcription factors |
| RNA polymerase III | tRNA | tRNA, rRNA 5S |
| Mitochondrial RNA polymerase | Transcribes RNA from mitochondrial genes | Inhibited by rifampin, more closely resembles bacterial RNA polymerase than eukaryotic RNA polymerase |

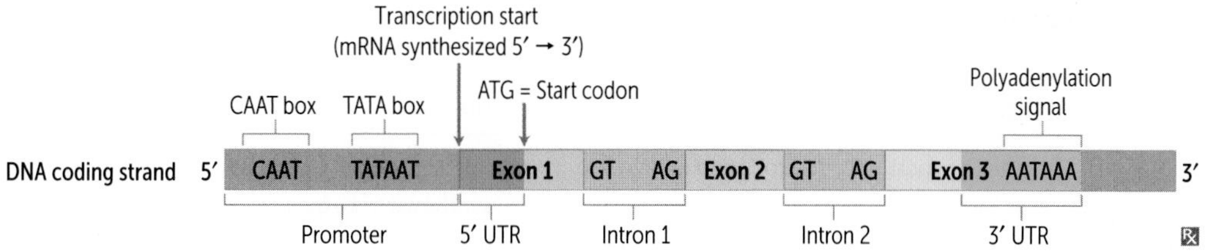

Transcription start
(mRNA synthesized 5′ → 3′)

| | CAAT box | TATA box | | ATG = Start codon | | | | | | | Polyadenylation signal | |
|---|---|---|---|---|---|---|---|---|---|---|---|---|

DNA coding strand  5′  | CAAT | TATAAT | | Exon 1 | GT | AG | Exon 2 | GT | AG | Exon 3 | AATAAA | 3′

Promoter          5′ UTR        Intron 1        Intron 2        3′ UTR

**FIGURE 2-13.** **Functional organization of a eukaryotic gene.** Eukaryotic genes are regulated by **enhancers,** DNA sequences that are relatively far away, and **promoters,** DNA sequences that are only several nucleotides upstream. Promoters often contain a TATA box, a sequence that helps to attract key transcriptional proteins.

## TRANSLATION

Translation is the process by which mRNA base sequences are translated into an amino acid sequence and protein. It involves all three types of RNA; mRNA is the template for protein synthesis. tRNA contains a three-base anticodon that hydrogen bonds to complementary bases in mRNA. Each tRNA molecule carries an amino acid that corresponds to its anticodon. rRNA—along with other proteins—comprises the ribosomes. Ribosomes coordinate the interactions among mRNA, tRNA, and the enzymes necessary for protein synthesis.

### Ribosomes

The site of protein synthesis. Composed of rRNA and protein. Consist of two subunits—one large, one small. The subunits in prokaryotes and eukaryotes differ in size (S values are usually not additive); eukaryotic ribosomes are larger.

| | (Small subunit) | | (Large subunit) | | |
|---|---|---|---|---|---|
| Prokaryote ribosome: | 30S | + | 50S | = | 70S |
| Eukaryote ribosome: | 40S | + | 60S | = | 80S |

### tRNA Structure

tRNA has a distinct structure designed to "translate" the mRNA sequence into the corresponding amino acid sequence (Figure 2-10). tRNA is composed of 75–90 nucleotides in a cloverleaf form. The anticodon end is opposite the 3′ aminoacyl end and is antiparallel and complementary to the codon in mRNA (Figure 2-9). All tRNAs—both eukaryotic and prokaryotic—have CCA at the 3′ end, in addition to a high percentage of chemically modified bases. The amino acid is covalently bound to the 3′ end of the RNA.

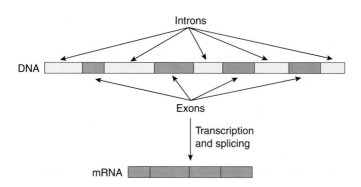

**FIGURE 2-14.** **Schematic representation of introns versus exons.**

**TABLE 2-9.**    **Types and Function of Post-transcriptional Modification**

| POST-TRANSCRIPTIONAL MODIFICATION | DESCRIPTION | FUNCTION |
|---|---|---|
| 5′ Capping | 7-Methyl-guanosine added to 5′ end of RNA | Prevents mRNA degradation, allows translation (protein synthesis) to begin |
| Poly-A tail | 40–200 adenine nucleotides added to 3′ end of RNA by polyadenylate polymerase | Stabilizes mRNA, facilitates exit from nucleus. Note: not all mRNAs have a poly-A tail (eg, histone mRNAs) |
| RNA splicing | Performed by the spliceosome, which is composed of small nuclear ribonucleoprotein particles (**snRNP**). Binds the primary transcript at splice junctions flanked by GU-AG | **Introns** (DNA sequences that do not code for protein) are removed and **exons** (coding sequences) are spliced together (see Figure 2-15). The excised intron is released as a lariat structure |

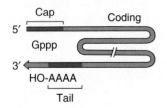

**FIGURE 2-15.**    **Structure of a typically processed mRNA in eukaryotes.**

### tRNA Charging

tRNA charging requires aminoacyl-tRNA synthetase, ATP, and tRNA. Each amino acid has a specific synthetase that transfers energy from 1 ATP to the bond between the amino acid and the 3′ hydroxyl (OH) group of the appropriate tRNA (Figure 2-16). This bond contains the energy that later forms the peptide bond when the amino acid is added to the growing peptide. If an amino acid is incorrectly paired with tRNA, aminoacyl-tRNA synthetase hydrolyzes the amino acid–tRNA bond. In other words, tRNA synthetases can proofread the charged tRNA, and if the incorrect amino acid is charged, it will be removed.

### tRNA Wobble

The code for certain amino acids relies only on the base sequence of the first two nucleotides in the codon. As described earlier, often the same amino acid has multiple codons that differ in the third "wobble" position. Therefore, < 61 tRNAs are needed to translate all 61 codons.

### Protein Synthesis

Proteins are assembled from the N- to the C-terminus, whereas the mRNA template is read from the 5′ to the 3′ end. The number of proteins that the mRNA can encode differs between prokaryotes and eukaryotes (Table 2-10). mRNA from eukaryotes encodes for only one protein, whereas prokaryotic mRNA can encode several different proteins. Protein synthesis occurs in three steps (**initiation, elongation,** and **termination**). Further changes, such as phosphorylation or glycosylation, are therefore referred to as **post-translational modifications.**

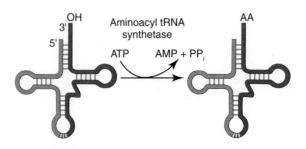

**FIGURE 2-16.**    **tRNA charging.**

**TABLE 2-10.    Prokaryotic Versus Eukaryotic Translation**

| PROKARYOTE | EUKARYOTE |
|---|---|
| > 1 coding region **(polycistronic)**, each of which is independently translated by ribosomes | RNA encodes only 1 polypeptide chain **(monocistronic)** |
| Each region has its own initiation codon and produces a separate polypeptide. Thus, the mRNA may code for multiple proteins | Each mRNA codes for only one protein |

## Initiation

In prokaryotes, the complex formed for initiation of translation consists of 30S ribosomal subunit, mRNA, f-Met tRNA, and three initiation factors. The formation of the initiation complex differs between prokaryotes and eukaryotes, as summarized in Table 2-11.

## Elongation

Three-step cycle in which tRNA delivers the appropriate amino acid to the ribosome, the amino acid forms a peptide bond to the growing peptide chain, and the ribosome shifts one codon so that the next codon can be translated (Figures 2-17 and 2-18).

- Aminoacyl-tRNA (charged tRNA) binds A site.
- Amino acid in A site forms peptide bond with peptide in P site. Reaction is catalyzed by peptidyl transferase and uses energy from the bond between the amino acid and tRNA. The peptide in the P site is effectively transferred to the amino acid–tRNA in the A site, leaving the tRNA in the P site empty.
- Ribosome translocates one codon (requires EF-2, GTP hydrolysis) toward the 3′ end of mRNA. Uncharged tRNA is now in the E site (where it exits), and tRNA with the growing peptide chain enters the P site.

## Termination

Occurs when one of three stop codons (**UGA, UAA, UAG**) is encountered. Peptide is released from ribosome via release factor (RF) protein and GTP.

## Post-translational Modification

Modification may result in the removal of amino acids or addition of molecules to make protein active and/or properly tag the protein for proper transport to its final destination.

**TABLE 2-11.    Prokaryotic Versus Eukaryotic Translation**

| | PROKARYOTES | EUKARYOTES |
|---|---|---|
| Ribosomal binding | 30S ribosomal subunit binds Shine-Dalgarno sequence, which is 6–10 nucleotides upstream (toward 5′ end) of AUG codon | No Shine-Dalgarno sequence, 40S ribosomal subunit binds 5′ cap and moves down mRNA until it encounters AUG codon |
| Initiator tRNA | fMet (methionine with a formyl group attached) | Met (methionine only) |
| Assembly of initiation complex | Facilitated by initiation factors (IF-1, IF-2, IF-3), 50S ribosomal subunit binds to make 70S complex | Initiation factors (eIF, and at least 10 other factors) |

**KEY FACT**

In both prokaryotic and eukaryotic cells, the small ribosomal subunit binds to the mRNA before the large ribosomal subunit.

**CLINICAL CORRELATION**

The differences in enzymes used for similar metabolic processes in eukaryotes and prokaryotes allows for selective targeting of prokaryotic enzymes by antibiotics and antivirals. As such, these drugs will selectively affect prokaryotic cells or viral infected eukaryotic cells, with minimal to no effects on healthy eukaryotic cells.

**FLASH FORWARD**

Drugs selective for prokaryotic protein synthesis machinery

| Drug | Site of Action |
|---|---|
| Tetracycline | Prevents initiation since charged tRNA cannot bind ribosome. |
| Streptomycin | Prevents initiation since code is misread. |
| Erythromycin | Inhibits translocation. |

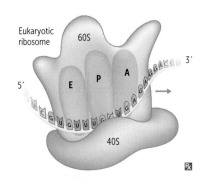

**FIGURE 2-17.    Schematic representation of eukaryotic ribosome and the sites involved in protein synthesis.** P (peptidyl) site initially binds initiator tRNA, later binds growing peptide chain. A (aminoacyl) site binds incoming tRNA molecule with activated amino acid (ie, bound amino acid with high-energy bond). E (exit) site receives uncharged tRNA once amino acid has been added to polypeptide.

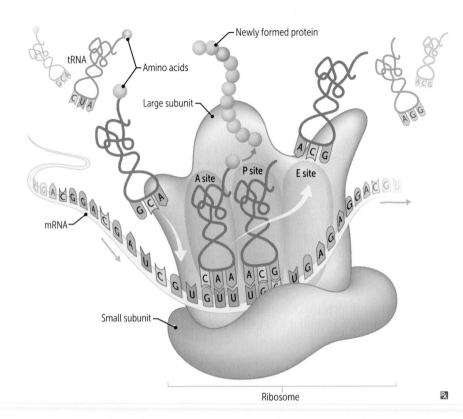

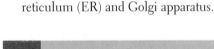

**FIGURE 2-18.**　**Schematic representation of elongation phase of protein synthesis.**

 **FLASH FORWARD**

Many digestive enzymes and proteins of the coagulation cascade are formed as zymogens that must be activated through cleavage (eg, trypsinogen, pepsinogen).

- **Trimming** (proteolysis) removes portions of the peptide chain to make the protein active (ie, zymogen, an inactive precursor of a secreted enzyme).
- Protein may be covalently modified through **phosphorylation** and **glycosylation.** Phosphorylation turns the protein on or off. Proteins that will be secreted or reside in the plasma membrane or lysosomes will be glycosylated in the endoplasmic reticulum (ER) and Golgi apparatus.

## Mutations and DNA Repair

DNA mutations and the intrinsic cellular mechanisms that act to minimize their occurrence play a very important role in health and disease. Not only do DNA mutations result in numerous pathologic conditions, they also form the basis for the evolution of novel traits in species.

### DEFINITIONS

 **CLINICAL CORRELATION**

In xeroderma pigmentosum (XP), an autosome recessive disorder involving defective nucleotide excision repair (NER) genes, DNA repair is impaired, preventing the ability of the cell to repair damage caused by ultraviolet light. Susceptible individuals are more likely to develop basal cell carcinomas, melanoma and squamous cell carcinomas. XP is more common among Japanese people.

#### Mutation

A mutation is any change in the sequence of DNA base pairs that is permanent and arises by chance. To be considered a mutation, the change in the base-pair sequence must not be a result of recombination.

#### DNA Repair

Several molecular mechanisms exist to ensure that most changes in the DNA sequence are repaired and thus do not become permanent mutations. It is estimated that between 1000 and 1,000,000 DNA sequence damaging events occur in each cell every day. However, most of these are quickly corrected by one of the DNA repair mechanisms. Note that DNA repair is independent of the proofreading action of DNA polymerase during DNA replication. Recall that the proofreading action of DNA polymerase is simply based on its 3′ to 5′ exonuclease activity, which excises the most recently added nucleotide if it is not complementary to the template strand.

## Types of Mutations

Mutated DNA includes DNA in which one nucleotide has changed (**point mutation**) and DNA in which one or more nucleotides have been added or removed. Since the DNA code is read in triplets (a **codon**, three consecutive nucleotides, encodes an amino acid), adding or removing one or two nucleotides will cause a **frame shift mutation.** Point mutations lead to one of three outcomes: the identity of the amino acid is unchanged (**silent mutation**); the amino acid is changed to another amino acid (**missense mutation**); or a stop signal is introduced (**nonsense mutation**). Because they prematurely end translation, nonsense mutations typically have the most devastating clinical consequences.

## Point Mutations

Point mutations occur when a single DNA nucleotide base is replaced by a different nucleotide. These are also known as **substitutions.**

There are three types of point mutations (Figure 2-19): missense mutations, nonsense mutations, and silent mutations.

- **Missense mutations:** The replacement of a single nucleotide base with a different one, resulting in a change in the codon so that it codes for a different amino acid. These are common types of mutations and cause several genetic diseases.
- **Nonsense mutations:** Mutation causes premature introduction of a STOP codon (TAA, TAG, or TGA). This causes the translation of the mRNA to stop, resulting in a truncated protein.
- **Silent mutations:** Mutation results in the same amino acid as the original. Because the genetic code is redundant (ie, several codons code for the same amino acid), in some cases a change in a single nucleotide base still codes for the same amino acid. Most often, this results from a base change in the **third** position of the codon (**wobble position**). The resulting protein is identical to the wild-type protein.

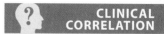
**CLINICAL CORRELATION**

In sickle cell anemia, a point mutation in the sixth codon of the β-globin gene from A to T results in a modified hemoglobin structure. The result is hemoglobin S (sickle), which polymerizes under low-$O_2$ conditions, causing distortion of red blood cells and leading to the associated clinical phenotype.

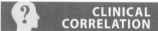
**CLINICAL CORRELATION**

One of the mutations causing **cystic fibrosis (CF)** results when T is substituted for C at nucleotide 1609 of the *CFTR* gene on chromosome 7. This converts a glutamine codon (CAG) to a STOP codon (TAG), thus stopping the translation of *CFTR* after the first 493 amino acids, instead of the normal 1480. (Note: the most common CF-causing mutation [ΔF508], which accounts for about 66% of cases worldwide, is actually not a nonsense mutation.)

**Point mutations**

| | Unmutated | Silent | Missense | | Nonsense |
|---|---|---|---|---|---|
| | | | Conservative | Nonconservative | |
| DNA | CTC | CTT | CTG | TTC | ATC |
| mRNA | GAG | GAA | GAC | AAG | UAG |
| Protein | Glu | Glu | Asp | Lys | Stop |

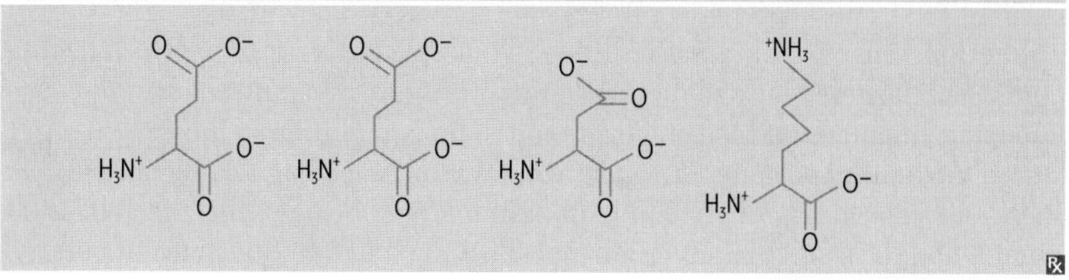

**FIGURE 2-19. Three types of point mutations.** Silent mutations do not alter the amino acid. Nonsense mutations erroneously introduce a premature stop codon. A truncated protein will result. Missense mutations alter the amino acid. If an amino acid with similar biochemical properties results—the mutation is said to be conservative (eg, from lysine to arginine—both are basic, cationic amino acids). If the new amino acid is biochemically different (eg, lysine to aspartate, which are oppositely charged), the missense mutation is said to be nonconservative.

With respect to their biochemical origin, point mutations can be one of five types: transition, transversion, tautomerism, depurination, or deamination.

- **Transition:** A mutation in which a pyrimidine is replaced by a pyrimidine, or a purine by a purine. For example, a replacement of a G-C pair by an A-T pair would result in a transition.
- **Transversion:** A purine replaced by a pyrimidine or vice versa. An A-T pair replaced by either a T-A or C-G pair would be a transversion.
- **Tautomerism:** The modification of a base caused by migration of a proton or a hydrogen bond, which results in switching of an adjacent single and a double bond.
- **Depurination:** Caused by a spontaneous hydrolysis of a purine base (A or G), in such a way that its deoxyribose-phosphate backbone remains intact.
- **Deamination:** A spontaneous reaction that can result in the conversion of cytosine into uracil (C to U), 5-methylcytosine into thymine, or adenine into hypoxanthine (A to HX). Of note, the deamination of C to U is the only one of these that can be corrected, since uracil can be recognized, whereas thymine and hypoxanthine are not detected as errant.

### Insertions

Insertions are mutations in which one or several base pairs are added to the DNA sequence. Most commonly, insertions of short DNA fragments called **transposons** (or transposable elements) are responsible. Insertions may result from errors in DNA replication of nucleotide repeats. Insertions can result in frameshift mutations and splice site mutations.

### Frameshift Mutations

Because codons are always read in triplets, adding or deleting any number of bases that is not a multiple of three shifts the reading frame during translation and greatly alters the amino acid sequence of the protein.

### Splice Site Mutations

At times, insertions of nucleotide bases in certain regions of a gene can alter the splicing of introns from the precursor mRNA. This results in mRNA that contains introns, resulting in significantly altered protein products.

### Deletions

Deletions refer to the loss of one or several nucleotides from the DNA sequence. Much like insertions described above, they can result in frameshift mutations and splice site mutations. They are generally irreversible.

### Amplifications

Amplifications are cellular events resulting in multiple copies of whole DNA segments, including all the genes located on them. Amplifications are usually caused by a disproportionately high level of DNA replication in a limited portion of the genome. In this manner, the multiplied genes are effectively amplified, leading to a higher number of copies of the encoded protein. This can alter the phenotype of the affected cell. For example, drug resistance in certain cancers is linked to amplifications of genes that confer resistance to chemotherapeutic agents by preventing their uptake into the cell.

### Chromosomal Translocations

A chromosomal translocation is defined as an exchange of genetic material between two nonhomologous chromosomes.

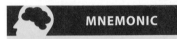

**MNEMONIC**

A **transition** is easy, **transversion** requires effort:

**Transition:** purine → purine; pyrimidine → pyrimidine.

**Transversion:** A purine is substituted for a pyrimidine or vice versa.

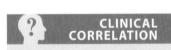

**CLINICAL CORRELATION**

A key example of a clinically relevant DNA amplification is in neuroblastoma, a tumor derived from primitive neural cells that affects children 1–2 years old. A key prognostic factor is the presence of an amplification of the *N-myc* gene—an important oncogene. The presence of *N-myc* portends a poor prognosis. Unopposed *N-myc* activity stimulates rapid cell proliferation.

- **Reciprocal (non-Robertsonian)** translocation: Results in a true exchange of DNA fragments between two chromosomes. This can lead to the formation of new fusion genes, or a changed level of expression of existing genes.
- **Robertsonian** translocation: A large fragment of a chromosome attaches to another chromosome, but no DNA is attached in return (Figure 2-20). Common Robertsonian translocations are confined to the acrocentric chromosomes (those in which the centromere is located very near to one of the ends, eg, 13, 14, 15, 21, and 22) because the short arms of these chromosomes contain no essential genetic material. A minority of cases of **Down syndrome** are caused by the Robertsonian translocation of approximately one third of chromosome 21 on to chromosome 14. The proportion of affected individuals due to trisomy, Robertsonian translocation and other causes are 95%, 3%, and 2%, respectively.

## Interstitial Deletions

Deletions of large DNA fragments on a single chromosome that results in the pairing of two genes that are not normally in sequence. Like chromosomal translocations, such events can lead to the formation of fusion oncogenes.

## Chromosomal Inversions

Chromosomal inversions refer to a large segment of a single chromosome becoming reversed within the same chromosome, usually resulting from a rearrangement following chromosomal breakage. Similar to translocations and interstitial deletions, chromosomal inversions can create fusion genes.

## ORIGINS OF MUTATIONS

Most mutations arise spontaneously, usually as a result either of errors in DNA replication (eg, point mutations and amplifications) or random cellular events (including

**CLINICAL CORRELATION**

The *bcr-abl* gene, associated with chronic myelogenous leukemia (CML), results from a translocation event between chromosomes 9 and 22 (Philadelphia chromosome). The chemotherapeutic imatinib mesylate (Gleevac) is a specific inhibitor of the tyrosine kinase domain in *abl* and c-kit and is a useful agent in the treatment of CML and gastrointestinal stromal tumors (GIST), respectively.

**KEY FACT**

The short arm of each chromosome is called the "p" arm because *petite* is French for *small*. The long arm is called the "q" arm, simply because q comes directly after p in the alphabet.

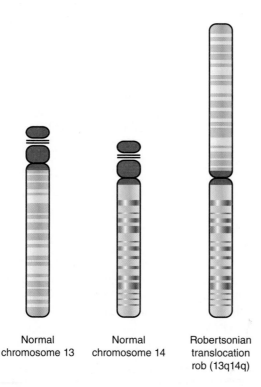

Normal chromosome 13    Normal chromosome 14    Robertsonian translocation rob (13q14q)

**FIGURE 2-20. Robertsonian chromosomal translocation.** A large fragment of a chromosome attaches to another chromosome, but no DNA is attached in return, resulting in the loss of a small amount of genetic material.

chromosomal translocations and inversions). However, many mutations are directly caused by specific agents, collectively known as **mutagens.** Some mutagens are external, whereas some are formed as by-products of cellular metabolism (eg, reactive oxygen species [ROS]).

The type of cell in which a mutation arises is also important. When a mutation arises in a germ cell, it is termed a **germline mutation.** These mutations can be passed to the offspring. Conversely, a mutation in a somatic cell is termed a **somatic mutation** and cannot be passed on to offspring. However, somatic mutations are passed on to the somatic daughter cells of the organism (ie, cancers resulting from somatic mutations).

## MUTAGENS

These are agents that directly cause or increase the likelihood of changes in the DNA sequence. Innumerable mutagens have been identified, and novel ones are continually discovered. Mutagens generally fall into two categories: **chemical agents** and **ionizing radiation.** Because mutations often give rise to cancer, they are often also **carcinogens.**

### Chemical Agents

#### Alkylating Agents

Chemical agents that transfer alkyl groups to other molecules, including DNA. Specifically, they cross-link guanine nucleotides in DNA, thus causing damage to the DNA that can lead to mutations in both replicating and nonreplicating cells. However, some alkylating agents are used as anticancer drugs because of their unique ability to introduce sufficient DNA damage to render a cell unable to divide.

Four classes of classic alkylating agents are used as chemotherapy. **Nitrogen mustards** are the oldest and are derived from mustard gases used in World War I. Cyclophosphamide is a prominent example. **Nitrosoureas** are similar to nitrogen mustards; several members of both classes, as a result, contain *mustine* in the drug name. As a class, nitrosoureas are extremely hydrophobic. Therefore, they cross the blood-brain barrier and were the first chemotherapy used against glioblastoma multiforme (GBM), a particularly devastating brain tumor. They have now been supplanted in the treatment of GBM by temozolimide, a newer, less-toxic alkylating agent. **Alkyl sulfonates** all end in the suffix *-sulfan* and were the mainstay of therapy for CML before the discovery of imatinib. The final class is the **aziridines.** Thiotepa is the only aziridine remaining in use. It was the first intravesicular agent used against bladder cancer. However, it is rarely used, because it has the adverse effects of all alkylating agents: short-term risk of bone marrow suppression, and long-term risk of secondary leukemia due to induction of mutations in hematopoietic stem cells. As a class, alkylating agents produce myelosuppression so reliably that when physicians want to destroy bone marrow before a hematopoietic stem cell transplant, they often use alkylating agents such as thiotepa, cyclophosphamide, or melphalan.

### Base Analogs

Chemical agents that are similar to one of the four nucleotide bases found in DNA and can thus be incorrectly incorporated into DNA during replication. However, they differ enough chemically that they cause mismatch during base pairing, thus introducing mutations in daughter DNA strands. An example of a base analog is bromodeoxyuridine (**BrdU**), which researchers often use to identify dividing cells because it is incorporated into the DNA during replication.

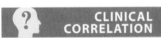

**CLINICAL CORRELATION**

The anthracycline class of chemotherapeutics (ending in -rubicin, such as doxo-, dauno-, epi-, idarubucin, or mitoxantrone) share a feared complication of **cardiomyopathy** leading to heart failure. As a result, baseline cardiac testing (echocardiogram) is usually obtained before initiating their use— patients with preexisting cardiac disease should not receive these chemotherapies. To further minimize cardiotoxicity, strict **maximum lifetime cumulative doses** have been established. Finally, **dexrazoxane** is a drug that reduces this cardiotoxicity and is used to prevent cardiomyopathy in patients receiving anthraquinones or anthracycline chemotherapy.

## DNA Intercalating Agents

Cause DNA damage by inserting themselves between two nucleotide base pairs. This physically interferes with DNA transcription and replication, leading to mutation events (Figure 2-21). Examples include **ethidium bromide,** a fluorescent DNA dye commonly used in research laboratories, and **aflatoxin,** a carcinogen produced by a fungus from the genus *Aspergillus.* Some DNA intercalating agents, such as **doxorubicin** and **daunorubicin,** are used as cancer chemotherapeutics. **Thalidomide,** a teratogen associated with numerous cases of phocomelia (very short or absent long bones and flipper-like appearance of hands and/or feet) in the 1960s, is also a DNA intercalating agent. It is now only used as a last resort anti-inflammatory agent in the treatment of erythema nodosum leprosum and sarcoidosis and as a salvage chemotherapeutic agent in patients with multiple myeloma.

## DNA Cross-Linking Agents

These chemical agents act as mutagens by forming covalent bonds between nucleotide bases in DNA, thus interfering with replication and transcription. A typical example is **platinum,** a derivative of which, **cisplatin,** is a chemotherapeutic agent commonly used to treat cancers.

## Reactive Oxygen Species

ROS are free radicals, molecular species that are rendered highly reactive by the presence of unpaired electrons. They damage DNA by "stealing" electrons from DNA to become more stable. Examples include **superoxide, hydrogen peroxide,** and **hydroxyl radicals.** These species are thought to be important in age-related cellular damage.

## Ionizing Radiation

Ionizing radiation, produced by radioactive materials, is electromagnetic radiation with energy high enough to ionize a molecule or atom by removing an electron from its orbit. This process causes significant DNA damage, resulting in mutations and eventual cell death. Although potentially very dangerous, this type of radiation can be used in targeted cancer treatment and radiography (x-rays).

## Ultraviolet Radiation

Ultraviolet (UV) radiation is a type of electromagnetic radiation with a shorter wavelength and higher energy than those of visible light. It causes DNA damage by inducing the formation of covalent bonds between adjacent thymine nucleotides, giving rise to bulky **thymine dimers.** This is the basis for increased risk of skin cancer resulting from sun overexposure (Figure 2-22). For example, DNA damage to melanocytes can result in loss of control mechanisms for cellular growth, creating uninhibited growth patterns seen in various types of melanomas.

## DNA REPAIR

DNA damage occurs almost constantly in living cells. When DNA damage surpasses a certain threshold, either because there is too much accumulated damage or because DNA repair mechanisms are no longer effective, a cell can have one of the following three fates:

1. **Senescence:** A cell enters a dormant state that is irreversible.
2. **Apoptosis:** A cell undergoes programmed cell death, or suicide, by activating specialized signal cascades.
3. **Cancer:** A cell starts undergoing unregulated cell division, resulting in neoplasia and tumor growth.

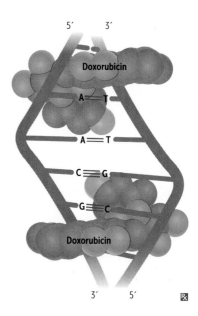

**FIGURE 2-21.    Doxorubicin.** DNA intercalating agents like doxorubicin squeeze between DNA base pairs, interfering with enzymes that need to interact with DNA during replication.

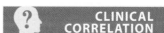

**CLINICAL CORRELATION**

Ionizing radiation (given by radiation oncologists) works by producing oxygen free radicals that cause DNA damage and trigger cancer cell apoptosis.

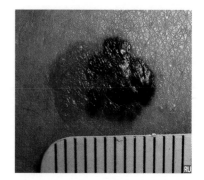

**FIGURE 2-22.    Skin cancer.** Clinical appearance of malignant melanoma, a skin cancer caused by UV radiation, often a consequence of sun overexposure.

DNA repair is thus extremely important for proper functioning of cells and the organism as a whole. A number of specialized DNA repair mechanisms have evolved, and are discussed below (Table 2-12 for an overview).

### Single-Strand Damage

When only one of the strands in the DNA double helix is damaged, the complementary base on the opposite strand can be used as a template for repair. Several DNA repair mechanisms rely on this principle.

**TABLE 2-12.** **DNA Repair Mechanisms**

| TYPE OF DAMAGE | HALLMARK LESION | REPAIR SYSTEM | HOW IT WORKS | DISEASE OF DEFECTIVE REPAIR | GENE IMPLICATED AND ITS FUNCTION |
|---|---|---|---|---|---|
| Single base oxidation, deamination, or alkylation | C deamination to U | Base excision repair | The individual base (not the entire nucleotide) is cleaved off by DNA glycosylase; the phosphodiester backbone remains intact. Now the involved nucleotide simply lacks a purine or pyrimidine base. Subsequently, AP endonuclease (so named because it excises apurinic/apyrimidinic bases) cleaves the phosphodiester backbone, severing the bond between the defective nucleotide and the rest of the polymer. DNA polymerase and ligase then replace the single nucleotide gap in the chain with the correct nucleotide. | Autosomal recessive familial adenomatous polyposis (hereditary colon cancer syndrome) | *MUTYH*; DNA glycosylase needed to cleave out damaged individual bases. |
| Two neighboring bases | UV-induced thymidine dimers | Nucleotide excision repair | After DNA surveillance enzymes detect the presence of bulky thymidine dimers, UV-specific endonucleases become activated and remove the thymidine dimer, as well as up to 30 adjacent bases. nDNA polymerase and ligase resynthesize the missing strand and fuse it to the existing phosphodiester backbone. | Xeroderma pigmentosum | Several genes involved in nucleotide excision repair. |
| Two normal nucleotides inappropriately base paired across the double helix | Any non-AT or GC pair | Mismatch repair | DNA surveillance proteins detect the mismatch and must assess which base is incorrect. Because DNA replication is semiconservative, one strand of a duplex is always old and the other new. It is assumed that the newly synthesized strand contains the erroneous nucleotide, so the mismatch repair pathway excises that nucleotide and several neighboring bases. The proteins involved can differentiate the old or parent strand from the newly synthesized strand, because the parent strand contains methylated adenine bases wherever the sequence GATC occurs. In the new strand, adenines within GATC sequences have not yet had a chance to undergo methylation, forming a convenient system for allowing mismatch repair to distinguish between the old strand and the new strand that requires repair. | Hereditary nonpolyposis colorectal cancer, aka Lynch syndrome | *MSH2* helps recognize mismatches within DNA; *MLH1* helps to excise the portion of the daughter strand containing the incorrect base. |

## Base Excision Repair

When **single** nucleotides are damaged by alkylation, deamination, or oxidation reactions, two enzymes, **DNA glycosylase** and **AP** endonuclease remove and repair the damaged bases. Endonuclease nicks the phosphodiester bond next to the base, releases deoxyribose, and creates a gap. **DNA polymerase** then inserts the correct nucleotide in its place (based on the complementary base), and the nick is sealed by **DNA ligase.** The most common DNA damage is the deamination of cytosine to uracil.

## Nucleotide Excision Repair (NER) (Figure 2-23)

A set of mechanisms similar to base excision repair, but used to excise and replace longer stretches of nucleotides (2–30 bases). UV-damaged DNA: dimers form between adjacent pyrimidines (eg, thymine), thus preventing DNA replication. **UV-specific endonuclease** (uvrABC excinuclease) recognizes the damaged base and makes a break several bases upstream (toward the 5′ side). Helicase removes the short stretch of nucleotides. The gap is filled in by DNA polymerase, and DNA ligase seals the nick.

## Mismatch Repair

Mismatch repair occurs when there is an error in the pairing of nucleotides secondary to DNA replication or recombination. The base pair mismatch repair system detects errors that escaped proofreading during DNA replication.

- **Identify the mismatched strand:** In newly synthesized DNA, adenine residues in GATC sequence motifs have not yet been methylated. Thus, the DNA parent strand, but not the newly synthesized strand, is methylated.
- **Repair damaged DNA:** The mismatched strand is nicked with endonuclease and the mismatched base(s) is/are removed. The sister strand is used as a template, and DNA polymerase fills in the gap.

> **KEY FACT**
>
> **Endonucleases** (aka restriction enzymes) only cut DNA in the middle of a sequence. By definition, **exonucleases** can only remove nucleotides from the 5′ or 3′ end.

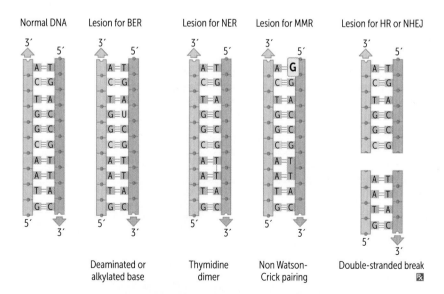

FIGURE 2-23. **DNA repair pathways and their hallmark lesions.** The pathway of DNA repair depends on the type of lesion present. Damaged purine or pyrimidine *bases* are repaired by simple **base excision.** If the entire nucleotide is damaged, **nucleotide excision** will be required. Mismatches are handled by **mismatch repair.** Double-stranded breaks (DSBs) are ideally repaired by **homologous recombination,** using the other copy of the genetic material from the **homologous chromosome** as a template. If the homologous chromosome cannot be used as a template, **nonhomologous end joining (NHEJ)** is used. NHEJ nonspecifically repairs the DSB without a template. This saves the cell from apoptosis, but never restores the DNA to its original sequence.

### Double-Strand Breaks

The situation is distinctly different when both strands of the DNA double helix are broken. In this case, no direct template exists to guide the cell's repair process. Double-stranded breaks (DSBs) can be repaired by either homologous recombination (recombinatorial repair or crossing over) or nonhomologous end joining (NHEJ). In NHEJ, specific proteins bring the ends of two DNA fragments together. However, this is error prone and mutagenic.

### Nonhomologous End Joining

When both strands of DNA are broken in a region that has not yet been replicated, there is truly no template for the cell to use to reconstruct the damaged DNA. However, because a complete break of the DNA double helix is highly deleterious for the cell, an attempt is made to fix the break using NHEJ. In this process, DNA ligase–containing complexes join the separated ends of the double helix, relying on microhomologies between the ends of the single-stranded fragments. However, by definition, NHEJ is always mutagenic.

### Homologous Recombination

Each cell has two copies of every chromosome (except X and Y). The homologous chromosome can serve as a backup copy or template if its counterpart experiences a **DSB.** The repair of DSBs using the homologous chromosome as a template is referred to as **homologous recombination.**

## CELL CYCLE CHECKPOINTS

When entering cell division or mitosis (M), the cell cycle enters the $G_1$ phase (growth phase 1). At this point, nonproliferating cells enter $G_0$, a quiescent phase, whereas active cells proceed to the synthesis (S) phase, which is characterized by DNA replication. Following the S phase is the $G_2$, or growth phase 2, a short period before the cell divides again (reenters the M phase).

Several checkpoints exist in the cell cycle for a damaged cell to prevent itself from proceeding to the next phase in the cycle (Figure 2-24).

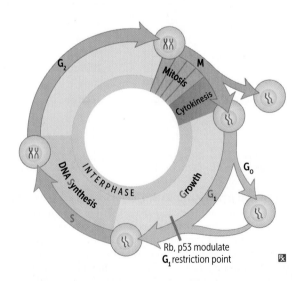

**FIGURE 2-24.    Cell cycle checkpoints.** At several points during the cell cycle, a dividing cell ensures that multiple criteria are satisfied before proceeding with the cycle. Most notably, these include the $G_1$, $G_2$, and M (mitosis or anaphase) checkpoints.

### G₁ Checkpoint

The first checkpoint takes place at the end of the $G_1$ phase. At this point, most eukaryotic cells decide whether to proceed with DNA replication (enter S phase) or become quiescent (enter the $G_0$ phase). The decision is made based on the availability of nutrients, the amount of DNA damage present, and surrounding conditions. This checkpoint is largely dependent on **p53** (a tumor suppressor protein), which can allow the cell to enter the S or the $G_0$ phase, or—if the amount of damage is too great—undergo apoptosis. Mutations in the *p53* gene are present in many cancers and are the basis for the **Li-Fraumeni syndrome.**

### G₂ Checkpoint

The second crucial checkpoint occurs at the end of $G_2$ just before mitosis. This is the final checkpoint before the cell divides. Two crucial molecules, the maturation promoting factor (**MPF**) and a **CDK,** regulate this step.

### M (Mitosis or Anaphase) Checkpoint

The final checkpoint in the cell cycle takes place in anaphase, when the action of CDK-1 triggers the destruction of **cyclins,** causing the cell to exit mitosis and initiate cytokinesis. The anaphase checkpoint is regulated by the attachment of chromosomes to the mitotic spindle. When all chromosomes are attached, the anaphase promoting complex (APC) is activated, which triggers the ubiquitination and proteolysis of the cyclin proteins.

Understanding the stages of the cell cycle helps to clarify the mechanisms of different chemotherapy drugs. Drugs that interfere with DNA **synthesis** act during S phase; classic examples are methotrexate, hydroxyurea, 6-mercapto**purine,** and 5-fluoro**uracil. Topo**isomerases untangle supercoils during DNA replication, so their inhibitors (**topo**tecan, **etopo**side) act during S phase as well. These drugs are preferentially toxic to **labile** cells that are rapidly dividing and frequently passing through S phase. This includes cancer cells, but also normal cells, such as hematopoietic stem cells and gastrointestinal (GI) epithelial cells, which explains the infamous GI and bone marrow toxicities of these medicines. Because **permanent** cells, like neurons, don't divide, they are relatively spared from the side effects of S-phase chemotherapeutics. However, drugs that directly damage DNA, such as alkylating agents, are toxic regardless of cell cycle stage. Finally, some chemotherapeutics act specifically during **M phase,** blocking stages of mitosis. For example, taxanes and vinca alkaloids interfere with microtubules, preventing normal mechanical partitioning of the DNA between the two daughter cells.

### PATHOLOGY

#### Xeroderma Pigmentosum

##### Cellular Characteristics

UV radiation causes DNA damage by inducing the formation of covalent bonds between adjacent thymine nucleotides, giving rise to bulky thymine dimers. Under normal circumstances, this damage is reversed by the **NER** mechanism. However, in XP, some of the proteins involved in NER are mutated, rendering the cell unable, or less able, to repair UV-induced damage. This leads to the accumulation of mutations and eventual development of skin cancers.

##### Genetics

XP is an autosomal recessive disease caused by mutations in one of the seven identified XP repair genes (XPA through XPG). Seven subtypes of XP are recognized (XPA–XPG, respectively), and occur with different frequencies. Different subtypes differ in their severity and clinical manifestations. The overall incidence of the disease is about 1 in 250,000 except in Japan, where it is as high as 1 in 40,000.

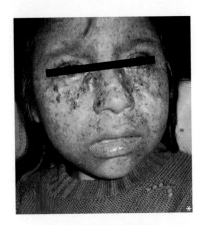

**FIGURE 2-25.** **Xeroderma pigmentosum.** Children born with defective **nucleotide excision repair (NER)** pathways develop **xeroderma pigmentosum** (XP). Because *xero-* means dry, the name simply means that patients develop dry, pigmented skin lesions. When exposed to sunlight, all of us develop **thymidine dimers** within our DNA. However, owing to deficient NER, patients with XP cannot repair them and are extraordinarily sensitive to sunlight. Mutations accumulate in exposed skin cells, leading to a variety of skin cancers. Patients are unable to venture outside in daytime and are sometimes referred to as "children of the night."

 **ANSWER**

During $G_1$, cells have not yet replicated their DNA. The main function of $G_1$ is to survey the existing DNA for mutations, and, where present, attempt to repair them. If an overwhelming number of mutations are present, healthy cells will opt for apoptosis rather than attempting to replicate badly damaged DNA.

In $G_2$, DNA replication has already occurred; the cell contains twice as much DNA as during $G_1$. Cells are now committed to division. The main goal becomes ensuring the newly duplicated chromosomes are paired off correctly in preparation for partitioning during mitosis.

### Clinical Features

XP is an autosomal recessive disorder caused by mutations that incapacitate the NER mechanism, rendering the cells unable to repair damage caused by UV radiation. Therefore, people with XP **cannot tolerate sunlight.**

Although patients are born with normal skin, the first signs of XP usually become apparent early in life (6 months of age) and include freckle-like increased pigmentation and diffuse erythema and scaling, especially in light-exposed areas. The second stage of disease usually involves the development of telangiectasias, skin atrophy, mottled irregular pigmentation, and other characteristics of poikiloderma. The final stage, which can occur in childhood, gives rise to malignancies, including malignant melanoma, squamous cell and basal cell carcinomas, and fibrosarcoma. In addition, patients exhibit generalized photosensitivity, photophobia, and conjunctivitis (80%) (Figure 2-25).

### Treatment and Prognosis

The only treatment for XP is the avoidance of sunlight. The main causes of mortality in XP are skin neoplasms, in particular, **malignant melanoma** and squamous cell carcinoma. Patients younger than 20 years have a 1000 times higher incidence of both melanoma and nonmelanoma, as compared to the general population. The average life span of a person with XP is reduced by about 40 years. Oral **retinoids** have been used to reduce the incidence of skin cancer, but they cause irreversible calcification of tendons and ligaments. **5-Fluorouracil** and topical **imiquimod** and **acitretin** have been used to treat keratoses. It has recently been discovered that topically applied bioengineered DNA repair enzymes lower the incidence of certain skin lesions during a year of treatment.

### Fanconi Anemia

#### Cellular Characteristics

At least 11 genes are involved in the Fanconi anemia (FA) pathway. Mutations in any of these genes render cells more susceptible to damage by $O_2$-free radicals. These mutations also cause deficiencies in DNA repair mechanisms and interfere with cell cycle control. Hematopoietic cells are particularly affected, and the risk of malignancy is increased in many tissues.

#### Genetics

FA is an autosomal recessive disorder that affects approximately 1 in 360,000 people worldwide; in Ashkenazi Jewish and Afrikaners populations, the incidence is approximately 10 times higher. The mutation can occur in any of the 11 genes involved in the pathway.

#### Clinical Features

FA is an autosomal recessive disease characterized by **bone marrow failure and DNA repair defects.** Patients often develop pancytopenia as a consequence of **aplastic anemia, leukemias,** and solid tumors. Pigmentation and **café-au-lait spots** are also often present. Signs of bone marrow failure include petechiae and bruising (due to thrombocytopenia), pallor and fatigue (due to anemia), and infection (due to leukopenia).

#### Treatment and Prognosis

There are no specific treatments for FA. The highest mortality and morbidity arise from bone marrow failure, leukemias, and solid cancers. Therefore, the treatments are focused on those specific clinical features.

### Cockayne Syndrome

#### Cellular Characteristics

The faulty NER mechanism leads to the inability of cells to repair DNA damage caused by exposure to UV light. This results in the accumulation of mutations and overall **accelerated aging of the cells.**

### Genetics

Both of the main types of Cockayne syndrome (CS) are autosomal recessive and are involved in NER. The incidence of the disorder is less than 1 in 250,000. It affects both genders and all races equally.

### Clinical Features

CS, like XP, is an autosomal recessive disorder caused by mutations that affect the **NER** mechanism, thus rendering the cells unable to repair damage caused by UV radiation. However, unlike XP, skin malignancies are uncommon. CS is characterized by birdlike facies, progressive retinopathy, dwarfism, and photosensitivity. Patients tend to have large ears, a thin nose, and microcephaly, with deeply set eyes, short stature, and long limbs. Skin hyperpigmentation, telangiectasia, and erythema are also common. Patients exhibit premature signs of aging and progressive neurologic deterioration.

### Treatment and Prognosis

There is no cure for CS, and treatment is largely supportive. It involves protecting the patients from sun exposure, using sunscreen, and treating neurologic deficiencies that arise, such as deafness.

## Trichothiodystrophy

### Cellular Characteristics

As in XP and CS, deficiencies in numerous proteins involved in NER result in the accumulation of UV light–induced DNA damage.

### Clinical Features

Trichothiodystrophy (TTD) is the rarest disorder arising from deficiencies in the NER mechanism. It is a heterogeneous group of autosomal recessive disorders characterized by sulfur-deficient brittle hair and nails; photosensitive, dry, thickened, scaly skin ("fish skin"); and both physical and mental retardation. Skin cancer is typically not associated with the disorder.

### Treatment and Prognosis

No cure exists for TTD, and much like in other NER disorders, the treatment is largely supportive.

## Ataxia-Telangiectasia

### Cellular Characteristics

The ATM protein is critical for detecting double-stranded breaks (DSBs) in DNA. When activated, it signals to p53 to initiate their repair. Therefore, when ATM is deficient, DSB repair is inadequate. Patients have higher frequencies of **chromosome and chromatid breaks and rearrangements,** disproportionately affecting chromosomes 7 and 14, which are responsible for T-cell receptor and immunoglobulin regulation.

### Genetics

Several genetic AT variants exist. The disease is inherited in an autosomal recessive pattern, and involves a mutation in the *ATM* gene (AT mutated), located on chromosome 11. It affects an estimated 1 in 100,000 people of all races and both sexes.

### Clinical Features

AT is typically characterized by progressive neurologic dysfunction, cerebellar ataxia, sinopulmonary infections, telangiectasias (**tel** = distant, **angio** = blood vessel, **ectasia** = dilated), increased risk of malignancy, and hypersensitivity to x-rays. Neurologically, it can progress to spinal muscular atrophy and peripheral neuropathies. Patients char-

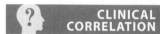

**CLINICAL CORRELATION**

Ataxia-telangiectasia mutated (*ATM*) and is the gene responsible for **ataxia-telangiectasia** (AT). *ATM* normally surveys DNA for DSBs and activates p53 to initiate repair. Because x-rays induce DSBs, AT patients must avoid radiologic tests that use x-rays, including CT scans. MRI is preferred. Recall that normal VDJ and class switch recombination rely on strategic induction and repair of DSWBs within lymphocytes, an ATM-dependent process. AT is also an immunodeficiency. Patients have low antibody levels and face significantly increased risk of recurrent pulmonary infections.

**QUESTION**

What is the difference between Fanconi anemia and Fanconi syndrome?

acteristically have dull, relaxed facies and oculomotor signs. About 30% of patients also have mild mental retardation. Skin and hair tend to show accelerated signs of aging.

### Treatment and Prognosis

The treatment of AT is aimed at controlling recurrent infections and malignancies. Supportive neurologic care is often required; the prognosis is very poor. Most patients survive until early or mid-adolescence, with the usual causes of death being broncho-pulmonary infections and cancer.

### Hereditary Nonpolyposis Colorectal Cancer (HNPCC)

#### Cellular Characteristics

Several genes involved in the **mismatch DNA repair** pathway are involved in pathogenesis in hereditary nonpolyposis colorectal cancer (HNPCC). This leads to significant **microsatellite instability** resulting in the accumulation of mutations that give rise to malignancies.

#### Genetics

HNPCC is an **autosomal dominant** disorder. It is caused by mutations in a number of genes, most notably *MSH2*, *MLH1*, and *PMS2*. In addition, *ras* gene mutations can be detected in the stool. HNPCC is thought to account for about 5% of all colorectal cancers.

#### Clinical Features

Affected individuals have a significantly increased risk of developing colorectal cancer in addition to other malignancies, such as cancers of the endometrium, ovary, stomach, and brain. HNPCC is also known as Lynch syndrome, and patients affected by this disorder have an **80% lifetime likelihood of developing colorectal cancer.** Female patients have an estimated 30–50% chance of developing endometrial cancer.

#### Treatment and Prognosis

Treatment is focused on the prevention and treatment of colorectal malignancies or other cancers. Some affected individuals elect to undergo prophylactic colectomy or hysterectomy. Common screening for cancers, including colonoscopy, pelvic exam, and urine cytology are recommended. According to the most recent guidelines, colonoscopy should be performed every two years beginning at age 25, or five years younger than the age of the earliest diagnosis in the family, whichever is earlier. Beginning at age 40, colonoscopy should be performed annually.

### Hereditary Breast Cancer

#### Cellular Characteristics

The genes involved in typical cases of hereditary breast cancer involve the DNA repair machinery. A higher frequency of *p53* mutations is seen in affected patients.

#### Genetics

Hereditary breast cancer is inherited as an **autosomal dominant** trait. It typically involves mutations of the *BRCA1* and *BRCA2* genes. Although it predominantly affects women, it is important to note that these mutations significantly increase the risk of breast tissue cancers in men as well. About 5% of all breast cancers are thought to be hereditary forms. Ashkenazi Jewish populations have increased frequencies of some common mutations in *BRCA1* and *BRCA2* genes.

#### Clinical Features

Patients affected with hereditary breast cancer have a 60 to 80% lifetime risk of developing breast cancer (compared with an average 11% lifetime risk in American women).

Characteristically, there is a strong family history of breast cancer, and the patients often develop cancer at an early age. They may also develop bilateral disease. The malignancies disproportionately include **serous adenocarcinomas.** Patients with *BRCA1* or *BRCA2* mutations face significantly increased risk of **both breast (including in men) and ovarian cancers.** Both genes are also (less strongly) associated with increased risk for cancers of the prostate, pancreas, and several other organs.

### Treatment and Prognosis

Primary interventions include breast cancer screening and mammography. Prophylactic mastectomy, oophorectomy, and chemoprevention remain controversial. The cancers are typically of higher histologic grade and are also more likely to be estrogen receptor and progesterone receptor negative, which carries implications for treatment and prognosis.

## Bloom Syndrome

### Cellular Characteristics

The mutation causing Bloom syndrome (BS) affects a gene coding for a protein with a helicase activity thought to be involved in the maintenance of genomic stability. A significantly higher frequency of sister chromatid exchanges and chromosomal instability is also seen and is thought to be due to consistent overproduction of superoxide radicals.

### Genetics

BS is an autosomal recessive disorder caused by a mutation in the *BLM* gene on chromosome 15. It is a very rare disorder (about 170 cases have been reported) that affects both sexes and all races, although it is somewhat more common in Ashkenazi Jews.

### Clinical Features

BS is a rare autosomal recessive disorder characterized by growth delay (usually of prenatal onset), a significantly increased risk of malignancy (approximately 300-fold), and recurrent respiratory and gastrointestinal infections due to compromised immunity. Telangiectatic erythema is often seen in a butterfly facial distribution. (In fact, the disease is also known as congenital telangiectatic erythema.)

### Treatment and Prognosis

Typically, there is no specific treatment for BS. Interventions are aimed at dealing with neoplasms, infection, and dermatologic manifestations. Sunscreen and sun avoidance are recommended. The highest risk of death is due to cancers, typically in the second and third decades of life.

## Werner Syndrome

### Cellular Characteristics

The gene involved in Werner syndrome (WS) codes for a DNA helicase involved in DNA repair mechanisms and general transcription and replication. WS particularly affects connective tissues, and overproduction of both collagen and collagenase has been reported. As in other diseases of this type, it is thought that the overall phenotype results from deficiencies in genome maintenance.

### Genetics

As noted, WS is a rare autosomal recessive disorder linked to a mutation in the WS gene, which codes for a helicase. It is estimated to affect 1 in 1,000,000 people. Even though no racial predilection is reported, more than 80% of the reported cases are found in Japan. It affects both men and women.

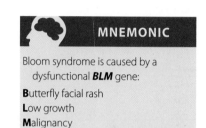

**MNEMONIC**

Bloom syndrome is caused by a dysfunctional **BLM** gene:
**B**utterfly facial rash
**L**ow growth
**M**alignancy

**QUESTION**

What are the key similarities and differences between XP and Cockayne syndrome?

### Clinical Features

WS is an autosomal recessive disease characterized by onset of accelerated aging, usually in the late teen years. The disease is also known as **progeria** of the adult. Affected individuals appear disproportionately aged, with signs including thin, tight, scleroderma-like skin, muscle atrophy, wrinkling, hyperkeratosis, gray, thinning hair, and nail dystrophy. Cataracts, osteoporosis, neoplasias, diabetes mellitus, and arteriosclerosis are generally the sources of morbidity and mortality. Of note, development is typically normal in the first decade of life.

### Treatment and Prognosis

There is no cure for WS, and the prognosis is grim. Treatments are aimed at conditions arising from the accelerated aging process, including cancers, diabetes mellitus, and arteriosclerotic complications. The mean survival for patients with WS is the middle of the fourth decade, with death usually resulting from malignancies and arteriosclerosis.

## Enzymes

### GENERAL

Enzymes are biologic polymers that catalyze chemical reactions, allowing them to proceed at rates that are compatible with life as we know it.

**KEY FACT**

Almost all enzymes are proteins. However, recent research has revealed that some RNA molecules can act as enzymes (known as ribo*zymes*).

**KEY FACT**

Apoenzyme + cofactor = holoenzyme.

**A    ANSWER**

Both XP and CS are caused by autosomal recessive defects in the NER pathway.

In XP,
- patients are hypersensitive to sunlight and at massively increased risk for skin cancer
- the minority of patients have mental retardation and neurologic deficits

In CS,
- patients are hypersensitive to sunlight, but are not at increased risk for skin cancer
- the majority of patients have dysmorphic features and severe neurologic deficits

### Nomenclature

The suffix "-ase" **always** indicates an enzyme (eg, DNA polymerase). Most enzyme names end with -ase.

Another common enzyme suffix is "-in" (eg, thrombin).

### Activity

Many enzymes are dependent on the presence of a cofactor. A **cofactor** is a small molecule that binds to an enzyme, affording that enzyme catalytic activity. Without the cofactor, the enzyme is inert (ie, it is an **apoenzyme**). All cofactors belong to one of two classes: metals (eg, $Mg^{2+}$, $Zn^{2+}$) or small organic molecules (eg, biotin, THF).

Vitamins are small organic molecules that serve as cofactors for many important enzymes. When patients become deficient in certain vitamins, the corresponding enzymes cannot catalyze reactions, eventually leading to clinical symptoms.

A given vitamin often serves as a cofactor for many distinct enzymes that catalyze similar or analogous chemical transformations. For example, vitamin $B_7$ (biotin) is a cofactor for several enzymes that add carboxyl groups to their substrates. $B_1$ (thiamine) is an essential cofactor for many enzymes that remove carboxyl groups; it is an essential participant in **decarboxylation** reactions. Therefore, when a patient has thiamine deficiency, many such enzymes cannot decarboxylate their targets.

For example, pyruvate dehydrogenase, $\alpha$-ketoglutarate dehydrogenase, and transketolase are all stuck in their inactive apoenzymatic forms. Key pathways relying on these enzymes are blocked, eventually producing the clinical syndrome of beriberi: a spectrum from "wet" beriberi, manifested by congestive heart failure and edema, to "dry" beriberi, in which neuromuscular dysfunction is most prominent.

## Thermodynamics

Enzyme activity can be quantified by several variables, as described in Table 2-13.

### Gibbs Free Energy Change

$$\Delta G = \Delta H - T\Delta S$$

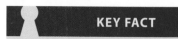

$\Delta G$ represents the difference in free energy state between the products and the reactants in a reaction. Systems favor low-energy states. Thus, a reaction proceeds in the direction that decreases the system's free energy.

If the reaction, $A + B \rightarrow C + D$, is characterized by $\Delta G = -3.0$ kJ/mol, then by definition, the reverse reaction, $C + D \rightarrow A + B$, is characterized by $\Delta G = +3.0$ kJ/mol.

In this example, $A + B \rightarrow C + D$ is said to be **exergonic.** It proceeds spontaneously (ie, no energy input is required to drive the reaction).

The reverse reaction, $C + D \rightarrow A + B$ is said to be **endergonic.** It does not proceed spontaneously but will occur if sufficient energy is added to the system.

For the reaction, $A + B \underset{\leftarrow}{\rightarrow} C + D$.

**TABLE 2-13. Thermodynamic Properties**

| | $\Delta G$ | $\Delta G_{ACT}$ | $\Delta H$ | $\Delta S$ |
|---|---|---|---|---|
| Represents | Change in free energy | Free energy of activation | Change in enthalpy (heat content) | Change in entropy |
| Information given | Direction and extent of a reaction. If negative, will proceed spontaneously. If positive, will not. These are not rules, just consequences of fact that energy must be invested to break strong chemical bonds | Rate of reaction | Whether heat is given off or absorbed | Level of disorder in system. If positive, will favor the reaction, reflecting nature's tendency toward disorder. For example, reactions that split one molecule into several (proteases, nucleases, or glycosylases) will have favorable entropy |
| Affected by enzymes | No | Yes—they lower it, which increases the reaction rate | No | No |
| If < 0 | Exergonic reaction—will proceed spontaneously | Does not occur | Exothermic reaction—heat is given off | Does not occur (except in isolated subsets of a system) |
| If = 0 | System is at equilibrium | Does not occur | No change in heat | The components of the system have neither absorbed nor given off energy |
| If > 0 | Endergonic reaction—energy input necessary to drive reaction | Energy of transition state—minimum energy required of reacting molecules for reaction to proceed | Endothermic reaction—heat is absorbed | Spontaneous reaction |

### The Equilibrium Constant

$$K'_{eq} = [C] [D] / [A] [B]$$

$K'_{eq}$ represents the ratio of the concentration of products to reactants when the reaction is at equilibrium (the rates of the forward and reverse reactions are equal, and there is no net change in the amounts of products or reactants).

When $K'_{eq} > 1$, the equilibrium lies to the right, and favors formation of products.

When $K'_{eq} < 1$, the equilibrium lies to the left and favors formation of reactants.

$\Delta G$ and $K'_{eq}$ are related by the expression:

$$\Delta G = \Delta G^{\circ\prime} + RT \ln K'_{eq}$$

$\Delta G^{\circ\prime}$ represents the **standard free-energy change,** or the change in free energy when the concentration of the reactants and products are each 1.0 M and the pH is 7. R is the gas constant (8.31 J/mol · K, but do *not* memorize it), and T is the absolute temperature.

## KINETICS

Many enzymes' kinetic properties can be explained by the Michaelis-Menten model. For the purposes of Step 1, you can assume Michaelis-Menten kinetics unless stated otherwise.

The Michaelis-Menten model states that:

$$E + S \underset{k_{-1}}{\overset{k_1}{\rightleftarrows}} ES \overset{k_2}{\rightarrow} E + P$$

- E (enzyme) + S (substrate) must combine to form an ES (enzyme-substrate complex), which then proceeds to E + P (product).
- $k_1$ represents the rate of complex formation, while $k_{-1}$ represents the rate of dissociation of the complex *back* to reactant.
- $k_2$ represents the rate of formation of product from the complex.

The concentration of enzyme-substrate complex is dependent on the rates of its formation ($k_1$) and dissociation ($k_{-1}$ and $k_2$).

$$\text{ES formation} = k_1[E][S]$$

$$\text{ES breakdown} = (k_{-1} + k_2) [ES]$$

Assuming steady-state conditions for the complex,

$$k_1[E][S] = (k_{-1} + k_2) [ES]$$

or

$$[E][S]/[ES] = (k_{-1} + k_2)/k_1$$

The familiar Michaelis-Menten constant, $K_m$, combines all of the rate terms.

$$K_m = (k_{-1} + k_2)/k_1$$

$K_m$ compares the rate of breakdown of the complex with the rate of formation, thus representing the affinity that an enzyme and substrate have for each other.

The lower the $K_m$, the higher the affinity.

The higher the $K_m$, the lower the affinity.

The rate of the enzymatic reaction, V, is defined as the rate of formation of P.

$$V = k_2[ES]$$

V, therefore, is directly related to [ES], and inversely related to $K_m$.

These relationships are summarized in Table 2-14 and are represented graphically in Figure 2-26.

As the substrate concentration increases, the rate of the reaction, V, increases. The asymptotic $V_{max}$ occurs at the substrate concentration that saturates the enzyme's active sites. At this [S], adding more substrate will not increase the rate of the reaction because there are no additional sites for the formation of the ES complex. Often, the relationship between V and S is plotted reciprocally as a **Lineweaver-Burk plot** to obtain a linear plot, as shown in Figure 2-27.

Inhibitors are molecules that bind to an enzyme and decrease its activity.

**Competitive** inhibitors **compete** for the active site. They bind at the same site as the substrate, thus preventing the substrate from binding.

**Noncompetitive** inhibitors bind at a site **distinct** from the active site. They reduce the enzyme's efficiency without affecting substrate binding. These differences are summarized in Table 2-15.

Clinically, the concept of **competitive inhibition** is extremely important when considering the toxicology of alcohol overdose. Three alcohols are commonly abused. Methanol is a common contaminant in home-brewed spirits or moonshine. Ethanol is the active ingredient in beer, wine, and spirits. Ethylene glycol is a component of antifreeze, often consumed accidentally by children owing to its sweet taste, or by alcoholics desperate for intoxication.

These three alcohols share a common metabolic fate in the liver (Figure 2-28). First, each alcohol is oxidized to the corresponding aldehyde by **alcohol dehydrogenase**, using oxidized nicotinamide adenine dinucleotide ($NAD^+$), an extremely common cofactor for enzymes catalyzing redox reactions. Specifically, methanol is converted to formaldehyde, which causes **blindness.** Ethanol becomes acetaldehyde, which is thought to be responsible for hangovers. Ethylene glycol becomes glycoaldehyde. Second, **aldehyde dehydrogenase** uses $NAD^+$ to oxidize these products to the corresponding carboxylic

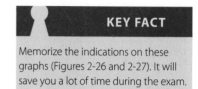

**KEY FACT**

Memorize the indications on these graphs (Figures 2-26 and 2-27). It will save you a lot of time during the exam.

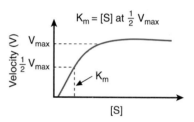

**FIGURE 2-26. Michaelis-Menten curve.**

**TABLE 2-14. $K_m$ Relationships**

| $K_m$ | INDICATES | IMPLICATION | V |
|---|---|---|---|
| Low | Low $k_1$ or $k_2$ <br> *or* <br> High $k_{-1}$ | High enzyme-substrate affinity because ES state is preferred over E and S | Fast |
| High | High $k_1$ or $k_2$ <br> *or* <br> Low $k_{-1}$ | Low enzyme-substrate affinity because E and S are preferred over ES state | Slow |

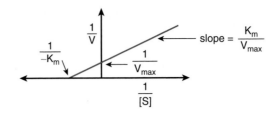

FIGURE 2-27.    **Lineweaver-Burk plot.**

acids. Most notably, glycoaldehyde is converted to oxalate, which can crystallize and cause nephrolithiasis, a feared complication of ethylene glycol poisoning. Therefore, a key principle in all three cases is that the **aldehyde metabolites produced by hepatic oxidation are more toxic than the original alcohol.** Therefore, in all three cases, a cornerstone of therapy is inhibition of alcohol dehydrogenase, the enzyme responsible for generating toxic metabolites.

Historically, methanol or ethylene glycol poisoning was treated with ethanol, because ethanol **competitively inhibits alcohol dehydrogenase,** thereby reducing aldehyde production. A newer alternative is **fomepizole,** another competitive inhibitor of alcohol dehydrogenase. Conversely, any compound that blocks **aldehyde dehydrogenase** will worsen toxicity by preventing aldehyde degradation. Some medications, most famously metronidazole, block aldehyde dehydrogenase. If patients consume even a small amount of alcohol while taking metronidazole, they can experience symptoms identical to those of a hangover, including flushing, nausea, and vomiting.

This effect can also be exploited therapeutically. If alcoholics take **disulfiram,** another **competitive inhibitor of aldehyde dehydrogenase,** they know to expect a horrific hangover, which discourages drinking. In honor of this infamous effect, any drug that causes an exaggerated hangover after alcohol consumption is said to produce a **"disulfiram-like reaction."**

## REGULATION

An enzyme's efficacy is regulated by many factors.

TABLE 2-15.    **Enzyme Inhibition**

|  | COMPETITIVE INHIBITORS | WHY | NONCOMPETITIVE INHIBITORS | WHY |
|---|---|---|---|---|
| Resemble substrate | Yes | — | No | — |
| Overcome by increasing [S] | Yes | Greater probability that substrate, rather than inhibitor, will bind active site | No | Inhibition is due to effect on enzyme alone, not enzyme-substrate interaction |
| Bind active site | Yes | — | No | — |
| Effect on $V_{max}$ | Unchanged | With maximal [S], inhibition is overcome[a] | Down | Enzyme cannot function at maximal efficiency |
| Effect on $K_m$ | Up | Presence of inhibitor decreases the likelihood of enzyme-substrate binding (affinity of the enzyme for the substrate) | Unchanged | Inhibitor does not affect likelihood of enzyme-substrate binding since it binds to the enzyme at a separate site |

[a]Although $V_{max}$ itself is unchanged, it occurs at a greater [S] than when no inhibitor is present.

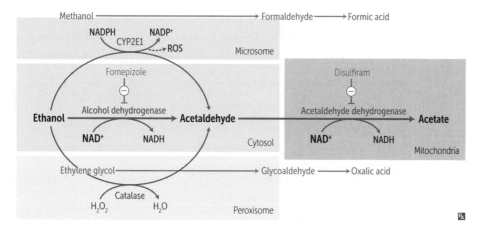

**FIGURE 2-28.** **Methanol, ethanol, and ethylene glycol metabolism.** The metabolism of methanol, ethanol, and ethylene glycol is analogous. In all three cases, alcohol dehydrogenase oxidizes the alcohol to an aldehyde, which is subsequently converted to a carboxylic acid (formate, acetate, or oxalate). Because the aldehyde metabolites are quite toxic, a cornerstone of treatment for methanol and ethylene glycol poisoning is alcohol dehydrogenase inhibition, using either fomepizole or ethanol. CYP2E1, cytochrome P450 2E1; NAD$^+$, oxidized nicotinamide adenine dinucleotide; NADP$^+$, oxidized nicotinamide adenine dinucleotide phosphate; NADPH, reduced nicotinamide adenine dinucleotide phosphate; ROS, reactive oxygen species.

## pH

The activity of enzymes is dependent on pH. Each enzyme has an optimal pH at which it is maximally active.

- The optimal pH varies by enzyme.
- The optimal pH often depends on the ionization state of the enzyme's side chain(s).
- The optimal pH often "makes sense" physiologically.
- Pepsin is an enzyme that breaks down protein in the stomach. Its optimal pH is about 2, which corresponds to the stomach's acidic environment.

### Temperature

In general, as temperature increases, an enzyme's activity also increases (the heat increases the kinetic energy in the system). In biology lab, you probably incubated many enzymatic reactions at 37°C or higher. At these temperatures, the enzyme-catalyzed reactions occur much more rapidly than they would have occurred at room temperature (22°C).

- Above a certain temperature, enzymatic activity rapidly decreases. This is due to protein denaturation.
- Each enzyme has a different optimum temperature.

### Concentration

- Increased enzyme concentration increases activity because more active sites are available for binding by reactants.
- Decreased enzyme concentration decreases activity because fewer active sites are available for binding by reactants.
- In the cell or the body, the concentration of any enzyme is determined by the relative rates of enzyme synthesis and enzyme degradation.
- Enzyme synthesis may be increased in the presence of an inducer or decreased in the presence of a repressor.
- Inducers and repressors act at the level of transcription by binding to DNA regulatory elements.
- Enzyme degradation is mediated by ubiquitination, which tags proteins for destruction by the proteasome.

## Covalent Modification

An enzyme's activity can be altered by the attachment or removal of other molecules. Such additions or subtractions may change the enzyme's structure or other properties, resulting in a change in enzyme activity.

### Phosphorylation and Dephosphorylation

Each of these processes can increase *or* decrease enzymatic activity, depending on the particular enzyme.

- Phosphorylation occurs at serine, threonine, and tyrosine residues.
- Kinases are enzymes that catalyze phosphorylation.
- Phosphatases are enzymes that catalyze dephosphorylation.

### Zymogens (Proenzymes)

Inactive precursors to enzymes that must be cleaved in some way to achieve their active form.

**Example:** The complement and coagulation cascades each consist of a chain of zymogens.

- Once activated, each zymogen cleaves and activates the next zymogen in the sequence.
- This mechanism allows large quantities of the complement and clotting proteins to be present at sites where they might be needed.
  - Because the factors are inactive, there is little risk of excessive immune response or thrombosis.
  - Because the factors are already synthesized and localized, the systems may be mobilized extremely quickly when needed.

### Allosteric Regulation

An enzyme's activity can be modified by the binding of a ligand to an allosteric site (a site **distinct from** the active site).

- The modulator may increase or decrease the enzyme's activity.
- The modulator may be the reactant or product itself, or it may be a distinct molecule.
- In many cases, the product of a reaction binds to its enzyme at an allosteric site to decrease further formation. This is a common mechanism of **feedback inhibition.**

Enzymes use allosteric regulation to sense the local environment and alter their activity accordingly. For example, end products of a metabolic pathway very frequently inhibit earlier enzymes in the pathway. A classic example is dATP, a final product of purine biosynthesis, allosterically inhibiting the earlier enzyme, ribonucleotide reductase (RR). RR senses sufficient dATP levels and reduces metabolic flux through the entire pathway. When levels of dATP fall, the allosteric inhibition is alleviated. RR activity increases and more dATP is made. Thus, **feedback inhibition through allostery is a fundamental principle of metabolic pathways. In sum, metabolites that signal success of a pathway, like dATP, inhibit earlier enzymes.**

On the other hand, **accumulation of precursor metabolites often causes allosteric activation.** A classic example from glycolysis is fructose 2,6-bisphosphate as a potent allosteric activator of phosphofructokinase. Its buildup signifies a backlog of glycolytic precursors, which logically causes activation of the rate-limiting enzyme.

An infamous example of deranged allosteric regulation occurs in SCID, due to deficiency of ADA. ADA normally degrades purines for subsequent recycling in the purine

**FLASH FORWARD**

Trypsin**ogen** is a **zymogen made in the pancreas and secreted into the duodenum.** Like a pinned grenade, zymogens (so named because eventually an en**zyme** will be **gen**erated from them) are inactive precursors that will become proteases only after proteolytic cleavage. Trypsinogen is cleaved into active trypsin only after reaching the intestine, where the protease that activates it, **enterokinase,** is uniquely expressed. Trypsin subsequently cleaves dietary peptides into smaller pieces, enabling their absorption. This **spatial regulation** is critical for preventing disastrous premature trypsin activation within the pancreas. This occurs during acute pancreatitis, when trypsin digests the pancreas itself, as do other pancreatic proteases that become inappropriately activated by trypsin.

**MNEMONIC**

**Allos** = other. An **allosteric** site is one *other* than the active site.

salvage pathway. When ADA is mutated, intact purines, like dATP, accumulate. As discussed, dATP allosterically inhibits RR, blocking de novo purine synthesis, particularly within lymphocytes, and leading to profound immunodeficiency.

# The Cell

## CELLULAR ORGANELLES AND FUNCTION

The **plasma membrane** is composed of a **lipid bilayer,** which separates the cytosol from the extracellular environment, maintains the structural integrity of the cell, and serves as an **impermeable barrier to water-soluble mole**cules (Figure 2-28). The lipid bilayer is a continuous double-sided membrane that is a dynamic, fluid structure. The membrane's fluidity allows movement of molecules laterally within a single membrane and can be influenced by the factors listed in Table 2-16.

There are two main functional groups within the lipid bilayer: **lipid molecules** and **membrane proteins.**

### Lipids

Membrane lipids fall into the following three classes:

1. **Phospholipids:** The most abundant lipid molecules. Phospholipids are **amphipathic,** having both a **hydrophilic (polar) head group** and typically two **hydrophobic (nonpolar) tails** (Figure 2-29). This amphipathic nature results in the spontaneous formation of a lipid bilayer when phospholipids are placed in an aqueous environment. There are four major phospholipids, arranged asymmetrically within the lipid bilayer (Table 2-17). This asymmetry has many important functional consequences for the cell and, if altered, can trigger inflammatory reactions in surrounding cells.
2. **Cholesterol:** Decreases the fluidity of the membrane (Table 2-16).
3. **Glycolipids:** Sugar-containing lipids found only on the outer membrane.

### Proteins

The second major component of the lipid bilayer is proteins, which carry out most membrane functions. The plasma membrane contains two main types of proteins: peripheral membrane proteins and transmembrane proteins (Figure 2-29).

#### Peripheral Membrane Proteins

- Have only hydrophilic amino acids exposed on their surfaces.
- Bind to either the inner or outer membrane via noncovalent interactions with other membrane proteins.
- Do **not** extend into the hydrophobic interior of the membrane.

**TABLE 2-16.    Factors That Affect Plasma Membrane Fluidity**

| INCREASE MEMBRANE FLUIDITY | DECREASE MEMBRANE FLUIDITY |
| --- | --- |
| ↑ Temperature | ↓ Temperature |
| ↑ Unsaturation of fatty acids (↑ no. of double bonds) | ↓ Unsaturation of fatty acids (↓ no. of double bonds) |
| ↓ Cholesterol content | ↑ Cholesterol content |

**FLASH FORWARD**

$G_q$ protein signaling involves the cleavage of inositol phospholipids (phosphatidylinositol 4,5 bisphosphate = $PIP_2$), which are present in the plasma membrane in smaller quantities than the four major phospholipids listed in Table 2-17.

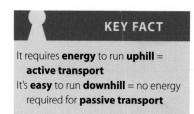

**KEY FACT**

It requires **energy** to run **uphill** = **active transport**

It's **easy** to run **downhill** = no energy required for **passive transport**

**TABLE 2-17.    Membrane Location of the Four Major Phospholipids**

| OUTER MEMBRANE | INNER MEMBRANE |
| --- | --- |
| Phosphatidyl-choline | Phosphatidyl-ethanolamine |
| Sphingomyelin | Phosphatidyl-serine |

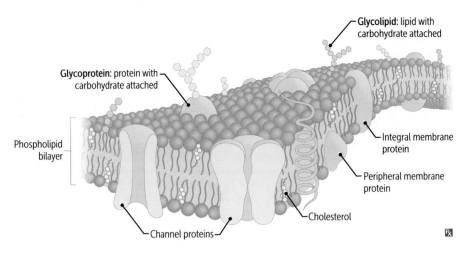

**FIGURE 2-29.** **Plasma membrane structure.** Phospholipid bilayer shown, with red circles representing polar hydrophilic groups, each contain two hydrophobic tails consisting of fatty acids.

### Transmembrane Proteins

- Are **amphipathic** (have both hydrophobic and hydrophilic regions).
- Hydrophobic regions pass through the hydrophobic interior of the membrane and interact with the hydrophobic tails of the lipid molecules.
- Hydrophilic regions are exposed to water on both sides of the membrane.

Membrane proteins play many important roles in the plasma membrane, including functioning in transport and as receptors and enzymes.

### Transport Proteins

Transmembrane proteins that allow small polar molecules (that would otherwise be inhibited by the hydrophobic interior of the plasma membrane) to cross the lipid bilayer. There are two main classes of transport proteins (Figure 2-30):

**FLASH FORWARD**

The $Na^+$-$K^+$ pump transports three positive ions out of the cell and only two positive ions into the cell, resulting in the creation of a relative negative charge inside the cell. This **electrical membrane potential** has many important functional consequences for the cell.

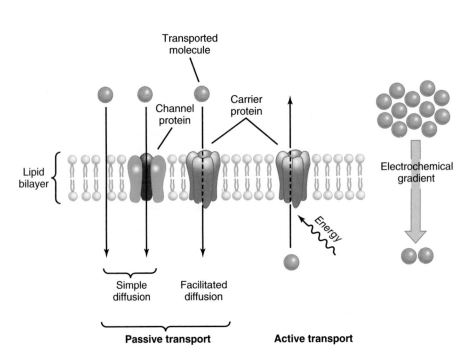

**FIGURE 2-30.** **Carrier proteins and channel proteins.**

- **Carrier proteins (transporters):** Undergo **conformational changes** to move specific molecules across the membrane.
- **Channel proteins (ion channels):** Form a narrow **hydrophilic pore** to allow passage of small inorganic ions.

Transport across the membrane can either be **active,** in which the solute is pumped "uphill" against its electrochemical gradient in an energy-dependent manner, or **passive,** in which the transport of a solute is driven by its electrochemical gradient "downhill" (Figure 2-31). Active transport can be driven either by ATP hydrolysis or by harnessing energy from the downhill flow of another solute. Transport via carrier proteins can be either active or passive, whereas transport by channel proteins is always passive.

## Carrier Proteins (Transporters)

There are three types of carrier proteins, most of which use active transport mechanisms:

- **Uniporters:** Transport a single solute from one side of the membrane to the other.
- **Symporters:** Transport two solutes across the membrane in the same direction.
- **Antiporters:** Transport two solutes across the membrane in opposite directions.

The most important carrier protein is the **$Na^+$-$K^+$ ATPase** or **$Na^+$-$K^+$ pump,** which is found in the basolateral membrane of nearly all cells. The $Na^+$-$K^+$ pump is an **antiporter** that utilizes the energy released from ATP hydrolysis to pump **three $Na^+$ ions out of the cell** and **two $K^+$ ions into the cell** with each cycle (Figure 2-32). The transport cycle depends on the phosphorylation and dephosphorylation of the $Na^+$-$K^+$ pump.

## Channel Proteins (Ion Channels)

Form **small, highly selective hydrophilic pores** that allow the **passive transport of specific inorganic ions** (primarily $Na^+$, $K^+$, $Ca^+$, or $Cl^-$) down their electrochemical gradients. Transport across ion channels (which do not need to undergo a conformational change) is much faster than transport via carrier proteins. Ion channels are selec-

**FLASH FORWARD**

**Ouabain** and the **cardiac glycosides (digoxin and digitoxin)** both bind and inhibit the $Na^+$-$K^+$ ATPase pump by competing for sites on the extracellular side of the pump. The binding of these inhibitors results in increased cardiac contractility through a $Ca^{2+}$-dependent mechanism.

**CLINICAL CORRELATION**

The ABC transporter superfamily is a clinically important class of carrier proteins. This family includes:

- The **multidrug resistance (MDR) protein,** which harnesses the energy from ATP hydrolysis to pump hydrophobic drugs out of the cell. This protein is **overexpressed in many human cancer cells,** conferring chemotherapeutic drug resistance to these cells.
- The **CF protein,** which harnesses the energy from ATP hydrolysis to pump $Cl^-$ ions out of the cell. CF results from a mutation in the *CFTR* gene on chromosome 7, which encodes the protein.

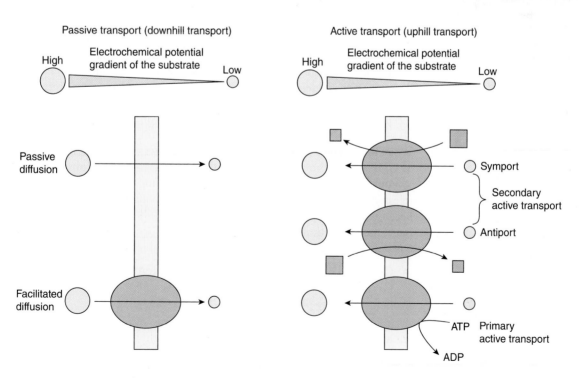

**FIGURE 2-31.    Comparison of passive and active transport.**

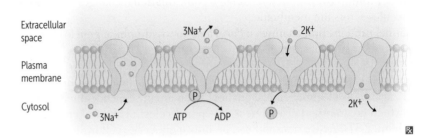

**FIGURE 2-32.**    **The Na$^+$-K$^+$ pump transport cycle.**

tively opened and closed in response to different stimuli, which determines the specific ion channel type:

- **Voltage stimulus** = voltage-gated ion channels
- **Mechanical stress stimulus** = mechanical-gated ion channels
- **Ligand binding stimulus** = ligand-gated ion channels

The activity of the majority of these channels is also regulated by protein phosphorylation and dephosphorylation.

The most common ion channels are the **K$^+$ leak channels,** which are found in the plasma membrane of almost all animal cells. K$^+$ leak channels are **open even when unstimulated or in a resting state,** which makes the plasma membrane much more permeable to K$^+$ than to other ions. This K$^+$-selective permeability plays a critical role in maintaining the negative intracellular membrane potential in nearly all cells.

### G-Protein Coupled Receptors

In addition to transporting small molecules, membrane proteins can also function as receptors. **G-protein coupled receptors,** the most important class of cell membrane receptors, are proteins that traverse the plasma membrane seven times (**seven-pass receptors**). They are **coupled to trimeric GTP-binding proteins (G proteins),** which are composed of **three subunits: α, β, and γ.** The G proteins are found on the cytosolic face of the membrane and serve as relay molecules. G-protein–coupled receptors have extremely diverse functions and respond to a vast array of stimuli. However, all G-protein–coupled receptor signaling is transduced via a similar mechanism (Figure 2-33).

When the receptor is **inactive,** the α subunit (active subunit) of the G protein is bound to **GDP.** When the receptor is **stimulated,** a change in conformation causes the α subunit to exchange GDP for **GTP,** thereby releasing itself from the βγ complex. Once released, it binds and activates target proteins. α Subunit activity is short-lived, however, because the **GTPase** quickly hydrolyzes GTP to GDP, resulting in its inactivation. The target proteins activated by the α subunit vary, depending on which of the three main types of G protein is involved.

- **Gs (stimulatory G protein)** = ↑ cyclic AMP (cAMP) levels
- **Gi (inhibitory G protein)** = ↓ cAMP levels
- **Gq** = activates phospholipase C (PLC)

### G$_s$- and G$_i$-Protein Signaling

Both the **G$_s$ and G$_i$ proteins** signal through the **adenylyl cyclase pathway.** Adenylyl cyclase is a plasma membrane bound enzyme that synthesizes cAMP from ATP. Receptors coupled to G$_s$ result in the **activation of adenylyl cyclase** and an **increase in cAMP.** Receptors coupled to G$_i$ result in the **inhibition of adenylyl cyclase** and a **decrease in cAMP.**

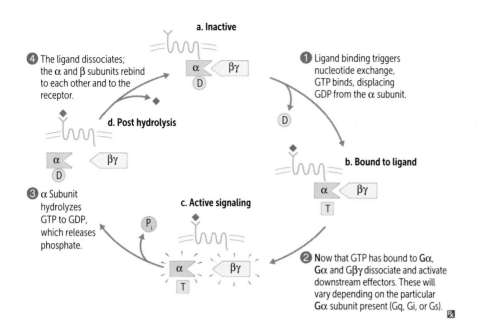

**a. Inactive**

❹ The ligand dissociates; the α and β subunits rebind to each other and to the receptor.

**d. Post hydrolysis**

❶ Ligand binding triggers nucleotide exchange, GTP binds, displacing GDP from the α subunit.

**b. Bound to ligand**

❸ α Subunit hydrolyzes GTP to GDP, which releases phosphate.

**c. Active signaling**

❷ Now that GTP has bound to Gα, Gα and Gβγ dissociate and activate downstream effectors. These will vary depending on the particular Gα subunit present (Gq, Gi, or Gs).

**FIGURE 2-33.** **G-protein–coupled receptor signaling.** GDP, guanosine diphosphate; GTP, guanosine triphosphate.

Increased concentrations of cAMP (in the case of $G_s$) result in the activation of cAMP-dependent PKA, which phosphorylates certain intracellular protein targets to cause a specific cellular response. A protein phosphatase dephosphorylates the protein targets, thus turning off their activity.

In $G_i$-protein signaling, the activated $\alpha_i$ subunit inhibits adenylyl cyclase, resulting in decreased cAMP and decreased PKA activity. Although this does elicit a cellular response, it is thought that the main effect of $G_i$ signaling is the activation of $K^+$ ion channels via the $\beta_i\gamma_I$ complex, which allows $K^+$ to flow out of the cell.

### $G_Q$-Protein Signaling

Occurs via the **PLC pathway.** PLC is a plasma membrane–bound enzyme that, when activated, cleaves the inositol phospholipid **$PIP_2$**, which is present in the inner leaflet of the plasma membrane in small amounts (see discussion of plasma membranes earlier under The Cell). This cleavage results in the formation of **inositol 1,4,5-triphosphate ($IP_3$)** and **diacylglycerol (DAG).** $IP_3$ causes **$Ca^{2+}$ release from the ER**, which activates the **$Ca^{2+}$/calmodulin-dependent protein kinase (or cAM-kinase).** cAM-kinase then phosphorylates certain intracellular proteins, resulting in a specific cellular response. DAG activates **protein kinase C (PKC)** directly, which also phosphorylates certain intracellular proteins, resulting in a specific cellular response (Figure 2-34).

## Connective Tissue

### CLASSIFICATION

One of the four basic tissue types, connective tissue serves as the structural support and internal framework of the body. There are many types of connective tissue (ie, bone, ligaments, tendons, cartilage, adipose tissue, and aponeuroses), but they all contain the same basic structural components: **few cells** and a large amount of **extracellular matrix (ECM)** that includes **ground substance and fibers.** Adult connective tissue can be classified based on the composition and function of each tissue type.

**G protein–linked 2nd messengers**

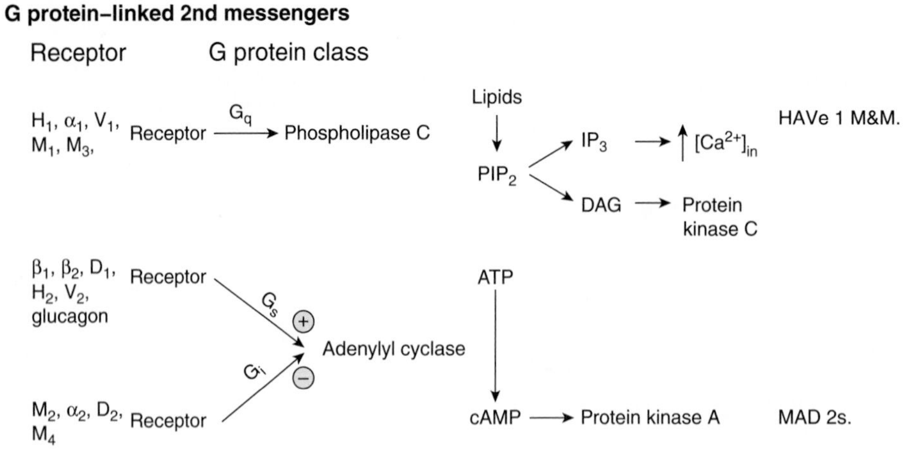

FIGURE 2-34.    **G-protein coupled receptor summary.** AMP, adenosine monophosphate; ATP, adenosine triphosphate; cAMP, cyclic adenosine monophosphate; DAG, diacylglycerol; IP$_3$, inositol triphosphate; PIP$_2$, phosphatidylinositol 4,5-bisphosphate.

### Composition

- **Loose connective tissue:** Loosely arranged fibers, abundant cells, and ground substance (ie, lamina propria).
- **Dense irregular connective tissue:** Irregularly arranged collagen fibers and few cells (ie, reticular layer of the dermis).
- **Dense regular connective tissue:** Densely packed parallel fibers with few cells packed in between (ie, tendons, ligaments, aponeuroses).

### Function

- **Structural:** Forms capsules around organs or adipose tissue that fills the spaces between organs.
- **Support:** Hard connective tissue with fibrous components arranged in parallel arrays (ie, bone, cartilage).
- **Nutrition:** Helps facilitate uptake of nutrients from extracellular space.
- **Defense:** The presence of phagocytic cells (ie, macrophages) and immunocompetent cells (ie, plasma cells and eosinophils) in the ECM is part of the body's defense mechanism against foreign objects.

### GROUND SUBSTANCE

Ground substance is a viscous, clear substance that occupies the space between the cells and fibers within connective tissue. Ground substance contains three main types of macromolecules:

- Proteogylcans
- Glycoproteins
- Fibrous proteins

The fibrous proteins and glycoproteins are embedded in a proteoglycan gel, where they form an extensive **ECM** that serves both structural and adhesive functions.

### Proteoglycans

These macromolecules consist of a **core protein** that is covalently attached to approximately 100 **glycosaminoglycan (GAG)** molecules and a **linker protein,** which binds hyaluronic acid (HA) and strengthens its interaction with the proteoglycan molecule (Figure 2-35). Proteoglycans are very large, highly negatively charged macromolecules

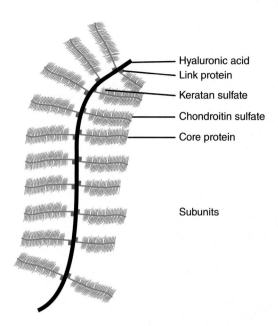

**FIGURE 2-35.**   **Proteoglycan structure.**

that attract water into the ground substance, giving it a gel-like consistency. This highly hydrated gel is able to resist compressive forces while allowing diffusion of $O_2$ and nutrients between the blood and tissue cells.

### Glycosaminoglycans

Glycosaminoglycans (GAGs) are long polysaccharide chains composed of repeating disaccharide units. One of the disaccharide units is always an **amino sugar** (N-acetylglucosamine or N-acetylgalactosamine), which is most often **sulfated** ($SO_4^{2-}$). The second sugar is usually an **uronic acid** (glucuronic or iduronic). GAGs are the most negatively charged molecules produced by animal cells because of the sulfate and carboxyl groups present on most of their sugars. These highly negatively charged molecules are essential for maintaining the high water content present in ground substance. Five types of GAGs are found in the human body (Table 2-18).

### Glycoproteins

Glycoproteins are large, multidomain proteins that help organize the ECM and attach it to surrounding cells. There are two main glycoproteins: **fibronectin** and **laminin,** both of which are present in the **basal lamina** of cells.

**FLASH FORWARD**

**Alport syndrome** results from a mutation in the α5 chain of type IV collagen, which destroys the ability of the glomerular basement membrane to properly filter blood in the kidney. Patients with Alport syndrome have kidney failure, sensorineural deafness, and ocular disorders (all organ sites where the α5 chain of type IV collagen are found).

**TABLE 2-18.**   **Glycosaminoglycans**

| GAG | LOCATION |
| --- | --- |
| Hyaluronic acid | Distributed widely throughout the connective tissues of the body |
| Chondroitin sulfate | Cartilage and bone; heart valves |
| Keratan sulfate | Cartilage, bone, cornea, and intervertebral disk |
| Dermatan sulfate | Dermis of skin, blood vessels, and heart valves |
| Heparan sulfate | Basal lamina, lung, and liver |

## FLASH FORWARD

**Bullous pemphigoid** is an autoimmune disorder in which an IgG antibody is directed against the **hemidesmosome,** which anchors the epidermis to the basement membrane. This results in detachment of the entire, intact epidermis from the basement membrane, causing **tense subepidermal bullae.** In contrast, in **pemphigus vulgaris,** autoantibodies are directed against the **desmosome,** which anchors cells together within the epidermis. This results in disintegration of the epidermis itself, causing **flaccid, intra-epidermal bullae.**

## KEY FACT

Collagen amino acid sequence = Gly-X-Y (X and Y commonly proline or hydroxyproline, respectively)

## CLINICAL CORRELATION

Peptides that are cleaved early in collagen synthesis include **p**rocollagen **i**ntact **N**-terminal **p**eptide, or **PINP.** This is measured clinically as a marker of bone formation.

On the other hand, peptide linkages between the ends of α collagen chains, referred to as **N** and **C** terminal **t**elopeptide crosslinks, or **NTX** and **CTX,** are only released later during local bone destruction. They are measured clinically as markers of bone turnover.

## FLASH FORWARD

During **wound healing,** type III collagen is laid down first in granulation tissue. As healing progresses, fibroblasts secrete type I collagen, which eventually replaces type III collagen in late wound repair.

## MNEMONIC

**Wound healing: Type III → Type I**
Three: owie (just scraped your knee).
One: it's all done.

### Basal Lamina (Basement Membrane)

Basal lamina is specialized ECM that underlies all epithelial cells and surrounds individual muscle, fat, and Schwann cells. It separates the cells from the underlying connective tissue, serves as a filter in the renal glomerulus, and functions as a scaffold during tissue regeneration/wound healing. The basal lamina is synthesized by the cells that rest on it and contains the following elements:

- Fibronectin
- Laminin
- Heparan sulfate
- Type IV collagen

### Fibronectin

Fibronectin is a dimer composed of two large subunits bound together by disulfide bridges that each contain domains specialized for binding a specific molecule (ie, integrins, collagen, or heparan) or cell. Fibronectin helps cells attach to the ECM via its different binding domains.

### Laminin

Laminin is composed of three long polypeptide chains (α, β, γ) arranged in the shape of an asymmetrical cross. Individual laminin molecules self-assemble and form extensive networks that bind to type IV collagen and form the major structural framework of basement membranes. Laminin also contains many functional domains that bind other ECM components and cell surface receptors, thus linking cells with the ECM.

## FIBERS

Fibers are present in varying amounts based on the structural and functional needs of the connective tissue type. **All fibers are produced by fibroblasts** present in the connective tissue and are composed of long peptide chains. There are three types of connective tissue fibers:

- Collagen fibers
- Reticular fibers
- Elastic fibers

### Collagen Fibers

Composed of collagen, the most abundant protein in the human body. Collagen fibers are flexible and provide high tensile strength to tissues. Collagen consists of **three polypeptide chains (α chains)** wound around each other to form a long, stiff **triple helical structure** (Figure 2-36). Collagen is **glycine** and **proline rich,** with glycine present as every third amino acid. The repeating amino acid sequence found in collagen is thus **gly-X-Y,** in which X and Y can be any amino acid (but X is commonly proline and Y is commonly hydroxyproline). One-third of the collagen amino acid structure is glycine; proline or hydroxyproline typically constitutes one-sixth of the amino acid content of collagen. This sequence is absolutely critical for triple-helix formation.

The α chains in each collagen molecule are not the same. They range in size from 600 to 3000 amino acids. At present, at least 42 types of α chains encoded by different genes have been identified, and 27 different types of collagen have been categorized based on their distinct α chain compositions. Depending on the specific type of collagen molecule, it may consist of three identical α chains (homotrimeric) or two or three genetically distinct α chains (heterotrimeric). The most important collagen types are described in Table 2-19.

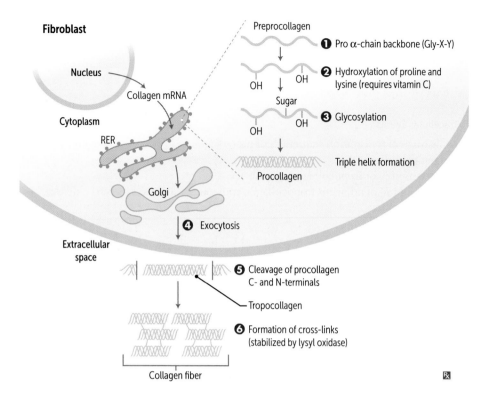

**FIGURE 2-36.** **Collagen structure and synthesis.** mRNA, messenger ribonucleic acid; RER, rough endoplasmic reticulum.

## Collagen Synthesis

Connective tissue cells or fibroblasts produce the majority of the collagen fibers. The biosynthesis process involves a series of both intra- and extracellular events (Figure 2-36).

### Intracellular Events

- Uptake of amino acids (proline, lysine, etc) by endocytosis.
- Formation of α chains (preprocollagen) mRNA in nucleus.
- Nuclear export of preprocollagen mRNA followed by entry into the rough ER (RER).
- Synthesis of preprocollagen α chains with registration sequences by ribosomes within the RER.
- Hydroxylation of proline and lysine within the RER catalyzed by peptidyl proline hydroxylase and peptidyl lysine hydroxylase. *This step requires vitamin C.*

**TABLE 2-19.** **Collagen Types, Composition, and Location**

| TYPE | COMPOSITION[a] | LOCATION |
|---|---|---|
| I | $[\alpha_1(I)]_2, \alpha_2(I)$ | Most abundant (90%) **Bone,** tendon, skin, dentin, fascia, cornea, late wound repair |
| II | $[\alpha_1(II)]_3$ | **Cartilage,** vitreous body, nucleus pulposus |
| III (reticulin) | $[\alpha_1(III)]_3$ | Skin, **blood vessels,** uterus, fetal tissue, **granulation tissue** |
| IV | $[\alpha_1(IV)]_2, [\alpha_2(IV)]$ | **Basal lamina** (basement membrane); kidney, glomeruli, lens capsule |
| X | $[\alpha_1(X)]_3$ | Epiphyseal plate |

[a]The Roman numerals simply indicate the chronological order of discovery and that each α chain has a unique structure that differs from the α chains with different numerals.

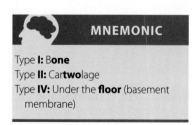

**MNEMONIC**

Type **I: B**one
Type **II:** Car**two**lage
Type **IV:** Under the **floor** (basement membrane)

- Glycosylation of hydroxylysine residues within the RER.
- Formation of α chain triple helix (procollagen) within the RER.
- Addition of carbohydrates within the Golgi network.
- Packaging into vesicles and movement to the plasma membrane.
- Exocytosis of procollagen.

### Extracellular Events

- Cleavage of registration sequences of procollagen to form tropocollagen by procollagen peptidases.
- Self-assembly of tropocollagen into fibrils.
- Cross-linking of adjacent tropocollagen molecules catalyzed by lysyl oxidase.

### Clinical Considerations

Many disorders are associated with defects in collagen synthesis.

### SCURVY

**Scurvy is caused by vitamin C deficiency** resulting in the inability to hydroxylate proline and lysine residues in α-chain polypeptides of collagen molecules. This results in **weakening of the capillaries** and the following complications:

- Ulceration of gums and gingival bleeding.
- Loose teeth (due to loss of periodontal ligaments, which are collagen rich).
- Tissue hemorrhage.
- Anemia.
- Poor wound healing.
- Impaired bone formation (in infants).

### OSTEOGENESIS IMPERFECTA

Primarily an **autosomal dominant** disorder, osteogenesis imperfecta (OI) is caused by a **variety of gene defects** leading to either **less collagen or less functional collagen** than normal (with the same amount of collagen present). Both conditions result in **weak or brittle bones.** The incidence is approximately 1:10,000 individuals. There are four types of OI, each with a range of symptoms. Type II is fatal in utero or in the neonatal period. The most common characteristics are:

- **Multiple fractures with minimal trauma** (may occur during the birthing process and is often confused with child abuse).
- **Blue sclerae** (due to the translucency of the connective tissue over the choroids) (Figure 2-37).
- **Hearing loss** (abnormal middle ear bones).
- **Dental imperfections** (defects in enamel synthesis = amelogenesis imperfecta).

### EHLERS-DANLOS SYNDROME

Ehlers-Danlos syndrome is actually a group of rare genetic disorders resulting in **defective collagen synthesis.** There are over 10 types, with disease severity ranging from mild to life-threatening, depending on the specific mutation. The most common symptoms are:

- Hyperextensible skin.
- Bleeding tendency (easy bruising), associated with berry aneurysms.
- Hypermobile joints.

**KEY FACT**

Defect in collagen synthesis:
- Collagen has three polypeptide chains that form a triple helix. Chains are made up of glycine-X-Y repeats.
- Point mutation in glycine prevents the formation of a triple helix.

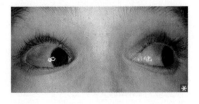

**FIGURE 2-37. Osteogenesis imperfecta.** Characteristic blue sclerae seen in osteogenesis imperfecta.

### Menkes Disease

Copper is a required cofactor for lysyl oxidase (LOX), that covalently links distinct collagen proteins, forming tough collagen fibrils. Therefore, copper deficiency results in weak collagen and kinky, breakable hair, as collagen is a major component of hair. A classic example is **Menkes disease,** an X-linked recessive copper deficiency due to lack of **ATP7A, a protein that absorbs copper from the gut.** Not surprisingly, the disease is also known as *kinky hair syndrome* (Figure 2-38).

An interesting contrast to Menkes disease is **Wilson disease,** an **autosomal recessive** deficiency of **ATP7B, a hepatic protein that excretes excess copper into the biliary tract.** These patients have **copper overload** leading to "**hepatolenticular degeneration,**" a combination of cirrhosis and neuropsychiatric disease, due to copper deposition in the liver and basal ganglia.

In sum, ATP7"**A**" absorbs copper. Deficiency causes Menkes disease, a congenital cause of copper **deficiency** that is treated with **parenteral** copper supplementation, because the gut cannot absorb copper. On the other hand, ATP7"**B**" **b**anishes copper. Deficiency causes Wilson disease, a congenital cause of copper **overload,** which is treated with copper chelators, such as penicillamine or trientine (triethylenetetramine).

### Reticular Fibers

**Type III collagen fibrils** arranged in a mesh-like pattern provide a supporting framework for cells in various tissues and organs. Reticular fibers contain a higher content of sugar groups (6–12% compared with 1% in collagen fibers) and are easily identified by the periodic acid–Schiff (PAS) stain. They are also recognized with silver stains and are thus termed **argyrophilic** (silver-loving) (Figure 2-39). Networks of reticular fibers are found in loose connective tissue in the space between the epithelia and connective tissue, as well as around adipocytes, small blood vessels, nerves, and muscle cells.

### Elastic Fibers

Elastic fibers, which allow tissues to stretch and distend, are found in skin, vertebral ligaments (ligamenta flava of the vertebral column and ligamentum nuchae of the neck), the vocal folds of the larynx, and elastic arteries.

Elastic fibers consist of two structural components: elastin and surrounding fibrillin microfibrils.

### Elastin

This highly hydrophobic protein, like collagen, is rich in proline and glycine. However, unlike collagen, elastin is poor in hydroxyproline and lacks hydroxylysine. The glycine molecules are randomly distributed, allowing for random coiling of its fibers. Elastin is produced by fibroblasts and smooth muscle cells, and its synthesis parallels collagen production. In fact, both processes can occur simultaneously within the same cell. Elastin synthesis entails two main steps:

- **Secretion of tropoelastin** (elastin precursor).
- **Cross-linking of tropoelastin** molecules via their two unique amino acids—**desmosine and isodesmosine**—to form extensive networks of elastin fibers and sheets.

Single elastin polypeptides adopt a loose "random coil" conformation when relaxed. When individual elastin proteins are cross-linked into an elastic fiber network, their collective random coil properties allow the network to stretch and recoil like a rubber band.

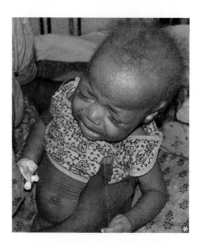

FIGURE 2-38. **Menkes disease.**

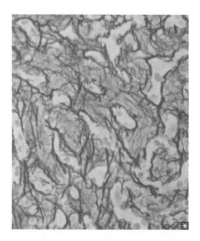

FIGURE 2-39. **Reticular fibers (silver stain).**

### Fibrillin-I

Fibrillin-I is a glycoprotein that forms fine microfibrils. Its microfibrils are formed first during elastic fiber genesis; elastin is then deposited on to the surface of the microfibrils. Elastin-associated fibrillin microfibrils play a major role in organizing elastin into fibers.

#### MARFAN SYNDROME

Marfan syndrome is a relatively common (1:3–5000) **autosomal dominant** connective tissue disorder caused by a **mutation in the fibrillin gene (*FBN1*)** (Table 2-20). In individuals with Marfan syndrome elastin-associated fibrillin microfibrils are absent, resulting in the formation of **abnormal elastic tissue.** The severity of the disease varies; affected individuals may die young or live essentially normal lives. Common symptoms include:

- **Bone elongation** (tall individuals with long, thin limbs).
- **Spider-like fingers** (arachnodactyly).
- **Hypermobile joints.**
- **Lens dislocation** (glaucoma and retinal detachment also common).
- **Cardiac abnormalities** (mitral valve prolapse is common).
- **Aortic rupture—most common cause of death** (due to loss of elastic fibers in tunica media).

## CELLS

Two different cell populations are found within connective tissue:

- Resident cells
- Transient cells

### Resident Cells

Relatively stable, permanent residents of connective tissue. These cells remain in the connective tissue and include:

- **Fibroblasts and myofibroblasts** (primary cells involved in collagen and ground substance secretion).

**TABLE 2-20.** **Key Differences Between Marfan Syndrome, Ehlers-Danlos Syndrome, and Homocystinuria**

|  | MARFAN | EHLERS-DANLOS | HOMOCYSTINURIA |
|---|---|---|---|
| Mutated gene | Fibrillin-1, which encodes a structural protein | Collagen, or related processing genes | Cystathionine β-synthase (most common), or other enzymes involved in conversion of homocysteine to cysteine or methionine |
| Inheritance | Autosomal dominant | Autosomal dominant | Autosomal recessive |
| Body habitus | Long limbs, tall stature, scoliosis, arachnodactyly, joint laxity | Hypermobile joints, distensible skin | Marfanoid habitus |
| Prototypical patient | Michael Phelps (does not have Marfan syndrome but perfectly illustrates the marfanoid habitus) | Extremely flexible circus contortionist | Has intellectual disability |
| Feared complication | Ascending aortic aneurysm and dissection | Subarachnoid hemorrhage due to ruptured cerebral aneurysm | Venous thromboembolism/hypercoagulability |
| Lens dislocation | Superiorly/laterally | Associated, but no clear anatomic pattern | Inferiorly/medially |

- **Macrophages** (arise from migrating monocytes).
- **Adipose cells.**
- **Mast cells** (arise from stem cells in the bone marrow).
- **Mesenchymal cells.**

## Transient Cells

Wandering cells that have migrated into the connective tissue from the blood in response to specific stimuli (usually during inflammation). This population is not normally found in connective tissue and is composed of cells involved in the immune response:

- Lymphocytes
- Plasma cells
- Neutrophils
- Eosinophils
- Basophils
- Monocytes

# Homeostasis and Metabolism

Various processes contribute to maintaining the energy, structure, and waste removal needs of living cells. These systems are intricate and interdependent, as summarized in Figure 2-40.

Metabolism converts four classes of substrate into energy or other usable products. These substrates include:

- Carbohydrates
- Lipids and fatty acids
- Proteins and amino acids
- Nucleotides

## CARBOHYDRATE METABOLISM

A process by which carbohydrates are broken down into water and carbon dioxide, accompanied by the generation of energy, mainly in the form of ATP. The overall reaction is relatively simple.

$$C_6H_{12}O_6 + 6O_2 \rightarrow 6H_2O + 6CO_2$$

However, the process is complicated by its relation to other metabolic cycles, namely, the fatty acid cycle, the urea cycle, Krebs cycle (tricarboxylic acid [TCA] cycle), and the hexose monophosphate (HMP) shunt.

### Intake and Absorption

Digestion of carbohydrates begins in the mouth and ends in the small intestine with absorption of the breakdown products. **Polysaccharides** (starch) and **oligosaccharides** are converted into **disaccharides** (sucrose and lactose) and **monosaccharides** (glucose and fructose).

- The monosaccharides are absorbed via transporters and carried to the liver through the portal vein.
- Ultimately, these are oxidized, stored as glycogen, transformed to fat (triglycerides), or transported as glucose via the circulation.

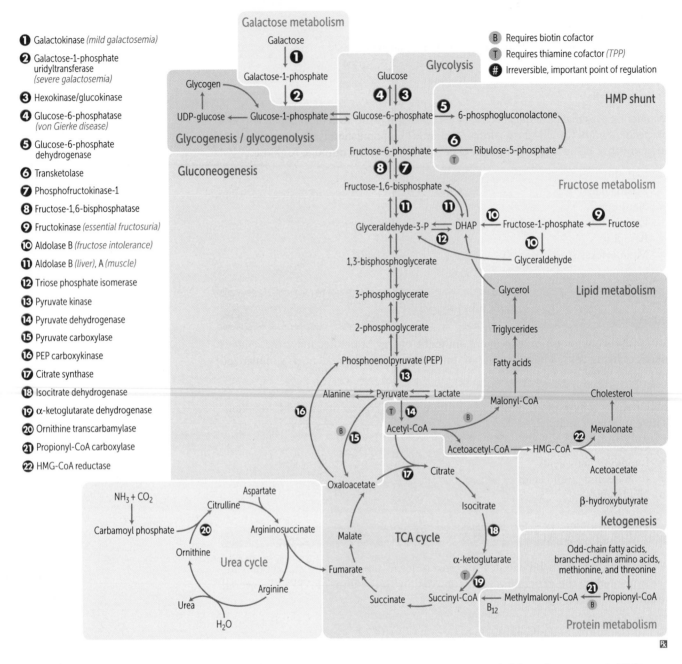

1. Galactokinase *(mild galactosemia)*
2. Galactose-1-phosphate uridyltransferase *(severe galactosemia)*
3. Hexokinase/glucokinase
4. Glucose-6-phosphatase *(von Gierke disease)*
5. Glucose-6-phosphate dehydrogenase
6. Transketolase
7. Phosphofructokinase-1
8. Fructose-1,6-bisphosphatase
9. Fructokinase *(essential fructosuria)*
10. Aldolase B *(fructose intolerance)*
11. Aldolase B *(liver)*, A *(muscle)*
12. Triose phosphate isomerase
13. Pyruvate kinase
14. Pyruvate dehydrogenase
15. Pyruvate carboxylase
16. PEP carboxykinase
17. Citrate synthase
18. Isocitrate dehydrogenase
19. α-ketoglutarate dehydrogenase
20. Ornithine transcarbamylase
21. Propionyl-CoA carboxylase
22. HMG-CoA reductase

B Requires biotin cofactor
T Requires thiamine cofactor *(TPP)*
\# Irreversible, important point of regulation

**FIGURE 2-40.** **Metabolic pathways.** DHAP, dihydroxyacetone phosphate; HMG-CoA, hydroxymethylglutaryl-coenzyme A; HMP, hexose monophosphate; TCA, tricarboxylic acid; UDP, uridine diphosphate.

### Glycolysis

#### Function

Initial step in the metabolism of glucose to produce energy for the cell. Glycolysis usually occurs in aerobic environments, but can occur under anaerobic conditions.

#### Location

Cytoplasm of all cells that utilize glucose.

#### Reactants

One molecule of glucose.

#### Products

**Aerobic** glycolysis: Two molecules of pyruvate, two ATP, two NADH. **Anaerobic** glycolysis: Two molecules of lactic acid (from pyruvate) and two ATP.

## Cycle

See Figure 2-41.

## Regulation

Phosphorylation of glucose to glucose-6-phosphate (G6P) blocks its ability to diffuse across the cell membrane, **trapping** it within the cell. Two kinases in the cytosol are

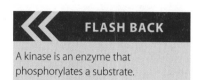

**FLASH BACK**

A kinase is an enzyme that phosphorylates a substrate.

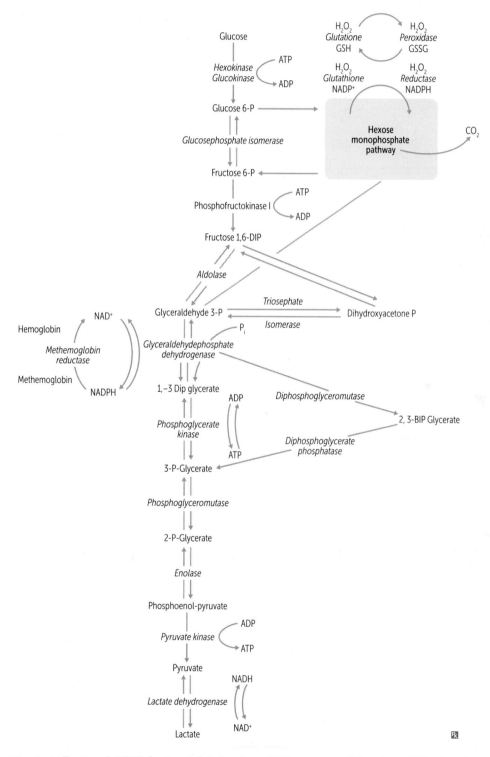

**FIGURE 2-41.** **Glycolysis.** Fructose 1,6-DIP, fructose 1,6-diphosphate. ADP, adenosine diphosphate; ATP, adenosine triphosphate; BIP, binding immunoglobulin protein; DIP, dipyridamole; GSH, reduced glutathione; GSSG, oxidized glutathione; NAD+, oxidized nicotinamide adenine dinucleotide; NADH, reduced nicotinamide adenine dinucleotide; NADP+, oxidized nicotinamide adenine dinucleotide phosphate; NADPH, reduced nicotinamide adenine dinucleotide phosphate.

involved. The process consumes one molecule of ATP per molecule of glucose phosphorylated.

- **Hexokinase:** Ubiquitous, nonspecific (phosphorylates many different six-carbon sugars), low $K_m$ (easily saturable), feedback inhibited by G6P.
- **Glucokinase:** Mainly in the liver, very specific for glucose, high $K_m$ (not easily saturable), feedback inhibited by fructose-6-phosphate (F6P, the product of the subsequent step in glycolysis).
- **Phosphofructokinase 1 (PFK-1):** The most important regulatory point in all of glycolysis, because after conversion of G6P to fructose 1,6, bisphosphate, the cell has committed to sending that molecule of glucose all the way through glycolysis. Before the action of PFK-1, it is still possible to re-route G6P into the HMP shunt, or into glycogen synthesis via transformation into glucose-1-phosphate. Thus, PFK-1 represents a key branch point between glycolysis, glycogen synthesis, and the HMP shunt. In general, PFK-1 regulation follows simple principles of allostery and negative feedback: It is inhibited by high concentrations of metabolites that are further downstream (eg, phosphoenolpyruvate, ATP, and citrate). The presence of these compounds indicates a high rate of successful completion of glycolysis and the TCA cycle, and therefore signifies reduced need for the action of PFK-1. Conversely, when fructose 2,6 bisphosphate and AMP accumulate, it signifies existence of high amounts of precursors that are built up behind PFK-1, and an overall depletion of ATP within the cell. Both clearly indicate the need to stimulate PFK-1, thereby increasing traffic through glycolysis. This will provide more fuel for subsequent ATP generation via the TCA cycle and electron transport chain.

### Pathophysiology

RBCs have no mitochondria and therefore cannot use the TCA cycle or electron transport chain to make ATP. They depend on anaerobic glycolysis entirely for ATP production. Consequently, deficiencies in glycolytic enzymes, most commonly pyruvate kinase, deplete ATP within RBCs, leading to hemolytic anemia. RBCs also face tremendous oxidative stress because they carry oxygen from the lungs to the tissues. They rely on glutathione for protection from ROS constantly generated within them. However, each time glutathione is used to quench ROS, it needs to be reduced again before it can be reused. This leads to a key point. **RBCs use the HMP shunt to generate NADPH, which is used by glutathione reductase to regenerate reduced glutathione, the major protection for RBCs against ROS** (Figure 2-42). Therefore, any defect in the HMP shunt will deplete RBC glutathione stores, leaving RBCs vulnerable to ROS and causing hemolytic anemia.

The classic example is deficiency of the first HMP shunt enzyme, glucose-6-phosphate dehydrogenase (G6PD), which is especially common among people of African, Asian, or Mediterranean descent. In this disease, ROS overwhelm the limited glutathione stores, causing hemoglobin to denature and resulting in **Heinz bodies,** inclusions consisting of unfolded hemoglobin. When splenic macrophages remove these bulky Heinz bod-

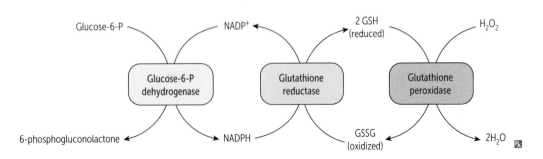

**FIGURE 2-42.** **Role of glucose-6-phosphate dehydrogenase.** 6GP, 6-phosphogluconate; G6P, glucose-6-phosphate; NADP, nicotinamide adenine dinucleotide phosphate; NADPH, reduced form of nicotinamide adenine dinucleotide phosphate.

ies, it appears as if RBCs have been bitten. As a result, blood smears will often show **degmacytes,** or "**bite cells.**"

In patients with G6PD deficiency, the consumption of foods or medications that generate ROS will exacerbate the stress on RBCs. For example, eating fava beans can precipitate attacks of hemolysis, a syndrome referred to as **favism.** Antimalarial and sulfa drugs can do the same. Finally, it is important to note that the gene for G6PD is on the X chromosome. Because this is an X-linked recessive disorder, the vast majority of patients will be male.

### Pentose Phosphate Pathway (HMP Shunt)

#### Function

Shunts G6P to form ribulose-5-phosphate for nucleotide synthesis. Generates NADPH as a reducing equivalent for GSH/GSSG (the premier antioxidant system in the cell) and NADPH for steroid and fatty acid biosynthesis.

#### Location

Cytoplasm of all cells.

#### Reactants

G6P.

#### Products

NADPH, which is used in steroid and fatty acid biosynthesis and regeneration of GSH in the GSH/GSSG antioxidant system; ribose-5-phosphate; $CO_2$.

#### Cycle

Summarized in Figure 2-43.

#### Regulation

The reaction consists of two parts:

- The first irreversible step is catalyzed by G6PD to produce NADPH from G6P (this step is oxidative).
- The second, reversible, step isomerizes the sugars so they can reenter glycolysis. This step is nonoxidative.

> **FLASH FORWARD**
>
> In healthy cells with intact mitochondria, cytochrome c should be confined within the mitochondria, helping to run the ETC. When mitochondrial damage occurs, cytochrome c leaks out, a key signal for initiating apoptosis.

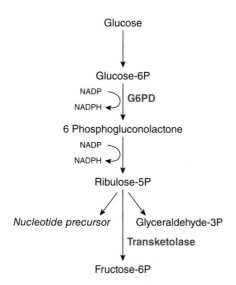

**FIGURE 2-43.    Pentose phosphate pathway (HMP shunt).** G6PD, glucose-6-phosphate dehydrogenase; NADP, nicotinamide adenine dinucleotide phosphate; NADPH, reduced form of nicotinamide adenine dinucleotide phosphate.

### KEY FACT

**Summary of HMP products and their roles:**
- NADPH: Oxidation, steroid synthesis, fatty acid synthesis.
- Ribulose-5-phosphate: Nucleotide synthesis, F6P, glyceraldehyde-3-phosphate (glycolysis intermediate).

### Pathophysiology

G6PD deficiency has a high prevalence among African-Americans. Please see discussion under Glycolysis.

## TCA (Krebs) Cycle

### Function

The Krebs cycle produces high-energy electron carriers (NADH, reduced flavin adenine dinucleotide [$FADH_2$]) for ATP generation in the mitochondria and completes the metabolism of glucose (final common pathway).

### Location

Mitochondria (inner matrix).

### Reactants

Pyruvate is the chief substrate. Proteins and fats enter the cycle after being converted to acetyl-CoA.

### Products

Three NADH, one $FADH_2$, two $CO_2$, and one GTP. Each NADH molecule ultimately yields three ATP. Each $FADH_2$ ultimately yields two ATP. The GTP is converted into ATP in a reaction that does not require energy. Each acetyl-CoA molecule yields 12 ATP molecules.

### Cycle

Summarized in Figure 2-44.

### Regulation

The cycle is controlled at three major steps:

- Acetyl-CoA + oxaloacetate (OAA) → citrate, catalyzed by citrate synthase (allosterically inhibited by ATP).

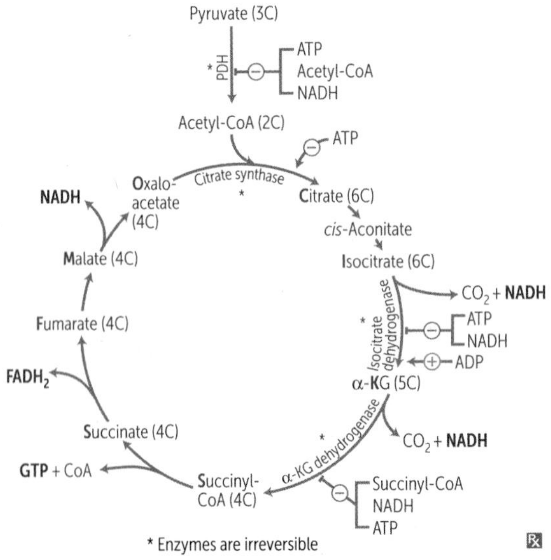

**FIGURE 2-44.  TCA (Krebs) cycle.** Steps with * indicate regulatory steps. α-KG, α-ketoglutarate. ADP, adenosine diphosphate; ATP, adenosine triphosphate; CoA, coenzyme A; $FADH_2$, reduced flavin adenine dinucleotide; GTP, guanosine triphosphate; NADH, reduced nicotinamide adenine dinucleotide.

- Isocitrate → α-ketoglutarate, controlled by isocitrate dehydrogenase (activated by ADP and inhibited by ATP and NADH).
- α-Ketoglutarate → succinyl-CoA, controlled by α-ketoglutarate dehydrogenase (inhibited by succinyl-CoA and NADH).

### Electron Transport Chain and Oxidative Phosphorylation

#### Function

High-energy electrons from NADH and $FADH_2$ are transduced to ATP.

#### Location

Mitochondria (inner membrane).

#### Reactants

High-energy electrons from NADH and $FADH_2$ are transferred onto complex 1 and complex 2, respectively. After electrons arrive at complex 4, they are transferred onto oxygen, the "final electron acceptor," a reaction that creates water.

As electrons travel down the ETC, they enable complexes 1 through 4 to expel protons from the mitochondrial matrix into the intermembrane space. This creates a pH gradient across the inner mitochondrial membrane (intermembrane space more acidic, ie, lower pH, and matrix less acidic with a higher pH). This gradient makes protons spontaneously "want" to enter the matrix. Conveniently, they can only do so via complex 5, the ATP synthase, providing it with the energy needed to phosphorylate ADP back to ATP.

Because NADH and $FADH_2$ which were generated in the cytosol, cannot physically cross the mitochondrial membrane, the electrons are shuttled into mitochondria by organ-specific shuttles.

- **Glycerol phosphate shuttle** → ubiquitous; transfers NADH electrons to mitochondrial $FADH_2$.
- **Malate-aspartate shuttle** → found in muscle, liver, and heart; transfers NADH electrons to mitochondrial NADH.

#### Products

ATP and $H_2O$.

#### Cycle

Summarized in Figure 2-45.

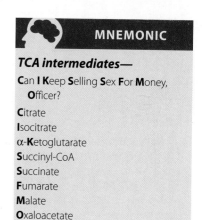

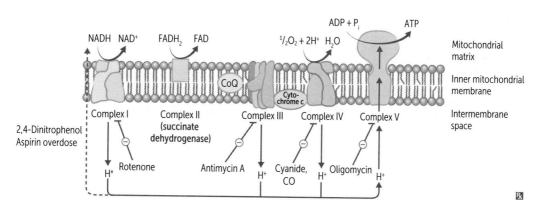

**FIGURE 2-45.** **Electron transport chain and oxidative phosphorylation.** ADP, adenosine diphosphate; ATP, adenosine triphosphate; CoQ, coenzyme Q; NADP, nicotinamide adenine dinucleotide phosphate; NADPH, reduced form of nicotinamide adenine dinucleotide phosphate; $P_i$, inorganic phosphate.

## Fructose Metabolism

### Function

Converts dietary fructose into a substrate for glycolysis.

### Location

Muscle, kidney, and liver.

### Reactants

Fructose and ATP.

### Products

Glyceraldehyde-3-phosphate.

### Cycle

See Figure 2-46.

- Dietary sucrose is broken down by sucrase in the small intestine to fructose and glucose.
- Fructose is phosphorylated by hexokinase to F6P in muscle and kidney.
- In the liver, fructose is converted to fructose-1-phosphate by fructokinase.
- Fructose-1-phosphate aldolase (also known as **aldolase B**) converts fructose-1-phosphate to dihydroxyacetone phosphate (DHAP) and glyceraldehyde. DHAP can be converted into glyceraldehyde-3-phosphate, which enters glycolysis. Glyceraldehyde is phosphorylated by triose kinase, also creating glyceraldehyde-3-phosphate, which enters glycolysis.

### Pathophysiology

- Deficiencies in fructokinase are benign, leading to **fructosuria** (essential fructosuria).
- Fructose-1-phosphate aldolase deficiency leads to **hereditary fructose intolerance,** characterized by severe hypoglycemia upon sucrose or fructose ingestion.

## Galactose Metabolism

### Function

Converts dietary galactose (from lactose) to a form that can enter glycolysis.

### Location

Kidney, liver, and brain.

### Reactants

Galactose and ATP.

> **CLINICAL CORRELATION**
>
> Fructose is not found in breast milk; therefore, disorders of fructose metabolism will not present until the infant is weaned from breastfeeding.

> **CLINICAL CORRELATION**
>
> Breast milk contains lactose, which consists of glucose and galactose, hence its name: Milk produced by **lac**tation contains **lac**tose. Recall that human breast milk does not contain fructose or sucrose. Therefore, classic galactosemia presents in **newborns,** as opposed to fructose intolerance, which presents at the time of weaning.

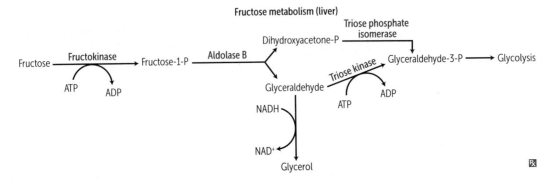

**FIGURE 2-46.    Fructose metabolism in the liver.** ADP, adenosine diphosphate; ATP, adenosine triphosphate; NADP, nicotinamide adenine dinucleotide phosphate; NADPH, reduced form of nicotinamide adenine dinucleotide phosphate.

Products

Glucose-1-phosphate.

Cycle

See Figure 2-47.

- Dietary lactose is broken down in the small intestine by lactase to galactose and glucose.
- Galactose is phosphorylated by galactokinase to galactose-1-phosphate.
- Galactose-1-phosphate is converted by galactose-1-phosphate uridyl transferase to glucose-1-phosphate.

Pathophysiology

- **Galactokinase deficiency:** Hereditary deficiency of galactokinase. An autosomal recessive, relatively mild overall condition. Galactose cannot be phosphorylated to galactose-1-phosphate, causing galactose to accumulate and be shunted towards galactitol. This occurs in the lens of the eye, leading to osmotic damage, and **early cataract formation** in this disease.
- **Classic galactosemia** is due to absence of **GALT,** or **gal**actose-1-phosphate uridyl transferase, and is inherited in an autosomal recessive fashion. This is a severe disease leading to failure to thrive and increased risk for *E coli* **sepsis** (a very important association for Step 1). Because the same pathway is blocked, just one step later, patients also have cataracts, and sometimes are born with them. Management requires elimination of **galactose and lactose** (the disaccharide consisting of glucose and galactose) from the diet.

### Anaerobic Metabolism and Cori Cycle

Function

Shuttles lactate from muscle into the liver, allowing muscle to function anaerobically when energy requirements exceed oxygen consumption.

Location

Muscle and liver.

Reactants

Anaerobic metabolism uses glucose. The Cori cycle begins with lactate and consumes six ATP.

Products

Anaerobic metabolism produces two net ATP and two pyruvates per glucose molecule. Lactate is converted to glucose in the Cori cycle.

Cycle

See Figure 2-48.

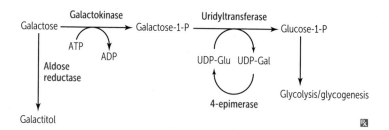

**FIGURE 2-47.** **Galactose metabolism.** ADP, adenosine diphosphate; ATP, adenosine triphosphate; Gal, galactose; Glu, glucose; UDP, uridine diphosphate.

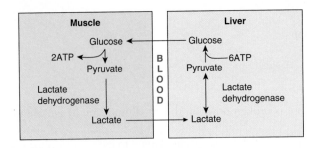

**FIGURE 2-48.    Cori cycle.** Transfers excess reducing equivalents from RBCs and muscle to liver, allowing muscle to function anaerobically (net 2 ATP).

## Gluconeogenesis

### Function

Gluconeogenesis simply means "new glucose production." It involves creation of brand-new molecules of glucose from **noncarbohydrate precursors,** including fatty and amino acids.

### Location

Cytoplasm and mitochondria of kidney, liver, and intestinal epithelium.

### Reactants

Pyruvate: Because it is the starting material for gluconeogenesis, any metabolite that can be converted to pyruvate can serve as raw material for generating glucose (Figure 2-49). The most commonly used are lactate (when derived from muscle, called the **Cori cycle**), glycerol (derived from triacylglyercols), alanine (converted directly to pyruvate via alanine transaminase [ALT]), and glutamine. Therefore, any compound that can be converted into pyruvate can be integrated into a glucose molecule via gluconeogenesis and is therefore said to be **glucogenic.** This entire paradigm is the reason starvation will cause muscle loss: When dietary intake is insufficient to support the blood glucose, muscles begin to break sarcomeric proteins into amino acids, transmitting them to the liver for conversion via gluconeogenesis into glucose to stave off hypoglycemia (and loss of consciousness). This extra burst of blood glucose is intended to allow for survival until the next meal.

### Products

Glucose.

### Cycle

See Figure 2-50.

### Regulation

Although some of the steps in glycolysis and the TCA cycle are irreversible, they can be bypassed by the use of ATP or GTP and four enzymes, found only in the kidney, liver, and intestinal epithelium.

- Pyruvate carboxylase converts pyruvate → OAA.
- PEP (phosphoenolpyruvate) carboxykinase converts OAA → PEP.
- Fructose-1,6-bisphosphatase converts fructose-1,6-bisphoshate → F6P.
- G6P converts glucose-6-phosphatase → glucose.

## Glycogen Metabolism

### Function

Helps maintain glucose homeostasis by forming (**glycogenesis**) or breaking down (**glycogenolysis**) glycogen. Crucial for the storage of energy derived from carbohydrate metabolism.

**A**    ANSWER

The liver exhausts NAD+ stores while metabolizing alcohol. The resulting NADH excess creates a reductive environment in the liver, causing reduction of pyruvate to lactate. Pyruvate depletion prevents adequate gluconeogenesis, leading to hypoglycemia. Hypoglycemia triggers a catabolic state, driven by counter-regulatory hormones, including epinephrine and glucagon. These activate lipolysis, releasing free fatty acids, which are subsequently converted to ketone bodies in the liver. In alcoholic ketoacidosis, β-hydroxybutyrate will be the predominant ketone. The same NADH excess that drives pyruvate's reduction causes reduction of acetoacetate, the only true ketoacid, to β-hydroxybutyrate, which no longer contains a ketone.

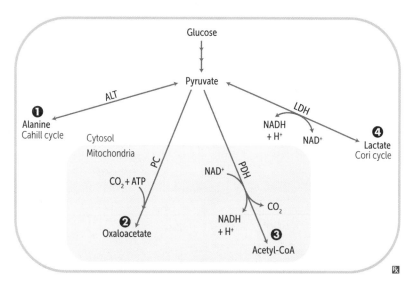

Functions of different pyruvate metabolic pathways (and their associated cofactors):

❶ Alanine aminotransferase ($B_6$): alanine carries amino groups to the liver from muscle

❷ Pyruvate carboxylase (biotin): oxaloacetate can replenish TCA cycle or be used in gluconeogenesis

❸ Pyruvate dehydrogenase ($B_1$, $B_2$, $B_3$, $B_5$, lipoic acid): transition from glycolysis to the TCA cycle

❹ Lactic acid dehydrogenase ($B_3$): end of anaerobic glycolysis (major pathway in RBCs, WBCs, kidney medulla, lens, testes, and cornea)

**FIGURE 2-49.    Pyruvate metabolism.** Pyruvate is a remarkably versatile metabolite that can be shunted into numerous other biochemical pathways, including the Cahill cycle (1), gluconeogenesis (2), tricarboxylic acid cycle (2 and 3), as well as anaerobic glycolysis and the Cori cycle (4). ALT, alanine transaminase; ATP, adenosine triphosphate; CoA, coenzyme A; LDH, lactate dehydrogenase; NAD, nicotinamide adenine dinucleotide; $NAD^+$, oxidized nicotinamide adenine dinucleotide; NADH, reduced nicotinamide adenine dinucleotide; PC, pyruvate carboxylase; PDH, pyruvate dehydrogenase; TCA, tricarboxylic acid.

### Location

Glycogenesis—liver and muscle. Glycogenolysis—heart, liver, and muscle.

### Reactants

Glucose/glycogen.

### Products

Glycogen/glucose.

### Glycogenesis

Glucose is polymerized into glycogen, its insoluble storage form. To increase storage efficiency, **branch points** are added by **branching enzymes** to allow for a more compact three-dimensional structure. Mainly stored in the liver and muscle tissue (Figure 2-51).

### Glycogenolysis

Release of glucose from glycogen stores. Serves to protect from hypoglycemia during periods of starvation or between meals. **Debranching enzymes** must be used to untangle the branches of glycogen created during glycogen synthesis. See Figure 2-51.

### Regulation

These opposing processes are regulated by the hormones insulin and glucagon. **Insulin** promotes the removal of glucose from the bloodstream, thereby increasing **glycogenesis** and decreasing glycogenolysis. Glucagon does the opposite.

### Pathophysiology

There are 12 types of glycogen storage diseases. All result in abnormal glycogen metabolism and an accumulation of glycogen within cells. See Table 2-21 for the most common types and Figure 2-52 and Table 2-22 for a summary of the metabolic cycles and pathways.

**KEY FACT**

Insulin release signifies a "well-fed" state and instructs cells to invest in creating energy stores for future use, eg, insulin encourages glycogen and lipid synthesis. These will be broken down during periods of starvation later. To ensure that glycogen and lipids aren't simultaneously synthesized and degraded (highly inefficient), insulin also blocks glycogenolysis and lipolysis.

**QUESTION**

A mother brings her baby to the ED after he started vomiting and crying inconsolably. The recently weaned baby tried apple juice for the first time this morning. Labs show severe hypoglycemia. What is the disorder? What is the mechanism for the hypoglycemia?

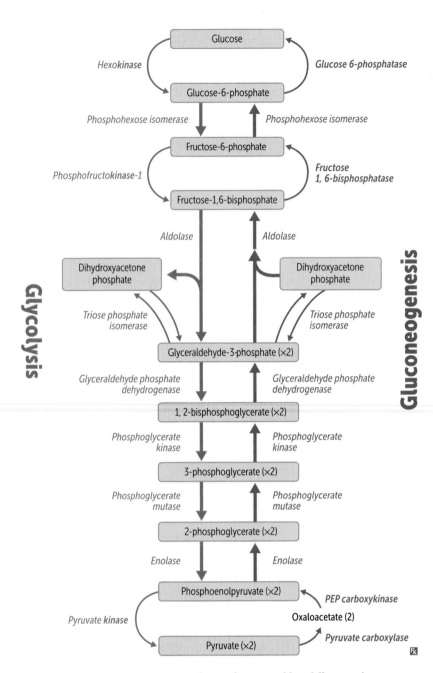

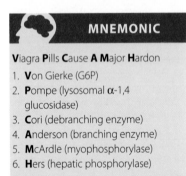

**A    ANSWER**

Hereditary fructose intolerance is an autosomal recessive disorder in which aldolase B is the missing enzyme. As a result, fructose-1-phosphate accumulates after fructose consumption, depleting hepatocytes of phosphate. Without free phosphate, the liver cannot perform gluconeogenesis and glycogenolysis, leading to hypoglycemia. Thus, fructose is toxic to these patients. They must avoid foods with both fructose and sucrose, because sucrose is simply a disaccharide composed of glucose and fructose.

**FIGURE 2-50.   Gluconeogenesis.** Note the similarities and key differences between glycolysis and gluconeogenesis. Glycolysis has three irreversible steps (catalyzed by hexo**kinase**, phosphofructo**kinase,** and pyruvate **kinase**). Gluconeogenesis uses four separate enzymes to bypass these unilateral steps, as shown with solid red *arrows*. These additional enzymes are only produced in the kidney, liver, and gut, hence these are the only tissues that are able to manufacture glucose during times of starvation (ie, to perform gluconeogenesis).

## Urea Cycle

### Function

Detoxification of $NH_4^+$ generated by amino acid metabolism (eg, de**amination** of alanine to pyruvate by alanine trans**aminase,** or ALT) releases ammonium. This free ammonium is subsequently incorporated into urea, which is excreted into the urine.

### Location

The urea cycle is a conversation between the mitochondria and cytoplasm of liver cells.

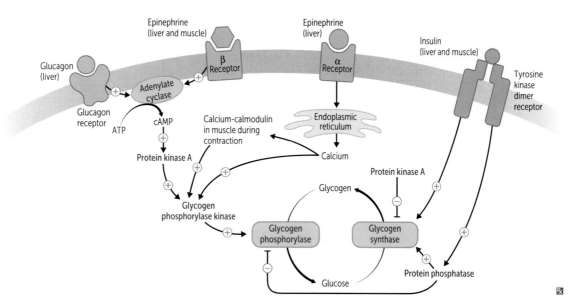

**FIGURE 2-51.** **Integration of glycogen metabolism.** The stress hormones glucagon and epinephrine ultimately induce glycogen breakdown so that glucose can be obtained for immediate use. Insulin, a hormone released after meals, causes liver cells to polymerize glucose into glycogen to prepare for future periods of starvation. ATP, adenosine triphosphate; cAMP, cyclic adenosine monophosphate.

### Reactants

$CO_2$, $NH_4^+$, and 3 ATP.

### Regulation

Carbamyl phosphate synthase catalyzes the formation of carbamoyl phosphate from $CO_2$ and $NH_4^+$. This enzyme, in turn, is activated by N-acetylglutamic acid.

### Products

Urea and fumarate (fumarate enters the TCA cycle).

### Pathophysiology

Disorders of the urea cycle involve enzymatic deficiencies that prevent detoxification of ammonia from protein catabolism into urea. Therefore, the **finding that unites them all is hyperammonemia that worsens with high protein intake.** The most common is the X-linked recessive ornithine transcarbamylase (OTCase) deficiency. Accordingly, it will virtually always present only in neonatal boys. Of note, all the other urea cycle disorders are inherited in an autosomal recessive fashion. Effectively, this means that if a female patient presents with hyperammonemia, OTCase deficiency is highly unlikely, even though it is by far the most common urea cycle disorder.

Key findings in OTCase deficiency include hyperammonemia and decreased blood urea nitrogen (BUN), due to inability to synthesize urea. A key differential for the USMLE is orotic aciduria, because orotic acid is increased in both disorders.

The urea cycle occurs in the liver, and its primary function is conversion of the toxic **ammonia** into the benign **urea.** Both are measured clinically: ammonia directly, and urea as the **BUN.** Elevated ammonia and low BUN signify liver dysfunction, specifically an inability to properly run the urea cycle, thereby failing to clear the normal ammonia load. Hyperammonemia can cause altered mental status and neurologic changes, including the classic **asterixis**, a loss of flexor tone, leading to "flapping" of the hands with wrists extended. Because there is neurologic dysfunction due to liver pathology, this condition is referred to as **hepatic encephalopathy.** On the other hand, elevated BUN often indicates volume depletion. The elevated urea is due to increased reabsorption by the nephron. **Uremia** refers to a constellation of electrolyte abnormalities due to renal insufficiency, the hallmark of which is elevated BUN, simply owing to inability

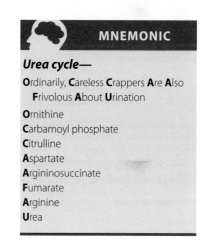

**MNEMONIC**

*Urea cycle—*

**O**rdinarily, **C**areless **C**rappers **A**re **A**lso **F**rivolous **A**bout **U**rination

**O**rnithine
**C**arbamoyl phosphate
**C**itrulline
**A**spartate
**A**rgininosuccinate
**F**umarate
**A**rginine
**U**rea

**CLINICAL CORRELATION**

In **diabetic ketoacidosis (DKA),** a state of absolute insulin deficiency, cells do not receive the signal to invest in glycogen and lipid synthesis. Fat cells, perceiving a state of starvation, induce lipolysis, which releases free fatty acids. **The liver will convert these into ketone bodies, exacerbating the patient's acidosis and anion gap.** Similarly, hepatocytes will upregulate gluconeogenesis and glycogenolysis, creating and releasing more glucose, respectively. This worsens the patient's hyperglycemia and **hyperosmolarity.**

**TABLE 2-21.    Glycogen Storage Diseases**

| DISEASE | FINDINGS | DEFICIENT ENZYME | GLYCOGEN APPEARANCE | COMMENTS |
|---------|----------|------------------|---------------------|----------|
| Von Gierke (type 1) | Severe fasting hypoglycemia, ↑↑ glycogen in liver, ↑ blood lactate, ↑ triglycerides, ↑ uric acid, and hepatomegaly. | Glucose-6-phosphatase | Normal. Glucose-6-phosphatase is not involved directly in synthesis or breakdown of glycogen. It dephosphorylates glucose-6-phosphatase already liberated from glycogen. | Autosomal recessive. Treatment: frequent oral glucose/cornstarch; avoidance of fructose and galactose. |
| Pompe (type 2) | Cardiomegaly, hypertrophic cardiomyopathy, exercise intolerance, and systemic findings leading to early death. | Lysosomal α-1,4-glucosidase (acid maltase) | Glycogen structure is normal, but lysosomes are unable to degrade it. | Autosomal recessive. **P**ompe trashes the **P**ump (heart, liver, and muscle). |
| Cori (type 3) | Milder form of type I with normal blood lactate levels. | Debranching enzyme (α-1,6-glucosidase) | Glycogen is excessively branched, owing to lack of debranching enzyme. | Autosomal recessive. Gluconeogenesis is intact. |
| Andersen (type 4) | Cirrhosis, esophageal varices, ascites, liver failure. | Branching enzyme | Long, linear strands (because no branching) that become insoluble and toxic. | Best treatment is a liver transplant. |
| McArdle (type 5) | ↑ glycogen in muscle, but muscle cannot break it down → painful muscle cramps, myoglobinuria (red urine) with strenuous exercise, and arrhythmia from electrolyte abnormalities. | Skeletal muscle glycogen phosphorylase (myophosphorylase) | Glycogen is normal, but muscles cannot liberate glucose from it. | Autosomal recessive. Blood glucose levels typically unaffected. **M**cArdle = **M**uscle. Treat with vitamin $B_6$ (cofactor). |
| Hers (type 6) | Significant hepatomegaly, mild hypoglycemia causing ketosis and growth retardation. | Hepatic phosphorylase | Normal, but in excess amounts, because glycogen can be synthesized but not degraded in Hers disease. | Overall relatively benign disease. Treatment is starch between meals to avoid hypoglycemia. |

Modified with permission from Le T, et al. *First Aid for the USMLE Step 1 2016.* New York, NY: McGraw-Hill Education; 2016: 99.

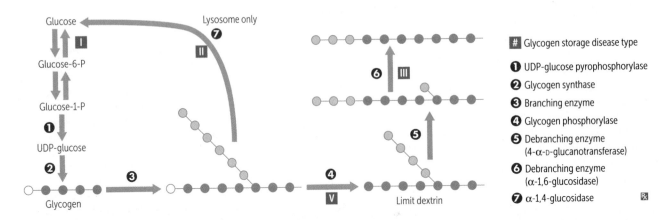

**FIGURE 2-52.    Glycogenesis.** Glucose can be polymerized into glycogen by specialized enzymes during the process known as glycogenesis. Distinct enzymes liberate glucose from glycogen in the process called glycogenolysis. Defects in either of these pathways are referred to as glycogen storage disorders. UDP, uridine diphosphate.

**TABLE 2-22.    Summary of Metabolic Cycles and Pathways**

| CYCLE/PATHWAY | FUNCTION | LOCATION | REACTANTS | PRODUCTS |
|---|---|---|---|---|
| Glycolysis | Breakdown of glucose into pyruvate, which either proceeds to lactate (anaerobic glycolysis) or the Krebs (TCA) cycle (aerobic glycolysis). | Cytoplasm of cells that use glucose | Glucose. | 2 Pyruvate, 2 ATP, and 2 NADH |
| Krebs cycle (TCA cycle) | Production of high-energy electron carriers for ATP generation in mitochondria. | Mitochondria | Pyruvate and acetyl-CoA derived from protein and fat breakdown. | 3 NADH, 1 $FADH_2$, 2 $CO_2$, 1 GTP. All equivalent to 12 ATP per acetyl-CoA |
| Electron transport chain/oxidative phosphorylation | Transduction of high-energy $e^-$ from NADH and $FADH_2$ to ATP. | Mitochondria | NADH, $FADH_2$, and $O_2$ as the final electron acceptor. | ATP and $H_2O$ |
| Pentose phosphate pathway (HMP shunt) | 1. Shunts G6P to form ribulose-5—for nucleotide synthesis. 2. Generation of NADPH for: ▪ Regeneration of GSH in the GSH/GSSG antioxidant system. ▪ Steroid and fatty acid biosynthesis. | Cytoplasm | G6P. | Ribulose-5-phosphate, NADPH, and $CO_2$ |
| Fructose pathway | Converts fructose to substrate for glycolysis. | Muscle, kidney, and liver | Fructose. | Glyceraldehyde-3-phosphate |
| Galactose pathway | Converts galactose to substrate for glycolysis. | Kidney, liver, and brain | Galactose and ATP. | Glucose-1-phosphate |
| Cori cycle/anaerobic metabolism | Cori cycle shuttles lactate from anaerobic metabolism in muscle to liver. | Shuttles lactate from muscle to liver | Lactate and 6 ATP. | Glucose |
| Gluconeogenesis | Generates glucose from glycolysis intermediates, fatty acid or TCA cycle. | Cytoplasm and mitochondria of kidney and liver, intestinal epithelium | All substrates end up as pyruvate/phosphoenolpyruvate → conversion to glucose. | Glucose |
| Glycogen metabolism | Maintains glucose homeostasis. | Glycogenesis (muscle and liver), glycogenolysis (heart, muscle, and liver) | Glycogen/glucose. | Glycogen/glucose |
| Urea cycle | Excretion of $NH_4^+$ from amino acid metabolism. | Partly in the mitochondria and partly in the cytoplasm | $CO_2$ and $NH_4^+$. | Urea and fumarate (enters TCA) |

ATP, adenosine triphosphate; CoA, coenzyme A; $FADH_2$, reduced flavin adenine dinucleotide; G6P, glucose-6-phosphate; GSH, reduced glutathione; GSSG, oxidized glutathione; GTP, guanosine triphosphate; NADH, reduced nicotinamide adenine dinucleotide; NADPH, reduced nicotinamide adenine dinucleotide phosphate; TCA, tricarboxylic acid.

## FLASH BACK

Now is a great time to return to the Clinical Correlation at Hereditary Orotic Aciduria and compare it with OTCase deficiency.

In OTCase deficiency, the urea cycle cannot proceed past ornithine, leading to **hyperammonemia, the hallmark of urea cycle disorders.** Furthermore, carbamoyl phosphate (CP) accumulates behind the enzyme blockage. Excess CP leaks out of the mitochondria and enters into pyrimidine biosynthesis, **which also uses CP as a carrier of toxic ammonia groups.** Once in the cytosol, CP is converted by **aspartate** transcarbamylase, or **ATCase,** into orotic acid and ultimately the pyrimidines C and U. Finally, recall that because OTCase is X-linked, this disorder will plague male neonates, who present with hyperammonemia. If patients don't respond to medical therapy, including ammonia "sponges," such as sodium phenylbutyrate or benzoate, liver transplantation is recommended. The patient's new hepatocytes will have a wild-type OTCase gene.

## MNEMONIC

Aspartic **ACID** and Glutamic **ACID** are the **acidic** amino acids.

## KEY FACT

All acidic and basic amino acids are polar, but not all polar amino acids are acidic or basic.

## KEY FACT

Leucine and lysine are strictly ketogenic.

---

to excrete urea in the urine. Elevated BUN can also result from increased protein absorption and catabolism, as classically seen during a **GI bleed.** The hemoglobin in the GI tract is digested into amino acids, absorbed, and deaminated, presenting the liver with additional ammonia to detoxify.

Cycle

See Figure 2-53.

## Amino Acids

### AMINO ACID METABOLISM

Metabolism utilizes various chemical reactions to extract energy and building blocks from food. Amino acids are extensively used in the synthesis of new proteins (eg, enzymes, hormones, growth factors) and can also be used as an energy source. To understand amino acids and their purpose in metabolism, it is always important to group them based on chemical properties and their role in medicine.

### AMINO ACID STRUCTURE

Amino acids consist of a carboxylic acid, an amine group, and a characteristic functional side group (Figure 2-54).

#### Acidic Amino Acids

Aspartic acid and glutamic acid contain an additional carboxylic acid group and are negatively charged at physiologic pH (7.4); this will yield a net charge of −1. An amino acid with a negative net charge can interact with metal cations in an enzyme. Remember that amino acids such as branched chain amino acids will have a net charge of 0.

#### Basic Amino Acids

Arginine, lysine, and histidine are polar and very hydrophilic. At physiologic pH (7.4), arginine and lysine are positively charged, whereas histidine has no net charge. In histones, a major component of chromatin, arginine and lysine are bound to negatively charged DNA.

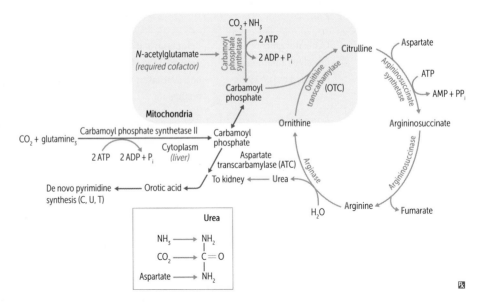

**FIGURE 2-53. Urea cycle.** ADP, adenosine diphosphate; AMP, adenosine monophosphate; ATP, adenosine triphosphate; PP$_i$, pyrophosphate.

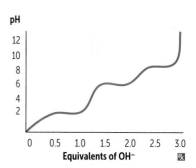

**FIGURE 2-54. Amino acid structure.** An amino acid consists of three main groups: (1) an amine group, (2) a functional side group, and (3) a carboxylic acid group. At physiologic pH, acidic amino acids are negatively charged, whereas basic amino acids, with the exception of histidine, have a net positive charge.

## THE AMINO ACID POOL

Amino acids are continually being used to synthesize proteins, and proteins are continually being broken down into amino acids. This dynamic pool of amino acids is in equilibrium with tissue protein.

### Replenishment

Takes place through:

- De novo synthesis
- Dietary supply
- Protein degradation

### Depletion

Occurs through:

- Protein synthesis
- Oxidation of excess amino acids

Remember, amino acids are not stored; they are converted into glycogen or fat if they are not used.

## ESSENTIAL AND NONESSENTIAL AMINO ACIDS

The 20 amino acids can be grouped into essential and nonessential. The following chart summarizes this grouping:

| Essential Amino Acid | Nonessential Amino Acid |
|---|---|
| Histidine | Alanine |
| Isoleucine | Serine |
| Leucine | Aspartic acid |
| Lysine | Cysteine |
| Methionine | Glutamic acid |
| Phenylalanine | Glutamine |
| Threonine | Glycine |
| Tryptophan | Proline |
| Valine | Tyrosine |
| Arginine | Asparagine |

Histidine and arginine are essential only for periods when cell growth demands exceed production, such as during childhood.

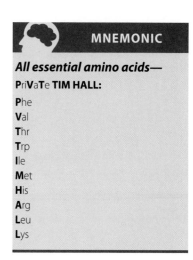

**FIGURE 2-55. Histidine titration curve.**

## CLINICAL CORRELATION

Asparagine synthesis is inhibited in leukemia cells. To compensate, they increase the uptake of this amino acid from the plasma. The chemotherapy drug L-asparaginase is used to lower plasma asparagine levels, thereby starving leukemia cells.

## FLASH FORWARD

Aminotransferases such as aspartate transaminase and alanine transaminase are important liver enzymes used in diagnostic testing. Elevated levels are suggestive of hepatocyte necrosis and liver pathology.

## KEY FACT

Vitamin $B_6$ and niacin deficiencies affect the functioning of transaminases.

## MNEMONIC

Amino acids that are ketogenic begin with an L. Amino acids that are both glucogenic and ketogenic are **FITTT** (**Ph**enylalanine, **I**soleucine, **T**hreonine, **T**ryptophan, **T**yrosine). All other amino acids are glucogenic.

## METABOLIC REACTIONS

Two simple reactions are the key to understanding amino acid metabolism: **transamination** and **oxidative deamination.**

### Transamination

#### Definition

Transfers an α-amino group to an α-keto acid group, creating a new amino acid (Figure 2-56).

- Transfer agent is an **aminotransferase/transaminase** (eg, aspartate transaminase [AST], ALT).
- Acceptor (usually α-ketoglutarate, can be pyruvate, oxaloacetate) becomes a new amino acid.
- Donor becomes a new α-keto acid.
- Reaction important for both synthesis and breakdown of amino acids.

#### Site

Cytosol and mitochondria.

#### Cofactors

All aminotransferases require the vitamin $B_6$ derivative **pyridoxal phosphate** (PLP).

### Oxidative Deamination

#### Definition

Removes an α-amino group, leaving a carbon skeleton (Figure 2-57).

- Ammonia released enters urea cycle.
- Carbon skeletons used as glycolytic and TCA cycle intermediates.
- **Glutamate,** with the assistance of glutamate dehydrogenase, is the only amino acid that **undergoes rapid oxidative deamination.**
- All other amino acids must be converted to glutamate by transamination prior to oxidative deamination.

#### Site

Mitochondria.

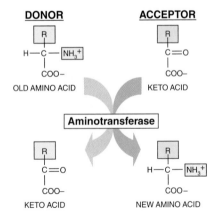

**FIGURE 2-56.** **Transamination reaction.** In this reaction, an α-amino group is being transferred from donor amino acid to the acceptor keto acid.

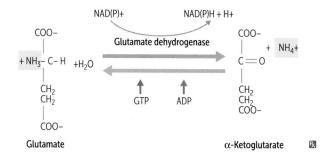

**FIGURE 2-57.** **Oxidative deamination reaction.** Glutamate is the only amino acid that undergoes rapid oxidative deamination. During this reaction, glutamate dehydrogenase catalyzes the removal of the α-amino group leaving an α-ketoglutarate carbon skeleton. The carbon skeleton serves as a TCA cycle intermediate while the released ammonia enters the urea cycle. ADP, adenosine diphosphate; GTP, guanosine triphosphate; NAD(P)⁺, oxidized nicotinamide adenine dinucleotide phosphate; NAD(P)H⁺.

## Control

Reversible reaction driven by need for TCA intermediates.

- **Low energy (GDP, ADP) activates.**
- **High energy (GTP, ATP) inhibits.** Remember the body will always regulate metabolism to favorable conditions. For instance, in states of high energy, the body will not require TCA intermediates.

> **KEY FACT**
>
> *Note:* During breakdown, all amino acid α-groups are transferred to α-ketoglutarate, since only glutamate undergoes rapid oxidative deamination.

## NONESSENTIAL AMINO ACID BIOSYNTHESIS

Nonessential amino acids can be synthesized in adequate amounts from essential amino acids and from intermediates of glycolysis and the TCA cycle (Figure 2-58).

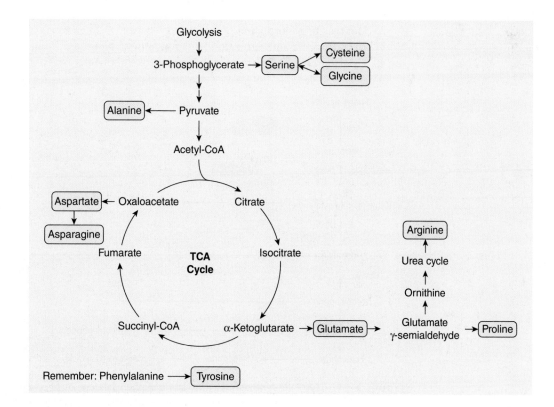

**FIGURE 2-58.** **Biosynthesis of nonessential amino acids.** This overview highlights the precursors and pathways used in nonessential amino acid synthesis. TCA, tricarboxylic acid.

### Tyrosine

**Precursor**

Phenylalanine.

**Synthesis**

Irreversible hydroxylation catalyzed by **phenylalanine hydroxylase** and its required cofactor **tetrahydrobiopterin** (Figure 2-59).

**Significance**

Tyrosine is the precursor for catecholamines (eg, dopamine, adrenaline, noradrenaline), melanin, and thyroxine. A genetic deficiency of phenylalanine hydroxylase causes **PKU** (discussed later), which results in the buildup of phenylalanine and an inability to produce tyrosine.

### Serine, Glycine, Cysteine

**Precursors**

Precursors for these amino acids are from glycolysis intermediates. Interestingly, serine can act as a precursor for glycine and cysteine. To synthesize cysteine from serine, the essential amino acid methionine is required.

**Synthesis**

- **Serine:** Mainly a three-step process from glycolytic intermediates in the cytosol. Can also be synthesized in a reversible reaction by transfer of a hydroxymethyl group from glycine in the mitochondria (Figure 2-60).
- **Glycine:** Mainly from $CO_2$, $NH_4^+$, and $N_5N_{10}$-methylene **tetrahydrofolate** in mitochondria. Can also be synthesized by the reverse of the serine synthesis reaction in the mitochondria (Figure 2-60).
- **Cysteine:** Synthesis is a multistep process with four main steps (Figure 2-61):
  1. Methionine activation.
  2. Homocysteine formation.
  3. Homocysteine and serine condensation to cystathionine.
  4. Cystathionine hydrolysis to cysteine and $\alpha$-ketobutyrate.

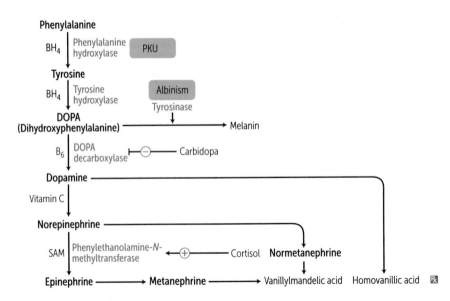

**FIGURE 2-59.** **Tyrosine synthesis.** Hydroxylation of phenylalanine by phenylalanine hydroxylase results in the formation of tyrosine. Tyrosine can then be used for the synthesis of other compounds. Deficiencies in either phenylalanine hydroxylase or its required cofactor tetrahydrobiopterin cause the disease phenylketonuria. A deficiency of $BH_4$ can also cause a buildup in phenylalanine and a deficiency in tyrosine.

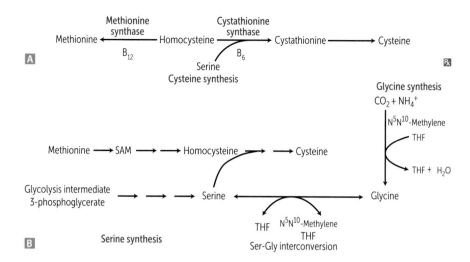

**FIGURE 2-60.  Serine, glycine, cysteine synthesis.** A Cysteine synthesis requires methionine and serine. B Serine (Ser) is mainly synthesized in a three-step process from the glycolytic intermediate 3-phosphoglycerate. Alternatively, serine can be formed from glycine (gly) by transfer of a hydromethyl carbon group. Glycine, in turn, can be synthesized from serine in a reversal of the previous reaction. However, it is mainly synthesized from $CO_2$, $NH_4^+$, and $N^5N^{10}$-methylene tetrahydrofolate. SAM, S-adenosyl methionine; THF, tetrahydrofolate.

## Significance

- Glycine is a component of collagen and also in the antioxidant glutathione, along with glutamate and cysteine. It also acts as an inhibitory neurotransmitter. The tetanus toxin produced by *Clostridium tetani* acts by inhibiting the release of glycine, thereby causing constant neurotransmitter release and producing generalized muscle spasms.
- Cysteine synthesis interruption can lead to a buildup of homocysteine in the urine known as **homocystinuria** (discussed later).

## Alanine

### Precursor

Pyruvate.

### Synthesis

One-step transamination of pyruvate (Figure 2-62).

> **KEY FACT**
>
> Folate is necessary for the DNA synthesis required from the growth of new cells. Tetrahydrofolates (THFs) are a series of derivatives of folate that participate in single-carbon transfer reactions. Folate is recommended for women wishing to conceive, as it reduces the risk of spinal cord defects in fetuses.

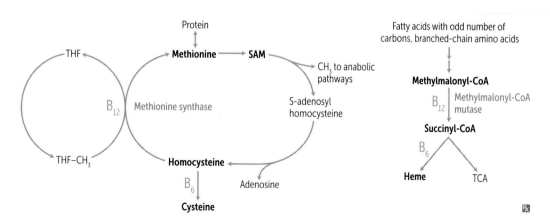

**FIGURE 2-61.  Regeneration of methionine.** The regeneration of methionine requires homocysteine and the enzyme methionine synthase. Methionine synthase transfers a methyl group from 5-methyltetrahydrofolate, which forms tetrahydrofolate, to homocysteine, to form methionine. CoA, coenzyme A; SAM, S-adenosylmethionine; TCA, tricarboxylic acid; THF, tetrahydrofolic acid.

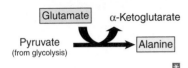

**FIGURE 2-62.** **Alanine synthesis.** Alanine is synthesized from the glycolytic intermediate pyruvate by a one-step transamination.

### KEY FACT

Transamination = transfer of amino group to new amino acid.
Deamination = removal of amino group.

### KEY FACT

The amino acid glutamine is the key amino acid that transfers ammonia in the blood. In the kidney, the enzyme glutaminase is used to regenerate glutamate and ammonia from glutamine.

### KEY FACT

Important amino acid derivatives:
Arginine → nitric oxide
Arginine + aspartate → urea
Glycine + succinyl CoA → heme
Glycine + arginine + SAM → creatine
Glutamate → GABA and glutathione
Glutamate + aspartate → pyrimidines
Glutamate + aspartate + glycine
  → purine
Histidine → histamine
Phenylalanine → tyrosine
Tryptophan → serine, niacin
Tyrosine → thyroxine, melanin

## Aspartate, Asparagine

### Precursor

TCA cycle intermediate oxaloacetate.

### Synthesis

- Aspartate: One-step transamination of oxaloacetate (Figure 2-63).
- Asparagine: Amide group transfer from glutamine (Figure 2-63).

### Significance

- Aspartate serves as an amino donor in the **urea cycle** and in **purine and pyrimidine synthesis.**
- Asparagine provides a site of carbohydrate attachment for N-linked glycosylation.

## Glutamate, Glutamine, Proline, Arginine

### Precursor

α-Ketoglutarate. Glutamate also serves as a precursor to glutamine, proline, and arginine.

### Synthesis

See Figure 2-64.

- **Glutamate:** Reductive amination of α-ketoglutarate. Also commonly from transamination of most other amino acids.
- **Glutamine:** Amidation (the addition of an amide group) of glutamate.
- **Proline:** Three-step synthesis from glutamate involving reduction, spontaneous cyclization, and another reduction.
- **Arginine:** Two-step synthesis from glutamate involving reduction and transamination to ornithine. Ornithine is then sent to the urea cycle where it is metabolized to arginine.

Although the details of these synthetic pathways can seem overwhelming, it is important to have a familiarity with the overall picture of nonessential amino acid synthesis and from where in the TCA cycle the precursors are obtained (Figure 2-58).

### AMINO ACID TISSUE METABOLISM

#### Amino Acid Transport

Protein digestion begins in the stomach, where gastric juice and pepsin break down proteins to form large peptides. Degradation continues in the small intestine to produce free amino acids, dipeptides, and tripeptides. These components are taken into epithelial cells via specific transporters and hydrolyzed into free amino acids. The concentration of amino acids inside the cell is greater than the concentration outside the cell; therefore, the transport of amino acids inside requires energy. Similar to glucose transport, luminal transport is sodium dependent, whereas contraluminal transport is

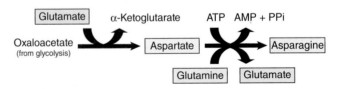

**FIGURE 2-63.** **Aspartate and asparagine synthesis.** Aspartate is formed in a one-step transamination from the TCA cycle intermediate oxaloacetate. Asparagine is then formed by amidation of aspartate. AMP, adenosine monophosphate; ATP, adenosine triphosphate; PPi, pyrophosphate.

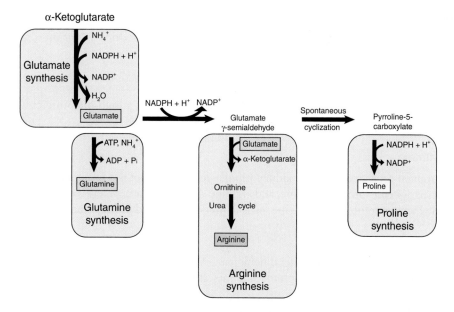

**FIGURE 2-64. Glutamate, glutamine, proline, and arginine synthesis.** These four amino acids are formed from α-ketoglutarate. (1) Glutamate is formed from a direct reductive amination. (2) Glutamine can then be formed from glutamate by amidation. At this branch point, either (3) proline can be formed in three steps or (4) ornithine can be formed in two and sent to the urea cycle, where it is metabolized to arginine. ADP, adenosine diphosphate; ATP, adenosine triphosphate; NADP, nicotinamide adenine dinucleotide phosphate; NADPH, reduced form of nicotinamide adenine dinucleotide phosphate.

sodium independent. The four main transport systems are based on their amino acid side chain specificity (Table 2-23).

## Amino Acid Transport Deficiency

### Hartnup Disease

This is a rare autosomal recessive defect in the intestinal and renal transporters for **neutral amino acids.** The symptoms are due to a **loss of tryptophan,** which is a nicotinamide precursor. Thus, many aspects of the presentation **mimic niacin (vitamin B₃) deficiency** (pellagra).

### Presentation

Patients exhibit pellagra-like skin lesions and neurologic manifestations ranging from ataxia to frank delirium.

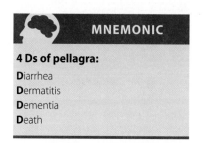

**MNEMONIC**

**4 Ds of pellagra:**
**D**iarrhea
**D**ermatitis
**D**ementia
**D**eath

**TABLE 2-23. Important Amino Acid Transport Systems**

| AMINO ACID SPECIFICITY | AMINO ACIDS TRANSPORTED | DISEASES RESULTING FROM DEFECTIVE CARRIER SYSTEM |
| --- | --- | --- |
| Small, aliphatic | Alanine, serine, threonine | Nonspecific |
| Large, aliphatic, aromatic | Isoleucine, leucine, valine, tyrosine, tryptophan, phenylalanine | Hartnup disease |
| Basic | Arginine, lysine, cysteine, ornithine | Cystinuria |
| Acidic | Glutamate, aspartate | Nonspecific |

**QUESTION**

A 6-year-old boy presents to the ED with flank abdominal pain and hematuria. The patient has a medical history of chronic renal stones. Urinalysis reveals the presence of renal stones that turn green when exposed to air. Microscopic examination shows the renal stones to be hexagonal. What is the most likely diagnosis for this patient?

### Diagnosis

Diagnosis is made by detection of neutral aminoaciduria, which is not present in pellagra.

### Treatment

Management is targeted at replacing niacin and providing a high-protein diet with nicotinamide supplements.

## Cystinuria

Autosomal recessive defect in kidney tubular reabsorption of the **basic amino acids,** such as cysteine, ornithine, lysine, and arginine—resulting in high levels of their excretion. The low solubility of cysteine leads to precipitation and **kidney stone** formation.

### Presentation

Patients may present with bilateral flank pain, hematuria, and, in severe cases, pyelonephritis, all of which are symptoms of kidney stones.

### Diagnosis

Microscopic examination of the stones, which show hexagonal crystals, can assist in the diagnosis, but quantitative urinary amino acid analysis confirms the diagnosis.

### Treatment

Management strives to eliminate precipitation and stone formation by increasing urine volume (high daily fluid ingestion) and urinary alkalization with citrate.

### Absorptive State Metabolism

Once amino acids are absorbed, most are transaminated to **alanine, the main amino acid secreted by the gut,** and released into the portal vein destined for the liver (Figure 2-65). Remember that amino acids can never be stored freely. They are either used for protein synthesis or transaminated to glutamate for rapid oxidative deamination and urea excretion. Excess amino acids are used for energy or converted to glycogen or fat.

## AMINO ACID DERIVATIVES

Amino acids serve as precursors to synthesis of many important compounds. Three simple reactions are the key to understanding amino acid derivatives: decarboxylation, hydroxylation, and methylation.

- **Decarboxylation:** Removal of a carboxyl group (–COOH) from a compound.
- **Hydroxylation:** Addition of a hydroxyl group (–OH) to a compound, thus oxidizing it.
- **Methylation:** Addition of a methyl group ($-CH_3$) to a compound.

### Methionine Derivative

#### S-Adenosyl-L-methionine

Main biosynthetic reaction methyl donor.

- **Synthesis location:** All living cells.
- **Synthesis reaction:** Methionine and ATP.

**KEY FACT**

Much like the amino acid pool, there exists a dynamic one-carbon pool. These one-carbon units are used for molecular synthesis and elongation, but require activation by a carrier (usually SAM or folate) to enable their transfer.

**A** **ANSWER**

The patient most likely has cystinuria. The patient has a history of renal stones that are hexagonal. Patients with this disease are also at risk for urinary tract infections, pyelonephritis, and hydronephrosis due to stone obstruction.

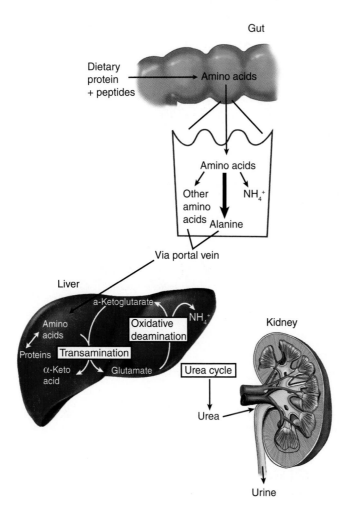

Gut

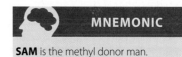

**FIGURE 2-65. Absorptive state amino acid metabolism.** When digested, protein is broken down into amino acids, most of which are converted to alanine and shuttled via the portal vein to the liver. The liver can use the amino acids for protein synthesis or lose the amino acids via entry to the urea cycle and excretion from the kidney.

## Tyrosine Derivatives

### Thyroid Hormones

Control the body's metabolic rate.

- **Synthesis location:** Thyroid follicle cells.
- **Synthesis reaction:** See Figure 2-66.
  - Tyrosine converted to the glycoprotein thyroglobulin.
  - Iodide oxidized to iodine ($I_2$) and incorporated into the tyrosine side chains of the thyroglobulin. (*Note:* Thyroid hormone also contains the 21st amino acid, selenocysteine.)
  - Tyrosine + one $I_2$ = monoiodinated tyrosine (MIT).
  - Tyrosine + two $I_2$ = diiodinated tyrosine (DIT).
  - DIT + DIT = thyroxine ($T_4$).
  - MIT + DIT = triiodothyroxine ($T_3$, [active form]).

### Melanin

Provides pigmentation, forms cap over keratinocytes for protection from UV rays.

- **Synthesis location:** Hair and skin melanocytes.
- **Synthesis reaction:** See Figure 2-67.

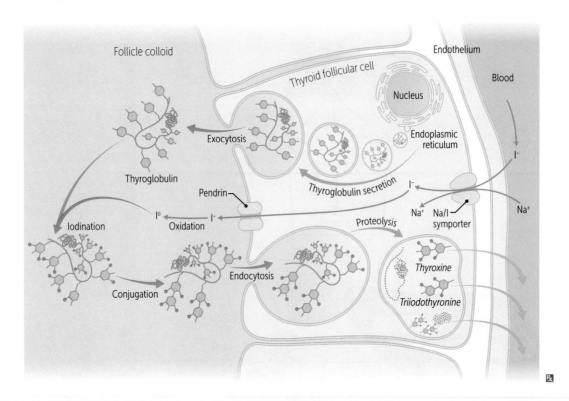

**FIGURE 2-66.** **Thyroid hormone synthesis.** Thyroglobulin, which is rich in tyrosine, is transported to the lumen, where its tyrosine residues are iodinated. The various forms of thyroid hormones ([T$_3$], thyroxine [ T$_4$]) produced can then be released in a regulated manner.

- Tyrosine hydroxylation at two sites.
- Catalyzed by **tyrosinase.**
- Requires cofactors copper and ascorbate.
- Reactive molecules variably polymerize to form different melanins.

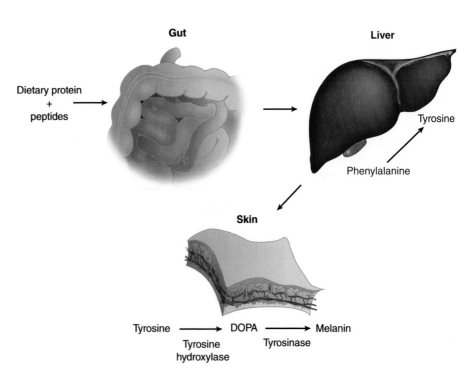

**FIGURE 2-67.** **Melanin synthesis.** Tyrosine can be converted by the enzyme tyrosine hydroxylase to a more active form that polymerizes to four different melanins.

## Catecholamines

Control body's stress responses acting as neurotransmitters or hormones.

- ▨ **Synthesis location:** CNS, adrenal medulla.
- ▨ **Synthesis reaction:** See Figure 2-68.
    - ▨ Tyrosine hydroxylation and decarboxylation to **dopamine.**
    - ▨ Dopamine hydroxylation to **norepinephrine.**
    - ▨ Norepinephrine methylation to **epinephrine** using the methyl donor SAM.

**CLINICAL CORRELATION**

Metabolism occurs through the enzymes catecholamine O-methyl-transferase (COMT) and monoamine oxidase (MAO). When treating diseases such as Parkinson disease, COMT and MAO are inhibited to increase the levels of dopamine.

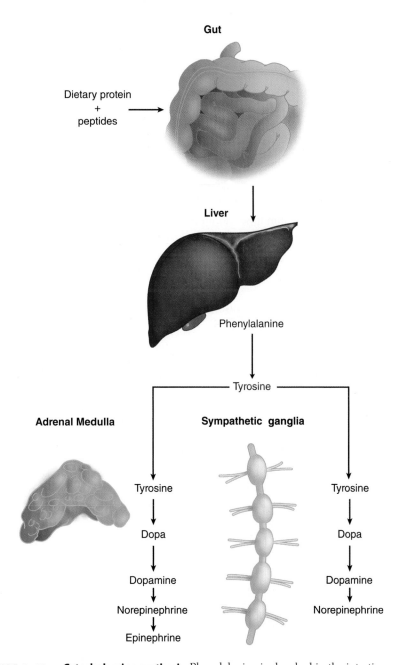

**FIGURE 2-68. Catecholamine synthesis.** Phenylalanine is absorbed in the intestine and converted to tyrosine in the liver. Tyrosine can then be converted to dopamine in the substantia nigra or further processed to norepinephrine in sympathetic ganglion neurons or to epinephrine in the adrenal medulla.

**QUESTION 1**

A patient presents to the ED with a blood pressure of 190/85. He has no history of high blood pressure. His past medical history is only significant for depression, for which he takes tranylcypromine regularly. He reports consuming a large amount of red wine and cheese during dinner. What is the most concerning feature of this patient's presentation?

**QUESTION 2**

A 43-year-old man has just begun a trial of duloxetine for his depression, as his previous medication, fluoxetine, did not provide any benefit. Moments after taking duloxetine, he becomes agitated and has diaphoresis and an increased heart rate. What is the most likely diagnosis? What would be the drug of choice for treatment?

## Tryptophan Derivatives

### Niacin (Vitamin B₃)

Forms essential redox reaction cofactors NAD+, NADP+.

- **Synthesis location:** Liver.
- **Synthesis reaction:** Requires cofactors pyridoxine (vitamin $B_6$), riboflavin (vitamin $B_2$), and thiamine (vitamin $B_1$).

### Serotonin

- **Synthesis location:** CNS serotonergic neurons, GI tract enterochromaffin cells.
- **Synthesis reaction:** Tryptophan aromatic ring hydroxylation and then decarboxylation (Figure 2-69).

Serotonin is present in platelets and is released when they bind to a clot; this promotes local vasoconstriction.

### Melatonin

Controls circadian rhythm functions.

- **Synthesis location:** Pineal gland pinealocytes.
- **Synthesis reaction:** See Figure 2-69.
  - Tryptophan conversion to serotonin (see earlier discussion).
  - Serotonin acetylation and methylation.

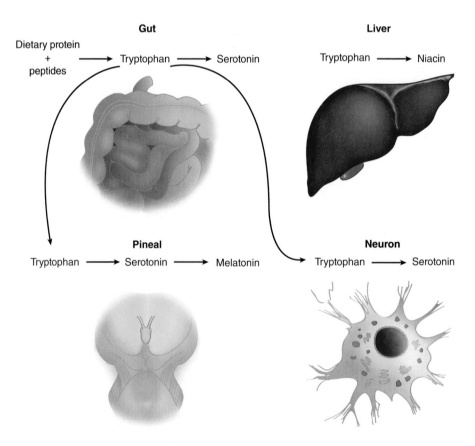

**FIGURE 2-69.** **Serotonin and melatonin synthesis.** Serotonin is derived from tryptophan via hydroxylation and decarboxylation cells of the aromatic ring, followed by decarboxylation. Melatonin can then be derived from serotonin via acetylation and methylation.

### Histidine Derivatives

#### Histamine

Mediates inflammatory responses, acts as neurotransmitter, stimulates gastric acid secretion.

- **Synthesis location:** Connective tissue mast cells, GI tract enterochromaffin cells.
- **Synthesis reaction:** Histidine decarboxylation.

### Glycine Derivatives

#### Heme

Electron carrier in cytochromes and enzymes, $O_2$ carrier in hemoglobin and myoglobin.

- **Synthesis location:** Mitochondria and cytosol of bone marrow erythroid cells (for hemoglobin), liver hepatocytes (for cytochromes).
- **Synthesis reaction:** See Heme Synthesis, later in this chapter, and particularly Figure 2-113.
  - Eight-step reaction with first three and last three occurring in the mitochondria.
  - δ-Aminolevulinic acid (ALA) synthesis—irreversible, rate-limiting step.
    - Glycine and succinyl-CoA condensation.
    - Catalyzed by ALA synthase, requires PLP cofactor. This step is inhibited in X-linked sideroblastic anemia.
  - Porphobilinogen (PBG) formation—dehydration of two ALA molecules. This step is inhibited in lead poisoning.
  - Uroporphyrinogen I (UROgen I) formation—condensation of four PBG molecules (inactive). This step is inhibited in acute intermittent porphyria.
  - Uroporphyrinogen III (UROgen III) formation—produces an active molecule. Coproporhyrinogen III is then formed. This step is inhibited in porphyria cutanea tarda.
  - Protoporphyrin IX formation, which alters side chains and porphyrin unsaturation degree. This step is inhibited by lead poisoning.
  - Heme formation—insertion of $Fe^{2+}$.

### Arginine Derivatives

#### Creatine

High-energy phosphate storage.

- **Synthesis location:** Liver, precursor formed in kidney.
- **Synthesis reaction:** See Figure 2-70.
  - Arginine and glycine formation of guanidoacetate in kidney.
  - Guanidoacetate methylation using SAM as methyl donor.

For storage, phosphate of ATP can be transferred to creatine, forming creatine phosphate. Phosphate transfer can be reversed in energy-depleted muscle, generating creatine and ATP. Creatine and creatine phosphate spontaneously cyclize, creating creatinine for excretion in urine.

#### Urea

Nontoxic disposable form of ammonia that is generated during amino acid turnover.

- **Synthesis location:** Liver.
- **Synthesis reaction:** Arginine cleavage to urea and ornithine in the urea cycle.
  - Urea travels via the blood to the kidneys, where it is excreted in the urine.

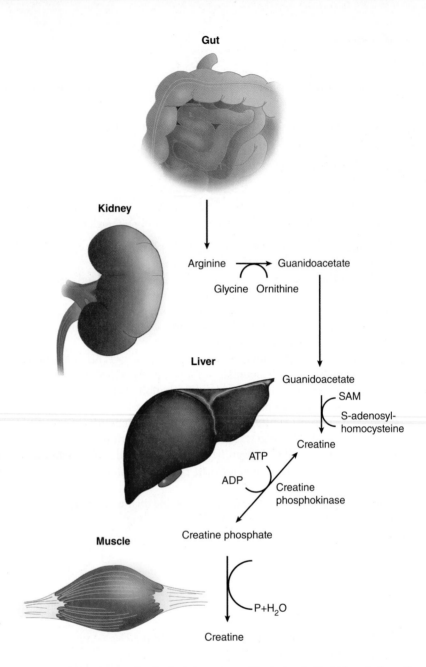

**FIGURE 2-70.** **Creatine synthesis.** Arginine reacts with glycine in the kidney to form the precursor guanidoacetate. Guanidoacetate is then methylated, using SAM, in the liver forming creatine. A high-energy phosphate group from ATP can then be transferred creating creatine phosphate. In muscle, when energy demand is high, the high-energy phosphate can be removed and creatine phosphate is converted back to creatine.

## Nitric Oxide

Positively regulates vessel dilation through smooth muscle relaxation.

- **Synthesis location:** Small-vessel endothelial cells.
- **Synthesis reaction:** Arginine oxidation.

## Glutamate Derivative

### γ-Aminobutyric Acid

Acts as an inhibitory neurotransmitter.

- **Synthesis location:** CNS.
- **Synthesis reaction:** Glutamate decarboxylation.

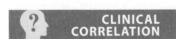

**CLINICAL CORRELATION**

During erection, nitric oxide (NO) is released in the corpus cavernosum of the penis, leading to smooth muscle relaxation. Sildenafil citrate, also known as Viagra, is a selective inhibitor of the phosphodiesterase that prolongs the effects of NO.

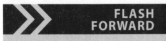

**FLASH FORWARD**

GABA analogs are used for anticonvulsant therapy and neuropathic pain.

## Review of Amino Acid Derivatives

A review of amino acid derivatives can be found in Figure 2-71.

## AMINO ACID BREAKDOWN

In states of excess amino acids, the body will recycle amino acids into components that will be used elsewhere. Two main steps are involved in this process: the removal of the α-amino group, followed by salvage of the carbon skeleton.

### Removal of the α-Amino Group

The removal of the α-amino group occurs via two possible routes, each beginning with the transamination to create glutamate (Figure 2-72). In the first route, glutamate undergoes oxidative deamination in the mitochondria, and the amino group is sent to the urea cycle for disposal. In the second route, the glutamate is transaminated a second time with a transfer of the α-amino group to oxaloacetate to form aspartate. This occurs mainly in the liver and is catalyzed by AST. The aspartate can then enter the urea cycle via condensation with citrulline and the amino group is again disposed of.

### Alanine-Glucose Cycle

As amino acids undergo catabolism, there is a net increase in the amount of ammonia produced. Each ammonia molecule is carried to the liver via alanine (Figure 2-73). In muscle tissue, there are two transamination reactions. The first transamination reaction creates glutamate. The second transfers the α-amino group to pyruvate, which then form alanine. Alanine is then released into the bloodstream, where it is taken up by the liver and the process is reversed, resulting in glutamate being regenerated in the liver.

### Disposal of the Carbon Skeleton

The remaining carbon skeleton can then be salvaged as TCA cycle and glycolytic intermediates. All 20 amino acids break down to seven common products: acetyl-CoA, acetoacetyl-CoA, pyruvate, oxaloacetate, fumarate, succinyl-CoA, and α-ketoglutarate

> ### KEY FACT
>
> Amino acids are converted to alanine for circulation and glutamate for rapid oxidative deamination and disposal.

> ### QUESTION
>
> A 27-year-old man is prescribed isoniazid prophylaxis after suspected TB exposure. The patient presents 3 weeks later with complaints of diarrhea and a general skin rash over his body. What should have been prescribed along with this medication to prevent these symptoms?

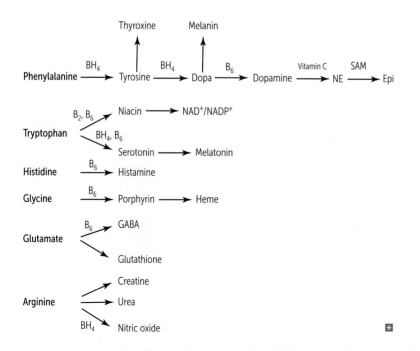

**FIGURE 2-71.    Amino acid derivatives.** Epi, epinephrine; GABA, γ-aminobutyric acid; NE, norepinephrine; SAM, S-adenosylmethionine.

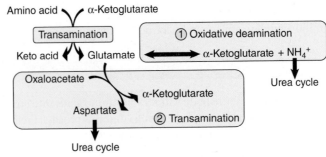

**FIGURE 2-72.** *α*-**Amino group disposal.** The first step in disposal is the transamination of amino acids to form a common pool of glutamate. This glutamate can undergo (1) oxidative deamination with the resulting amino group sent to the urea cycle or (2) a second transamination with aspartate being sent to the urea cycle.

(Figure 2-74). Ketogenic amino acids are those that are broken down into the **ketone body formers acetyl-CoA and acetoacetyl-CoA.** Glucogenic amino acids are those that are broken down to **pyruvate or TCA intermediates** that can be channeled into gluco-neogenesis. Only leucine and lysine are considered to be purely ketogenic. **Isoleucine, phenylalanine, tyrosine, threonine, and tryptophan are both ketogenic and gluco-genic.** Histidine, methionine, and valine are glucogenic.

**AMINO ACID METABOLIC DISORDERS**

### Phenylketonuria

**Autosomal recessive** deficiency of **phenylalanine hydroxylase,** also known as classic PKU (Figure 2-75). The lack of this enzyme causes a **buildup of phenylalanine** and an **inability to produce tyrosine.** In some cases, there is a deficiency in dihydrobiopterin reductase, which is called atypical PKU. Dihydrobiopterin reductase is used for the conversion of phenylalanine to tyrosine and also to dopa. To distinguish classic PKU from atypical PKU, one must remember that patients with classic PKU get better when tyrosine is introduced into their diet. Patients with atypical PKU will remain symp-tomatic, because they lack tetrahydrobiopterin, which is needed to convert tyrosine to dopa. Last, patients with atypical PKU can have a deficiency of serotonin because the same enzyme, dihydrobiopterin reductase, is used for the conversion of tryptophan to serotonin. Excess phenylalanine is converted into the phenylketones: phenylpyruvate, phenyllactate, and phenylacetate.

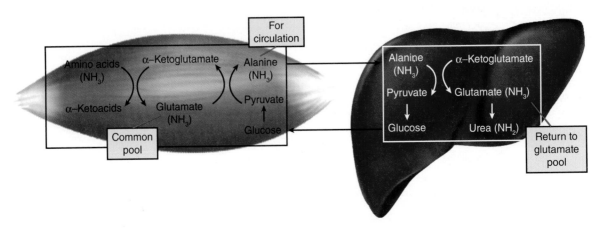

**FIGURE 2-73.** **Alanine-glucose cycle.** Alanine is used as a carrier to transport *α*-amino acid groups from the skeletal muscle to the liver for disposal via the urea cycle. This cycle allows carbon skeletons to be converted between protein and glucose.

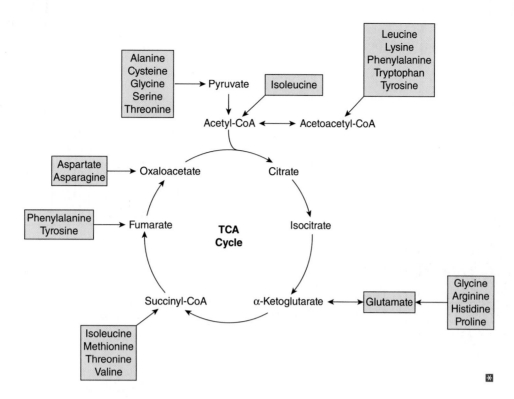

**FIGURE 2-74.** **Amino acid carbon skeleton recycling.** The 20 amino acids can be broken down to seven common carbon skeletons, which can be feed into the tricarboxylic acid (TCA) cycle. Depending on the energy needs of the cell, these products can also be used to synthesize fat or glycogen. CoA, coenzyme A.

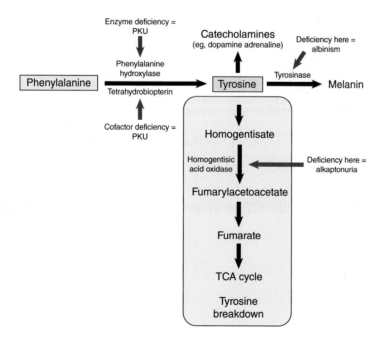

**FIGURE 2-75.** **Phenylalanine derivative disorders.** Blockades in the metabolism of phenylalanine lead to the enzyme deficiencies alkaptonuria, albinism, and phenylketonuria. PKU, phenylketonuria; TCA, tricarboxylic acid cycle.

### Incidence

PKU is one of the most common amino acid deficiencies, with an incidence of 1 in 13,500–19,000 live births.

### Presentation

If untreated, infants present at 6–12 months with CNS symptoms of developmental delay, seizures, and failure to thrive. Patients also exhibit characteristics of hypopigmentation such as fair hair, blue eyes, and pale skin. Hypopigmentation occurs because tyrosine, a derivative of phenylalaline, is the precursor for melanin.

### Diagnosis

In the United States all neonates are screened for increased blood levels of phenylalanine.

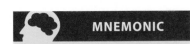

**MNEMONIC**

**PKU:** Disorder of **aromatic** amino acid metabolism—musty body **odor.**

### Treatment

Classically, management of the condition is accomplished by **restriction of dietary phenylalanine,** which is contained in aspartame (eg, NutraSweet), and an increase in dietary tyrosine along with monitoring of blood phenylalanine levels. Newer treatments, such as enzyme substitution therapy, are in development.

## Alkaptonuria

Congenital deficiency of **homogentisic acid oxidase,** an enzyme used in the conversion of tyrosine to fumarate (Figure 2-75). This deficiency results in a buildup of homogentisate that polymerizes to a black-brown pigment. This pigment deposits in connective tissue, including cartilage.

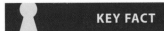

**KEY FACT**

Although patients with alkaptonuria may have disabling features, such as arthritis and joint pain, life expectancy is not affected.

### Presentation

Alkaptonuria is one of the few inborn errors of metabolism that does not manifest until **adulthood.** In this disease, patients will have joint pain, decreased range of motion, arthritis, and pigmentation in the eyes. However, it may be detected at an earlier age, since **urine and sweat may turn black** upon standing, owing to the formation of alkapton.

### Diagnosis

This condition may be diagnosed by allowing the patient's urine to stand and monitoring for colorimetric change. The results can be confirmed quantitatively with a measurement of homogentisate in the urine.

### Treatment

There is no specific treatment for alkaptonuria, and the clinical effects of dietary restriction are limited.

## Albinism

Deficiency of the enzyme **tyrosinase,** which catalyzes conversion to melanin, or defective **tyrosine transporters.** The disorder can also result from lack of migration of neural crest cells.

### Presentation

Neonates present with amelanosis (whitish hair, pale skin, gray-blue eyes), nystagmus, and photophobia (low pigment in iris and retina leads to failure to develop fixation reflex).

### Diagnosis

Iris translucency and other fundal findings are pathognomonic signs.

### Treatment

Tinted contact lenses and high sun protection are important in management.

### Prognosis

Disease prognosis is affected by the **increased risk of skin cancer.**

## Homocystinuria

Excess homocystine in the urine can result from **cystathionine synthase deficiency, decreased affinity of cystathione synthase for PLP,** or **methionine synthase (homocysteine methyltransferase) deficiency** (Figure 2-60).

### Presentation

Patients can present with mental retardation, osteoporosis, tall stature, kyphosis, lens sublaxation (downward and inward), and atherosclerosis (stroke and myocardial infarction).

### Diagnosis

Diagnosis consists of measuring excess homocystine in the urine of a patient without vitamin $B_{12}$ deficiency.

### Treatment

The management depends on the underlying cause of the homocystinuria. For cystathionine synthase deficiency, treatment is a dietary decrease in methionine and an increase in cysteine, $B_{12}$, and folate. For decreased affinity of PLP, treatment is increased vitamin $B_6$ and cysteine. For methionine synthase (homocysteine methyltransferase) deficiency, treatment is increased methionine.

## Maple Syrup Urine Disease

Deficiency of the enzyme **α-keto acid dehydrogenase,** which catalyzes degradation of the branched-chain amino acids (**isoleucine, valine, leucine**). This leads to an increase of leucine and α-keto acids in the blood.

### Presentation

Affected infants appear healthy at birth but develop a characteristic odor caused by isoleucine, lethargy, feeding difficulties, coma, and seizures. The amino acid leucine is responsible for the neurotoxicity, which leads to coma and seizures. If untreated, this leads to CNS defects, mental retardation, and death.

### Diagnosis

High levels of branched-chain amino acids in the urine and blood are used for diagnosis.

### Treatment

Dietary restriction of branched-chain amino acids. Thiamine supplementation can also improve symptoms, as branched-chain α-keto acid dehydrogenase requires thiamine.

### Prognosis

If untreated, the infant dies in the first month of life.

**CLINICAL CORRELATION**

It can be difficult to distinguish homocystinuria and Marfan syndrome. A key feature to distinguish the two is looking at lens subluxation. In homocystinuria, the lens sublaxation occurs downward and inward, while with Marfan, it occurs upward. Also remember that Marfan is inherited in an autosomal-dominant pattern, whereas homocystinuria is inherited in an autosomal-recessive pattern. Last, patients with Marfan syndrome are at risk of developing aortic aneurysms, whereas patients with homocystinuria get recurrent thromboembolisms.

**MNEMONIC**

**Branched-chain amino acids that build up in maple syrup urine disease—**

**I L**ove **V**ermont maple syrup:

**I**soleucine
**L**eucine
**V**aline

**KEY FACT**

Amino acid deficiencies are autosomal recessive disorders, present in the neonatal period (except for alkaptonuria) and are usually treated with dietary restrictions.

**KEY FACT**

**Propionyl-CoA Carboxylase Deficiency**
- Inability to convert propionyl-CoA to methylmalonyl-CoA → development of propionic acidemia
- Propionyl-CoA is derived from amino acids (Val, Ile, Met, & Thr), odd-number fatty acids, and cholesterol
- **Presentation:** Lethargy, vomiting, and hypotonia (usually during the first few days of life)
- **Findings:** Anion-gap metabolic acidosis, ketosis, and hypoglycemia

## Nutrition

### VITAMINS

Vitamins are ubiquitous to enzymatic processes. Both anabolic (formation) and catabolic (breakdown) reactions require vitamins.

Vitamins are divided into those that are **soluble in water** and those that are **soluble in fat.** Water-soluble vitamins include the B vitamins, and vitamin C. Fat-soluble vitamins include vitamins A, D, E, and K.

**Water-soluble vitamins** are readily absorbed from the gut by a variety of specific carrier-mediated processes. It should be noted that water-soluble vitamins are less likely to achieve toxic levels, because they are readily excreted in the urine. Patients are therefore more likely to be deficient in them, as there is limited storage in the body for water-soluble vitamins.

**Fat-soluble vitamins** dissolve in dietary fats and migrate through the lymphatic system before entering the blood via the thoracic duct. In the blood, they are bound to protein carriers, such as albumin. These vitamins are stored in adipose and other fatty tissues and accumulate, making it possible to reach toxic levels. Patients are less likely to be deficient in fat-soluble vitamins because of their ability to accumulate in lipid. However, patients with malabsorptive diseases, such as celiac disease, cystic fibrosis, and pancreatic insufficiency, or short-gut syndrome (after gastric bypass), are much more likely to suffer from deficiencies in fat-soluble vitamins.

### Water-Soluble Vitamins

#### Vitamin B₁—Thiamine

Thiamine is a water-soluble vitamin found in grains, meats, and legumes. It is used as a coenzyme in many biochemical reactions involving **carbohydrate metabolism.** The biologically active form, thiamine pyrophosphate (TPP, also called thiamine diphosphate), is found in liver, kidneys, and leukocytes.

TPP, as its name implies, is formed from the transfer of a pyrophosphate group from ATP to thiamine. Once formed, it is used in the cell as a coenzyme for:

- Transketolation reactions found in the pentose phosphate pathway.
- Conversion of pyruvate to acetyl-CoA.
- Conversion of $\alpha$-ketoglutarate to succinyl-CoA.
- Decarboxylation of branched-chain amino acids leucine, isoleucine, and valine.

In the United States, thiamine deficiency is most commonly due to chronic alcoholism. Absence of thiamine decreases the amount of acetyl-CoA available to enter the TCA cycle and increases the amount of pyruvate available for anaerobic oxidation. This leads to increased lactic acid production.

Clinically, signs of thiamine deficiency include:

- Muscle cramps
- Paresthesias
- Irritability
- Beriberi (wet or dry)
- Wernicke-Korsakoff syndrome (described below)

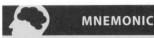

**MNEMONIC**

**VOMIT**
**V**aline, **O**dd-chain fatty acids, **M**ethionine, **I**soleucine, and **T**hreonine

**CLINICAL CORRELATION**

Vitamin B₁ deficiency leads to necrosis of mammillary bodies and periaqueductal gray matter. This is why patients presenting with severe alcoholism should be repleted with high dose IV thiamine.

Beriberi is divided into wet and dry. Wet beriberi involves the cardiovascular system, whereas dry beriberi involves the peripheral nervous system.

**Wet beriberi** is characterized by heart failure, which may be high output, and includes a **triad** of **peripheral vasodilation, biventricular failure,** and **edema.** It is often brought on by physical exertion and increased carbohydrate intake.

**Dry beriberi** occurs with little physical exertion and decreased caloric intake and may affect peripheral nerves (motor and sensory neuropathy). **Wernicke-Korsakoff syndrome** occurs in chronic alcoholics with thiamine deficiency. **Wernicke** encephalopathy is caused by neuronal damage in the most thiamine-dependent brain regions, predominantly in the medial thalamus. Mamillary body atrophy is specific to this pathology. Clinically, Wernicke encephalopathy presents with a triad of ophthalmoplegia (and nystagmus), truncal ataxia, and confusion. Untreated encephalopathy progresses to **Korsakoff** syndrome, which is characterized by both anterograde and retrograde amnesia. This is caused by demyelination in the limbic system. Patients will present with an **impaired short-term memory and confabulation,** with otherwise grossly normal cognition. Remember that Wernicke encephalopathy can be reversible with high doses of thiamine, whereas Korsakoff syndrome is irreversible.

### Vitamin B$_2$—Riboflavin

Riboflavin is a cofactor in the oxidation and reduction of various substrates. It is commonly found in liver, dairy products, nuts, soybeans, and green, leafy vegetables. It serves as a precursor to the **coenzymes flavin mononucleotide (FMN)** and **flavin adenine dinucleotide (FAD).**

Both riboflavin and ATP are used in the formation of FMN and FAD. Riboflavin reacts with a single ATP, yielding FMN and ADP. FAD is formed next, via FMN's reacting with a second ATP molecule, yielding FAD and pyrophosphate (PPi) as byproducts.

FMN and FAD are required in fatty acid oxidation, amino acid oxidation, and the TCA cycle, as they are able to add or subtract two hydrogen atoms. Riboflavin is also important for **erythrocyte integrity,** through erythrocyte glutathione reductase, and also for the conversion of **tryptophan to niacin.**

Deficiencies in riboflavin, leading to deficiencies in FMN and FAD, clinically cause **glossitis, cheilosis, and corneal vascularization.** They may also cause angular stomatitis, seborrheic dermatitis, and weakness. Riboflavin is required for erythrocyte glutathione reductase; therefore deficiency also results in erythrocyte lysis and hemolytic anemia.

### Vitamin B$_3$—Niacin

Niacin, found in liver, milk, and unrefined grains, is another coenzyme used in oxidation and reduction reactions. Niacin appears in the diet as its precursor tryptophan or as **nicotinamide adenine dinucleotide (NAD)** or its phosphorylated form, **nicotinamide adenine dinucleotide phosphate (NADP),** both of which are hydrolyzed by intestinal enzymes to form nicotinamide.

Pharmacologically, nicotinic acid can be a treatment option to decrease total and LDL cholesterol (and has some effects to raise HDL). Its side effects include flushing, pruritus (both of which are treated with aspirin), hives, nausea, and vomiting. Excess niacin intake can lead to intrahepatic cholestasis.

**KEY FACT**

It is important to give thiamine before glucose to alcoholic patients to avoid precipitating Wernicke encephalopathy and, more importantly, worsening metabolic acidosis via an increase in lactic acid. If glucose were given first, pyruvate would be formed via glycolysis, which would then form lactic acid owing to a deficiency in the coenzyme thiamine pyrophosphate.

**MNEMONIC**

Wernicke encephalopathy: "Eyes lies capsize": nystagmus, confabulation, ataxia

**KEY FACT**

Absence of vitamin B$_2$ causes the two **C**'s:
**C**heilosis
**C**orneal vascularization

**CLINICAL CORRELATION**

Pellagra can be caused by niacin deficiency or tryptophan deficiency. Patients who lack tryptophan in their diet or have underlying diseases, such as Hartnup disease or malignant carcinoid syndrome, are at risk for pellagra. Tryptophan, with vitamin B$_6$ as a cofactor, is used to synthesize niacin.

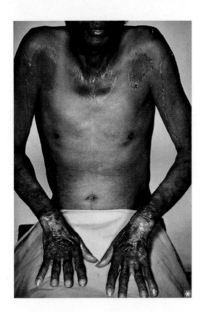

**FIGURE 2-76.    Pellagra.** Signs of pellagra include hyperpigmented, brittle, cracked, and scaly skin.

**Pellagra** is the name of niacin deficiency. Patients can get pellagra from lack of dietary niacin, isoniazid use, Hartnup disease, or malignant carcinoid syndrome. Corn-based diets are also known to cause pellagra, as they lack both niacin and tryptophan. Pellagra is characterized by **diarrhea, dermatitis,** and **dementia** (Figure 2-76). If untreated, pellagra can be fatal. Dietary replacement of both tryptophan and niacin is the treatment.

**Hartnup disease** is a genetic defect in tryptophan membrane transport that causes small intestinal malabsorption and poor renal resorption. Therefore, simple replacement therapy is insufficient. Similarly, in **malignant carcinoid syndrome,** tryptophan is used for excessive 5-hydroxytryptamine (5-HT) production and is less available for NAD synthesis, causing pellagra that is nonresponsive to therapy as well as symptoms of serotonin excess.

### Vitamin B$_5$—Pantothenic Acid

Pantothenic acid is the major constituent of CoA, and it is found in most foods. It is a cofactor for acyl transfers (pantothen-A is in the CoA complex). These reactions take place in the TCA cycle, fatty acid oxidation, acetylations, and cholesterol synthesis. Deficiency of vitamin B$_5$ is rare in humans, but may result in paresthesias or dysesthesias, and gastrointestinal distress.

### Vitamin B$_6$—Pyridoxine

A pyridine derivative, pyridoxine, along with pyridoxal and pyridoxamine, serves as a building block for **PLP,** which is the coenzyme involved in **amino acid metabolism** (eg, conversion of serine to glycine). These molecules are found in wheat, egg yolk, and meats. The coenzyme is responsible for numerous processes including transamination, deamination, decarboxylation, and condensation and creation of the liver enzymes **AST** and **ALT.** Specifically, vitamin B$_6$ is involved in heme synthesis and neurotransmitter synthesis.

Although clinical manifestations are rare, a deficiency of vitamin B$_6$ can result in **convulsions,** peripheral neuropathy, and sideroblastic anemia, as well as **hyperirritability.** Decreased concentrations of vitamin B$_6$ deficiency may occur after use of oral contraceptives, isoniazid, cycloserine, penicillamine, or chronic alcoholism. Pyridoxine can also treat some types of cystathionine synthase deficiency as it is a cofactor for the deficient enzyme and helps convert homocysteine to cystathionine. Too much vitamin B$_6$ can cause sensory neuropathy that is unrelieved when toxicity is corrected.

### Vitamin B$_{12}$—Cobalamin

Animal products (meat or dairy) are the only dietary source of vitamin B$_{12}$. Absorption of cobalamin starts in the stomach after ingestion. Vitamin B$_{12}$, bound to animal protein, is released by mechanical and chemical digestion, and by amylase from saliva. The parietal cells, located primarily at the gastric fundus, secrete both hydrochloric acid and **intrinsic factor** in response to a meal. As the cobalamin is released by salivary gland enzymes, it is unbound from the animal protein, and it is bound by R binder (haptocorrin) from the salivary glands, which forms a stable complex in the low pH. **The R binder–cobalamin complex** and the secreted intrinsic factor move into the duodenum, where pancreatic enzymes degrade R binder. The R binder–cobalamin complex is broken down and allows intrinsic factor to bind B$_{12}$. **The intrinsic factor–cobalamin complex** formed in the duodenum moves toward the distal ileum and binds to the **intrinsic factor–cobalamin receptor** expressed on the enterocytes. Once bound, the entire unit is internalized by the enterocyte. Intrinsic factor is degraded in the enterocyte, freeing cobalamin. The available cobalamin is bound to plasma **transcobalamin II** (TCII), forming yet another complex. The TCII–cobalamin complex then migrates through the basolateral side of the enterocyte into circulation, stored in the liver, and made available for $B_{12}$-dependent enzymes.

$B_{12}$-dependent enzymes:

- Methylmalonyl-CoA mutase (converts propionyl-CoA to methylmalonyl-CoA and then to succinyl-CoA)
- Leucine aminomutase
- Methionine synthase

Cobalamin is used as a cofactor for **methionine synthase** and **methylmalonyl-CoA synthase.** Methionine synthase catalyzes the conversion of homocysteine to methionine via a one-carbon transfer from methyl-THF to create THF (Figure 2-77). These one-carbon transfers are necessary for **de novo synthesis of purines** and require folate as a cofactor. Deficiency in cobalamin causes a buildup of methyl-THF (unconjugated form), which eventually leaves the cell and can lead to a corresponding folate deficiency.

**Vitamin $B_{12}$ deficiency** can be caused by a myriad of disorders. **Dietary deficiency** is rare, because the liver stores large quantities of vitamin $B_{12}$, but it can be seen in vegans. **Pernicious anemia** is the most common cause of megaloblastic anemia (mean corpuscular volume [MCV] > 100 fL). It is typically caused by an autoimmune attack on gastric parietal cells, which leads to decreased production of intrinsic factor (accompanied by achlorhydria and atrophic gastritis). This condition also puts patients at risk for gastric adenocarcinoma. **Gastrectomy** and gastric bypass surgery disrupt secretion of intrinsic factor by gastric parietal cells, leading to decreased absorption of vitamin $B_{12}$. **Infectious** causes include *Helicobacter pylori*, which causes chronic gastritis; *Diphyllobothrium latum*, in which the fish tapeworm competes for vitamin $B_{12}$ absorption in the intestine; and in blind loop syndrome, in which bacterial overgrowth competes for vitamin $B_{12}$ absorption in the intestine. **Structural abnormalities of the terminal ileum,** such as Crohn disease and surgical resection, can cause decreased absorption of vitamin $B_{12}$. **Pancreatic insufficiency** leads to a decrease in enzymes necessary to break down the R protein–cobalamin complex, which prevents cobalamin from binding with intrin-

**KEY FACT**

Methylmalonyl-CoA is formed in the catabolism of valine or isoleucine.

**KEY FACT**

Methotrexate inhibits dihydrofolate reductase and is used to treat Hodgkin lymphoma, non-Hodgkin lymphoma, lung cancer, breast cancer, and osteosarcomas as well as rheumatoid arthritis.

**CLINICAL CORRELATION**

Vitamin $B_{12}$ deficiency can lead to megaloblastic anemia, just like folate deficiency. A hallmark finding in megaloblastic anemia is hypersegmented neutrophils on peripheral smear (Figure 2-78).

**FLASH FORWARD**

Pernicious anemia is a type II hypersensitivity disorder.

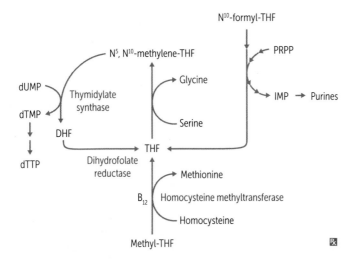

**FIGURE 2-77. Tetrahydrofolate metabolism.** DHF, dihydrofolate; dTMP, deoxythymidine monophosphate; dTTP, deoxythymine triphosphate; dUMP, deoxyuridine monophosphate; THF, tetrahydrofolate.

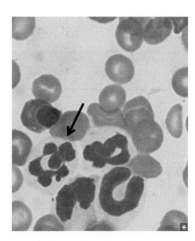

**FIGURE 2-78. Hypersegmented neutrophil (arrow).**

sic factor. Finally, **deficiency of transcobalamin II** prevents cobalamin from entering systemic circulation.

Clinical signs of vitamin $B_{12}$ deficiency include a neuropathy characterized by defective myelin formation and consequent subacute combined degeneration of the posterior column and lateral corticospinal tracts. This results in symmetrical paresthesias and ataxia, loss of proprioception and vibration senses, and, in severe cases, spasticity, clonus, paraplegia, and fecal and urinary incontinence. The mechanism for this defect occurs from the lack of vitamin $B_{12}$, which causes a decrease in folate, which in turn decreases methylmalonic acid and leads to impaired myelin production.

The most evident sign of vitamin $B_{12}$ deficiency, however, is megaloblastic change of the RBCs (seen on a peripheral blood smear) and MCV. **Elevated MCV** (> 110 fL) and **hypersegmented neutrophils** (lobe count ≥ 5) indicate deficiency. The megaloblastic changes due to vitamin $B_{12}$ deficiency and folate deficiency can be difficult to distinguish. Both will have megaloblastic anemia with hypersegmented neutrophils and an increased homocysteine level, which will increase a risk for thrombosis. $B_{12}$ deficiency, however, will have an increase in methylmalonic acid, as well as neurologic symptoms.

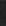
### Folic Acid (Vitamin B₉)

Present in fruits and vegetables, folic acid is required for erythropoiesis and one-carbon transfers. It is responsible for the conversion of homocysteine to methionine (where vitamin $B_{12}$ is a cofactor), conversion of serine to glycine (where $B_6$ is a cofactor), and conversion of deoxyuridylate to thymidylate for DNA synthesis, and it is indirectly responsible for purine ring formation (through its derivatives) (Figure 2-77).

Folate is maintained in the body via the **folate enterohepatic cycle.** Dietary folate (available as polyglutamates) undergoes hydrolysis and reduction from enzymes on mucosal cell membranes to form monoglutamate. **Dihydrofolate reductase** found in the duodenal mucosa methylates the folate and allows it to be absorbed by enterocytes in the jejunum. Folate then joins with plasma-binding proteins and travels systemically or to the liver, where it is converted and secreted in bile back to the duodenum to repeat the cycle.

Causes of folate deficiency include **inadequate dietary intake; malabsorptive diseases; liver dysfunction; medications,** such as anticonvulsants; and states of **increased folate use.** Inadequate dietary intake is seen in alcoholics or persons who do not consume a lot of raw vegetables. Malabsorptive diseases that affect the jejunum, celiac sprue, and biliary diseases alter the folate enterohepatic cycle. Liver dysfunction, seen in patients with alcoholic cirrhosis, also interferes with the enterohepatic cycle and may interfere with production of plasma-binding proteins. Medications such as **methotrexate** and **trimethoprim** inhibit dihydrofolate reductase and decrease absorption of dietary folate. Other medications that cause folate deficiency is 5-FU, which inhibits thymidylate synthase, and phenytoin, which interferes with absorption. Finally, states that require high consumption of folate, such as pregnancy, hemolytic anemias, and malignancy, can deplete folate stores and create a deficiency.

Clinical manifestations of folate deficiency consist of megaloblastic anemia, glossitis, decreased serum folate, increased serum homocysteine, and normal methylmalonic acid. However, there are no neurologic sequelae from folic acid deficiency in adults, in contrast to what occurs with vitamin $B_{12}$ deficiency, which consists of a megaloblastic anemia and neurologic symptoms. Note that folic acid deficiency in pregnant women is associated with increased rate of neural tube defects.

## Biotin (Vitamin B₇)

Biotin is a water-soluble vitamin found in peanuts, cashews, almonds, and other foods. Intestinal flora also synthesize biotin. Raw egg whites contain **avidin,** which binds to biotin, forming a nonabsorbable complex. The biotin coenzyme **carries carboxylate** and is involved in carboxylation reactions important for carbohydrate and lipid metabolism. Biotin participates in several key carboxylation reactions, including conversion of **pyruvate to oxaloacetate** (by pyruvate carboxylase in the TCA cycle), conversion of propionyl-CoA to methylmalonyl-CoA (by propionyl-CoA carboxylase, in synthesis of odd-chain fatty acids), and conversion of acetyl-CoA to malonyl-CoA (via acetyl-CoA carboxylase). A congenital defect of propionyl-CoA decarboxylase leads to an increased consumption of valine, isoleucine, and threonine, which then leads to nausea, vomiting, and metabolic acidosis.

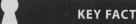

**MNEMONIC**

**Avidin** in egg whites **avid**ly binds to biotin.

## Vitamin C—Ascorbic Acid

Vitamin C, or ascorbic acid, is found in citrus fruits. Dietary vitamin C is taken up in the ileum. It provides reducing equivalents for several enzymatic reactions, particularly those catalyzed by **copper- and iron-containing enzymes.** Vitamin C is necessary for proper hydroxylation of proline and lysine used in **collagen synthesis.** It also serves as an antioxidant and facilitates iron absorption in the duodenum by keeping iron in its reduced state. Many copper-containing or iron-containing hydroxylases require ascorbic acid to maintain normal metabolism. The copper-containing enzyme dopamine β-hydroxylase, which converts dopamine to norepinephrine, requires ascorbate as a cofactor to maintain copper in a reduced state. Likewise, **proline and lysine hydroxylase** are required for the posttranslational modification of procollagen to form collagen, because hydroxylated residues are required for the formation of stable triple helices and for cross-linking of collagen molecules to form fibrils.

**KEY FACT**

Genetic disorders of collagen synthesis include osteogenesis imperfecta and Ehlers-Danlos syndrome.

**Scurvy** results from vitamin C deficiency. Swollen gums, bruising, anemia, "corkscrew hair," and poor wound healing are signs of scurvy and are due in part to impaired collagen formation (Figure 2-79). **Excess vitamin C** can result in uric acid–based renal calculi formation.

### Fat-Soluble Vitamins

### Vitamin A—Retinoids

Vitamin A (eg, retinol, retinaldehyde, retinoic acid) is found in fish oils, meats, dairy products, and eggs. β-Carotene, a precursor of vitamin A, which is metabolized by intestinal mucosal cells into retinaldehyde, is found in green vegetables. Vitamin A in the form of retinol is absorbed into the **intestinal mucosal cells** and is transported **to the liver via chylomicrons.** In the liver, vitamin A is stored in Ito cells, which are located in the space of Disse. Ito cells contribute to cirrhosis by secreting transforming growth factor beta (TGF-β) and promoting fibrosis. Vitamin A is delivered to the rest of the body via prealbumin and retinol-binding protein.

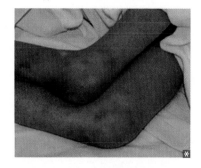

**FIGURE 2-79. Ecchymosis secondary to vitamin C deficiency.**

Vitamin A combines with opsin in the eye to form rhodopsin in the rod cells of the retina. A similar reaction produces iodopsin in cone cells. These proteins play a crucial role in sensing light in the retina and are essential for vision. Vitamin A also has a role in the differentiation and proliferation of epithelial cells in the respiratory tract, skin, cornea, conjunctiva, and other tissues.

**CLINICAL CORRELATION**

Vitamin A derivatives such as isotretinoin are commonly used to treat acne. They have been linked to birth defects such as facial abnormalities. As such, common practice requires simultaneous use of two forms of contraception while taking these medications.

Deficiency of vitamin A, therefore, causes vision problems, disorders of epithelial cell differentiation and proliferation, and impaired immune response. Visual symptoms are usually the first sign of vitamin A deficiency, which include loss of green light sensitivity, poor adaptation to dim light, and night blindness (loss of retinol in rod cells). **Xerophthalmia** (squamous epithelial thickening), **Bitot spots** (squamous metaplasia), and **keratomalacia** also occur in vitamin A deficiency. Keratomalacia is metaplasia of the conjunctival lining, which leads to a change from a thin squamous lining to a keratinized, stratified squamous epithelium. Metaplasia of respiratory epithelia is seen (often common in cystic fibrosis due to failure of fat-soluble vitamin absorption), as well as frequent respiratory infections (secondary to respiratory epithelial defects).

Because vitamin A is stored in the liver and is lipophilic, the body can store large amounts of the vitamin. Toxicity can occur acutely, chronically, or as a teratogenic effect. Acute toxicity can be caused from a large, single dose of vitamin A and results in nausea, vertigo, and blurry vision. Chronic toxicity can manifest as ataxia, alopecia, hyperlipidemia, edema, or hepatotoxicity. Excess vitamin A also can turn the skin yellow, but this can be distinguished from jaundice because the sclera remain white.

### Vitamin D—Cholecalciferol

Vitamin D plays an important role in bone metabolism by regulating plasma calcium concentrations. Vitamin D is absorbed from dietary sources (saltwater fish and egg yolks) and is also synthesized in the skin. Vitamin D absorption is regulated by serum calcium concentrations.

In the presence of UV light, 7-dehydrocholesterol present in the skin is converted to previtamin D. Once previtamin D is formed, it is converted to cholecalciferol, which enters the circulation. Activation of cholecalciferol takes place in the liver and the kidney. The **liver** converts **cholecalciferol** to **25-hydroxycholecalciferol.** The **kidney** converts 25-hydroxycholecalciferol into **1,25-hydroxycholecalciferol (1,25 OHD, calcitriol),** its active metabolite. The kidney also converts 25-hydroxycholecalciferol into 24,25-hydroxycholecalciferol, an inactive metabolite (Figure 2-80). Vitamin D–binding globulin stores vitamin D and is also responsible for its transport in the circulation.

Vitamin D maintains the plasma calcium concentration by increasing intestinal absorption of calcium, minimizing calcium excretion in the distal renal tubules, and mobilizing bone mineral in bones. It also stimulates osteoblasts and improves calcification of bone matrix (and, hence, bone formation).

Activated vitamin D binds to a nuclear receptor in cells (intestinal cells, renal cells, and osteoblasts) and induces gene expression. It is regulated by a series of feedback mechanisms involving parathyroid hormone (PTH), calcium, and phosphate. Low levels of calcium stimulate PTH synthesis and secretion, which in turn prompt the conversion of 25-hydroxycholecalciferol to 1,25-hydroxycholecalciferol. In turn, 1,25-hydroxycholecalciferol has a

**KEY FACT**

Calci**TRI**ol works on the **TRI**ad of intestines, kidneys, and bone to maintain plasma calcium levels.

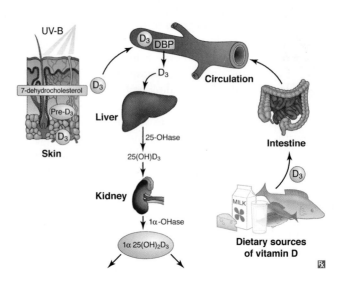

**FIGURE 2-80.** **Pathways of vitamin D formation.** DBP, vitamin D binding protein.

negative feedback effect on its own production and PTH production. In excess, 1,25-hydroxycholecalciferol also promotes the production of 24,25-dihydroxyvitamin D.

In the presence of excess calcitriol and thus calcium from either bone or intestinal absorption, high levels of calcium act to decrease PTH production, and high levels of phosphate act to decrease conversion of 25-hydroxycholecalciferol to 1,25-hydroxycholecalciferol by blocking the 1α-hydroxylase enzyme (found in the kidney) involved in the activation of the 25-hydroxy derivative (Figures 2-81 and 2-82).

Deficiency of vitamin D leads to **rickets** in children and **osteomalacia** in adults, with the differences being open (in children) and closed (in adults) epiphyseal plates. Rickets results from not receiving enough calcium and phosphate at the sites where bone mineralization is taking place.

Clinically, children with rickets show signs of hypocalcemia, bowing of the lower extremities, and poor dentition. Other signs include pigeon breast deformity, frontal bossing, rachitic rosary (knobs of bone at costochondral joints), and bowing of the legs. The treatment for vitamin D–deficient rickets and osteomalacia is vitamin D therapy.

**KEY FACT**

Malabsorption syndromes can lead to deficiencies in vitamins A, D, E, and K. This can be confirmed with a 24-hour stool collection for quantification of stool fat.

**CLINICAL CORRELATION**

With any renal disease, the patient's calcium and phosphate levels may be altered. Therefore, always check these two electrolytes in any patient with suspected renal disease.

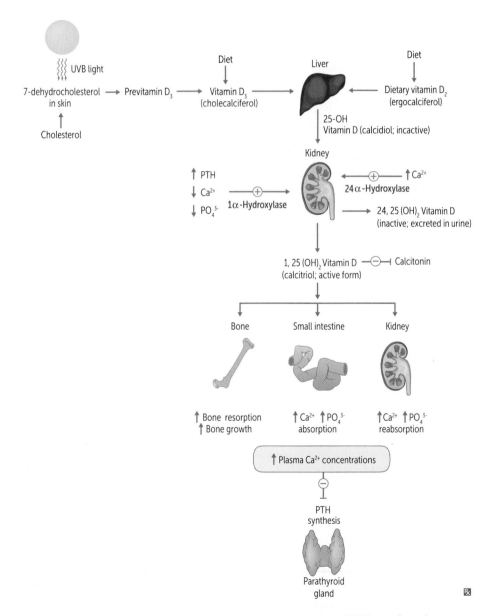

**FIGURE 2-81.** **Vitamin D target organs and consequent effects.** PTH, parathyroid hormone.

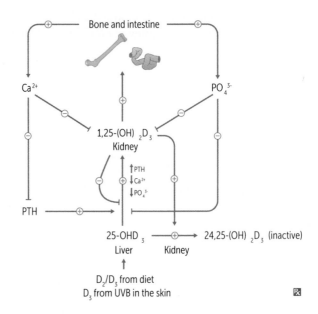

**FIGURE 2-82.** **Vitamin D regulation.** PTH, parathyroid hormone.

In vitamin D–resistant rickets, vitamin D repletion does not treat the syndrome, and a genetic abnormality may be present.

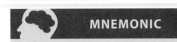

- **Type I vitamin D–resistant rickets** occurs when there is a genetic mutation of $1\alpha$-hydroxylase. This can be treated with 1,25-hydroxycholecalciferol bypassing the conversion of 25-hydroxycholecalciferol in the kidney. If supplementation of 1,25-hydroxycholecalciferol does not treat the underlying problem, then the patient has **type II vitamin D–resistant rickets.**
- Type II vitamin D–resistant rickets occurs when the 1,25-hydroxycholecalciferol receptor is mutated and therefore unresponsive to both vitamin D and calcitriol.
- **X-linked rickets** is entirely due to renal phosphate wasting. In this condition, 1,25-hydroxycholecalciferol levels are normal or low.

Excess vitamin D leads to hypercalcemia and all of the sequelae associated with it (eg, kidney stones, dementia, constipation, abdominal pain, depression). Sarcoidosis can lead to excess vitamin D, because there is increased production of $1\alpha$-hydroxylase by macrophages, which completes the production of vitamin D. Similarly, lymphoma can produce calcitriol.

### Vitamin E—$\alpha$-Tocopherol

Vitamin E is a lipid-soluble antioxidant found in sunflower oil, corn oil, soybeans, meats, fruits, and vegetables. It can be found in cell membranes and serves as an antioxidant like glutathione and vitamin C. It is used to react to the radicals formed by peroxidation of fatty acids. Like other fat-soluble vitamins, vitamin E is absorbed in the intestine and travels to the liver via chylomicrons. Fat malabsorption diseases (cystic fibrosis, liver disease) decrease the amount of vitamin E available. Deficiency of vitamin E is uncommon, but can cause hemolytic anemia, peripheral neuropathy and ataxia due to degeneration of the spinocerebellar tract, and ophthalmoplegia. In excess, vitamin E can interfere with vitamin K metabolism, which can lead to hemorrhagic stroke in adults and necrotizing enterocolitis in infants.

### Vitamin K—Phylloquinone

Vitamin K is found in either vegetable or animal sources (phylloquinone) or through bacterial flora (menaquinone). It is used by the liver in the carboxylation of glutamate residues during post-translational modification of coagulation factors. Prothrombin and coagulation factors II, VII, IX, and X, and the antithrombotic proteins C and S all require $\gamma$-carboxylation

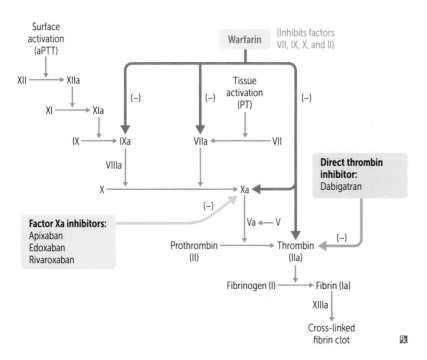

**FIGURE 2-83.** **Procoagulation and thrombolytic coagulation pathways.** aPTT, activated partial thromboplastin time; PT, prothrombin time.

of glutamate residues for function (Figure 2-83). γ-carboxyglutamate acts as a chelator, trapping calcium ions and thereby allowing the clotting proteins to bind to negatively charged phospholipids at the surface of platelets and to function at these membranes.

The reduced form of vitamin K is oxidized by γ-glutamyl carboxylase (and epoxidase) to form the γ-carboxyglutamate (Gla) in the postsynthetic modification. The oxidized form of vitamin K, or **vitamin K epoxide,** is converted back to its reduced form by 2,3-epoxide reductase. **Warfarin** inhibits this enzyme, thereby preventing adequate recycling of vitamin K and the γ-carboxylation of coagulation factors (Figure 2-84).

Vitamin K deficiency is rare in otherwise healthy adults, but can be present when broad-spectrum antibiotics are taken, as they kill gut bacteria. Vitamin K deficiency can predispose patients to GI bleeding, intracranial bleeding, ecchymoses, epistaxis, and hematuria. Laboratory signs include prolonged prothrombin time (PT/INR) and partial thromboplastin time (PTT).

## Zinc

Zinc is found in foods such as beef, crab, and cashews. One of the most notable uses of zinc is structural stabilization of zinc finger proteins, which have diverse functions including DNA sequence recognition, transcriptional regulation, and protein folding. A common cause of zinc deficiency is consumption of food grown in soil lacking zinc. Common manifestations include delayed wound healing, hypogonadism, anosmia, and acrodermatitis enteropathica (characterized by well-demarcated, scaly plaques in the intertriginous area).

**KEY FACT**

Supratherapeutic levels of warfarin lead to bleeding (intracranial, GI, intraperitoneal), and ecchymoses.

**CLINICAL CORRELATION**

Warfarin overdose resulting in excess anticoagulation (a supratherapeutic INR) is reversed with high dose vitamin K and replenishment of coagulation factors with fresh frozen plasma. Interestingly, one of the main ingredients of rat poison is warfarin.

**CLINICAL CORRELATION**

Newborns lack bacterial colonization of the gut and cannot synthesize vitamin K. They need a vitamin K injection at birth to prevent hemorrhagic disease of the newborn.

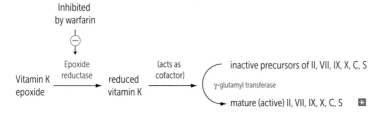

**FIGURE 2-84.** **Warfarin prevents conversion of vitamin K epoxide to vitamin K.**

## Fed Versus Unfed State

The fed and unfed states can be understood by first understanding the "metabolic priorities" of the body. The sole purpose of metabolism is to take a variety of carbon-containing compounds (carbohydrates, lipids, and peptides, or "fuel") and subject them to enzymes that can generate ATP or other molecules like NADH and $FADH_2$ that are used in ATP-forming reactions (Figure 2-85). In all tissues except the brain, **insulin directs how fuel is utilized.** In the unfed and starvation states, the body catabolizes carbohydrate, lipid, and, finally, protein sources to generate the ATP required to ward off organ failure.

### The Brain

ATP is used in all important cellular and molecular processes. The most important ATP-consuming processes, however, are those occurring in the brain. The body does everything possible to ensure the brain receives the carbon-containing compounds it needs to function. The brain is unable to store **fats as triglycerides** or **glucose as gly-**

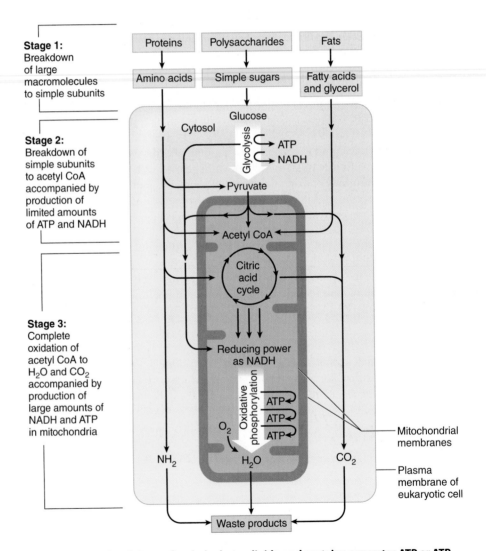

**FIGURE 2-85.** **Breakdown of carbohydrates, lipids, and proteins generates ATP or ATP equivalents.** The body has evolved enzymatic processes that are capable of producing ATP from a variety of carbon-containing compounds. ATP, adenosine triphosphate; CoA, coenzyme A; NADH, reduced nicotinamide adenine dinucleotide.

**cogen** as other tissues do. Therefore, it requires a constant blood supply, which is why ischemic conditions can be so damaging. Glucose is the brain's preferred fuel source. Ketone bodies such as β-hydroxybutyrate can traverse the blood-brain barrier and be used as fuel too.

Metabolic homeostasis is predominantly regulated by three tissues: muscle, adipose, and liver. Each is discussed briefly.

### Muscle Tissue

Skeletal muscle can adapt to a wide variety of fuel sources, as it contains all the enzymes needed to catabolize glucose, fatty acids, and ketones to produce ATP. **When insulin levels are high,** a glucose transporter (GLUT) known as GLUT4 is displayed on the cell membrane, allowing myocytes to take up glucose from the blood (Table 2-24). **When insulin levels are low,** myocytes break down stored glycogen to generate glucose. In fact, the majority of glycogen in the body is made and stored by muscle tissue, with the liver being responsible for the rest.

### Adipose Tissue

Adipose tissue is the main storage site for fatty acids in the form of triacylglycerides. It uses glucose as fuel, but it is an unimportant source of fatty acid synthesis. The liver not only synthesizes fatty acids but also delivers them to adipose tissue in the form of very low density lipoproteins (VLDLs).

**When stimulated by insulin,** an enzyme known as **lipoprotein lipase** releases fatty acids from VLDL particles, making them available for uptake by adipocytes. At the same time, insulin promotes the display of GLUT4 transporters on the adipocyte membrane, permitting the entry of glucose. Glucose is then converted into glycerol-3-phosphate and combined with fatty acids to form triacylglycerides (Figure 2-86). **In the absence of insulin,** an intracellular enzyme known as **hormone-sensitive lipase** mediates the breakdown of stored fats into fatty acids that can be released into the blood. The enzyme, hormone-sensitive lipase can be activated by epinephrine during exercise or by adrenocorticotropic hormone (ACTH).

**KEY FACT**

Both lipoprotein lipase and hormone-sensitive lipase are produced by adipocytes. While hormone-sensitive lipase remains within the cell, lipoprotein lipase is released and associates with capillary endothelial cells. This allows it to act on VLDL particles floating in the blood.

**TABLE 2-24.** **The Four "Metabolic" Organs and Their Features**

| ORGAN | FUEL STORAGE | EFFECT OF INSULIN | FUEL SOURCES[a] | TRANSPORTER | COMMENTS |
|---|---|---|---|---|---|
| Brain | None | None | **Glucose** and **ketone bodies** from blood | GLUT3 | GLUT3 has the **highest affinity** for glucose (it is saturated even when blood glucose is low) |
| Muscle | Glycogen | Glucose uptake by GLUT4; glycogen synthesis | **Glucose** (from blood and stored glycogen), **fatty acids**, **ketone bodies** | GLUT4 | GLUT4 is only present on the cell membrane **when stimulated by insulin** |
| Adipose | Triacylglyceride | Glucose uptake by GLUT4; triacylglyceride synthesis | **Glucose** | GLUT4 | Same as above |
| Liver | Glycogen | Glycogen synthesis; fatty acid synthesis | α-Ketoacids | GLUT2 | Because GLUT2 is **constitutively expressed** on the cell membrane, the liver is always "monitoring" blood glucose |

[a]Fuel sources are listed from most to least preferred for each organ.

GLUT, glucose transporter.

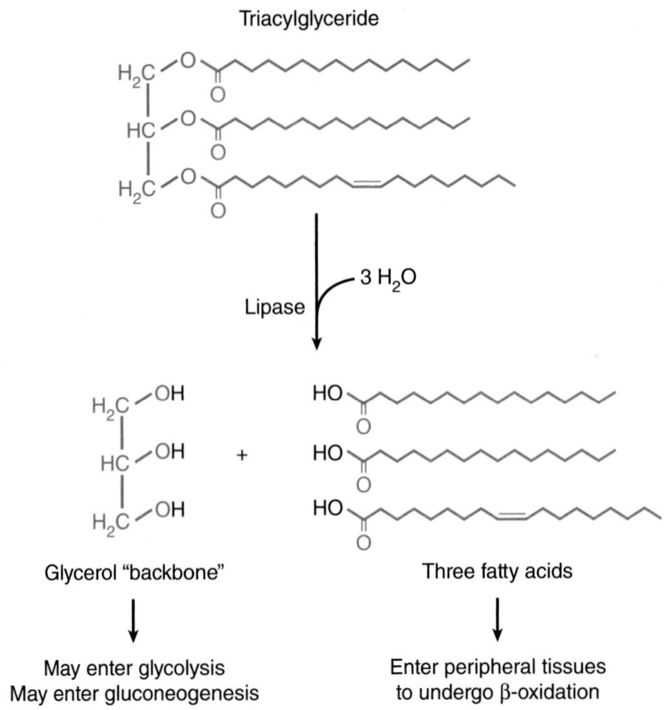

**FIGURE 2-86.** **Components of triacylglyceride.** A triacylglyceride is composed of a glycerol backbone (green) and three "acyl" or fatty acid tails (red). Cells that use triacylglycerides as fuel can catabolize glycerol using glycolysis or, in the liver, glycerol can be used to generate glucose via gluconeogenesis. Each fatty acid may undergo β-oxidation to generate reduced form of nicotinamide adenine dinucleotide (NADH), reduced form of flavin adenine dinucleotide (FADH$_2$), and acetyl-CoA, which in turn are used to produce adenosine triphosphate (ATP).

## Glucose Transporters

Glucose is driven into cells via a concentration gradient. Different glucose transporters (GLUTs) exist in the body and can be classified based on their location, affinity for glucose, and regulation (Table 2-25). Although many GLUTs have been identified and characterized, types 1–4 are most important to understand. GLUT-1 transporters are found in most cell types but more notably in erythrocytes and the blood-brain barrier. This transporter is responsible for basal uptake of glucose. Because this transporter, along with GLUT-3, has a high affinity for glucose, it ensures that glucose will be delivered, even in periods of hypoglycemia. GLUT-2 transporters are found in the liver and in the β cells of the pancreas. The dual role of GLUT-2 makes it unique in that in the liver, it acts on excess glucose for storage, whereas in the pancreas, it serves as a glucose sensor for insulin release. GLUT-3 transporters are similar to GLUT-1 in that it has a high affinity for glucose, and its role is basal glucose uptake. These transporters are found

**TABLE 2-25.** **GLUT Transporters**

| TRANSPORTER | TISSUES | FUNCTION |
| --- | --- | --- |
| GLUT-1 | RBC, blood-brain barrier | Basal uptake of glucose |
| GLUT-2 | Liver, pancreas | Manages surplus of glucose, facilitates insulin release |
| GLUT-3 | Neurons, brain | Basal uptake of glucose |
| GLUT-4 | Skeletal muscle, adipose tissue | Insulin-stimulated glucose uptake, stimulated by exercise |

GLUT, glucose transporter; RBC, red blood cell.

in neuronal tissue, including the brain. GLUT-4 transporters are found in adipose and skeletal muscle tissue. This transporter is unique in that it responds to insulin, which enables additional transporters to move to the surface membrane.

## The Liver

The liver is capable of metabolizing the three major fuel sources:

- **Carbohydrates:** Glucose can be synthesized into glycogen, which then can be broken down into glucose. Glucose may be further broken down via glycolysis or, more commonly, released into the blood.
- **Lipids:** Fats obtained from the diet are metabolized differently depending on whether the body is in a fed or unfed state. If the body is in a fed state, they can be synthesized into triglycerides and packaged into VLDLs. If the body is in an unfed state, they are catabolized to ketone bodies. The liver also uses fats to synthesize cholesterol and bile acids. Lastly, fats can be broken down into acetyl-CoA, which will be fed into the TCA cycle for ATP.
- **Proteins:** Amino acids are used last because they form the structural (cytoskeletal) and functional (enzymatic) basis of all cells; when amino acid catabolism does occur, the α-amino group is removed and excreted as **urea.**

Since a primary function of the liver is to generate fuel sources for other tissues, it tends not to use glucose or fatty acids for its own metabolic needs. Instead it relies on **α-ketoacids,** such as pyruvate and oxaloacetate, which are created when amino groups are removed from amino acids.

> **KEY FACT**
>
> α-Ketoacids, such as pyruvate and oxaloacetate, are substrates in the TCA cycle.

## INSULIN AND THE FED STATE

Insulin is an anabolic hormone used by the body to **maximize the storage of dietary glucose in the fed state.** Its actions serve to decrease serum glucose levels. It targets tissues responsible for glucose storage and utilization, such as the liver, muscle, and adipose tissues (Figure 2-87).

In the **liver,** insulin:

- Inhibits gluconeogenesis
- Inhibits breakdown of glycogen
- Promotes glycogen synthesis

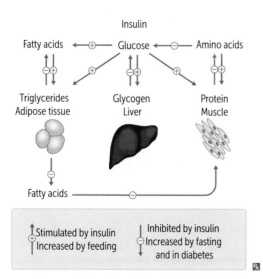

**FIGURE 2-87.    Targets of insulin.** Pathways in blue indicate targets that are stimulated by insulin. Pathways in red indicate targets that are inhibited by insulin. The blue pathways are increased by feeding, whereas the red pathways are increased by fasting.

In **muscle** cells, insulin:

- Promotes glycogen synthesis
- Increases glucose entry into cells (mediated by GLUT4)
- Stimulates the entry of amino acids (desirable for protein synthesis)

In **adipose** tissue, insulin:

- Increases glucose uptake into cells (mediated by GLUT4)
- Increases triacylglycerol synthesis
- Decreases triacylglycerol degradation
- Inhibits activity of hormone-sensitive lipase
- Increases lipoprotein lipase activity

### STAGES OF STARVATION

The effects of starvation can be described by their effects on four tissues: brain, skeletal muscle, adipose, and liver. Starvation is discussed for each organ in the following sections.

#### Early Starvation (1–3 days)

Homeostasis functions to prevent blood glucose levels from becoming too high (by releasing insulin) and from falling too low (by releasing glucagon). When blood glucose drops below 70 mg/dL, glucagon begins to be released from the α-cells of the pancreas. If blood glucose gets too low (< 50 mg/dL), the brain will not have enough fuel to generate the ATP it needs, and permanent damage can occur.

The main target of glucagon is the liver, where it **promotes the release of glucose** into the blood by:

- Inhibiting **glycogen synthase,** which synthesizes glycogen, and activating **glycogen phosphorylase,** which promotes glycogenolysis and glucose release
- Promoting gluconeogenesis
- Increasing uptake of amino acids, such as alanine, thereby providing additional carbon skeletons for **gluconeogenesis**
- Promoting ketone body formation
- Switching fuel use from glucose to free fatty acids (in muscle and liver)

In the liver, glucagon also inhibits fatty acid synthesis by inhibiting the action of acetyl-CoA-carboxylase, the enzyme that mediates the first committed step. In muscle, glucagon **has no effect** on glycogen stores.

In adipose tissue, glucagon stimulates release of free fatty acids.

Glucagon mediates each of the previously mentioned effects by stimulating the production of **cAMP,** which then activates **protein kinase A.**

Because glucagon and insulin oppose one another, when glucagon is high, insulin is low. In the absence of insulin, neither muscle nor fat displays the GLUT4 transporter, the net effect being **maximum delivery of glucose to the brain** and preferential utilization of fatty acids by muscle.

As the liver's glycogen stores are depleted, it must begin to supply the brain with the other source of fuel that neurons can use, such as **ketone bodies** (Table 2-26). Recall, when insulin levels are low, **lipoprotein lipase** is not active; when glucagon levels are high, **hormone-sensitive lipase** is active. The net result is **the release of fatty acids into the blood,** which can be converted into ketone bodies by the liver.

**TABLE 2-26.    Summary of Action of Insulin and Glucagon**

| ORGAN | ↑ BY INSULIN | ↓ BY INSULIN | ↑ BY GLUCAGON |
|---|---|---|---|
| **Adipose tissue** | Glycogen uptake<br>Fatty acid synthesis | Lipolysis | Lipolysis |
| **Liver** | Fatty acid synthesis<br>Glycogen synthesis<br>Protein synthesis | Ketogenesis<br>Gluconeogenesis | Glycogenolysis<br>Gluconeogenesis<br>Ketogenesis |
| **Muscle** | Glycogen uptake<br>Glycogen synthesis<br>Protein synthesis | | |

### Late Starvation (3 days or more)

With prolonged starvation, the body's ability to produce adequate glucose for the brain diminishes, as glycogen reserves are depleted after approximately 1 day. Though muscle continues to store glycogen, it is unable to contribute to the glucose pool because muscle tissue (unlike the liver) does not contain **G6P,** the enzyme that dephosphorylates G6P to free glucose that can leave the cell and be utilized by other tissues.

As glycogen stores are depleted, the liver begins to produce ketone bodies from fatty acids. And as fatty acid stores are also depleted, and the liver begins to rely more on proteins as a source of carbon. This compromises the integrity of tissues and ultimately, leads to organ failure and death (Figure 2-88).

### ENDOCRINE PANCREAS

The pancreas has both exocrine and endocrine functions. The **exocrine** function of the pancreas is to secrete **digestive enzymes** and bicarbonate-rich fluids into the duodenum. The **endocrine** function of the pancreas is to release **insulin, glucagon,** and **somatostatin.**

Insulin is an anabolic polypeptide hormone, as it induces growth of muscle, fat, and other tissues. It is produced by the β-cells of the **islets of Langerhans** (Figure 2-89). The **α-cells** secrete glucagon, whereas δ-cells secrete somatostatin. The β-cells are typically located centrally with α-cells and δ-cells located around them, allowing for **paracrine regulation.**

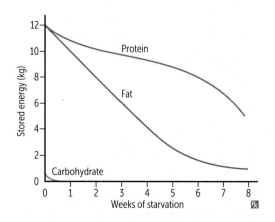

**FIGURE 2-88.    Use of all three fuel sources during starvation.**

**KEY FACT**

Because the body relies on fatty acid stores before it draws on protein sources, the amount of fat a person has largely determines how long he or she can survive during starvation.

**KEY FACT**

**Multiple endocrine neoplasia (MEN) type 1,** or **Wermer syndrome,** consists of parathyroid, pituitary, and enteropancreatic tumors. Among the pancreatic tumors are **insulinomas** (causing fasting hypoglycemia), **glucagonomas** (causing migratory necrolytic erythema and symptoms of hyperglycemia and weight loss), and **somatostatinomas** (also causing a diabetes-like condition, steatorrhea, achlorhydria, and cholelithiasis).

**MNEMONIC**

A useful way to remember MEN type 1 is **PPP: P**ancreatic, **P**arathyroid, and **P**ituitary.

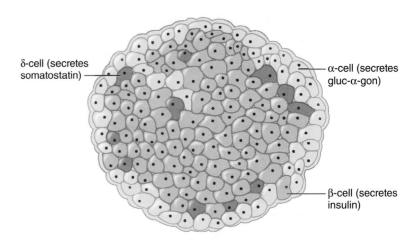

**FIGURE 2-89.** **Islet of Langerhans.** Note that β-cells predominate and are located centrally. α-cells are the next most prevalent cell type and form the periphery of the islet. δ-cells are scattered throughout the islet tissue.

## Insulin

The hormone insulin is actually derived from a much larger polypeptide that undergoes several cleavage steps. Figure 2-90 explains these steps in detail. Although not part of the biochemically active hormone, these cleaved segments allow insulin to fold properly (Figure 2-91).

Insulin secretion is **stimulated** by the ingestion of carbohydrates, proteins, and fats. It is **inhibited** by epinephrine, norepinephrine, and glucocorticoids, as well as growth hormone.

## Insulin Secretion

Insulin secretion starts with glucose entering the β-islet cells through the **GLUT2 transporter.** Glucose is then phosphorylated by glucokinase and is trapped in the β-cells.

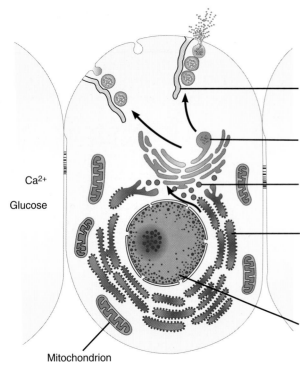

5. After a meal, entry of glucose into β-cells results in calcium influx, which causes secretory vesicles to fuse with the cell membrane and release their contents (insulin and C-peptide) into the bloodstream.

4. In the **Golgi apparatus,** enzymes cleave proinsulin to produce **insulin** and **C-peptide,** which bud from the Golgi as secretory vesicles.

3. Small vesicles containing proinsulin bud from the ER and travel toward the Golgi apparatus.

2. The mRNA is delivered to the cytosol, where translation begins, but because the developing polypeptide contains an N-terminal signal sequence, the entire mRNA-ribosome-polypeptide complex is shuttled to the ER. There, the remainder of the polypeptide **(preproinsulin)** is produced and is "threaded" into the ER lumen. The N-terminal signal sequence is snipped off to produce **proinsulin.**

1. In the nucleus, the gene encoding insulin is transcribed to produce mRNA.

**FIGURE 2-90.** **Formation and secretion of insulin.**

Glucose is then metabolized to form ATP, which inhibits the ATP-sensitive potassium channels that are used to pump potassium out of the cell. Retention of intracellular potassium causes the cell membrane to depolarize, and then the influx of extracellular calcium through voltage-sensitive calcium channels. The rise in intracellular calcium triggers the exocytosis of vesicles containing insulin and C-peptide (Figure 2-92).

## Mechanism of Action of Insulin

Insulin binds to the insulin receptor, a tyrosine kinase. Once insulin binds to the external part of the receptor, tyrosine residues on the internal part of the receptor become autophosphorylated. Once activated, the tyrosine kinase phosphorylates insulin receptor substrate (IRS) proteins. The newly activated IRS proteins in turn, activate cellular kinases and phosphatases that vary depending on the type of cell. After insulin binds to its receptor, both are taken up into the cell. Although insulin is then degraded, its receptor may return to the cell membrane.

## Insulin and Hyperkalemia

Insulin is used to treat **hyperkalemia** (serum K$^+$ > 5.5 mEq/L), a serious electrolyte abnormality that predispose patients to cardiac arrythmias. When serum K$^+$ levels are too high, the electrochemical gradient that usually drives K$^+$ out of cells is reduced. More K$^+$ remains within the cell, which causes a slight baseline depolarization in the **resting membrane potential**. Clinically, the following tissues are most affected:

- Skeletal muscle and nerves: fatigue, weakness, and, ultimately, paralysis
- Cardiac muscle: loss of coordinated contractions, causing arrhythmias and death; ECG may show peaked T waves as well as PR shortening
- Smooth muscle, such as the GI tract: paralysis or "ileus"

Because insulin **stimulates K$^+$ entry into cells, it can be used to treat severe hyperkalemia. Glucose, however, must be given simultaneously to avoid hypoglycemia.** These are important clinical considerations when treating diabetic ketoacidosis (DKA) with intravenous insulin. Potassium follows glucose into cells through a "solvent drag" mechanism.

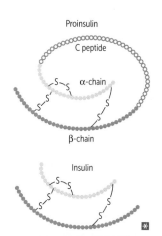

**FIGURE 2-91.   Structure of proinsulin and insulin.** Proinsulin contains the "C peptide" segment, which links the insulin α- and β-chains and allows the protein to fold properly during its formation.

**CLINICAL CORRELATION**

C-peptide levels are used to distinguish insulinoma versus exogenous insulin use. If a patient is using exogenous insulin, C-peptide levels will be low; if the patient has an insulin-producing tumor, both insulin and C-peptide levels will be high.

**FLASH FORWARD**

Exenatide is an incretin mimetic approved by the FDA in 2005 to improve glycemic control in patients already using insulin for the treatment of type 2 diabetes.

**MNEMONIC**

**BRICK-L** (insulin-independent glucose uptake):
**B**rain, **R**BCs, **I**ntestine, **C**ornea, **K**idney, **L**iver

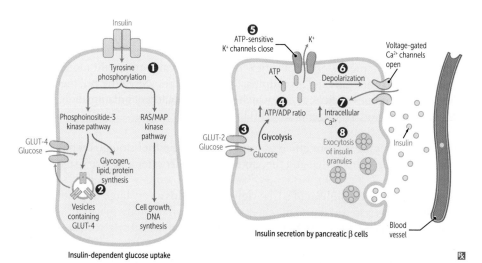

**FIGURE 2-92.   Pancreatic β-cell insulin secretion.** Glucose enters β cells ❸ → ↑ ATP generated from glucose metabolism ❹ closes K$^+$ channels (target of sulfonylureas) ❺ and depolarizes β cell membrane ❻. Voltage-gated Ca$^{2+}$ channels open → Ca$^{2+}$ influx ❼ and stimulation of insulin exocytosis ❽. ADP, adenine diphosphate; ATP, adenosine triphosphate; GLUT, glucose transporter.

### Glucagon

Glucagon is a polypeptide hormone secreted by **α-cells of the pancreatic islets.** Glucagon regulates the actions of insulin and **maintains serum glucose levels.** It does so by activation of hepatic glycogenolysis and gluconeogenesis.

Stimuli for glucagon release include:

- Hypoglycemia (primary stimulus)
- Amino acids
- Epinephrine

Release of glucagon is inhibited by:

- Insulin
- Hyperglycemia

### Somatostatin

Somatostatin is a peptide hormone that is released from pancreatic D cells in response to meal ingestion or gastric acid secretion. The overall effect of this hormone is inhibition and downregulation of several biochemical processes. In regard to metabolism, somatostatin decreases GI hormones, such as gastrin, cholecystokinin, and motilin, to name a few. Somatostatin acts on the anterior pituitary to inhibit the release of hormones such as thyroid-stimulating hormone (TSH), prolactin (PL), growth hormone (GH).

### Molecular Pathways

Insulin and glucagon oppose one another in glycogen metabolism by acting on two key enzymes. **Glycogen synthase** is responsible for forming glycogen. **Phosphorylase kinase** breaks it down. Since insulin signals the well-fed state, glucose is preferentially stored as glycogen. As expected, insulin **activates** glycogen synthase and **inhibits** phosphorylase kinase. This occurs because insulin initiates a transduction pathway that relies on **protein phosphatase 1.**

Glucagon does the exact opposite by initiating a transduction pathway that relies on **protein kinase A.** These effects are summarized in Table 2-27.

### Fatty Acid Metabolism

Fatty acids are the precursors for a variety of physiologically important molecules. In the form of **phospholipids** and **glycolipids,** they are components of the cell membrane. They act as **hormones** or **eicosanoids,** which serve as mediators of inflammation. Finally, they can be catabolized **to generate ATP** for the body.

Triacylglycerides are a more efficient form of metabolic fuel storage than glycogen because they are hydrophobic and therefore can exclude water and save space.

Also recall that **the catabolism of a triacylglyceride yields a very large number of ATP equivalents.** This is in part due to the sheer number of carbon atoms in a triacylglyceride molecule and in part due to the fact that no component of the triacylglyceride—neither

**KEY FACT**

Insulin tends to promote **dephosphorylation** via protein phosphatase 1 to exert its effects. Glucagon, on the other hand, promotes **phosphorylation** via protein kinase A. A good way to remember this is to recall that during glycogen breakdown, glycogen must be phosphorylated before it can be cleaved to generate glucose.

**KEY FACT**

- **Amino acids** cause the release of **both** insulin and glucagon. The release of glucagon opposes the action of secreted insulin on cellular intake of serum glucose.
- **Catecholamines** released in the sympathetic nervous system "fight or flight" response allow for an increase in serum glucose for use by muscles, the brain, and other critical tissues.

**KEY FACT**

Roughly 6.5 ATP molecules per carbon atom in **palmitate** are generated from β-oxidation. Compare that with the 5 ATPs per carbon atom produced after complete oxidation of **glucose.**

**TABLE 2-27.**   **Molecular Effects of Insulin and Glucagon**

| | TRANSDUCTION PATHWAY | GLYCOGEN SYNTHASE | PHOSPHORYLASE KINASE | OVERALL EFFECT |
|---|---|---|---|---|
| Insulin | Protein phosphatase 1 (removes phosphate groups) | **Activated** by dephosphorylation | **Inhibited** by dephosphorylation | Production of glycogen |
| Glucagon | Protein kinase A (adds phosphate groups) | **Inhibited** by phosphorylation | **Activated** by phosphorylation | Glycogen breakdown |

the glycerol "backbone" nor the fatty acid constituents—goes unused (Figure 2-86). Glycerol can enter **glycolysis** or **gluconeogenesis**. Each of the three fatty acid tails may undergo β-**oxidation**. As an example, the complete oxidation of **palmitate,** a common 16-carbon fatty acid, generates enough acetyl-CoA, $FADH_2$, and NADH to produce the equivalent of 106 ATP molecules.

## Fatty Acid Synthesis

Fatty acid synthesis occurs in the brain, liver, kidney, lung, and adipose tissue. Though it appears complicated, synthesis of a fatty acid occurs by repetition of the steps shown in Figure 2-93. The most important features of fatty acid synthesis are as follows:

- **Activation:** The enzyme **acetyl-CoA carboxylase** adds carbon dioxide to **acetyl-CoA** (a 2-carbon molecule) to form **malonyl-CoA** (a 3-carbon molecule).
- **Elongation:** Each step of elongation uses the 3-carbon malonyl-CoA molecule. **Two carbons are added to the growing fatty acid and one carbon is lost as carbon dioxide.**
- **Termination:** Malonyl-CoA donates 2 carbons to the growing fatty acid chain until the chain is 16 carbons in length (**palmitate**). Sixteen is common stopping point because the enzyme **thioesterase recognizes and cleaves 16-carbon fatty acids.** Addition of more carbon units, or the introduction of double bonds, is carried out by enzymes associated with the ER.

## Fatty Acid Synthase

All the reactions involved in elongation and termination are carried out by a single 260-kilodalton polypeptide known as **fatty acid synthase.** Fatty acid synthase has multiple enzymatic domains in proximity, allowing for coordination between the many synthetic steps.

The exact chemical reactions are less important than understanding how the domains of fatty acid synthase interact with one another. In Figure 2-93, the domain marked as "1" is the area of initiation. The domain marked as "2" is the elongation end. The steps summarized here refer to Figure 2-93:

- Domain 1 is added with acetyl-CoA (step 1a), and domain 2 is combined with malonyl-CoA (step 1b).
- The acetyl group of domain 1 is transferred to domain 2 (step 2), and $CO_2$ is released from the malonyl group, resulting in a 4-carbon chain.
- The 4-carbon chain undergoes a series of chemical reactions (steps 3, 4, and 5) carried out by domain 2 to produce the final 4-carbon fatty acid.
- The fatty acid is then transferred from domain 2 to domain 1 so that domain 2 can be "reloaded" with another malonyl group in preparation for the next cycle.

Note that in the second cycle, domain 1 no longer accepts an acetyl group as illustrated by step 1a. This is because domain 1 is now combined with the growing fatty acid chain. The fatty acid on domain 1 is transferred to domain 2, $CO_2$ is released, and this time the result is a 6-carbon chain.

## Fatty Acid Oxidation

The enzymes involved in fatty acid oxidation are found in the **mitochondrial matrix,** whereas enzymes of fatty acid synthesis are in the **cytosol.** This separation ensures that fatty acids are not consumed by the cell as soon as they are created. Fatty acids enter the mitochondria via the **carnitine translocase** or **carnitine transport system (CTS).**

The outer mitochondrial membrane is relatively permeable, but the inner mitochondrial membrane is not. The CTS is essentially a channel for fatty acids that employs **carnitine,** an ammonium compound, to handle large molecules like fatty acids. If carnitine is not available for synthesis, such as in carnitine deficiency, carnitine acetyltransferase

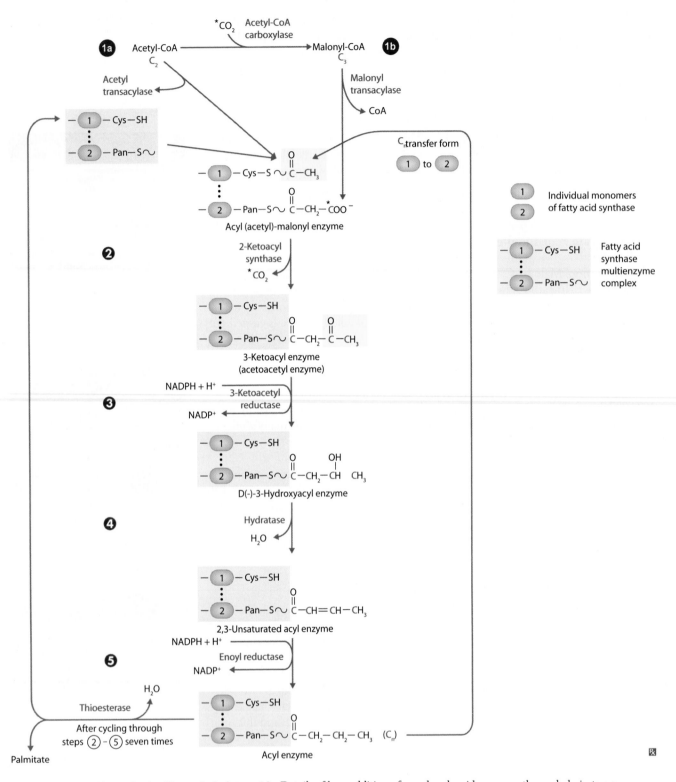

**FIGURE 2-93.** **Biosynthesis of long-chain fatty acids.** Details of how addition of a malonyl residue causes the acyl chain to grow by two carbon atoms. CoA, coenzyme A; Cys, cysteine residue; SH, sulfhydryl; NADP⁺, oxidized nicotinamide adenine dinucleotide phosphate; NADPH, reduced nicotinamide adenine dinucleotide phosphate; Pan, 4′-phosphopantetheine.

will not be synthesized. This enzyme is used in the rate-limiting step for β-oxidation of fatty acids. Glucose will be the only energy source, which will lead to a hypoketotic hypoglycemic state.

Once inside the matrix, the fatty acid chain is broken at the bond between the α and β carbons and is appropriately titled β-oxidation (Figure 2-94). The process of β-oxidation removes two carbon units as acetyl-CoA per cycle. A 16-carbon fatty acid like palmitate yields a total of eight acetyl-CoA molecules following complete β-oxidation.

In addition, the FADH$_2$ and NADH formed from β-oxidation are used in the **electron transport chain** for the generation of ATP. As mentioned in the beginning of this section, the complete β-oxidation of palmitate into acetyl-CoA, FADH$_2$ and NADH produces 106 ATP equivalents.

## KETONES

The body is unable to convert free fatty acids (FFA) into glucose. Therefore, **the liver must convert fatty acids (and ketogenic amino acids) into ketone bodies, which can be utilized by the brain** (Figure 2-95).

The two ketone bodies made by the liver are **acetoacetate** and **β-hydroxybutyrate**.

### Anabolism

**Low insulin/glucagon ratio stimulates the ketogenic pathway:**

- All the material for ketone body synthesis comes from acetyl-CoA, the breakdown product of most fatty acids and ketogenic amino acids (Figure 2-96).
- Two molecules of acetyl-CoA unite with the help of β-ketothiolase, forming acetoacetyl-CoA.
- There is no hydrolase to split this molecule into acetoacetate and CoA, so a two-step detour must be taken:
  1. β-Hydroxy-β-methylglutaryl-CoA combines acetoacetate-CoA with another molecule of acetyl-CoA, forming HMG-CoA. This is the rate-limiting step of ketone body synthesis. A subsequent cleavage by HMG-CoA lysase yields the ketone body acetoacetate.
  2. Reduction with NADH-dependent β-hydroxybutyrate dehydrogenase provides the second ketone body, β-hydroxybutyrate.

Formation of β-hydroxybutyrate requires NADH. Hence, the ratio of [β-hydroxybutyrate]/[acetoacetate] in the blood reflects the ratio of [NADH]/[NAD$^+$] in the mitochondria.

- Blood tests are the most reliable gauge of ketone levels, because urine tests such as nitroprusside strips only detect acetoacetate. Routine tests do not typically screen for β-hydroxybutyrate.
- Alcohol (ethanol) consumption leads to NADH accumulation, which drives the conversion of acew toacetate to β-hydroxybutyrate. Hence, ketone levels in alcoholics may be underestimated if nitroprusside strips are used.
- High ketone concentrations often manifest a fruity smelling breath; acetoacetate decomposes into acetone, which has a low vapor pressure and is therefore largely cleared by the lungs.

### Catabolism

- Once β-hydroxybutyrate and acetoacetate reach the mitochondria of the target organ, the former is converted to the latter by β-hydroxybutyrate dehydrogenase.

**KEY FACT**

Fatty acids with an odd number of carbon atoms that undergo β-oxidation produce acetyl-CoA, until they are shortened to **propionyl-CoA** (3 carbons). Propionyl-CoA can be converted to succinyl-CoA to enter the TCA cycle.

**CLINICAL CORRELATION**

Zellweger syndrome is an autosomal recessive disorder of peroxisomes in which very-long-chain fatty acids and branched-chain fatty acids cannot be broken down and accumulate in peroxisomes. Symptoms include jaundice, hepatomegaly, seizures, hypotonia, and facial abnormalities.

**FLASH FORWARD**

Statins block HMG-CoA reductase, the committed step in cholesterol synthesis.

**FLASH FORWARD**

Ethanol is metabolized to acetaldehyde and then acetate by **alcohol dehydrogenase** and **aldehyde dehydrogenase,** respectively (Figure 2-97). Both steps consume NAD$^+$ and generate NADH. The increase in NADH favors the conversion of pyruvate to lactate (since NADH serves as a reactant). This depletes the pool of pyruvate available for the TCA cycle and, consequently, oxidative phosphorylation. This effectively places the alcoholic into a **constant state of anaerobic glycolysis,** seriously impairing his or her ability to generate ATP. Furthermore, the increase in NADH will favor fatty acid synthesis, which is why hepatic steatosis or fatty liver occurs. This, compounded by general malnutrition, may explain why alcoholics are far more vulnerable to metabolic derangements in times of stress and illness.

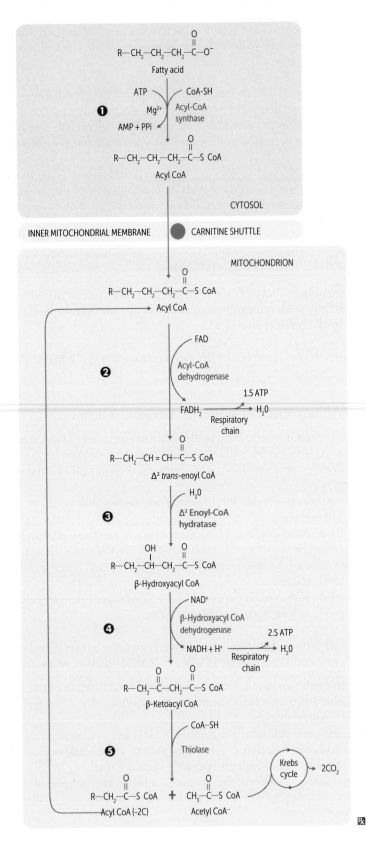

FIGURE 2-94.    **Fatty acid oxidation.** β-Oxidation of fatty acids. Long-chain acyl-CoA is cycled through reactions 2–5, acetyl-CoA is split off, each cycle, by thiolase (reaction 5). When the acyl radical is only four carbon atoms in length, two acetyl-CoA molecules are formed in reaction 5. AMP, adenosine monophosphate; ATP, adenosine triphosphate; CoA, coenzyme A; FAD, flavin adenine dinucleotide; FADH$_2$, reduced flavin adenine dinucleotide; NAD$^+$, oxidized nicotinamide adenine dinucleotide; NADH, reduced nicotinamide adenine dinucleotide; PPi, pyrophosphate; SH, sulfhydryl.

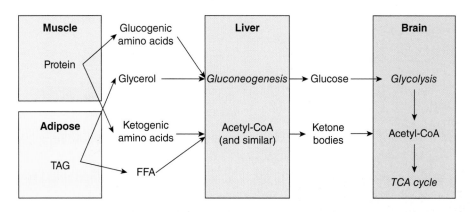

**FIGURE 2-95. Brain energy supply in the prolonged fasting state.** CoA, coenzyme A; FFA, free fatty acid; TAG, triacylglycerol; TCA, tricarboxylic acid.

- Eventually all ketone bodies will form acetoacetate. Succinyl-CoA transferase subsequently attaches coenzyme A to acetoacetate, making it a ready substrate for β-ketothiolase.
- Each ketone body therefore delivers two units of acetyl-CoA to the target organ; β-hydroxybutyrate also provides an NADH. Note that synthesis and subsequent degradation of one acetoacetate molecule results in net energy loss due to cleavage of one succinyl-CoA molecule.

### Ketosis

**Fasting ketosis** refers to an increase in the concentration of ketone bodies when liver glycogen is diminished. An overnight fast or high-intensity exercise is enough to result in ketosis, which becomes more prominent if the subject is on a low-carbohydrate diet and thus has low liver glycogen stores. Ketosis alone is not a pathologic process, and replenishing glucose stores is the fastest remedy.

**Alcoholic ketoacidosis** manifests in chronic alcoholics. $NAD^+$ is depleted due to oxidation of ethanol to acetate. Hypoglycemia results from depleted glycogen and lack of gluconeogenesis (blocked by **high $NADH/NAD^+$**), which prompts mobilization of fat stores and their conversion to ketones. The resulting acidosis is usually not life-threatening.

**Diabetic ketoacidosis (DKA)** is a life-threatening condition, which may occur in type 1 diabetics with poorly controlled blood glucose. Without sufficient insulin, glucagon and other stress hormones are unopposed and begin to rise, despite high blood glucose levels. The liver produces exceptional amounts of ketone bodies, which make the blood more acidic. As acidemia worsens (and, by definition, protons in the blood increase),

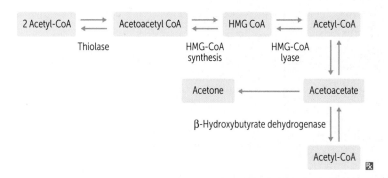

**FIGURE 2-96. Ketone body synthesis.** CoA, coenzyme A; HMG CoA, 3-hydroxy-3-methylglutaryl coenzyme A.

>> **FLASH FORWARD**

The conversion of acetaldehyde to acetate by aldehyde dehydrogenase is inhibited by **disulfiram.** The antibiotic metronidazole has some disulfiram-like activity. Patients on metronidazole must refrain from drinking alcohol because the inability to clear acetaldehyde from the body can result in **nausea, flushing, and respiratory difficulties.** This is the basis for prescribing disulfiram to recovering alcoholics: the nausea is meant to deter relapse. Drugs that cause a disulfiram-like reaction are metronidazole, some cephalosporins, procarbazine, and first-generation sulfonylureas.

**? CLINICAL CORRELATION**

Fomepizole inhibits alcohol dehydrogenase and serves as an antidote for methanol or ethylene glycol poisoning.

**? CLINICAL CORRELATION**

Diabetes mellitus (DM) type 1 is an autoimmune disease in which β-cells in the pancreas are attacked. There is virtually no insulin produced.
In type 2 DM, the pancreas often produces more insulin than is normal, but peripheral tissues are relatively resistant to insulin action.

**? CLINICAL CORRELATION**

Medium-chain acyl-CoA dehydrogenase deficiency is an autosomal recessive disorder of fatty acid oxidation. In this disease, there is an impairment in the ability to break down fatty acids into acetyl-CoA. This leads to an accumulation of 8- to 10-carbon fatty acylcarnitines in the blood, and a hypoketotic hypoglycemic state ensues. Symptoms include vomiting, lethargy, seizures, coma, and hepatomegaly.

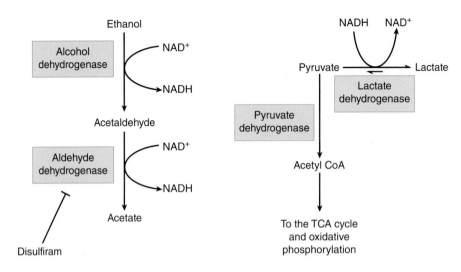

**FIGURE 2-97. Production of NADH during ethanol metabolism drives the conversion of pyruvate to lactate.** NAD, nicotinamide adenine dinucleotide; NADH, reduced form of nicotinamide adenine dinucleotide.

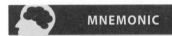

**MNEMONIC**

The common causes of **high anion gap metabolic acidosis** (meaning that acids are present in blood that are not detected by routine lab tests) are **I am SLUMPED:**
**I**sopropyl alcohol
**S**alicylates
**L**actate
**U**remia
**M**ethanol
**P**araldehyde (paint sniffing)
**E**thylene glycol (antifreeze)
**D**iabetic ketoacidosis

cells of the body begin to exchange one cation for another: protons are taken up from the blood and K$^+$ is released, resulting in **hyperkalemia.** Hyperkalemia lasts only for a short time, as total body stores of potassium greatly diminish, which in turn will result in hypokalemia. Additionally, there is significant water and sodium loss via osmotic diuresis.

Typical causes of DKA include not taking insulin (common in teenagers with DM), infection, and other physiologic stressors that raise cortisol and consequently blood sugar in type 1 diabetics. Treatment includes:

- IV 0.9 normal saline until blood glucose is ≤ 200 mg/dL. Dextrose solution is then used as a maintenance fluid.
- IV insulin infusion, but must be used with caution, especially if the patient is already hypokalemic.
- K$^+$ replacement (high blood [K$^+$], but low total body K$^+$ due to diuresis).
- HCO$_{3-}$ is given if pH is less than 6.9.

Patients often present with increased respiratory rate and tidal volumes (**Kussmaul** respirations) that is driven by attempted respiratory compensation to metabolic acidosis. Patients also present with dehydration, nausea, vomiting, mental status changes, and fruity-smelling breath.

DKA is rare in type 2 diabetics. This is because the pancreas is still able to produce small amounts of insulin and therefore inhibit glucagon secretion and significant ketone body production.

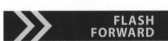

**FLASH FORWARD**

Intravenous fluids are the first-line treatment for many acute disorders and should be administered even before starting an "actual medication." Extra caution is warranted in patients with heart conditions, however, since the blood volume ejected with each contraction may be much lower than normal. The excess fluid can "back up" into the lungs (impairing gas exchange) and myocardial stretch causing arrhythmias and death.

Patients with type 2 DM, however, do suffer from **hyperosmolar hyperglycemic nonketotic syndrome (HHNS).** In this condition, serum glucose levels frequently exceed 1000 mg/dL (normal is about 100 mg/dL). The presenting symptoms of HHNC are caused by **the gradual increase of blood glucose,** leading to blood hyperosmolarity:

- Excessive urination (**osmotic diuresis**) occurs because nephrons are unable to keep up with glucose reabsorption, and free water is lost by osmosis
- Increased thirst (**polydipsia**) due to free water depletion
- Weight loss due to dehydration

If hyperglycemia continues, the high osmolarity of the blood draws away intracellular fluid, most notably from the brain. The accompanying "cellular shrinking" disrupts normal brain function as manifested by neurologic deficits delirium, confusion, somnolence, lethargy, and ultimately coma and death.

## LIPOPROTEINS

### Function and Structure

Because fat is hydrophobic and does not dissolve in blood, lipids require carrier molecules to enter the circulation.

- **Albumin** can carry fat in the form of free fatty acids from adipose tissue. Fatty acids are "free" in that they are not covalently attached to glycerol, but they are noncovalently bound to albumin in blood.
- Dietary fat from the intestine and fat from the liver associates with specialized amphiphilic (detergent-like) proteins, called **apolipoproteins.** Together with various lipids (cholesterol, cholesterol esters [CE], triglycerides [TG], and phospholipids [PL]), the apolipoproteins form **lipoproteins.**
- Lipoproteins are spherical. Like a cell, their shell is formed by PL, cholesterol, and protein, whereas the core is composed of the more hydrophobic lipids.

Most lipoproteins are named according to their density. From low to high density: **Chylomicrons < VLDL < IDL < LDL < HDL.**

In general, higher density implies more protein, more cholesterol, more CE content, less TG, and smaller particle size. HDL is an exception in that its cholesterol content is only moderately high.

### Chylomicrons and Remnants

- The dietary lipids (mostly TG, some cholesterol) in the cytoplasm of enterocytes enter the ER, where they assemble along with a freshly translated, large apolipoprotein, called **ApoB-48,** and a smaller protein **ApoA-1.** The resulting lipoprotein is called a **chylomicron.** "Chylo-," because these particles enter the lymphatic (chyle) vessels and the thoracic duct before actually reaching blood (Figure 2-98).
- When a chylomicron meets an HDL particle, they exchange ApoA-1 for **ApoC-2** (Figure 2-98).
- ApoC-2 is a cofactor for lipoprotein lipase (**LPL**), so that when chylomicrons reach **muscle** and **adipose tissue,** LPL cleaves the TG content (Figure 2-98). The resulting fatty acids are taken up by muscle or adipose cells then either stored or β-oxidized. Donation of ApoC-2 to chylomicrons can be regarded as an "activation step" since without it LPL would not actv and chylomicrons would continue to float in the blood unchanged.
- As TG, but not PL leave the lipoprotein, a relative buildup of PL results in a large amount of surface shell and a small core. To avoid rupture of an enzyme, phospholipid transfer protein (**PLTP**) moves PL from chylomicrons to HDL.
- In addition, blood contains cholesterol ester transfer protein (**CETP**), which moves TG from chylomicrons to HDL, and CE in the opposite direction.
- Once most TGs have been removed by LPL, the chylomicron returns ApoC2 to an HDL particle, so that no further cleavage takes place. In exchange, HDL provides yet another apolipoprotein, called **ApoE.** The resulting shrunken, TG-depleted, CE-enriched, ApoE-labeled lipoprotein is known as the **chylomicron remnant** (Figure 2-98).
- The remnants are ready to leave the circulation by entering the liver (Figure 2-98). Hepatocytes have two receptors for chylomicrons. **The LDL receptor** requires both ApoE and ApoB-48 (or B-100) to bind. The low-density lipoprotein-related protein (**LRP**) receptor is specific for ApoE-labeled chylomicrons. So even when LDL

**KEY FACT**

Albumin is a negatively charged protein that binds cations, especially calcium. In states of hypoalbuminemia, the calcium level must be **corrected.** For every 1 unit albumin below normal, calcium must be increased by 0.8.

**KEY FACT**

Without **ApoB-48,** chylomicrons cannot be released into the blood from intestinal cells. **ApoE** is recognized by hepatocytes and allows the liver to remove **chylomicron remnants** from the blood.

**KEY FACT**

Although LPL is produced by peripheral tissues, it is found on the apical membranes of the blood vessel **endothelium.** LPL, therefore, has access to chylomicrons in the blood.

**CLINICAL CORRELATION**

Familial hypercholesterolemia is an autosomal dominant disorder that is caused by dysfunctional LDL receptors. LDL cannot be removed, cholesterol levels spike, and patients suffer from premature atherosclerosis.

**CLINICAL CORRELATION**

Abetalipoproteinemia is an autosomal recessive disorder that is caused by a deficiency of ApoB-48 and B-100. VLDL and LDL will be absent in plasma because they require ApoB-100. There will also be malabsorption of lipids due to defective chylomicron formation, which requires B48. Other symptoms include steatorrhea, acanthocytosis, ataxia, and night blindness.

| Chylomicron flow | Schema of main event | Description |
|---|---|---|

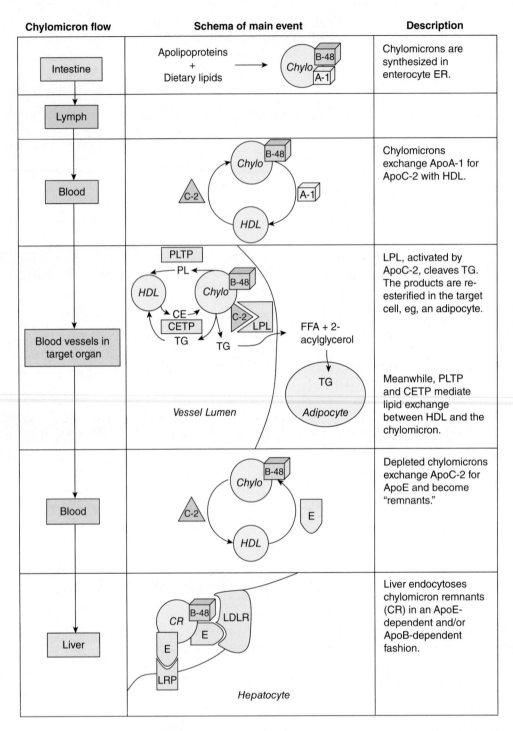

**FIGURE 2-98.** **Chylomicrons and important events in their life cycle.** Apo, apolipoprotein; ER, endoplasmic reticulum; CE, cholesterol ester, CETP, cholesterol ester transfer protein; Chylo, chylomicron; CR, chylomicron remnant; FFA, free fatty acid; HDL, high-density lipoproteins; LDLR, low-density lipoprotein receptor; LPL, lipoprotein lipase; LRP, low-density lipoprotein-related protein; PL, phospholipids; PLTP, phospholipid transfer protein; TG, triglyceride.

receptors are not functional, as in familial hypercholesterolemia, chylomicron remnants do not accumulate, because of sufficient LRP activity.

### VLDL, IDL, and LDL

Like the intestine, the liver packages all of its would-be secreted lipids into lipoproteins, called very-low-density lipoproteins (**VLDL**). VLDL is the hepatocyte's analog to the enterocyte's chylomicrons, with a few differences:

- The main VLDL apolipoprotein is the larger ApoB-100 (not ApoB-48).
- Although VLDL still contains more TG than cholesterol, it has a higher cholesterol content than do chylomicrons.
- The lipids packaged into VLDL are synthesized in the liver. This contrasts with the lipids in chylomicrons, which are from the diet.
- The VLDL remnants are called intermediate-density lipoproteins (**IDL**).
- Although IDL can be taken up by the liver, it often loses some of its ApoE and shrinks even further, resulting in **LDL.**
- Liver's LDL receptors can still recognize LDL. However, LDL also tends to cross the endothelium into various tissues. In capillaries, this is not a problem, but in large arteries, LDL can get trapped and oxidized in the vessel intima. Oxidation of LDL renders it recognizable by macrophages, resulting in endocytosis and formation of foam cells, which initiates **atherosclerosis.**

## HDL

High-density lipoproteins (HDLs) differ from the other lipoproteins in that HDL contains no large apolipoprotein (eg, ApoB-48 or B-100). ApoA-1 is the most characteristic protein.

HDL, commonly referred to as the "good cholesterol," has multiple functions (Figure 2-99):

- **Cholesterol collection:** Cells secrete cholesterol using a pump called **ABC1.** HDL then collects this peripheral cholesterol, using the plasma enzyme lecithin-cholesterol acyl transferase (**LCAT**).
- **LPL activation:** HDL supplies ApoC-2 to chylomicrons and VLDL in exchange for ApoA-1. Hence, the TGs in these large lipoproteins can be digested by LPL.
- **Lipoprotein size control:** Takes up excess phospholipids from other lipoproteins via phospholipid transfer protein.

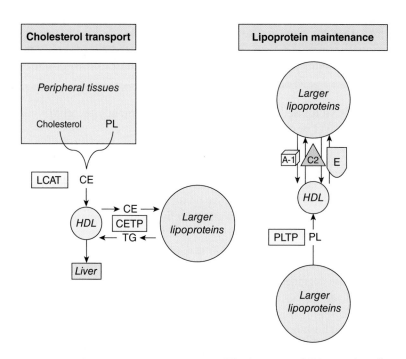

FIGURE 2-99. **High-density lipoproteins (HDL).** The functions of HDL can be split into two main categories: cholesterol transport and maintenance of other lipoproteins. CE, cholesterol ester; CETP, cholesterol ester transfer protein; HDL, high-density lipoproteins; LCAT, lecithin : cholesterol acyl transferase; PL, phospholipids; PLTP, phospholipid transfer protein; TG, triglyceride.

**CLINICAL CORRELATION**

High **LDL** is correlated with increased coronary heart disease (CHD) risk, whereas high **HDL** is correlated with a lower risk.

Causes of higher HDL:

- Estrogen. High HDL is expected in all premenopausal women (especially those taking oral contraceptives).
- Moderate alcohol consumption.
- Niacin, fibrates.

**CLINICAL CORRELATION**

**Orlistat** is a weight-reducing drug that inhibits pancreatic lipase and therefore prevents the conversion of dietary fat (triglycerides) into absorbable fatty acids. As a result, considerable steatorrhea (fatty, foul-smelling stools) can occur. Because it exerts its effects in the gut lumen, it need not enter the systemic circulation.

**CLINICAL CORRELATION**

Elevated pancreatic **lipase** is a more specific sign for acute pancreatitis than is elevated pancreatic amylase. Other causes of elevated amylase include esophageal rupture, perforated ulcer, and mesenteric ischemia.

**FLASH FORWARD**

**Fibrates** (clofibrate, gemfibrozil, fenofibrate) are a class of lipid-lowering drugs that activate peroxisome proliferator–activated receptor-α (PPAR-α), causing an increase in LPL activity. Therefore, fibrates decrease blood TG, but have little effect on plasma cholesterol levels. Common side effects include upset stomach, myopathy, and gallstones.

**CLINICAL CORRELATION**

Sporadic early onset of Alzheimer disease is related to the ApoE gene. More specifically, ApoE2 decreases the risk of developing this disease, whereas having ApoE4 increases the risk of developing this disease.

- **Refills lipoproteins with CE:** HDL supplies CE to other lipoproteins in exchange for TG via CETP.
- **Enables lipoproteins to leave circulation:** HDL supplies ApoE to depleted chylomicrons and VLDL in exchange for ApoC-2. Hence, the remnant lipoproteins (chylomicron remnants and IDL) can leave circulation because ApoE is recognized and taken up by hepatocytes.

HDL mediates a net flow of cholesterol from peripheral tissues into the liver, because a portion of HDL particles are degraded and endocytosed by the liver. This is referred to as "**reverse cholesterol transport.**" Notice that the enzyme CETP bypasses this transport, by feeding the HDL cholesterol back into the tissue targeted lipoproteins. Consequently, drugs inhibiting CETP can be expected to lower peripheral cholesterol and are currently in clinical trials.

### Lipases

**Lingual and gastric lipases** only partially digest dietary TG. Their primary purpose is to emulsify the lipids for further digestion.

**Pancreatic lipase,** present in the small intestine, cleaves TG to FFA and 2-monoacylglycerol. These products then enter the enterocyte and re-esterify into a TG that can be exported in a chylomicron.

**Lipoprotein lipase (LPL)** mediates the same reaction as pancreatic lipase. However:

- LPL is present on the vascular endothelium of adipose and muscle.
- It requires ApoC-2 as a cofactor.
- LPL activity increases when insulin levels rise.
- The TG substrate comes from VLDL and chylomicrons.

To reiterate, the products of LPL digestion (FFA and 2-acylglycerol, which then become FFA and glycerol) enter the target cells. The myocytes use the FFA to fuel their β-oxidation, whereas adipocytes re-esterify them back to TG for storage. During re-esterification, the adipocyte uses endogenously synthesized glycerol phosphate from adipocyte carbohydrate metabolism. The glycerol from the LPL cleavage actually travels back to the liver.

**Hormone-sensitive lipase** is an intracellular enzyme, mainly present in adipocytes, where it degrades TG stores.

- It is induced in response to stress hormones such as glucagon, adrenocorticotropic hormone (ACTH), epinephrine, and norepinephrine.
- These hormones raise intracellular cAMP concentrations, and hence PKA activity.
- PKA phosphorylates hormone-sensitive lipase, thus activating the cleavage of stored TG into FFA and glycerol. These then enter the bloodstream and, mostly attached to albumin, travel back to the liver.
- Insulin inhibits this activation by favoring dephosphorylation of the enzyme.

**Hepatic TG lipase** degrades TG from IDL and chylomicron remnants previously endocytosed by the liver.

Note that LPL and hormone-sensitive lipase both respond to insulin, though in opposite ways. However, their roles in diabetes are still being elucidated (Tables 2-28 and 2-29).

### Dyslipidemias

A standard lipid profile measures LDLc (LDL cholesterol), HDLc (HDL cholesterol), total cholesterol, and TG in blood. Any significant difference from normal values constitutes a **dyslipidemia.**

**TABLE 2-28.** Key Proteins Involved in Lipoprotein Turnover

| PROTEIN | LOCATION | FUNCTION |
|---|---|---|
| ApoB-48 | Chylomicrons | Structural, chylomicron transport from small intestine → lymph → blood to bind LDLR |
| ApoB-100 | VLDL, IDL, LDL | Structural, transports liver apoliprotein (VLDL) → peripheral LDLR |
| ApoA-1 | HDL | Cholesterol collection and activation of LCAT |
| ApoC-2 | VLDL, chylomicrons | Lipoprotein lipase cofactor, release FA/glycerol from chylomicrons, VLDL, LDL |
| ApoE | IDL, chylomicron remnants | Binds to LDLR, helps lipoproteins exit blood into liver |
| PLTP | Blood | Moves phospholipids from large lipoproteins to HDL |
| CETP | Blood | Exchanges CE for TG between HDL and large lipoproteins |
| LCAT | Blood | Allows HDL to collect cholesterol |
| ABC1 | Cellular membrane | Secretion of cholesterol by tissues |

CE, cholesterol esters; HDL, high-density lipoproteins; IDL, intermediate-density lipoproteins; LCAT, lecithin-cholesterol acyl transferase; LDL, low-density lipoproteins; LDLR, low-density lipoprotein receptor; TG, triglycerides; VLDL, very-low-density lipoproteins.

- High LDLc and low HDLc are well-established risk factors for atherosclerosis and coronary artery disease. High TG is probably less important.
- Very high LDLc may also cause cholesterol to be deposited in skin or tendons (xanthomas; Figure 2-100), eyelids (xanthelasma), and cornea (arcus senilis).
- In most dyslipidemias, LDLc, HDLc, and TG are altered simultaneously. Isolated changes in one lipid are less common and are usually indicative of familial dyslipidemias.

Primary causes of elevated blood lipids (genetic or innate problems):

- Polygenic hypercholesterolemia (ie, family history)
- Familial dyslipidemias (often present with isolated lipid elevations)
- Gender (male > female) and age (increase with age)

Secondary causes of elevated blood lipids (acquired problems):

- Saturated fat, *trans* fat, cholesterol, and carbohydrates in diet
- Lack of exercise (low HDLc)
- High body mass index (BMI)
- Metabolic syndrome and diabetes (low HDLc, high TG, LDLc usually normal)
- AIDS (high TG owing to HIV infection *and* to treatment)
- Smoking (low HDLc)
- Hypothyroidism (due to reduced LDL receptors)

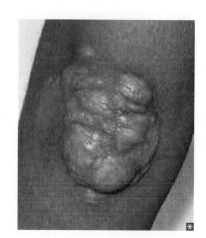

**FIGURE 2-100. Xanthoma on elbow.**

**TABLE 2-29.** Important Lipases

| | | |
|---|---|---|
| Lingual, gastric lipases | Saliva, stomach | Fat emulsification |
| Pancreatic lipase | Pancreatic juice | Fat absorption by intestine |
| Lipoprotein lipase | Endothelium | Fat absorption by muscle and adipose |
| Hormone-sensitive lipase | Adipocyte cytoplasm | Release of fat during fast |
| Hepatic TG lipase | Hepatocyte cytoplasm | Remnant TG IDL digestion |

IDL, intermediate-density lipoproteins; TG, triglycerides.

**FLASH FORWARD**

Smoking may cause a decrease in HDLc, which is a risk factor for coronary artery disease. However, smoking also causes damage to vessel walls, which is an **independent risk factor** for coronary artery disease.

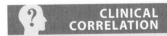

**CLINICAL CORRELATION**

**Xanthomas** are accumulations of lipid-laden macrophages in tissues.
Eruptive xanthoma = high TG
Tendinous xanthoma = high cholesterol
Palmar xanthoma = dysbetalipoproteinemia

**KEY FACT**

LDL receptor mutations are either **null** (complete absence of the gene product) or affect receptor **trafficking** (either to or from the membrane). The actual affinity for LDL tends not to be affected.

- Nephrotic syndrome
- Anorexia nervosa and stress

Causes of decreased lipid levels are:

- Infections, malignancies, hematologic disorders
- Liver disease
- Hyperthyroidism
- Genetic disorders (Tangier disease and abetalipoproteinemia)

Selected pathologic states are discussed later.

**Diabetes** (types 1 and 2) can cause hyperglycemia, which in turn causes:

- Increased VLDL synthesis, and impaired VLDL and chylomicron removal. Therefore, TG accumulates in the plasma.
- Decreased turnover of lipoproteins causes HDLc levels to decrease.
- LDLc usually stays normal.
- First treat diabetes. If that fails to correct lipid levels, start lipid-lowering drugs.

See Table 2-30 for a summary of familial hyperlipidemias.

**Familial hyperchylomicronemia** (type I) is a rare disease.

- Autosomal recessive disorder in which there is an increase in chylomicrons in childhood and increased VLDL in adulthood.
- Lack of LPL or its cofactor, ApoC-2, prevents the breakdown of chylomicrons and their TG content, in particular. Hence, TG accumulates in blood, resulting in **turbid** plasma.
- Since no treatment is available, patients must avoid fatty food for life.
- Acute pancreatitis and eruptive xanthomas are major complications, whereas atherosclerosis is usually **not** a problem.

**TABLE 2-30.**     **Characteristics of Familial Dyslipidemias**

| FAMILIAL DYSLIPIDEMIA | LIPOPROTEINS ELEVATED | LIPIDS ELEVATED | PATHOPHYSIOLOGY | MAIN COMPLICATION |
|---|---|---|---|---|
| Type I: Hyperchylomicronemia | Chylomicrons | Cholesterol: +<br>TG: +++ | ApoC-2 or LPL deficiency | Pancreatitis, no atherosclerosis |
| Type IIa: Hypercholesterolemia | LDL | Cholesterol: +++<br>TG: no change | LDL receptor deficiency | Atherosclerosis |
| Type IIb: Combined hyperlipidemia | VLDL, IDL | Cholesterol: +++<br>TG: +++ | VLDL overproduction | Atherosclerosis |
| Type III: Dysbetalipoproteinemia | IDL, chylomicron remnants | Cholesterol: ++<br>TG: ++ | ApoE deficiency | Atherosclerosis |
| Type IV: Hypertriglyceridemia | VLDL | Cholesterol: +<br>TG: +++ | VLDL overproduction | Atherosclerosis |
| Type V: Mixed hypertriglyceridemia | VLDL, chylomicrons | Cholesterol: +<br>TG: +++ | VLDL overproduction | Pancreatitis, no atherosclerosis |

FA, fatty acids; IDL, intermediate-density lipoproteins; LDL, low-density lipoproteins; LPL, lipoprotein lipase; TG, triglycerides; VLDL, very-low-density lipoproteins.

**Familial hypercholesterolemia** (type IIa) is an autosomal dominant disease.

■ Usually results from an absent or defective LDL receptor (or ApoB-100). The cholesterol-laden LDL particles cannot be reclaimed by the liver (unlike chylomicron remnants, which are still recognized by the LRP receptor).

■ Not only does LDL accumulate in the blood, but liver cholesterol synthesis is deprived of negative feedback, which further contributes to high cholesterol levels.

■ **Homozygous** patients have extreme levels of blood LDL cholesterol (LDLc > 600 mg/dL) and suffer from severe premature atherosclerosis and coronary artery disease, which tends to be the cause of death before age 30 (without treatment).

■ **Heterozygotes** have a slightly better prognosis, with LDLc of 200–400 mg/dL.

■ Tendon xanthomas (Figure 2-101), particularly on Achilles tendon and **corneal arcus,** are fairly pathognomonic.

■ Treatment consists of:
  ■ Healthy diet
  ■ Cholesterol-lowering drugs (statins, niacin, cholestyramine but not fibrates)
  ■ LDL apheresis (a weekly plasmapheresis, used in homozygous patients)
  ■ Portocaval anastomosis (mechanism unknown)
  ■ Liver transplantation (the ultimate measure)

**Familial combined hyperlipidemia** (type IIb) is a fairly common autosomal dominant disease.

■ Liver overproduces VLDL. Consequently, VLDL, LDL, or both accumulate in blood.

■ As a result, TG, cholesterol, or both can be elevated.

■ As with type IIa, patients can get atherosclerosis, coronary artery disease, and pancreatitis.

■ Likewise, the treatment consists of diet, exercise, and lipid-lowering drugs, which may include fibrates to lower TG (unlike with type IIa, for which their application is of little usefulness).

**Dysbetalipoproteinemia** (type III) is an autosomal dominant disease.

■ It is also known as **remnant removal disease** because lipoproteins lack functional ApoE and cannot "exit" the bloodstream.

■ This is not sufficient to cause any pathology, but a concomitant condition (eg, obesity) can cause dysbetalipoproteinemia to manifest itself.

■ Both blood TG and cholesterol become high, because chylomicron remnants and VLDL remnants (ie, IDL) accumulate.

■ Patients present with palmar xanthomas (fairly pathognomonic) and atherosclerosis. Remember that in this disease, there is a risk of peripheral vascular disease, whereas in type II, there is no risk of vascular disease.

■ Exercise, diet modification, and lipid-lowering drugs, such as fibrates, reduce the risk of atherosclerosis.

**Familial hypertriglyceridemia** (type IV) is a common autosomal dominant disorder.

■ As in type IIb, there is an elevation in VLDL production, but TG accumulates in preference to cholesterol.

■ There is some association with insulin resistance and eruptive xanthomas.

■ Risk for ischemic heart disease (IHD) and atherosclerosis can be reduced with TG-lowering drugs, diet change, and exercise.

**Familial mixed hypertriglyceridemia** (type V) is an uncommon mixture of types I and IV familial dyslipidemias.

■ VLDL and chylomicrons are elevated, probably as a result of overproduction. TG levels are high, whereas cholesterol concentration increases only moderately.

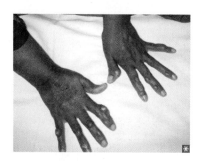

**FIGURE 2-101.    Multiple tendon xanthoma.**

**FLASH FORWARD**

There are three types of lipid-lowering drugs:
■ Drugs that lower cholesterol: Resins and ezetimibe
■ Drugs that lower TG: Fibrates
■ Drugs that lower cholesterol *and* TG: Niacin and statins

**FLASH FORWARD**

Think of **niacin** as the opposite of hyperlipidemia type IIb. This drug lowers TG and cholesterol by **inhibiting VLDL secretion.**

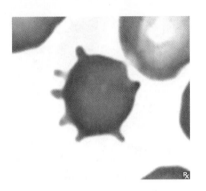

**FIGURE 2-102.** **Acanthocyte ("spur cell").**

- Like type I, but unlike type IV, there is no major risk of atherosclerosis, so that pancreatitis and eruptive xanthomas remain the main complications.

**Tangier disease** is a rare autosomal recessive disorder.

- Tangier disease is due to lack of *ABC1* cholesterol transporter gene.
- Cholesterol accumulates inside cells.
- Blood HDL and cholesterol are low.
- The disease is characterized by atherosclerosis (compare with other dyslipidemias), hepatosplenomegaly, polyneuropathy (compare with metabolic storage diseases), and pathognomonic **orange tonsils.**
- Although there is no specific treatment, enlarged organs are sometimes excised.

**Abetalipoproteinemia** is a rare autosomal recessive disease.

- Cells are unable to make functional ApoB-48 and ApoB-100, resulting in a deficiency of most lipoproteins.
- Lipids and lipid-soluble vitamins (especially **A** and **E**) are poorly absorbed **(steatorrhea).**
- CNS disease—vitamin deficiency causes progressive neurologic disease, ataxia, and optic degeneration.
- Hemolytic anemia—lipid imbalance causes RBC membranes to pucker (**acanthosis;** Figure 2-102).
- No treatment other than vigorous vitamin supplementation.

## SPECIAL LIPIDS

### Cholesterol

The highly lipophilic core of cholesterol contains four carbon rings and very few polar hydroxyl substituents; hence, it is poorly soluble in water. Cholesterol is found in:

- Plasma in the core of VLDL and LDL. It is mostly esterified to a fatty acid.
- In all plasma membranes, conferring rigidity (lipid rafts).
- In bile, where it is solubilized by phospholipids and bile salts.

Although all cells can synthesize cholesterol, some cells are able to further process it to other derivatives, such as:

- **Steroids** (adrenal cortex, ovary/testes, placenta)
- **Vitamin D** (skin, then liver and kidney)
- **Bile acids** (liver, then intestinal bacteria)

### Anabolism

Cholesterol synthesis can be characterized by a few major enzymatic conversions (Figure 2-103):

- Cholesterol synthesis begins with conversion of three molecules of **acetyl-CoA** into **HMG-CoA.** The reactions are the same as in ketone body synthesis except that they occur in the **cytoplasm.**
- **HMG-CoA reductase,** the **rate-limiting** enzyme in cholesterol synthesis, converts HMG-CoA to **mevalonic acid.** It is inhibited by an increase in AMP and by leptin. This enzyme is anchored to the ER and utilizes two molecules of NADPH per reduction.
- Mevalonic acid then gives rise to either isopentenyl pyrophosphate (IPP) or dimethylallyl pyrophosphate (DPP). IPP and DPP are known as **activated isoprene units.**
- IPP and DPP combine, forming geranyl pyrophosphate (GPP).

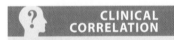

**CLINICAL CORRELATION**

Statins are HMG-CoA reductase inhibitors.

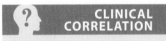

**CLINICAL CORRELATION**

**Terbinafine** inhibits the conversion of squalene to lanosterol in fungi. It is a useful antifungal, especially for treating onychomycosis.

**Imidazole and triazole antifungals** (fluconazole, ketoconazole, etc) inhibit conversion of lanosterol to ergosterol in fungi. An important adverse effect is cytochrome P450 inhibition. Any inhibitors of P450 should be used with caution as they can interfere with the metabolism of other drugs (eg, warfarin, resulting in supratherapeutic INR and increased bleeding risk).

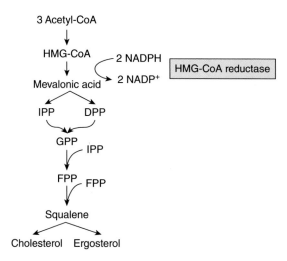

**FIGURE 2-103.** **Cholesterol synthesis.** DPP, dimethylallyl pyrophosphate; FPP, farnesyl pyrophosphate; GPP, geranyl pyrophosphate; HMG CoA, 3-hydroxy-3-methylglutaryl coenzyme A; IPP, isopentenyl pyrophosphate; NADP, nicotinamide adenine dinucleotide phosphate; NADPH, reduced form of nicotinamide adenine dinucleotide phosphate.

- GPP and IPP combine, forming farnesyl pyrophosphate (FPP).
- Two FPP molecules combine, forming **squalene.**
- Squalene then cyclizes, forming **lanosterol.**
- Finally, lanosterol is converted (via several steps) into cholesterol.

Plants and fungi convert lanosterol to **ergosterol,** a cholesterol analog.

## Cholesterol Derivatives

Most cholesterol in the body actually exists in the form of **CE.** These are usually formed with a fatty acid.

Steroid hormones are derivatives of cholesterol (Figure 2-104). The main adrenal cortical hormones are **dehydroepiandrosterone** and its sulfate (DHEA and DHEA-S, respectively), **cortisol,** and **aldosterone.** It should be noted that DHEA-S is only produced from the adrenal gland, and an elevated amount is suspicious for adrenal hyperplasia. **Androstenedione** and **testosterone** are produced by theca and Leydig cells. In women, granulosa cells along with several extraovarian tissues use aromatase to convert these androgens to **estrogens.** Similarly, in men, Sertoli cells convert testosterone to **dihydrotestosterone** (DHT) via 5α-reductase.

Additional steroid hormones, especially **estriol** (E3) are produced by the placenta, which uses fetal DHEA as its substrate.

Deficiencies in 11β-hydroxylase, 17α-hydroxylase, and 21β-hydroxylase result in characteristic clinical signs that can be predicted from the relative excess or deficiency of the steroids they normally produce.

Another cholesterol derivative, **7-dehydrocholesterol,** is converted to **cholecalciferol** (vitamin D₃) in skin on exposure to UV light. Subsequent hydroxylations in liver and kidney produce the biologically active 1,25-dihydroxycholecalciferol, known as **calcitriol** (Figure 2-105). Note that irradiation of the plant lipid **ergosterol** produces vitamin D₂, which can undergo the same set of hydroxylations, but displays lower activity than vitamin D₃.

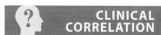

**CLINICAL CORRELATION**

The **quad screen** (an assay of blood α-fetoprotein, inhibin A, β-human chorionic gonadotropin, and estriol) detects congenital abnormalities in a second-trimester fetus.

**Estriol** can also be detected in urine during third-trimester gestation and indicates general well-being of the fetus. A low E3 level can indicate serious congenital diseases, including Down syndrome and Edwards syndrome.

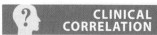

**CLINICAL CORRELATION**

Congenital deficiency in any of the "numbered" enzymes in Figure 2-104 leads to serious disease. Missing enzymes 3, 11, 17, or (most commonly) 21 manifest as the various forms of **congenital adrenal hyperplasia** (CAH). **5α-reductase deficiency** in genetic males results in ambiguous genitalia that virilize during puberty.

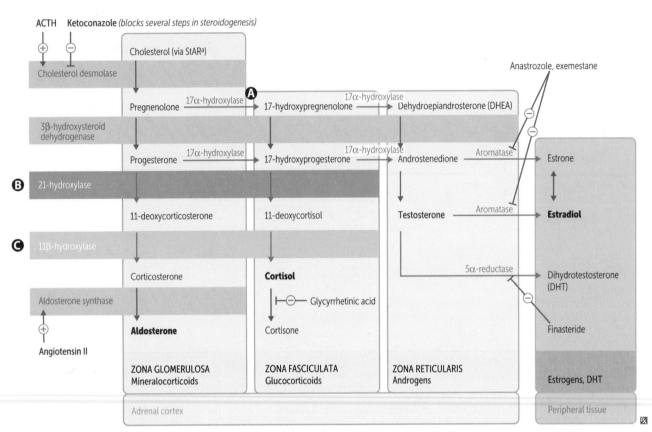

aRate-limiting step.

| ENZYME DEFICIENCY | MINERALOCORTICOIDS | CORTISOL | SEX HORMONES | BP | [K+] | LABS | PRESENTATION |
|---|---|---|---|---|---|---|---|
| **A** 17α-hydroxylasea | ↑ | ↓ | ↓ | ↑ | ↓ | ↓ androstenedione | XY: ambiguous genitalia, undescended testes XX: lacks 2° sexual development |
| **B** 21-hydroxylasea | ↓ | ↓ | ↑ | ↓ | ↑ | ↑ renin activity ↑ 17-hydroxy-progesterone | Most common Presents in infancy (salt wasting) or childhood (precocious puberty) XX: virilization |
| **C** 11β-hydroxylasea | ↓ aldosterone ↑ 11-deoxycorti-costerone (results in ↑ BP) | ↓ | ↑ | ↑ | ↓ | ↓ renin activity | XX: virilization |

aAll congenital adrenal enzyme deficiencies are characterized by an enlargement of both adrenal glands due to ↑ ACTH stimulation (in response to ↓ cortisol) and by skin hyperpigmentation.

Modified with permission from Le T, et al. *First Aid for the USMLE Step 1, 2017*. New York: McGraw-Hill, 2017.

**FIGURE 2-104.    Adrenal steroid synthesis and the manifestations of certain enzyme deficiencies.**

The liver also converts cholesterol into **bile salts.** These detergents are secreted into the intestine (in bile) and render dietary fat more absorbable. Although the intestine reclaims most bile salts (enterohepatic circulation), some are excreted. Therefore, bile excretion is one of the body's ways of reducing cholesterol load. Figure 2-106 demonstrates the components of bile and how they influence the formation of gallstones.

- **Liver** forms the primary bile salts, **cholate** and **chenodeoxycholate,** in its smooth ER and mitochondria. The primary salts are secreted only after **conjugation** to **taurine** or **glycine,** which improves their solubility.
- After cecal and colonic **bacteria deconjugate** the primary salts, they proceed to modify them into secondary and tertiary bile salts. Cholate becomes **deoxycholate,** whereas chenodeoxycholate turns into **ursodeoxycholate** and the highly insoluble **lithocholate.**
- Most bile salts are reclaimed and **reconjugated** by the liver. In addition, sulfation of lithocholate also occurs in hepatocytes. The resulting **sulfolithocholate** is not reclaimed by the intestine, which enables it to go back into the enterohepatic circulation.

## Glycerophospholipids and Sphingolipids

### Structure and Function

Glycerophospholipids and sphingolipids can be thought of as substituted glycerol molecules. Fatty acids usually attach to two of the glycerol carbons, leaving the third carbon with a polar group. Therefore, most of these lipids are amphiphilic and consequently ideal constituents of lipid bilayers. See Figure 2-107 for a summary of their structures.

### Glycerophospholipids

- $C_2$ and $C_3$ carry **esterified fatty acids.**
- $C_1$ carries a **polar head group,** consisting of a phosphate coupled to a polar molecule such as choline, ethanolamine, serine, or inositol. The resulting phospholipids are named accordingly: phosphatidylcholine, phosphatidylethanolamine, and so on.
- The synthetic pathways vary depending on the phospholipid. Note that the phosphate group is often derived from cytidine triphosphate (**CTP**), rather than ATP.

### Sphingolipids

- $C_3$ carries a **carbon chain** (attached directly, not as an ester).
- The alcohol group on $C_2$ is changed into an **amine.** In some sphingolipids, this amine condenses with a fatty acid, thus becoming an **amide.**
- A glycerol molecule with the above modifications (carbon chain on $C_3$ and $C_2$ alcohol changed to amine) is called **sphingosine.**
- $C_1$ carries a polar head group, which varies widely among the different sphingolipids:
  - **Ceramides** use a plain alcohol group as their polar heads.

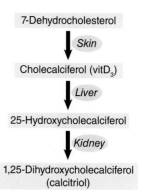

7-Dehydrocholesterol

*Skin*

Cholecalciferol (vitD$_3$)

*Liver*

25-Hydroxycholecalciferol

*Kidney*

1,25-Dihydroxycholecalciferol (calcitriol)

**FIGURE 2-105. Vitamin D metabolism.**

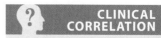

**CLINICAL CORRELATION**

Bile salt deficiency leads to malabsorption. Conditions that cause it include cirrhosis, hepatic blockage, bacterial overgrowth, and Crohn disease.

**CLINICAL CORRELATION**

**Ursodeoxycholate (ursodiol) is** used in treatment of radiolucent gallstones or primary biliary cirrhosis. It not only solubilizes cholesterol, but also inhibits its production. However, cholecystectomy is usually the preferred treatment, so ursodiol is reserved mostly for poor surgical candidates.

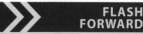

**FLASH FORWARD**

**PIP$_2$** is an important membrane phospholipid, cleaved by **PLC** into **IP$_3$** and **DAG.** PLC responds to **G$_q$,** a G-protein subunit activated by: muscarinic, angiotensin, $\alpha_1$-adrenergic, 5-HT$_{1c}$, 5-HT$_2$, TRH, and vasopressin V$_1$ receptors.

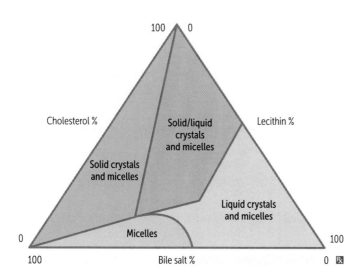

**FIGURE 2-106. Gallstone formation.** Can be due to increased cholesterol or decreased bile salts. A perfect balance must be obtained to prevent stone formation.

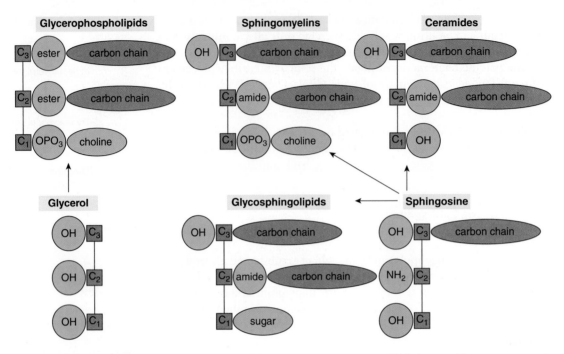

**FIGURE 2-107.** **Glycerophospholipids, sphingolipids, and their backbone molecules.** Choline is used here as an example of a polar head group component and can be replaced by several others, such as ethanolamine, inositol, and serine. Polar groups are blue, and lipophilic groups are brown.

- Just like glycerophospholipids, **sphingomyelins** use a phosphate coupled to another polar molecule, including choline, ethanolamine, and others.
- **Glycosphingolipids** carry a sugar on their C1 and are subdivided into **cerebrosides** and **gangliosides.**

### Lysosomal Storage Diseases

These diseases include **sphingolipidoses, mucopolysaccharidoses, mucolipidoses,** and the **type II glycogen storage disease** (Pompe disease). The diseases are summarized in Figure 2-108.

Note that only the sphingolipidoses result from defects in lipid metabolism. Other lysosomal storage diseases are included in this chapter because of their clinical similarity; however, their etiology is not related to lipid metabolism.

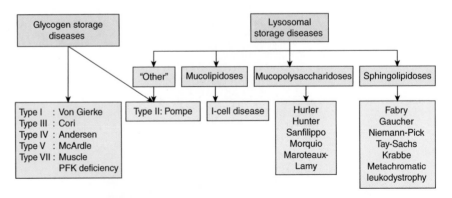

**FIGURE 2-108.** **The storage diseases.** Pompe disease can be classified as both a glycogen and a lysosomal storage disease.

## Sphingolipidoses

These are rare, autosomal recessive diseases (except Fabry disease, which is X-linked recessive). They share the following characteristics:

- A missing enzyme leads to the accumulation of its substrates in lysosomes (Figure 2-109).
- As with many autosomal recessive diseases, the incidence is higher in certain ethnic groups (eg, Tay-Sachs disease among Ashkenazi Jews).
- Each disease has many subtypes, usually organized by age of onset. Gaucher and Fabry diseases often present in adulthood, whereas most other sphingolipidoses are diagnosed in early infancy.
- Variable expressivity is often present (especially Gaucher disease). The early-onset diseases often include neurodegeneration.
- There is usually no effective treatment for the sphingolipidoses, and individuals who have early-onset disease die early.

Table 2-31 summarizes the sphingolipidoses.

The syndromes associated with these diseases tend to be complex and variable, with no "typical presentation." The following shows hypothetical presentations to differentiate between the different sphingolipidoses:

- **Fabry:** A young man presents with a stroke. History reveals recurring pain in his hands and feet. Physical exam is significant for raised dark-red lesions all over his body and mitral valve prolapse.
- **Gaucher:** A girl of Ashkenazi Jewish heritage presents with chronic fatigue due to anemia. History reveals painful bone crises and pathologic fractures. Physical exam shows massively enlarged spleen and liver.
- **Niemann-Pick:** A 3-month-old infant presents with hepatosplenomegaly. Initially hypotonic, the infant later becomes spastic, rigid, and eventually unresponsive. He fails to meet developmental milestones and dies at age 2.
- **Tay-Sachs:** A 6-month-old infant becomes unresponsive and paralyzed and dies at age 3. Autopsy reveals microcephaly.
- **Christensen-Krabbe:** A 3-month-old infant will not feed and is irritable. He gradually becomes hypertonic, suffers from seizures, and assumes decerebrate posture. Eventually, he stops responding to all stimuli and dies.
- **Metachromatic leukodystrophy:** A 6-year-old girl's performance in school is declining. She becomes clumsy and unable to walk. She dies at age 16.

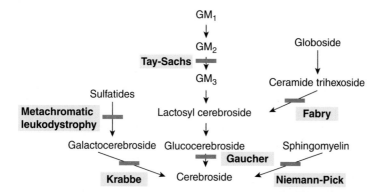

**FIGURE 2-109.** **Sphingolipidoses.** Several sphingolipid catabolic pathways are shown. Steps affected by sphingolipidoses are designated with a red bar. GM, gangliosides.

**TABLE 2-31.** **Sphingolipidoses**

| DISEASE | FINDINGS | DEFICIENT ENZYME | ACCUMULATED SUBSTRATE | INHERI-TANCE |
|---|---|---|---|---|
| SPHINGOLIPIDOSES | | | | |
| Fabry disease  | Early: Triad of episodic peripheral neuropathy, angiokeratomas A, hypohidrosis. Late: progressive renal failure, cardiovascular disease | α-galactosidase A | Ceramide trihexoside | XR |
| Gaucher disease | Most common. Hepatosplenomegaly, pancytopenia, osteoporosis, aseptic necrosis of femur, bone crises, Gaucher cells B (lipid-laden macrophages resembling crumpled tissue paper) | Glucocerebrosidase (β-glucosidase); treat with recombinant glucocerebrosidase | Glucocerebroside | AR |
| Niemann-Pick disease | Progressive neurodegeneration, hepatosplenomegaly, foam cells (lipid-laden macrophages) C, "cherry-red" spot on macula D | Sphingomyelinase | Sphingomyelin | AR |
| Tay-Sachs disease | Progressive neurodegeneration, developmental delay, "cherry-red" spot on macula D, lysosomes with onion skin, no hepatosplenomegaly (vs Niemann-Pick) | Hexosaminidase A | $GM_2$ ganglioside | AR |
| Krabbe disease | Peripheral neuropathy, developmental delay, optic atrophy, globoid cells | Galactocerebrosidase | Galactocerebroside, psychosine | AR |
| Metachromatic leukodystrophy | Central and peripheral demyelination with ataxia, dementia | Arylsulfatase A | Cerebroside sulfate | AR |

Modified with permission from Le T, et al. *First Aid for the USMLE Step 1, 2017*. New York: McGraw-Hill, 2017.

**A** ANSWER

This child has Tay-Sachs disease, which is caused by a lack of hexosaminidase A, which leads to a buildup of $GM_2$ ganglioside.

## Mucopolysaccharidoses

Table 2-32 summarizes a subset of lysosomal storage diseases, called **mucopolysaccharidoses** (MPS). These result from lysosomal enzyme defects that lead to accumulation of GAGs, the principal glycopeptide components of ECM in connective tissue.

The four most important GAGs are heparan sulfate, dermatan sulfate, chondroitin sulfate, and keratan sulfate.

- In general, accumulation of GAGs causes **skeletal deformities** (usually leading to coarse facial features), **corneal clouding, cardiovascular disease** (especially valvulopathies), and **excessive hair.**
- Heparan sulfate accumulation is particularly deleterious to the nervous tissue, causing **cognitive defects.**

**TABLE 2-32. Some Major Mucopolysaccharidoses**

| DISEASE | SYMPTOMS | ENZYME DEFECT | ACCUMULATED SUBSTRATE | INHERITANCE PATTERN |
|---------|----------|---------------|----------------------|---------------------|
| Hurler syndrome | Developmental delay<br>Gargoylism<br>Corneal clouding<br>Hepatosplenomegaly | α-L-iduronidase | Heparan sulfate<br>Dermatan sulfate | AR |
| Hunter syndrome | Mild Hurler symptoms +<br>    aggressive behavior<br>Hearing loss<br>No corneal clouding | Iduronate sulfatase | Heparan sulfate<br>Dermatan sulfate | XR |

- Keratan sulfate accumulation damages mostly corneal and cartilaginous tissues, while sparing the brain.

Note the following:

- All the listed MPS are autosomal recessive except **Hunter** syndrome.
- Multiple subtypes exist for each disease.

## Mucolipidoses

**I-cell disease** is an autosomal recessive disease.

- Caused by a defect in the enzyme N-acetylglucosamine-1-phosphotransferase. This Golgi enzyme targets newly synthesized enzymes to the lysosome by "labeling" them with mannose-6-phosphate. With a defective targeting system, these enzymes never reach the lysosome, thus preventing the organelle from working properly.
- Similar presentation to Hurler syndrome.
- Pathology significant for many membrane-bound inclusion bodies in fibroblasts.

## Other Lysosomal Storage Diseases

**Pompe disease** is an autosomal recessive disorder that can also be classified as a type II glycogen storage disease. It has several subtypes (here we discuss the infantile form).

- It is caused by defective lysosomal α-1,4-glucosidase, a glycogen-breakdown enzyme.
- Unlike most other glycogen storage diseases, Pompe disease does not severely violate the cell's energy economy. This is because the main glycogenolytic pathway (eg, phosphorylase) is intact to break down most of the glycogen. However, the accumulation of glycogen in the lysosomes causes pathology (the glycogen storage diseases associated with energy economy are most frequently defects in the synthesis or degradation of glycogen granules in liver and muscle cytosol).
- Death occurs by 8 months of age.
- Pompe disease is characterized by cardiomegaly, hepatomegaly, macroglossia, hypotonia, and other systemic findings.
- As in most systemic diseases, several blood lab values tend to be abnormal. However, glucose, lipids, and ketones tend to be normal (in contrast to other glycogen storage diseases).

## Eicosanoids

Eicosanoids are derivatives of polyunsaturated long-chain fatty acids, synthesized from the cell's own membrane lipids. Whereas steroid hormones serve as systemic, long-term messengers, eicosanoids serve as **local (autocrine or paracrine) signals.**

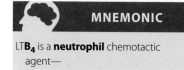

**MNEMONIC**

LTB$_4$ is a **neutrophil** chemotactic agent—
**Neutrophils** arrive **"B4"** others

PGI$_2$ inhibits platelet aggregation and promotes vasodilation—
**P**latelet-**G**athering **I**nhibitor

**KEY FACT**

Remember that although Tay-Sachs and Niemann-Pick present similarly, Niemann-Pick patients will have hypotonia and hepatosplenomegaly, whereas Tay-Sach patients will have hyperreflexia, not hepatosplenomegaly.

**KEY FACT**

Sanfilippo disease is associated with severe intellectual disability but few somatic symptoms. Morquio and Maroteaux-Lamy syndromes are the opposite.

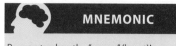

**MNEMONIC**

Pompe trashes the "pump" (heart)!

Eicosanoids are divided into four subfamilies:

- Leukotrienes
- Prostacyclins
- Prostaglandins
- Thromboxanes

Arachidonic acid is the major precursor in eicosanoid synthesis. It is a 20-carbon poly-unsaturated fatty acid that resides in membranes as part of phospholipids, and is released by the action of **phospholipase A$_2$ (PLA$_2$)**.

Arachidonic acid is then modified by several different pathways:

- **Cyclooxygenase (COX)** 1 and 2 lead to the production of prostaglandin G$_2$ (PGG$_2$) and subsequently PGH$_2$, from which most other prostaglandins, prostacyclin (PGI$_2$), and thromboxane A$_2$ (TXA$_2$) are synthesized.
- **5-Lipoxygenase (5-LOX)** converts arachidonic acid into 5-hydroperoxyeicosatetrae-noic acid (5-HPETE) and is later transformed into leukotrienes.
- **12-Lipoxygenase (12-LOX)** converts arachidonic acid into lipoxins.

The main synthetic pathways of the arachidonic acid–derived eicosanoids are summarized in Figure 2-110. Note that not all eicosanoids are derived from arachidonic acid. For example, TXA$_3$, a thromboxane that prevents platelet aggregation, is a derivative of **omega-3 fatty acids**. For this reason, consuming fish oil (high in omega-3 fatty acids) is thought to reduce one's risk of **coronary artery disease**.

**FLASH FORWARD**

The inflammatory pathway is critical to the pathophysiology of a variety of diseases and is an important target in their management, ranging from stroke prevention (aspirin) to asthma (leukotriene receptor antagonists, 5-lipoxygenase inhibitors) to pain (NSAIDs).

**CLINICAL CORRELATION**

To keep the patent ductus arteriosus (PDA) open in a neonate, use PGE$_1$ (alprostadil), PGE$_2$, or PGI$_2$. To promote closure of a PDA, use a COX inhibitor, such as indomethacin.

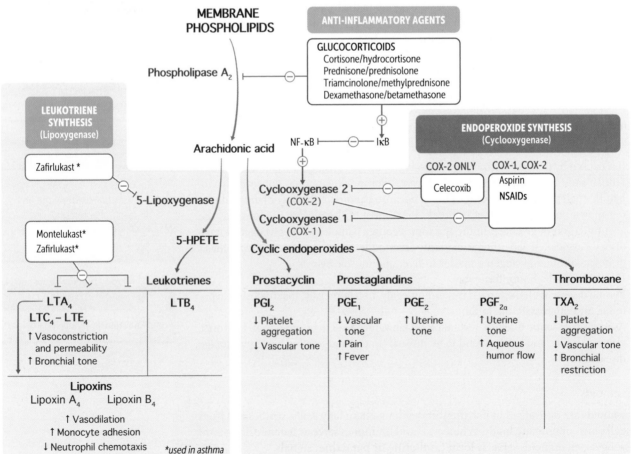

**FIGURE 2-110.    Targets of pharmacologic intervention in eicosanoid synthesis and function.** COX, cyclooxygenase; 5-HPETE, 5-hydroperoxyeicosatetraenoic acid; LTB, leukotriene B; LTC, leukotriene C; LTD, leukotriene D; LTE, leukotriene E; NSAIDs, nonsteroidal anti-inflammatory drugs; PGE, prostaglandin E; PGF, prostaglandin F; PGI, prostaglandin I; TXA, thromboxane A.

The important eicosanoids and their diverse roles in various organ systems are summarized in Figure 2-110. Synthetic analogs of several prostaglandins are employed in clinical medicine (Table 2-33).

## HEME

### Structure

Heme is a cofactor composed of an aromatic ring (known as protoporphyin IX) and a ferrous ion ($Fe^{2+}$) (Figure 2-111). Heme itself is not a peptide, although it is associated with peptides as a prosthetic group.

### Heme Proteins

The heme cofactor can associate with **hemoglobin** and **myoglobin,** where it binds to $O_2$ for both storage and transport. Both hemoglobin and myoglobin proteins share the same basic structural unit: a globin peptide plus heme moiety. A single hemoglobin protein consists of four total globin peptides, whereas a single myoglobin protein consists of one globin peptide. The globin chains hold the heme in place with two histidine residues. The proximal histidine binds $Fe^{2+}$, and the distal histidine associates with $O_2$ to form something of a "heme sandwich" (Figure 2-112).

Heme's function is not limited to $O_2$ storage and transport. Because heme is an excellent means of transporting electrons, it is used in a variety of biological reactions. It is found in **peroxidase,** in the mitochondrial electron transport system as part of **cytochrome c,** and in detoxification reactions as a part of the **cytochrome P450** system.

### Heme Synthesis

- Heme synthesis predominately occurs in the bone marrow (**erythroid cells**) and liver (**hepatocytes**). This is consistent with heme's role in oxygen storage and drug metabolism described earlier.
- The building blocks of heme are **succinyl-CoA** and **glycine.** The $Fe^{2+}$ is introduced at the very end of the pathway (once the large porphyrin ring is ready to "catch it").

Figure 2-113 summarizes the pathway.

In the **liver,** the rate of heme synthesis is highly regulated through feedback inhibition. Because δ-aminolevulinic acid (δ-ALA) synthase catalyzes the first committed step of

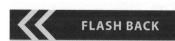

**FLASH BACK**

Knowing that succinyl-CoA is a product of the TCA cycle, it's easy to remember that heme synthesis begins in the mitochondrion. It also ends there, but several intermediate steps occur in the cytosol.

**TABLE 2-33. Clinical Use of Prostaglandins**

| MEDICATION | PROSTAGLANDIN ANALOG | CLINICAL USE |
|---|---|---|
| Alprostadil | PGE$_1$ | Keeps the PDA open |
| | | Treats male erectile dysfunction |
| Misoprostol (synthetic) | PGE$_1$ | Prevents NSAID-induced peptic ulcers |
| | | Induces labor (in combination with mifepristone) |
| Dinoprostone | PGE$_2$ | Induces labor |
| Latanoprost, carboprost | PGF$_2$ | Treats open-angle glaucoma |

NSAID, nonsteroidal anti-inflammatory drug; PDA, patent ductus arteriosis; PGE, prostaglandin E; PGF, prostaglandin F.

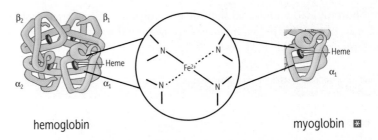

**FIGURE 2-111.    Hemoglobin.** The hemoglobin protein consists of two globular alpha subunits and two globular beta subunits. Each subunit has a heme moiety that can bind $O_2$.

heme synthesis, it is also the main target for regulating heme synthesis. This enzyme is feedback-inhibited by:

- Its own product (δ-ALA).
- The final pathway product (**heme**).
- Oxidized heme (**hematin,** which is heme carrying $Fe^{3+}$ rather than $Fe^{2+}$).

In the **bone marrow,** this regulation is absent, so that all primordial RBCs produce heme without inhibition.

### Defects in Heme Synthesis

#### Porphryias

Porphyrias are hereditary or acquired conditions of defective heme synthesis that leads to accumulation of heme precursors. The precise precursor accumulated and subsequent disease manifestation depends on the specific enzyme deficiency (Figure 2-113).

Because heme is generally made in the blood and liver, porphyrias tend to affect these two systems preferentially. However, accumulation of heme precursors ultimately affects every organ system and leads to the following systemic manifestations.

- **Encephalopathy:** Particularly in children, who present with confusion, inability to maintain attention, and behavioral changes.
- **Photosensitivity rash:** Due to the accumulation of the large aromatic ring precursors of heme, which absorb light.

The intermittent, or seemingly sporadic nature of porphyria symptoms make their diagnosis difficult. Generally, symptoms are triggered by events that increase heme synthesis. This includes medications that up-regulate the production of P450 enzymes (which use heme as a cofactor). Family history can aid in diagnosis, as inheritable forms are generally autosomal dominant, with the exception of erythropoietic porphryia, which is recessive.

Table 2-34 describes and compares the porphyrias.

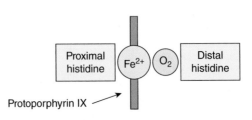

**FIGURE 2-112.    Heme in hemoglobin (or myoglobin).** In this figure, the flat aromatic ring of protoporphyrin IX ring is seen from the side.

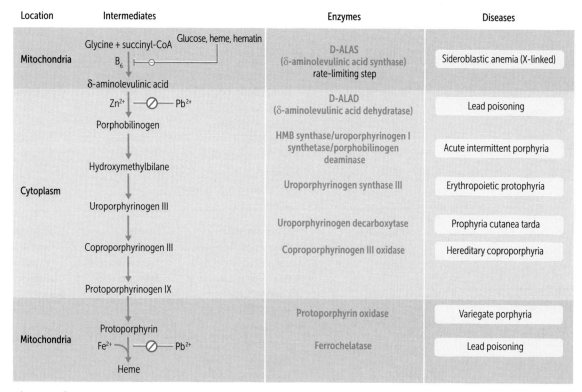

| Location | Intermediates | Enzymes | Diseases |
|---|---|---|---|

Mitochondria — Glycine + succinyl-CoA → (Glucose, heme, hematin) B₆ → δ-aminolevulinic acid
- D-ALAS (δ-aminolevulinic acid synthase) rate-limiting step → Sideroblastic anemia (X-linked)

Zn²⁺ ⊘ Pb²⁺ → Porphobilinogen
- D-ALAD (δ-aminolevulinic acid dehydratase) → Lead poisoning

Porphobilinogen → Hydroxymethylbilane
- HMB synthase/uroporphyrinogen I synthetase/porphobilinogen deaminase → Acute intermittent porphyria

Cytoplasm — Hydroxymethylbilane → Uroporphyrinogen III
- Uroporphyrinogen synthase III → Erythropoietic protophyria

Uroporphyrinogen III → Coproporphyrinogen III
- Uroporphyrinogen decarboxytase → Prophyria cutanea tarda
- Coproporphyrinogen III oxidase → Hereditary coproporphyria

Coproporphyrinogen III → Protoporphyrinogen IX → Protoporphyrin

Mitochondria — Protoporphyrin
- Protoporphyrin oxidase → Variegate porphyria
- Fe²⁺ ⊘ Pb²⁺ → Heme
- Ferrochelatase → Lead poisoning

↓ heme → ↑ ALA syntase activity
↑ heme → ↓ ALA syntase activity

**FIGURE 2-113.   Heme synthesis.**

## Lead Poisoning

Lead poisoning occurs both in children (**GI exposure** via chewing on objects with lead-based paint) and adults (eg, battery, ammunition, radiator, or pipe factory workers). Although best known as a heme synthesis inhibitor, lead can affect virtually every organ.

- Lead is chemically similar to calcium and zinc. This has two main consequences:
  - Lead is better absorbed when calcium or zinc are lacking in the diet. For this reason, it is especially important for children's diet to be replete in calcium and zinc.
  - Lead inhibits zinc-dependent enzymes and can replace calcium in two places: (1) bones, and (2) neurons, which impairs brain physiology.
- Lead impairs heme synthesis in two ways:
  - It inhibits δ-**aminolevulinic acid** (δ-**ALA**) **dehydratase** (which relies on zinc), leading to the accumulation of δ-ALA. ALA chemically resembles γ-aminobutyric acid (GABA), which may explain acute lead poisoning psychosis.
  - It inhibits **ferrochelatase,** leading to the accumulation of protoporphyrin.
- Chronic lead exposure leads to accumulation places in kidneys, causing interstitial nephritis and eventually renal failure.

Clinically, lead poisoning can be subdivided into three categories, depending on timing and chronicity of exposure:

1. **In utero exposure** even at very low concentrations has primarily **neurologic** consequences. It is an independent risk factor for spontaneous abortion.
2. **Acute lead posioning** can present in days or weeks after exposure, with the symptomatic triad of **abdominal colic, CNS symptoms (with cerebral edema),** and **sideroblastic anemia.** CNS symptoms can range from nonspecific cognitive problems and headache to frank encephalopathy with seizures.

**MNEMONIC**

Porphyria cutanea **tarda** (PCT) is **"tardy"** compared with acute intermittent porphyria (AIP). (The enzyme defective in AIP precedes the enzyme defective in PCT in the synthetic pathway.)

**FLASH FORWARD**

When RNA precipitates in RBCs, it appears as blue dots in the cytosol (on a stained blood smear). This **basophilic stippling** (Table 2-34, Image A) is commonly associated with lead poisoning, although it can be seen in several other anemias.

**CLINICAL CORRELATION**

Dimercaprol requires intramuscular injection, which is often painful. Succimer is a water-soluble form of dimercaprol that can be given by mouth. This makes it the preferred drug, particularly when treating children (unless lead poisoning is very severe).

**TABLE 2-34.    Summary of Diseases of Hemoglobin Synthesis**

| CONDITION | AFFECTED ENZYME | ACCUMULATION SUBSTRATE | HALLMARK SYMPTOMS | DIAGNOSIS | TREATMENT |
|---|---|---|---|---|---|
| Lead poisoning | Ferrochelatase and ALA dehydratase | Protoporphyrin, δ-ALA (blood) | ▪ Microcytic anemia with basophilic stippling **A**, GI and kidney disease<br>▪ Children → mental deterioration<br>▪ Adult → headache, memory loss, demyelination (foot/wrist drop) | Elevated blood lead level | EDTA, penicillamine, dimercaprol |
| Acute intermittent porphyria (AIP) | PBG deaminase | PBG, δ-ALA, coporphobilinogen (urine) | 5 **P**s (no skin rash):<br>▪ **P**ainful abdomen (without abdominal tenderness)<br>▪ **P**ort-wine colored urine (on standing)<br>▪ **P**olyneuropathy<br>▪ **P**sychological disturbances<br>▪ **P**recipitated by drugs (cytochrome P450 inducers), alcohol, and starvation | Elevated porphobilinogen in urine (**Watson-Schwartz** test) | Glucose and heme arginate (to inhibit ALA synthase)<br>Note: If misdiagnosed, use of barbiturates to "treat" psychosis can exacerbate attack |
| Porphyria cutanea tarda (PCT) | Uroporphyrinogen decarboxylase | Uroporphyrin (tea-colored urine) | Blistering cutaneous photosensitivity **B**, usually presents after exposure to medications (P450 inducers), fasting, viral, infection (HCV or HIV), or hepatocellular carcinoma | Elevated porphyrin in urine, tea-colored urine that turns pink on **Wood lamp** illumination (PBG levels are normal) | Treat underlying cause, but manage with repeated phlebotomy to reduce Fe$^{2+}$ levels |
| Coproporphyria | Coproporphyrinogen III oxidase | PBG | Similar to AIP, but with additional symptom of photosensitivity skin rash and blisters (similar to PCT) | Elevated porphyrin in the **stool** (better sensitivity than in urine) | Same as AIP |
| Erythropoietic porphyria | Uroporphyrinogen III synthase | Protoporphyrin IX | Severe photosensitivity rash, hemolytic anemia, port-wine colored urine | Elevated porphyrin in the **urine** (**Watson-Schwartz** test), blood smear may reveal hemolytic anemia | Prevention: total avoidance of sun exposure. Severe cases are treated with blood transfusion and possibly bone marrow transplantation |

ALA, aminolevulinic acid; HCV, hepatitis C virus; PBG, porphobilinogen.

Modified with permission from Le T, et al. *First Aid for the USMLE Step 1 2017.* New York, NY: McGraw-Hill Education, 2017.

3. **Chronic lead poisoning** can present with the same symptoms, but is often less clear cut. More chronic manifestations include **renal insufficiency,** gout, and **growth retardation** (in children). Peripheral motor neuropathy may be present with characteristic **wrist drop.** Heart disease and **hypertension** can also occur.

Diagnosis of lead poisoning is established by directly measuring elevated lead levels in blood. Bone X-ray fluorescence can demonstrate chronic lead exposure (X-ray shows "lead lines" on epiphyseal bones [Figure 2-114]).

Blood tests show **sideroblastic anemia** (microcytic, hypochromic RBCs) (Figure 2-78), and **basophilic stippling** of RBCs (Table 2-34, Image A). Erythrocyte protoporphyrin IX is increased.

Severe symptoms (eg, encephalopathy) should be treated with ethylenediaminetetraacetic acid **(EDTA) calcium disodium, dimercaprol,** and **succimer.** Mild symptoms and prophylaxis may only require succimer.

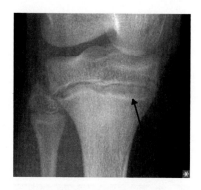

**FIGURE 2-114.** **Lead lines on the metaphysis of long bone.**

**FLASH BACK**

Most chelating drugs non-selectively trap divalent metal ions. In addition to toxins (eg, lead, mercury, arsenic), they can remove important physiologic ions (eg, zinc), resulting in deficiency.

**CLINICAL CORRELATION**

In sideroblastic anemia, developing RBCs are unable to insert iron into hemoglobin. Free iron accumulates in mitochondria, causing them to stain as blue dots around the nucleus. Remember that these **ringed sideroblasts** are seen only on bone marrow smears, in contrast to **basophilic stippling,** which appears on peripheral blood smears and represents ribosomal RNA.

## Heme Catabolism

### Pathway

- Senescent RBCs are destroyed by the spleen, where their heme is released and degraded to **biliverdin** and subsequently converted into **indirect bilirubin,** a linearized molecule devoid of iron (Figure 2-115).
- Indirect bilirubin is poorly water-soluble, but it attaches to albumin and is transported to the liver, where it is conjugated to glucuronic acid molecules. The resulting **direct bilirubin** is water-soluble.
- Conjugated bilirubin then enters the intestine via bile.
- Colonic bacteria deconjugate bilirubin.
- A small portion of urobilinogen is reabsorbed, enters the blood, and is filtered into urine. The resulting urobilin also lends its color to urine.
- Note that in jaundice, bilirubin (not urobilin) causes yellow skin discoloration.

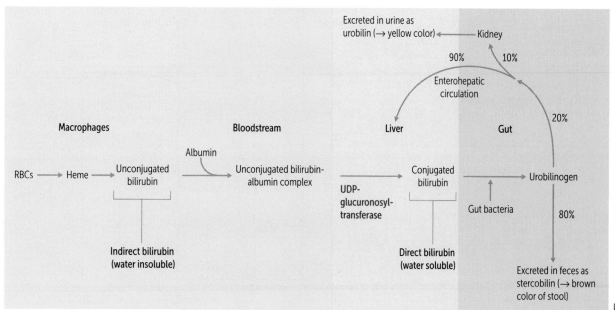

**FIGURE 2-115.** **Heme catabolism.** UDP-glucuronosyltransferase, uridine diphospho-glucuronosyltransferase.

### Causes of Elevated Bilirubin

Elevated **indirect (unconjugated) bilirubin** is caused by defects of heme catabolism prior to and including conjugation:

- Overabundance of heme: mainly due to hemolytic anemia
- Defects in bilirubin conjugation in the liver (Gilbert syndrome, Crigler-Najjar syndrome, and neonatal hyperbilirubinemia)

**Direct (conjugated) bilirubin** elevation results from dysfunctional steps down the excretion pathway:

- Defects of bilirubin secretion from the liver (Dubin-Johnson and Rotor syndromes)
- Obstruction of the biliary pathway (variety of hepatic and biliary disorders, including hepatitis, cirrhosis, choledocholithiasis, pancreatic carcinoma, cholangiocarcinoma, or infection with *Clonorchis sinensis*)

### Hemoglobin

#### Structure

Hemoglobin is the chief $O_2$-binding protein in RBCs. In adults, it exists as a **tetramer,** mostly consisting of two $\alpha$ and two $\beta$ subunits ($\alpha_2\beta_2$). Each subunit contains one heme molecule, each of which may bind one $O_2$ atom (Figure 2-111).

With no $O_2$ bound, the tetramer remains in a taut (T) conformation, notable for its low $O_2$ affinity. Once an $O_2$ molecule binds to one of the subunits, the entire tetramer twists into a relaxed (R) conformation, which is more willing to accommodate second, third, and fourth $O_2$ molecules. In other words, the more $O_2$ is around, the more likely the transition from T to R, and the higher the $O_2$ affinity of hemoglobin.

- This is an example of **cooperative binding,** in which affinity of a protein increases as more ligand is bound.
- Cooperative binding is a subtype of **allostery,** a more general concept, in which binding of one molecule to a protein somehow affects the binding of another molecule.

Cooperative binding results in a sigmoidal hemoglobin binding curve (Figure 2-116). At low partial pressures of $O_2$ (P$O_2$), such as in peripheral tissues, the affinity of hemoglobin for $O_2$ is low. This allows hemoglobin to release its cargo $O_2$ to supply tissues. Conversely, at high P$O_2$ (as in the lungs), $O_2$ binding is enhanced.

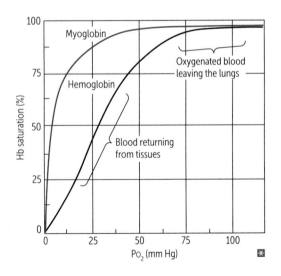

**FIGURE 2-116.** **Hemoglobin binding curve.** Myoglobin curve is included for comparison.

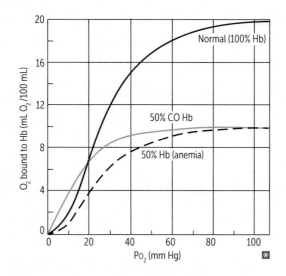

**FIGURE 2-117.** **Carboxyhemoglobin binding curve.**

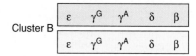

**FIGURE 2-118.** **Hemoglobin genes.** Clusters are shown in duplicates to emphasize the availability of two copies of each gene in a diploid cell. Refer to Figure 2-119 to see which forms predominate throughout development.

Compare this with **myoglobin,** the $O_2$-binding protein in muscles. The amino acid sequence of myoglobin is similar to that of a hemoglobin subunit, except it does not form tetramers. As a result, the monomeric protein does not show allosteric binding, and its binding curve is therefore hyperbolic.

### Hemoglobin Isotypes

Two gene clusters encode hemoglobin subunits: A and B (Figure 2-118). Ideally, two chains from cluster A and two chains from cluster B form the hemoglobin tetramer. For example, the major adult hemoglobin isotype (called $HbA_1$) comes in the form $\alpha_2\beta_2$, in which $\alpha$ chains come from cluster A and $\beta$ chains come from cluster B.

Figure 2-119 and Table 2-35 describe some normal and pathologic hemoglobin isotypes, respectively.

### Allosteric Effectors

Several molecules can bind to hemoglobin (at sites distinct from $O_2$) and alter the stability of the R conformation. This results in changes in the net affinity of hemoglobin for $O_2$, visualized as horizontal shifts in the sigmoidal binding curve. Molecules that stabilize the R conformation increase $O_2$ affinity and therefore cause a **left shift.** As a result, the partial pressure at which 50% hemoglobin capacity is saturated ($P_{50}$) **decreases.** Conversely, stabilization of the T conformation results in lower affinity, **right shift** of the binding curve, and **higher $P_{50}$** (Figure 2-120).

>> **FLASH FORWARD**

One of the major complications in thalassemias is iron overload. Hence, pharmacologic treatment includes iron chelation with **deferoxamine.** Sickle cell disease can be managed with **hydroxyurea,** which moderately augments HbF levels.

? **CLINICAL CORRELATION**

$HbA_{1c}$ has a long half-life and undergoes glycosylation in proportion to blood glucose concentration. As a result, its levels reflect blood sugar control in over the past 6–8 weeks. In the treatment of diabetes mellitus, the goal is to keep $HbA_{1c} < 7\%$.

Q **QUESTION**

What are the differences and the similarities between Dubin-Johnson and Rotor syndrome?

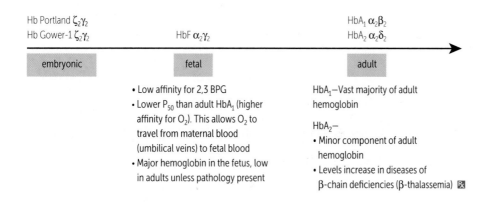

- Low affinity for 2,3 BPG
- Lower $P_{50}$ than adult $HbA_1$ (higher affinity for $O_2$). This allows $O_2$ to travel from maternal blood (umbilical veins) to fetal blood
- Major hemoglobin in the fetus, low in adults unless pathology present

$HbA_1$—Vast majority of adult hemoglobin

$HbA_2$—
- Minor component of adult hemoglobin
- Levels increase in diseases of β-chain deficiencies (β-thalassemia)

**FIGURE 2-119.** **Hemoglobin isotypes.**

**TABLE 2-35.    Blood Dyscrasias and Abnormal Hemoglobin Isotypes**

| DISEASE | | GENOTYPE | HEMOGLOBIN EXPRESSED |
|---|---|---|---|
| α-Thalassemia | Hydrops fetalis | Loss of function of all **four** α genes | Hb Barts ($\gamma_4$). Death in utero |
| | HbH disease | Loss of function of **three** α genes | HbH ($\beta_4$) and Hb Barts, some HbA$_2$. Death by age 8 |
| | α-Thalassemia minor | Loss of function of **two** α genes | Normal HbA$_1$ content. May have mild anemia |
| | Carrier | Loss of function of **one** α gene | Normal HbA$_1$ content. Silent phenotype |
| β-Thalassemia | Thalassemia major | Both β genes affected by a severe mutation (so that no or little β produced) | HbF and HbA$_2$ are the main isotypes available. HbA$_1$ reduced or absent |
| | Thalassemia intermedia | Both β genes affected by a mild mutation | As in thalassemia major, but more HbA$_1$ |
| | Thalassemia minor | Only one β gene affected by a mutation (mild or severe) | Normal HbA$_1$, but increased HbA$_2$ |
| Sickle cell anemia | | Both β genes have a mutation at position 6 (glutamate → valine) | HbSS present, no HbA$_1$. HbF increased |
| Sickle cell anemia carrier | | One β gene with the above mutation | HBSS present along with HbA$_1$ |
| Diabetes | | Normal hemoglobin genes | Normal hemoglobin pattern in addition to HbA$_{1c}$, a glycosylated form of HbA$_1$ |

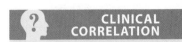

**CLINICAL CORRELATION**

Sickle cell anemia carriers are resistant to malaria.

**A    ANSWER**

Although both present as an asymptomatic elevation in conjugated bilirubin and normal LFTs, they can be differentiated by

- Hepatocyte defect:
  - Dubin-Johnson: Hepatocytes cannot excrete conjugated bilirubin into the *apical biliary cannaliculi.*
  - Rotor: Hepatocytes cannot take up previously conjugated bilirubin from the *basolateral sinusoidal membrane.*
- Liver color:
  - Dubin-Johnson: Liver is *black,* due to accumulation of pigment within hepatocytes.
  - Rotor: liver is normal in color.

Allosteric effectors producing a **left shift** in the $O_2$-binding curve include:

- Low partial pressure of $CO_2$ (P$CO_2$)
- Low temperature
- Alkaline environment (low H$^+$ concentration, high pH)
- Low 2,3-bisphosphoglycerate (2,3-BPG)
- Carbon monoxide poisoning
- Fetal hemoglobin (HbF; note that HbF is a hemoglobin variant, not an allosteric effector, its binding curve is left-shifted compared with the adult variant)

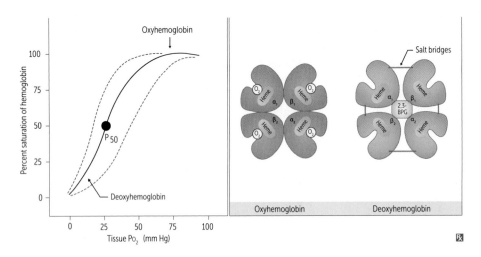

**FIGURE 2-120.    Hemoglobin allostery.** 2,3-BPG, 2,3-bisphosphoglycerate.

Allosteric effectors producing a **right shift** in the $O_2$-binding curve include:

- High $P_{CO_2}$
- High temperature
- Acidic environment (high [H$^+$], low pH)
- High 2,3-BPG

## Methemoglobinemia

In methemoglobinemia (Table 2-36), an unusually high percentage of hemoglobin contains iron in the ferric ($Fe^{3+}$) rather than ferrous ($Fe^{2+}$) state, thus preventing $O_2$ from binding. Normally, the methemoglobin reductase system is responsible for restoration of the $Fe^{2+}$ state.

- In the uncommon, **congenital** forms of methemoglobinemia, methemoglobin reductase is faulty or there is a defect in hemoglobin itself that makes the reductase less effective.
- More commonly, methemoglobinemia is **acquired** by exposure to strong oxidants that overwhelm the reductase system. Such oxidants include **nitrates** (typically from fertilizer-contaminated water), **aniline** dyes, **naphthalene** (in mothballs), **local anesthetics** (lidocaine), **vasodilators** (nitric oxide, nitroprusside), **antimalarials** (chloroquine, primaquine), **sulfonamides, dapsone,** and others.
- Laboratory tests usually show normal partial arterial pressure of oxygen ($Pao_2$), but decreased saturated level of oxygen in hemoglobin ($Sao_2$). Direct tests for methemoglobin detection are available.
- Cyanosis is usually the chief sign. Blood is dark and "chocolate-colored" and does not turn bright red on exposure to $O_2$.
- Treatment consists of removal of the offending toxin by using **methylene blue,** and sometimes **ascorbic acid.**
- Because methylene blue utilizes NADPH which is formed by G6PD in the pentose phosphate pathway, it is ineffective (and may even precipitate hemolysis) in patients with G6PD deficiency.

## Carbon Monoxide Poisoning

Carbon monoxide (CO) is a colorless, odorless gas. Intoxication occurs either directly by inhalation of fumes from incompletely combusted fuel (car exhaust, heaters) or by inhalation of certain organic solvents (methylene chloride, a paint stripper), which are metabolized to CO in the liver.

CO binds to heme in hemoglobin with much higher affinity than does $O_2$. As a result (Table 2-36):

- CO diminishes the $O_2$ carrying capacity of hemoglobin by competing for the binding sites.
- CO shifts the $O_2$-binding curve of hemoglobin to the left. In other words, binding of a CO molecule to one hemoglobin subunit increases the affinity of the other

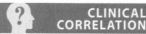

**CLINICAL CORRELATION**

Patients suffering from methemoglobinemia or CO poisoning display normal $Pao_2$, but have low $Sao_2$. Because the heme of patients with methemoglobinemia cannot bind *any* gas, their blood is dark red. On the other hand, the heme of CO poisoned victims avidly binds CO, and their blood becomes bright red.

In CO poisoning, the apparent $Sao_2$ on a conventional probe is normal due to the similar structure of CO-Hb and $O_2$-Hb.

**FLASH FORWARD**

**Amyl nitrite** and **sodium nitrite** work as an antidote for cyanide poisioning by inducing methemoglobinemia.

**MNEMONIC**

Treat **meth**emoglobinemia with **meth**eylene blue

**TABLE 2-36.    Forms of Hemoglobin**

| FORMS OF HEMOGLOBIN | MODIFICATION | AFFINITY FOR $O_2$ | $O_2$ SATURATION | CLASSIC SYMPTOM | TREATMENT |
|---|---|---|---|---|---|
| Methemoglobin | Oxidized hemoglobin ($Fe^{3+}$) | Reduced | Normal $PaO_2$, decreased $SaO_2$ | Cyanosis, chocolate-colored blood | Methylene blue, ascorbic acid |
| Carboxyhemoglobin | Hb bound by CO | Unchanged (but CO occupies $O_2$-binding site on Hb with 200× greater affinity) | Normal $PaO_2$, decreased $SaO_2$ | Cherry-red discoloration of skin | 100% $O_2$ supplementation, hyperbaric $O_2$ |

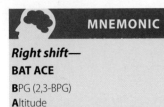

**MNEMONIC**

*Right shift—*
**BAT ACE**
**B**PG (2,3-BPG)
**A**ltitude
**T**emperature
**A**cid
**C**O$_2$
**E**xercise

three subunits for $O_2$. Although this results in better $O_2$ uptake in the lungs, it also prevents $O_2$ unloading in the tissues.

- Symptoms of CO poisoning are usually very **nonspecific.** Cherry-red discoloration of skin is specific but not sensitive (pale skin is more common).
- As with methemoglobinemia, arterial blood gas tests show normal $Pao_2$ but diminished $Sao_2$. Direct CO detection tests are available. Note that smokers often present with values indicative of mild CO poisoning as a result of the CO in inhaled cigarette smoke.
- Treatment consists of 100% $O_2$ supplementation. Patients with severe cases may require hyperbaric $O_2$.

### Carbon Dioxide

Although hemoglobin is primarily known for its $O_2$-carrying capacity, it is also an important transporter of $CO_2$. There are three main mechanisms by which this occurs (Figure 2-121):

**KEY FACT**

Hemoglobin's ability to bind and release $O_2$ at appropriate locations is facilitated by two main and distinct phenomena: cooperative binding of $O_2$ and the Bohr-Haldane effect.

- **Isohydric transport** accounts for 90% of $CO_2$ movement. As $CO_2$ diffuses into an RBC, the enzyme **carbonic anhydrase** combines it with water, yielding carbonic acid ($H_2CO_3$). As the word *acid* implies, $H_2CO_3$ tends to lose a proton, leaving behind the bicarbonate ion ($HCO_3^-$). The proton can bind to several **histidine** residues on hemoglobin, whereas $HCO_3^-$ leaves the RBC in exchange for chloride ion ($Cl^-$) (the chloride shift). Note that in isohydric transport, the $CO_2$ is not directly carried by hemoglobin.
- In **carbamino-hemoglobin transport,** which carries up to 5% of $CO_2$, the $CO_2$ molecule reacts directly with amino groups on hemoglobin. This reaction produces one free proton.
- The remaining 5% of $CO_2$ is dissolved in the plasma.

**MNEMONIC**

**B**ohr effect in the **B**ody (tissue).
**H**aldane effect "**h**igher up" (respiratory tract).

The reactions involved are allosteric effectors of hemoglobin, both causing an increase in $P_{50}$ and thus lower affinity for and increased release of $O_2$. In other words, the presence of $CO_2$ and protons is a signal for the hemoglobin molecule that it has reached the periphery and that its time to release its $O_2$ cargo. This is called the **Bohr effect.** Conversely, as blood returns to the lungs it faces high $Po_2$, which prompts the release of protons and $CO_2$. This is the **Haldane effect.**

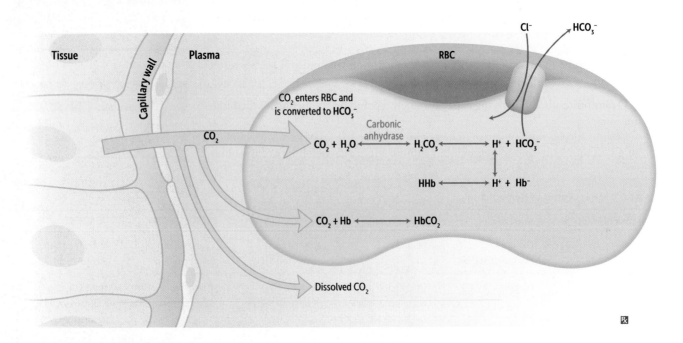

**FIGURE 2-121.** **$O_2$/$CO_2$ exchange in peripheral tissues.**

## Laboratory Tests and Techniques

Hospital laboratories often use basic techniques of molecular biology and biochemistry to analyze clinical samples from patients. Although these tests are often developed and used in basic science research, they aid in diagnosis and help guide clinical decision making (Table 2-37).

Choice of a specific laboratory test for diagnosis depends on the level and the magnitude of change expected in patient samples as compared to controls. Table 2-37 outlines these key tests, with a detailed discussion of each test to follow.

Across these levels of analyses, two common core techniques are frequently used in clinical laboratory testing: **gel electrophoresis** and **detection.**

**Gel electrophoresis** is used to separate charged samples of interest according to size. This is commonly done for DNA and RNA (based on length) and proteins (based on mass), and will be discussed in more detail. After separation, samples can be either analyzed on the gel itself, or transferred to a membrane for downstream analysis.

Another frequently used core technique is **detection,** whereby antibodies or nucleic acids specific to an epitope or nucleic acid sequence (respectively) are used to demonstrate its presence or absence in a sample. This can be done both qualitatively and quantitatively. For detection to occur, we must be able to (1) **specifically** identify the target of interest, and (2) **visualize** its presence or absence using a probe. In the case of proteins, specificity is conferred by using primary antibodies. In the case of nucleic acids, specificity is conferred by using complementary nucleic acid sequences. The signal is visualized by tagging these probes with various reporters that allow for chemiluminescence, fluorescence, or radioactivity.

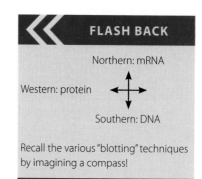

**FLASH BACK**

Northern: mRNA

Western: protein

Southern: DNA

Recall the various "blotting" techniques by imagining a compass!

### DNA-BASED LAB TESTS

#### DNA Gel Electrophoresis

Principle

Because DNA carries an **overall negative charge** (due to its phosphate backbone), it migrates toward the positive cathode in an electric field. When loaded into an agarose gel, the internal structure of the gel provides a physical barrier for the movement of DNA. The **rate of movement is inversely proportional to the size of the DNA fragment**

**TABLE 2-37.** **Key Laboratory Tests**

| LEVEL OF ANALYSIS | MAGNITUDE OF CHANGE | TEST OF CHOICE |
|---|---|---|
| **DNA** | Single to several nucleotides<br>Chromosomal level | DNA electrophoresis, sequencing, PCR, Southern blot<br>Karyotyping, FISH |
| **RNA** | Qualitative expression levels<br>Quantitative expression levels | Northern blot, RT-PCR<br>qRT-PCR |
| **Protein** | Qualitative expression levels | **Overall:** protein gel electrophoresis, western blot, radioimmunoassay<br>**Localization** within a sample: ICC, IHC |

FISH, fluorescent in situ hybridization; PCR, polymerase chain reaction; q, quantitative; RT, reverse transcription.

(smaller moves faster), making it possible to separate and visualize DNA fragments of different sizes from a clinical sample. The DNA fragments are visualized by adding fluorescent dye to the gel, called ethidium bromide. This dye intercalates between the two DNA strands and fluoresces with UV-illumination.

### Use

Many of the DNA-based tests discussed here use DNA electrophoresis as a **step** in DNA analysis. This general technique has wide applications, from separating amplified polymerase chain reaction (PCR) products to separating digested fragments of genomic DNA for Southern blotting. Examples of how this technique is used in clinical medicine will follow in subsequent sections.

### Polymerase Chain Reaction

#### Principle

PCR is an important method for amplifying DNA, making it possible to exponentially increase the amount of DNA available for analysis from a small clinical sample. The original double-stranded DNA serves as a template. This reaction also requires a thermally stable DNA polymerase, primers flanking the region that needs to be amplified, and nucleotides. The mixture then undergoes the following procedure in an automated cycle (Figure 2-122). Of note, the polymerase usually used is Taq polymerase, which was first isolated from **Thermus aquaticus,** a bacterium found in hot springs.

> **≪ FLASH BACK**
>
> Recall that guanosine-cytosine base pairs have more hydrogen bonds than adenosine-thymidine base pairs, so GC-rich DNA sequences require higher temperatures to denature (see Figure 2-4).

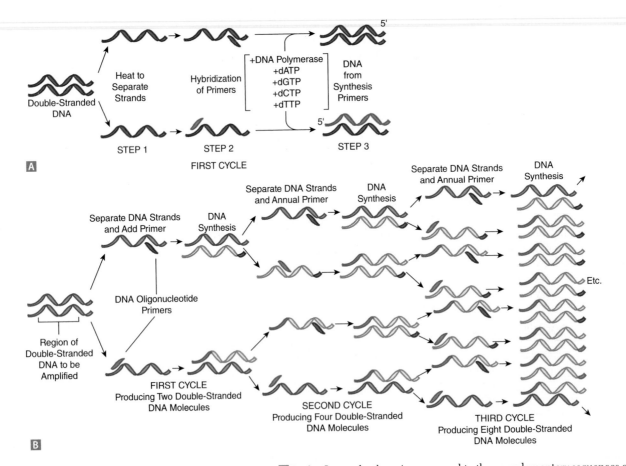

**FIGURE 2-122.** **Cycles of the polymerase chain reaction.** **A** In the first cycle, the primers anneal to the complementary sequences on the DNA in the sample, and the polymerase extends the strands. **B** In each of the subsequent cycles, the newly synthesized strands are separated from the template, the primers reanneal, and the steps are repeated. The result is an exponential rise in the number of DNA fragments synthesized between the positions of the two original primers. Typically, about 30 cycles are conducted. d, deoxynucleotides.

- **Denaturing:** Heating to approximately 95°C separates the double-stranded DNA.
- **Annealing:** Cooling to approximately 45°C causes the primers to attach to single strands of DNA in sequence-specific complementary regions.
- **Elongation:** Heating to approximately 72°C causes Taq polymerase to synthesize a complementary DNA strand, starting at the primer.

This cycle is usually repeated approximately 30 times, resulting in an exponential increase in the number of synthesized copies of the original DNA fragment. The DNA is then available for further analysis.

### Use

PCR is widely used to genotype specific mutations, detect hereditary diseases, diagnose viral diseases, and in genetic fingerprinting and paternity testing. It is now also used in clinical microbiology to identify pathogenic microorganisms, often after initial antibody-based approaches.

PCR detects the actual presence of the virus by amplifying its DNA, even in the absence of the host's antibody response. Although PCR is most widely used for identification of microbial pathogens, it is also used to measure various endogenous host processes as well, as indicated in the examples in Table 2-38.

### DNA Sequencing

#### Principle

Two major approaches to DNA sequencing will be discussed here: the **classic chain-termination Sanger** sequencing, or first-generation sequencing, and **next-generation** sequencing.

In the classic chain-termination Sanger sequencing, a single-stranded DNA fragment from a clinical sample is used as a template in the presence of DNA polymerase, a fluorescent-labeled 5′ short primer, four standard deoxynucleotides (dATP, dTTP, dGTP, dCTP), and a small amount of dideoxynucleotides. Although these dideoxynucleotides are otherwise identical to the standard A, T, G, and C deoxynucleotides, they cause **chain termination** when incorporated into a synthesizing DNA molecule.

Statistically, this random incorporation of the dideoxynucleotides produces a sample with DNA fragments of different sizes, corresponding to each of the positions of a particu-

 **QUESTION**

Why use Taq polymerase for PCR instead of human DNA polymerase enzyme?

**TABLE 2-38.** **Use of Polymerase Chain Reaction in Clinical Settings**

| MICROBIAL PATHOGENS | | |
|---|---|---|
| VIRUSES | BACTERIAL INFECTION | ENDOGENOUS |
| ▪ HBV | ▪ Group A Strep | ▪ Tumor factors |
| ▪ HCV | ▪ Legionella spp | ▪ Cytokines |
| ▪ HIV | ▪ Bordetella | ▪ Gene expression |
| ▪ VZV | ▪ Bordetella pertussis | ▪ Genetic testing |
| ▪ HSV | ▪ VRE | |
| ▪ CMV | | |
| ▪ EBV | | |
| ▪ Parvovirus B19 | | |
| ▪ Influenza | | |

CMV, cytomegalovirus; EBV, Epstein-Barr virus; HBV, hepatitis B virus; HCV, hepatitis C virus; HSV, herpes simplex virus; VRE, vancomycin-resistant Enterococcus; VZV, varicella zoster virus.

lar nucleotide in the DNA chain. Repeating this process for each of the four nucleotides and separating the resulting fragments using DNA gel electrophoresis makes it possible to determine the sequence of nucleotides in the DNA sample fragment because the relative positions of the fragments on the DNA gel reveal the order of the nucleotides in the DNA molecule (Figure 2-123). In the last few years, genomic sequencing tools have advanced tremendously. Now, a patient's entire genome can be sequenced using so-called next-generation sequencing platforms. In this technique, first, an amplified library of a patient's DNA is generated using polymerase chain reaction (PCR). Then, the DNA is sequenced during synthesis (as opposed to via chain termination) using techniques such as pyrosequencing, which detects the release of pyrophosphate upon nucleotide incorporation during strand synthesis. The nucleotide identity is known because only one (dATP, dTTP, dGTP, or dCTP) is added at a time. This sequencing occurs on a large parallel scale that uses a variety of sequencing platforms.

### Use

DNA sequencing is used to confirm or exclude known sequence variants or to fully characterize a defined DNA region. It is most commonly used to detect specific mutations to diagnose genetic diseases.

In patients with a clinical diagnosis of **osteogenesis imperfecta,** a blood sample can be analyzed for mutations in *COL1A1* or *COL1A2* genes. Similarly, DNA of patients with **Ehlers-Danlos syndrome (EDL)** is analyzed for mutations in *COL5A1, COL5A2,* and several other genes. Genotyping is also used to diagnose cystic fibrosis (*CFTR*), Duchenne and Becker muscular dystrophy (*DMD*), as well as in many cancers for the identification of targetable mutations.

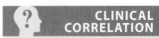

**ANSWER**

Human enzymes are sensitive proteins that function best at our specific physiologic body temperature. The high temperatures required to denature DNA (72°C) would also denature the human enzyme, rendering it nonfunctional. Taq polymerase, on the other hand, is ideally suited to withstand these high temperatures.

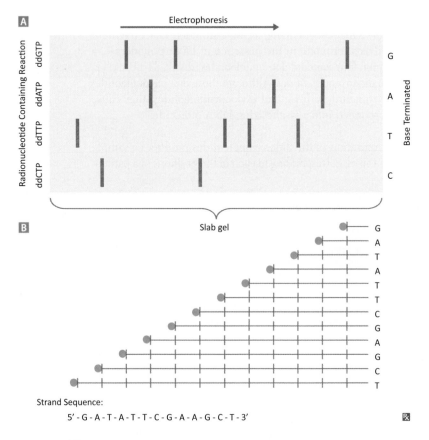

**FIGURE 2-123.    DNA sequencing.** A DNA fragments formed in each of the four reactions containing one of the four nucleotides are run on a DNA gel and separated by size. B Fluorescently labeled 5′ primer (red asterisk) allows for the visualization of the fragment. The order of individual nucleotides is deduced from the length of the fragment and the distinct dideoxynucleotides added to the reaction for each distinct lane. dd, dideoxynucleotides.

## Karyotyping

### Principles

Karyotyping is the cytogenetic technique whereby the **number** and **morphology** of chromosomes in the nucleus of any cell type can be analyzed. This technique allows us to visualize any gross complete chromosomal absence/gain, or gross translocations and inversions. Cells of interest are isolated from a patient and stained with **Giemsa**, which is a dye that binds specifically to the phosphate backbone of DNA. Tightly packed chromosomal regions (heterochromatin) stain darkly, and loosely packed chromosomal regions (euchromatin) stain lightly, producing a "banding" pattern characteristic of each chromosomal pair (Figure 2-124).

A normal karyotype reveals 22 pairs of autosomes and one pair of sex chromosomes (either XX or XY). This technique is limited because it relies solely on chromosomal *morphology* for identification of an abnormality. This limitation can be overcome with fluorescent in-situ hybridization (FISH), which specifically binds to target genetic sequences, as discussed in the next section.

### Use

Karyotyping is often used to diagnose **aneuploidies** (abnormal chromosome number). Entire chromosomal duplications, as seen in the various trisomy conditions (trisomies 13, 18, and 21) can be diagnosed via karyotyping the cells in a mother's amniotic fluid or sampling her chorionic villi. The abnormal duplication or deletion of sex chromosomes, as seen in Klinefelter syndrome (47 XXY), Turner syndrome (45 XO), double Y males (XYY), and true hermaphroditism (46 XX or 47 XXY), can also be diagnosed via karyotyping.

## Fluorescence In Situ Hybridization (FISH)

### Principle

In the cytogenetic technique known as fluorescence in situ hybridization (FISH; Figure 2-125), a specific region of a chromosome is identified by a **complementary DNA sequence** tagged to a fluorophore. This technique allows for both detection and localization of a specific sequence.

- Single-stranded DNA that has been tagged with a fluorophore, antibody epitope, or biotin is added to a preparation of nuclear DNA, either in intact nuclei (interphase FISH) or chromosomes arranged on a slide (fiber FISH).
- After binding to the complementary sequence in the sample, the excess unbound probe is washed away.
- The sample is then imaged using fluorescence microscopy.

### Use

FISH is used to map specific DNA sequences such as genes or rearrangements to a particular position on a chromosome. It plays a particular role in detecting chromosomal abnormalities such as inversions or translocations at the molecular level, which are too small to see via karyotyping. When using labeled primers for the 16S rRNA region of specific bacteria as probes, it can also determine the presence of microorganisms in clinical samples.

FISH can be used in place of karyotyping for aneuploidies, such as trisomy 13, 18, 21, or sex chromosome number abnormalities (eg, Klinefelter, Turner, and triple X syndromes), as it provides the added benefit of **specificity** to nucleic acid sequences on the chromosomes themselves. It can be used on tissue samples, as well as amniotic fluid. It is also used in the diagnosis of certain **cancers,** such as the Philadelphia chromosome (ie, *BCR-ABL* t(9,22) translocation) in chronic myelogenous leukemia (CML). Furthermore, it can be used for detection of **microdeletions,** such as 5p– in cri du chat,

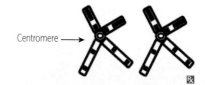

**FIGURE 2-124.   Karyogram.** A schematic representation of a single chromosomal pair from a karyogram, a banding pattern unique to the specific pair of chromosomes.

**FLASH FORWARD**

Trisomy 13: Patau syndrome
Trisomy 18: Edward syndrome
Trisomy 21: Down syndrome

**FLASH FORWARD**

**Cri du chat**—partial deletion of the **short arm of chromosome 5,** which may be visualized by FISH or karyotyping → characteristic **cry similar to the mewing of kittens.** Patients exhibit failure to thrive and severe cognitive and motor delays, but typically are able to communicate socially. Often present are microcephaly and coarsening of facial features.

**FLASH FORWARD**

**Angelman syndrome (AS)**—loss of **maternal 15q11** (both copies of paternal origin) → mental retardation, seizures, wide-based gait, inappropriate outbursts of laughter.
**Prader-Willi syndrome (PWS)**— loss of **paternal 15q11** (both copies of maternal origin) → mental retardation, hyperphagia, obesity, hypogonadism, hypotonia, weak cry. AS and PWS are examples of **genomic imprinting,** in which the expression of a particular allele and the associated phenotype are exclusively determined by parental origin of the allele.

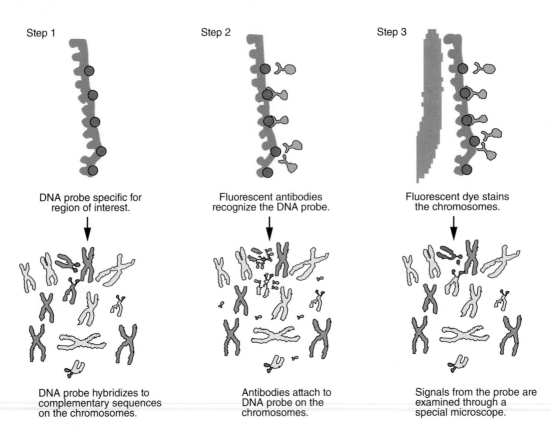

Step 1

Step 2

Step 3

DNA probe specific for
region of interest.

Fluorescent antibodies
recognize the DNA probe.

Fluorescent dye stains
the chromosomes.

DNA probe hybridizes to
complementary sequences
on the chromosomes.

Antibodies attach to
DNA probe on the
chromosomes.

Signals from the probe are
examined through a
special microscope.

**FIGURE 2-125.** **Fluorescence in situ hybridization.** Step 1: A DNA probe complementary to the gene of interest is added to the chromosomal preparation. Step 2: A fluorescent antibody against the epitope that was used to tag the DNA probe is added, and it binds to the DNA probe. Step 3: Chromosomes are counterstained with a fluorescent dye of a color different from that of the antibody. This enables clear visualization of the regions of interest under a fluorescent microscope.

15q11.2–q13 in Prader-Willi and Angelman syndromes, 7q11.23 deletion in Williams syndrome, and 22q11.2 deletion in DiGeorge and velocardiofacial syndrome.

### Southern Blot

#### Principle

Southern blotting refers to a technique whereby a **DNA sample is separated according to fragment size** (number of base-pairs) using gel electrophoresis and is then transferred on to a nitrocellulose or nylon membrane, where it is fixed in place. Much like FISH, a single-stranded DNA probe, usually labeled with a radioactive isotope, is allowed to incubate with the membrane containing the sample. This **radioactive DNA probe binds to complementary sequences** in the DNA sample. After the nonbound probe has been washed away, X-ray film is placed on top of the membrane. The radioactivity from the bound probe exposes the X-ray film in the exact position of the radiolabeled probe. This indicates the presence, and the position of the sequence of interest, within a particular DNA fragment from the original sample (Figure 2-126).

#### Use

Southern blots are no longer routinely used in clinical medicine, but can be used on a case-by-case basis to detect trinucleotide expansion in **fragile X syndrome, Friedreich's ataxia,** and **myotonic dystrophy,** as well as methylation or deletion of the SNRPN locus in **Prader-Willi/Angelman syndromes.** Southern blotting has also been used to directly detect malaria parasites (*Plasmodium* spp) in the blood of patients. Her2+ breast cancer specifically caused by *HER2* gene amplification can also be detected by Southern blot, as measured by increased band intensity.

**≪  FLASH BACK**

Recall that trinucleotide expansions occur because DNA polymerase is **error prone,** especially when replicating repetitive strings of nucleotides. Nucleotide expansions in coding regions of DNA are transcribed and translated into a repetitive string of amino acids that can cause abnormal protein aggregation, as seen in Huntington disease. However, trinucleotide repeats in noncoding regions of DNA can also lead to disease (as seen in Fragile X syndrome or Friedrich ataxia).

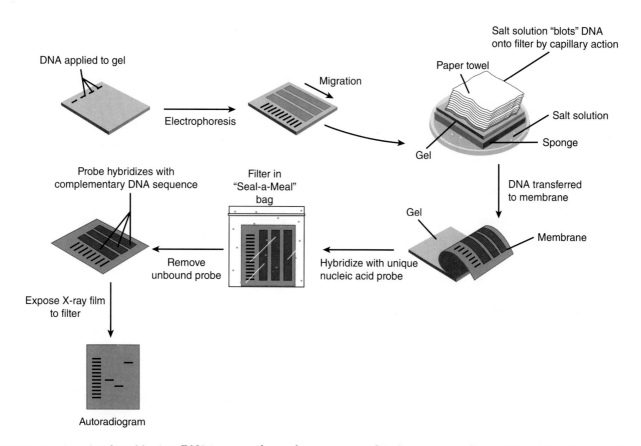

**FIGURE 2-126.** **Southern blotting.** DNA is separated according to size, transferred on to a nitrocellulose filter, and hybridized with radiolabeled probes specific for the sequence of interest. Exposure of the X-ray film reveals the position and size of the DNA fragments that contain the sequence of interest.

## RNA-BASED LAB TEST

### Northern Blot

#### Principle

Northern blotting is similar to Southern and Western blotting, except that the substance being analyzed is **RNA,** rather than DNA or protein. In Northern blotting, a sample of RNA is run on an agarose gel and is then transferred to a nitrocellulose membrane. A radiolabeled RNA or single-stranded DNA is used as a probe. Finally, an X-ray film is exposed to the membrane, revealing the location of the RNA sequences of interest. These identical steps were described for Southern blotting (Figure 2-126), with the main difference being that RNA is used for Northern blotting (whereas DNA is used for Southern blotting).

#### Use

Northern blotting is usually used in special laboratory studies to detect the levels of gene expression for specific genes in clinical samples, as measured by intensity of the band's signal.

## PROTEIN-BASED LAB TESTS

### Protein Gel Electrophoresis

#### Principle

Sodium dodecyl sulfate-polyacrylamide gel electrophoresis, or SDS-PAGE, is a fundamental technique for **separating proteins based on mass.** It is the protein counterpart to DNA agarose gel electrophoresis. Proteins are coated with a uniform negative charge using SDS, denatured via boiling, and then loaded onto a polyacrylamide gel. The buffer used in this technique gives the denatured proteins an **overall negative charge.** Therefore, when placed into an electric field, the proteins move through the gel matrix toward the positive electrode. Because the internal gel structure serves as a barrier for the movement of proteins, their migration toward the positive electrode is indirectly proportional to the size of the protein, with the **smallest proteins migrating farthest** (closest to the positive electrode). A standard mix of proteins of known sizes (ladder) is also run on the gel for comparison (Figure 2-127).

### Use

Gel-separated proteins can be visualized with Coomassie or silver staining, or used in conjunction with other methods to analyze clinical samples. One of the most common uses is as part of Western blot analysis.

### Western Blot

#### Principle

Western blotting is a technique by which protein separated in a gel is transferred to a protein-binding membrane for subsequent analysis. First, protein samples are separated via electrophoresis on a polyacrylamide gel (see SDS-PAGE in preceding text). The second step involves using an electrical field perpendicular to the gel to **transfer the proteins from the gel on to a polyvinylidene fluoride (PVDF) membrane.** To prevent nonspecific antibody binding to the membrane, it is **blocked** by incubating in a solution of bovine serum albumin (BSA) or nonfat dry milk. The membrane is then incubated with a **primary antibody** specific for the protein of interest. After washing off the excess unbound primary antibody, a **secondary antibody** is added. This secondary antibody is conjugated to a reporter; it is also specific for the primary antibody that was used in the previous step. If the protein of interest is contained in the sample, its presence will be indicated by the secondary reporter via chemiluminescence or fluorescence (Figure 2-128).

### Use

Western blotting is used to detect the presence of a protein in a clinical sample, indicating an infection with a specific agent. This may refer to both antigens native to the pathogen (eg, in the case of **bovine spongiform encephalopathy** or **BSE**) or to the actual host antibodies that have developed in response to the infection (eg, **HIV** and **Lyme disease** [*Borrelia burgdorferi*]). Note that Western blots can also be used for relative quantification of the amount of protein present.

Western blotting is a confirmatory test performed when an initial ELISA (see below) test is positive for HIV antibodies.

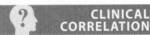

### CLINICAL CORRELATION

**Serum protein electrophoresis (SPEP)** is used in clinical laboratories to diagnose monoclonal gammopathies, such as **multiple myeloma, Waldenström macroglobulinemia,** and **primary amyloidosis.** A patient's serum is run through gel electrophoresis, and proteins are identified based on size. The relative quantities are estimated based on band intensity. If the SPEP suggests abnormal proliferation of a particular immunoglobulin, **immunofixation** is performed, whereby separated serum proteins are subsequently probed for specific monoclonal immunoglobulins.

### KEY FACT

Western blot is a confirmatory test **(high specificity)** performed when the results of an ELISA test are positive for HIV antibodies **(high sensitivity).**

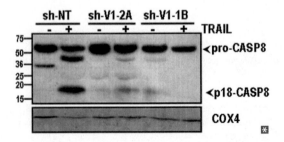

**FIGURE 2-127.     Example of SDS-PAGE.** Protein cleavage products of caspase-8 are separated by mass as the positively-charged anode causes migration through the polyacrylamide gel. Following separation, proteins can be transferred to a membrane by applying a potential *en face.* These can then be stained using tagged antibodies for identification.

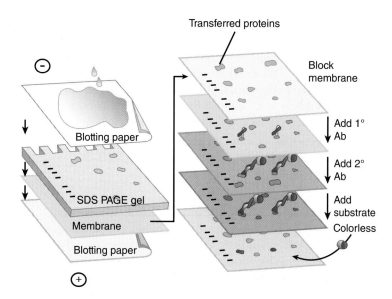

**FIGURE 2-128.** **Western blotting.** After they are separated by size using SDS-PAGE (sodium dodecyl sulfate-polyacrylamide gel electrophoresis), the proteins are transferred on to a membrane with the aid of an electric field. The membrane is then blocked and incubated with the primary and the secondary antibodies. Using a substrate, a color signal is produced showing the fragments that contain the protein of interest. 1° Ab, primary antibody; 2° Ab, secondary antibody.

## Enzyme-Linked Immunosorbent Assay (ELISA)

### Principle

ELISA is an immunologic technique widely used for the detection of antigens and antibodies in clinical samples (Figure 2-129). There are two types of assays, **direct** and **indirect**:

- **Direct ELISA:** Patient sample (often blood serum) is probed with a **test antibody** to see if a **specific antigen** is present. The antibody itself is coupled to a reporter (colorimetric or fluorescent) to detect the antigen.
- **Indirect ELISA:** Patient's blood sample is probed with either **test antigen** or **test antibody** to see if a **specific antibody** or **antigen** (respectively) is present. Then, a **secondary antibody** coupled to a reporter (color-generating, or fluorescent) is added to detect the antibody-antigen complex.

ELISA is used for the detection of antibodies against many pathogens, as a means of establishing present or past infection with the pathogen. It is also sometimes used by the food industry to detect the presence of certain common allergens.

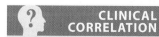

**CLINICAL CORRELATION**

The CDC recommends diagnosing HIV using fourth-generation laboratory assays, which detect **HIV p24 antigen** and **HIV antibodies.** Positive tests are then followed by confirmatory **HIV antibody differentiation immunoassays.** Early in infection, HIV can be detected by measuring viral load using reverse-transcriptase-PCR **(RT-PCR).** This is helpful in managing patients who present soon after infection, prior to antibody formation.

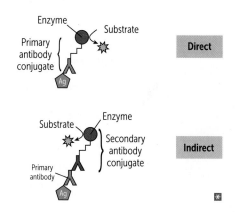

**FIGURE 2-129.** **ELISA.** See text for a step-by-step explanation.

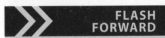
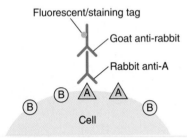

**FIGURE 2-130.**
**Immunohistochemical detection.**
An antibody specific to the protein of interest is incubated with a clinical sample and allowed to bind to it. Then a secondary antibody is used to provide a visual signal, which identifies and localizes the protein of interest if it is present in the sample.

## Use

ELISA test for antibodies to HIV (eg, anti-gp120) was considered the most *sensitive* screening test for HIV infection. A positive result would then be followed up by the more *specific* confirmatory Western blot assay. Now, combined antigen/antibody tests are recommended for HIV diagnosis. ELISA is also used to screen for other viral pathogens, such as the West Nile virus. Indirect ELISA is also used to detect the presence of Rh antigen on red blood cells using anti-Rh test antibody when evaluating for a possible Rh mismatch.

## Immunohistochemistry

### Principle

Similar to ELISA and Western blotting, immunohistochemistry (IHC) is a general technique that relies on visual detection of proteins in a sample using antibodies. The main difference is that IHC refers to the detection of antigens in **native tissue samples,** as opposed to lysates or other biochemical preparations. Immunocytochemistry (ICC) is a related technique by which antigens are detected in **cells** grown in culture. Both IHC and ICC look at antigens in situ on samples treated with a fixative (eg, formaldehyde).

In both techniques, an antibody specific for the protein of interest is incubated on the tissue sample; the tissue is subsequently washed to remove unbound primary antibody. If the antigen is present in the tissue, bound antibodies stay attached. A secondary antibody with reporter (enzyme-conjugated or fluorophore-conjugated) is added to the reaction, which binds to the primary antibody. This reporter secondary is ultimately visualized, either directly via fluorescence (in the cause of fluorophore-conjugated antibodies) or indirectly, via colorimetric or luminescence reactions (in the case of enzyme-conjugated antibodies) (Figure 2-130).

## Use

In the clinical setting, IHC is commonly used in histopathology, often to detect a specific cancer antigen in a tissue sample, thus confirming the tumor type. Tissue can come from diagnostic biopsies or tumor samples following resection.

Examples of such tumor markers can be found in Table 2-39.

## Radioimmunoassay

### Principle

Radioimmunoassay (RIA) is used to **quantitatively** measure **small** amounts of antigen in clinical samples. The protein of interest is first labeled with a **radioactive isotope** and allowed to bind to the antibody against that protein until the point of saturation. The clinical sample is then added to the mix, **causing any antigen in the sample to displace the radioactively labeled one from the antibodies.** This free radiolabeled

**TABLE 2-39.    Immunohistochemistry (IHC) Markers and Associated Tumors**

| IHC-DETECTABLE MARKER | TUMOR TYPE |
| --- | --- |
| Carcinoembryonic antigen (CEA) | Adenocarcinoma |
| CD15, CD30 | Hodgkin disease |
| α-Fetoprotein | Yolk sac tumors, hepatocellular carcinoma |
| CD117 | Gastrointestinal stromal tumors (GISTs) |
| Prostate-specific antigen (PSA) | Prostate cancer |

antigen is then measured in the solution, making it possible to calculate the amount of the antigen in the original sample.

### Use

RIA is used most commonly to measure various hormone levels in patients. It is also sometimes used to measure the amounts of vitamins, enzymes, and drugs in clinical samples.

RIA is routinely used to measure the levels of thyroid-stimulating hormone (**TSH**), $T_3$, and $T_4$ as part of a thyroid disease workup, as well as **insulin** levels in patients with suspected diabetes mellitus or insulinomas.

# Genetics

## HARDY-WEINBERG GENETICS

Humans carry two copies of each gene in every somatic cell (one inherited from each parent). These copies, known as alleles, each can be dominant or recessive. Dominant alleles are phenotypically expressed over recessive alleles. **Hardy-Weinberg genetics** are used to describe the frequency of these alleles in large populations.

The percentage of each of the two alleles ($p$ and $q$) in the population must total 100%.

$$p + q = 1.00$$

### Example

In a sample population, there are only two eye colors: brown and blue. If 90% of the alleles in the population are for brown eyes ($p = 0.90$), then the other 10% must be for blue eyes ($q = 0.10$).

To determine the number of people with each combination of alleles:

$$p^2 + 2pq + q^2 = 1.00$$

where $p^2$ and $q^2$ are the fractions of the population homozygous for $p$ and $q$, respectively, and $2pq$ is the fraction heterozygous for $p$ and $q$ (Figure 2-131).

Using the previous example of eye color, if $p = 0.90$ and $q = 0.10$, then:

| | |
|---|---|
| $p^2 = 0.90^2 = 0.81$ | 81% homozygous for brown eyes |
| $2pq = 2 \times 0.90 \times 0.10 = 0.18$ | 18% heterozygous for eye color |
| $q^2 = 0.10^2 = 0.01$ | 1% homozygous for blue eyes |

Disease inheritance depends on the number of copies of the mutant gene required to produce the condition and on which chromosome the gene is located.

### Non–Sex Chromosome Diseases

**Autosomal dominant** and **autosomal recessive** diseases are caused by genes carried on chromosomes other than the X and Y sex chromosomes.

- **Autosomal dominant** diseases require the presence of only one mutant gene (or allele), often resulting in a defective structural gene. These individuals are termed heterozygotes. Affected persons may be of both sexes and appear in most generations (Figure 2-132A).

|  | $pA$ | $qa$ |
|---|---|---|
| $pA$ | $AA$ $p \times p = p^2$ | $Aa$ $p \times q$ |
| $qa$ | $Aa$ $p \times q$ | $aa$ $q \times q = q^2$ |

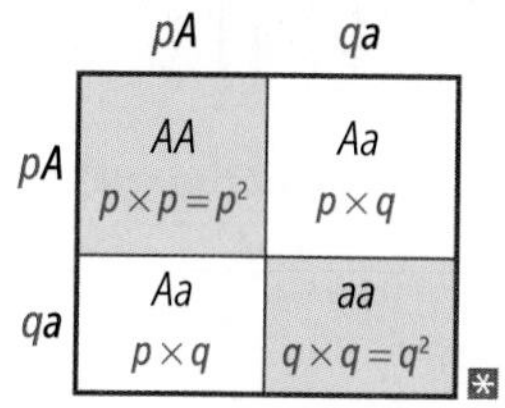

**FIGURE 2-131. Hardy-Weinberg formula.** A Punnett square can be used to visualize and derive the Hardy-Weinberg formula ($p^2$ + 2pq + $q^2$), whereby each box represents a fraction of the population with a given genotype, and the sum total of the four boxes must equal one.

- **Autosomal recessive** diseases require the presence of two mutant genes (homozygous), often resulting in an enzyme deficiency. Affected persons are of both sexes, but autosomal recessive diseases appear sporadically and infrequently throughout a family tree (Figure 2-132B).

### Sex Chromosome Diseases

**X-linked recessive** diseases affect males because they carry one X chromosome that is always inherited from the mother. Sons of heterozygous mothers have a 50% chance of being affected, and there is no male-to-male transmission. Because they have only one allele for each gene on the X-chromosome, the recessive mutant gene is always expressed (there can be no second, dominant allele to disguise the recessive allele) (Figure 2-132C).

**X-linked dominant** diseases affect both sexes. An affected male has only one X chromosome and thus always passes the disease to daughters, but cannot pass it down to a son. Affected mothers have a 50% chance of passing on the disease to offspring of either sex (Figure 2-132D).

### Mitochondrial Diseases

Mitochondria carry their own DNA, which is inherited from the mother. (Only the oocyte contributes mitochondria to the zygote; the sperm neck and tail, which carry mitochondria of the sperm, never penetrate the oocyte.) Any mutation present in the maternal mitochondria will be passed to offspring (Figure 2-132E). Not all mutations cause disease, however. Even within a single individual, mitochondrial DNA is heterogenous (due to heteroplasmy), and often a defect in one or many mitochondria can be compensated for by others.

These modes of inheritance are summarized in Table 2-40.

### Inheritance Properties

- **Incomplete penetrance** occurs when a person with a mutant genotype does not show signs of the **disease** (phenotype).
- **Variable expression** occurs when the severity and nature of the disease phenotype varies between individuals with the same mutant **genotype.**

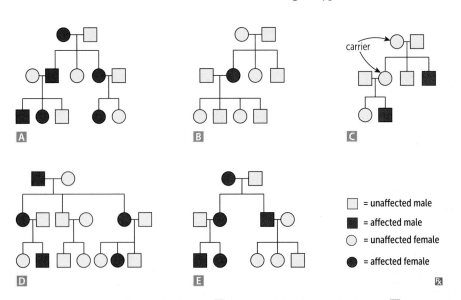

**FIGURE 2-132. Modes of inheritance.** A Autosomal dominant inheritance. B Autosomal recessive inheritance. C X-linked recessive inheritance. D X-linked dominant inheritance. E Mitochondrial inheritance.

**TABLE 2-40.** **Modes of Inheritance**

| MODE | CHROMOSOME CARRIED ON | SEX AFFECTED | GENERATIONS AFFECTED | PARENT WHO TRANSMITS | TYPES OF DISEASE | HINTS WHEN LOOKING AT PEDIGREE TREE |
|------|----------------------|--------------|---------------------|---------------------|------------------|-------------------------------------|
| Autosomal dominant | Autosome | Both equally | Multiple sequential generations | Parent who is also affected. | Often structural and not fatal at early age | Most generations affected. |
| Autosomal recessive | Autosome | Both equally | Usually multiple offspring of one generation | Both parents are carriers. | Most metabolic diseases and cystic fibrosis | Often sporadically appears in one generation. |
| X-linked recessive | X chromosome | Males | Variable depending on presence of male offspring | Mother. | Fragile X, muscular dystrophy, hemophilias, Lesch-Nyhan syndrome | Mostly males. |
| X-linked dominant | X chromosome | Females > males | Multiple serial generations | Both parents can give gene to a female, only mother gives to male offspring. | Hypophosphatemic rickets, Rett syndrome, Alport syndrome, fragile X syndrome | All female children of affected male are affected. |
| Mitochondrial | None (carried in mitochondrial DNA) | Both equally | Multiple serial generations | Mother. | Leber's optic neuropathy, MELAS, many myopathies | Only affected mothers can pass mutant alleles to offspring. |

MELAS, mitochondrial encephalomyopathy with lactic acidosis and stroke-like episodes.

## TRISOMIES

**Trisomies** occur when three homologous chromosomes are present in a zygote.

### Nondisjunction

Either the sperm or the egg carries the extra chromosome, as shown in Figure 2-133.

### Chromosomal Translocation

Trisomy can also occur when a piece of one chromosome attaches to another and "hitches a ride" during meiosis. As a result, two homologous chromosomes can be sorted to the same zygote, as shown in Figure 2-134.

### Common Trisomies

All trisomies are characterized by mental retardation, abnormal facies, and often heart disease (Figure 2-135, Table 2-41). Few fetal trisomies survive to birth (ie, most terminate in spontaneous abortion).

**Trisomy 21 (Down syndrome)** is the most common trisomy (1:700) and the most common cause of mental retardation. Ninety-five percent of cases are due to meiotic nondisjunction, 4% of cases are due to Robertsonian translocation, and 1% of cases are due to mosaicism (postfertilization mitotic error). Mothers may express **low α-ferroprotein and high** levels of **beta human chorionic gonadotropin (β-hCG)** during pregnancy and ultrasound may show **nuchal translucency.** Patients are characterized by:

- Epicanthal folds
- Simian crease
- Flat facies

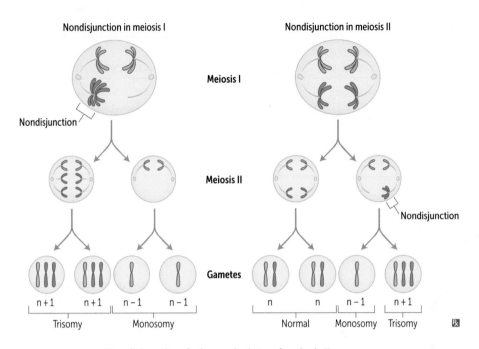

**FIGURE 2-133.** **Nondisjunction during meiosis I and meiosis II.**

- Gaps between first two toes
- Atrial septal defect (ASD) or other congenital heart disease
- Acute lymphocytic leukemia (ALL)
- Duodenal atresia

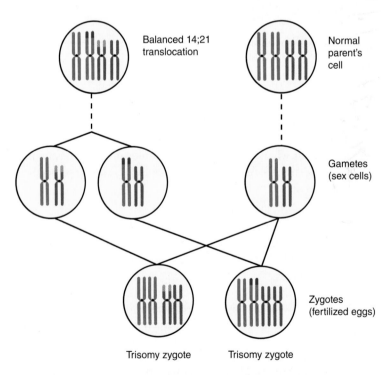

**FIGURE 2-134.** **Robertsonian translocation resulting in Down syndrome.** Key: *Green:* region of blue chromosome translocated onto red chromosome; *purple:* region of red chromosome translocated onto blue chromosome.

**TABLE 2-41.** Laboratory Findings in Trisomies 21, 18, and 13

| TIMING OF TEST | IMAGING/LABORATORY TEST | TRISOMY 21 DOWN SYNDROME | TRISOMY 18 EDWARD SYNDROME | TRISOMY 13 PATAU SYNDROME |
|---|---|---|---|---|
| First trimester | Ultrasound | Nuchal translucency & hypoplastic nasal bone | | Nuchal translucency |
| | Serum PAPP-A | ↓ | ↓ | ↓ |
| | β-HCG | ↑ | ↓ | ↓ |
| Second trimester | α-Fetoprotein | ↓ | ↓ | |
| | β-HCG | ↑ | ↓ | |
| | Estriol | ↓ | ↓ | |
| | Inhibin A | ↑ | Normal or ↓ | |

β-HCG, beta-human chorionic gonadotropin; PAPP-A, pregnancy-associated plasma protein A.

- Celiac disease
- Brushfield spots
- **Associated with:**
  - Early-onset Alzheimer disease
  - Increased risk of ALL and AML

**Trisomy 18 (Edward syndrome;** 1:8000) is often fatal by < 1 year of age. Patients are characterized by:

- Micrognathia
- Overlapping, clenched fingers
- Rocker-bottom feet
- Large occiput
- Congenital heart disease

**Trisomy 13 (Patau syndrome;** 1:15,000) is often fatal by < 1 year of age. Patients are characterized by:

- Microphthalmia
- Polydactyly
- Cleft lip/palate
- Holoprosencephaly
- Cutis aplasia

## IMPRINT DISORDERS

**Imprinting** occurs when identical genes are expressed differently, depending on the parent from which the gene is inherited.

Prader-Willi and Angelman syndromes are both due to mutations on chromosome 15. The two distinct phenotypes depend on the exact **locus** that is mutated.

### Prader-Willi Syndrome

This syndrome occurs when a specific locus of chromosome 15, which is normally **imprinted** at the **maternal** chromosome, is **deleted** in the **paternal** chromosome. This results in:

- Neonatal hypotonia and failure to thrive
- Later childhood hyperphagia and obesity

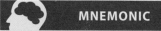

**MNEMONIC**

Think **"Edward Scissorhands"** when you read **Edward** syndrome/trisomy 18, to recall the classic overlapping fingers

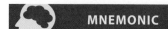

**MNEMONIC**

**D**rink at 21, **E**lection age is 18, **P**uberty at 13.
**D**own = Trisomy 21
**E**dward = Trisomy 18
**P**atau = Trisomy 13

**KEY FACT**

**Trisomy 8** is rare, but can also result in live births. **Trisomy 16** is a common cause of miscarriage.

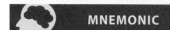

**MNEMONIC**

**A**FP, or α-feto-**Patau,** is the main condition in which AFP is elevated on the quad screen.

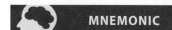

**MNEMONIC**

**P**rader-Willi = **P**aternal deletion
Angel**M**an = **M**aternal deletion

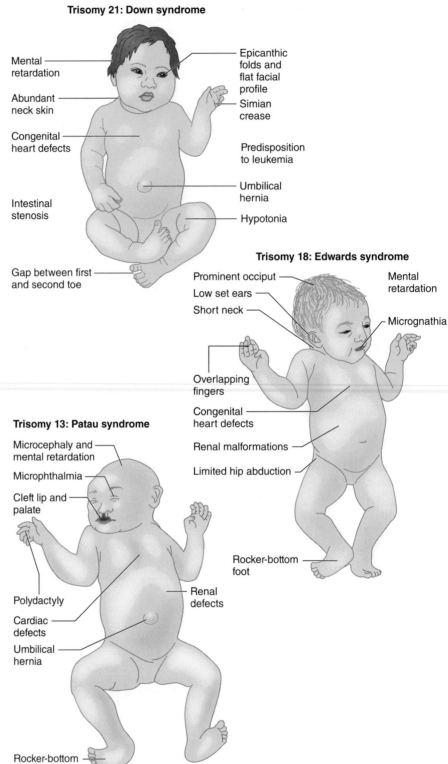

**Trisomy 21: Down syndrome**

- Mental retardation
- Abundant neck skin
- Congenital heart defects
- Intestinal stenosis
- Gap between first and second toe
- Epicanthic folds and flat facial profile
- Simian crease
- Predisposition to leukemia
- Umbilical hernia
- Hypotonia

**Trisomy 18: Edwards syndrome**

- Prominent occiput
- Low set ears
- Short neck
- Overlapping fingers
- Congenital heart defects
- Renal malformations
- Limited hip abduction
- Mental retardation
- Micrognathia
- Rocker-bottom foot

**Trisomy 13: Patau syndrome**

- Microcephaly and mental retardation
- Microphthalmia
- Cleft lip and palate
- Polydactyly
- Cardiac defects
- Umbilical hernia
- Renal defects
- Rocker-bottom foot

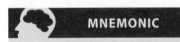

**MNEMONIC**

In the quad screen for Down syndrome/ trisomy 21, remember β-hCG and inhibin are **high,** or **HI = high.**

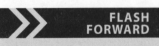

**FLASH FORWARD**

Both **Turner** syndrome and **Down** syndrome have the **same** quad screen findings.

FIGURE 2-135.    **Dysmorphic features and other abnormalities seen in trisomies 13, 18, and 21.**

- Mild mental retardation
- Aggressive/psychotic behavior
- Short stature, with small hands, feet, and gonads

Twenty-five percent of cases of Prader-Willi syndrome are due to maternal uniparental disomy (two maternally imprinted genes are inherited; no paternal gene).

## Angelman Syndrome

Occurs when a specific locus of chromosome 15 (normally imprinted in the **paternal** chromosome) is **deleted** in the **maternal** chromosome. This results in:

- Inappropriate laughter (also known as happy puppet syndrome)
- Jerky, flexed movements
- Microcephaly
- Minimal speech
- Severe mental retardation and seizures
- Sleep disturbance

Five percent of cases of Angelman syndrome are due to paternal uniparental disomy (two paternally imprinted genes are inherited; no maternal genes).

**NOTES**

# Immunology

## Principles of Immunology

The immune system distinguishes foreign molecules and potential **pathogens** from the body's own cells and removes these pathogens from the body. Cells of the immune system respond to **antigens,** molecular structures (eg, peptides) capable of producing an immune response.

### CONCEPTS OF IMMUNITY

Immune processes can be divided into those that are present at birth (**innate immunity**) and those that require antigen exposure before forming a precise response (**adaptive immunity**).

### Innate Immunity

Innate immunity is composed of rapid, nonspecific immunologic processes that recognize and destroy certain common pathogens. The protein receptors (eg, Toll-like receptors) involved in recognizing these pathogenic danger signals (ie, pathogen-associated molecular patterns [PAMPs]) are germline encoded, so they do not require prior exposure for shaping the response. Some components of innate immunity include:

- Physical barriers, such as skin (with help of the tight junctions between cells) and mucous membranes
- Cells, such as **neutrophils, macrophages,** and **dendritic cells**
- The **complement** system

### Adaptive Immunity

Adaptive immunity encompasses a set of highly specific immune processes that have a delayed response on first exposure. Unlike innate immunity, this response has the capacity for memory. Cells of adaptive immunity have the ability to undergo genetic rearrangements, resulting in a highly specific and powerful response to pathogens. Key components of adaptive immunity include:

- Cellular components, such as T lymphocytes (**cell-mediated immunity**), also referred to as T cells.
- Antibody-producing B lymphocytes (**humoral immunity**), also referred to as B cells.

Apart from classifying immunity based on how the body detects and responds to insults, immune processes can be classified based on how immune protection is acquired, that is, **passive immunity or active immunity.**

### Passive Immunity

Passive immunity is provided by preformed antibodies from a source outside the body. Exposure to virulent pathogens or toxins can result in serious illness or death if the body's own immune system is unable to mount an adequate response. Preformed antibodies can be administered therapeutically to quickly neutralize the pathogens. While exhibiting antigen specificity, the antibodies are short-lived, and the body is unable to respond to a subsequent exposure (ie, lack of immune memory). Some examples of passive immunity include:

- Antibodies in mothers' milk for breast-fed infants
- Administered **antitoxins** for tetanus or botulinum toxins
- Administered **antibodies** to the hepatitis B or rabies virus

Table 3-1 summarizes the characteristics of each subset of immunity.

**KEY FACT**

The innate immune system uses nonspecific markers to prime the body for an adaptive response. Subsequently, lymphocytes are responsible for the two key features of adaptive immunity: specificity and memory.

**TABLE 3-1. Subsets of Immunity**

|  | INNATE | ADAPTIVE | PASSIVE |
|---|---|---|---|
| Means of acquisition | Innate | Exposure to foreign antigens | Receiving preformed antibodies |
| Onset | Rapid | Delayed | Rapid |
| Duration | Initial response | Long-lasting protection | Short span of antibodies (half-life ~3 wk) |
| Specificity | Nonspecific | Specific | Specific |
| Memory | No | Yes | No |
| Cells and proteins involved | Neutrophils<br>Macrophages<br>Dendritic cells<br>Complement | T lymphocytes<br>B lymphocytes | Foreign antibodies |
| Examples | Acute infection | Natural infection, vaccines, toxoid | IgA in breast milk, monoclonal antibodies, maternal IgG crossing the placenta |

## ANATOMY OF THE IMMUNE SYSTEM

The immune system is composed of both primary and secondary lymphoid organs, as summarized in Table 3-2. The primary or central lymphoid organs include the bone marrow and thymus and are involved in lymphocyte production and development. The spleen and lymph nodes are considered secondary, or peripheral, lymphoid organs and are important sites of antigen interaction with cells of the immune system.

### Bone Marrow

The bone marrow is the location of **hematopoiesis,** or production of white and red blood cells. The maturation of B cells also occurs in the bone marrow, whereas the maturation of T cells occurs in the thymus. Some immunodeficiency syndromes can be treated by bone marrow transplantation, thus providing a source of functional cells to protect the body.

### Thymus

This encapsulated primary lymphoid organ is located in the anterior mediastinum. The thymus is derived from the third branchial pouch during development and is the site of **T-cell differentiation,** maturation, and selection. The thymus increases in size until adolescence, when it begins to atrophy and accumulate fat.

Following production in the bone marrow, immature T cells migrate to the thymic **cortex** early in their development to undergo positive and negative selection (see section on Anergy and Tolerance later in chapter). Selection begins in the cortex as the

**FLASH FORWARD**

Chemotherapy or radiation treatment may result in leukopenia (low white blood cell count) and therefore immunosuppression due to bone marrow damage.

**CLINICAL CORRELATION**

Many types of tumors can induce an autoimmune disorder. For example, 30% of patients with a thymoma (tumor of the thymus) develop an associated autoimmune disorder, such as myasthenia gravis.

**TABLE 3-2. Organs of the Immune System**

|  | ORGAN | FUNCTION |
|---|---|---|
| Primary | Bone marrow<br>Thymus | Production of immune cells, maturation of B cells<br>Maturation of T cells |
| Secondary | Spleen<br>Lymph nodes<br>Tonsils<br>Peyer patches | Interaction of immune cells with antigen |

**QUESTION**

Patients without a spleen have an increased susceptibility to encapsulated bacteria. This includes patients with surgical splenectomies and sickle cell anemia. Which specific vaccines must be offered to these patients?

cells reach the **corticomedullary junction** and continues as the T cells move into the inner **medulla.** Mature T cells are finally released into the bloodstream and travel to peripheral sites (Figure 3-1).

Microscopically, the cortex stains darkly owing to the density of lymphocytes. The medulla is lighter, with fewer lymphocytes and a higher concentration of dendritic and epithelial reticular cells.

### Spleen

The spleen is a secondary lymphoid organ located in the upper left quadrant of the peritoneal cavity. It contains many blood-filled sinuses that filter antigens and cells from the blood. Microscopically, the splenic parenchyma is divided into the red and white pulp. The **red pulp** is the location of red blood cell storage and turnover; it contains rich vasculature with splenic cords (cords of Billroth) and fenestrated capillaries (sinusoids). The sinusoid structure allows blood cells to freely pass through capillary walls.

The **white pulp** is the location of immune cell interaction. Blood flows into the white pulp through the central arteriole, which is surrounded by the **periarterial lymphatic sheath (PALS)** of T cells. Follicles of B cells are found more distant from the central arteriole; they have pale germinal centers when B cells are activated. The marginal zone surrounds both the PALS and lymphocytic follicle, in addition to separating the white and red pulp. Antigen-presenting cells (**APCs**) in the marginal zone ingest pathogens by phagocytosis and present them to nearby lymphocytes. Blood is drained through the **marginal sinus** located within the marginal zone. The microscopic structure of the spleen is shown in Figure 3-2.

### Lymph Nodes

Lymph nodes are encapsulated secondary lymphoid organs that receive lymph from multiple afferent vessels, providing the opportunity for interaction between the stored immune cells and the lymphatic fluid. The fluid is returned to the lymphatic ducts through the efferent vessel after the antigens and pathogenic cells contained in the fluid encounter APCs, B cells, and T cells.

The tissue architecture of lymph nodes is maximized for antigen recognition and response, as shown in Figure 3-3.

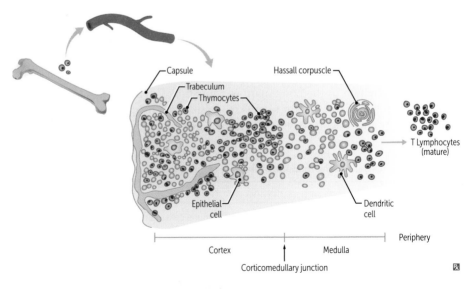

**FIGURE 3-1. Microscopic structure of the thymus.**

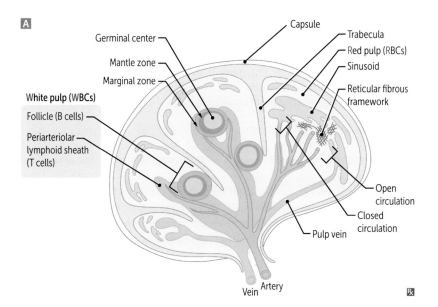
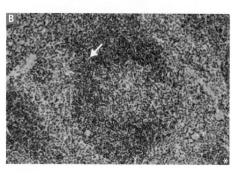
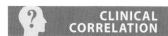

FIGURE 3-2.    **The spleen.** A Anatomy of the spleen. B Normal spleen showing red pulp (red arrow) and white pulp (white arrow).

- Primary, or inactive, follicles are dense with stored lymphocytes awaiting antigen presentation.
- Secondary, or active, follicles have pale **germinal centers** within the cluster of lymphocytes. Here, B cells proliferate and produce antibodies in response to antigens.

T cells are found in the **paracortex** between the follicles and the medulla. The paracortex may become enlarged in severe infections, such as viral infections, that result in a cellular immune response.

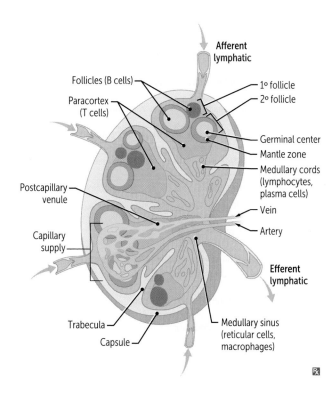

FIGURE 3-3.    **Lymph node architecture.**

Lymph nodes are supplied by their own capillary system. B and T lymphocytes enter lymph nodes via high endothelial venules. From there, chemokines will guide T cells to the paracortex and B cells to lymphoid follicles. Afterward, both B and T cells will exit via the efferent lymphatic vessels. The medullary sinus drains cells and fluid in the medulla into the efferent lymphatic duct. APCs within the sinus filter the lymph by engulfing pathogens and presenting them to lymphocytes.

### Lymphatic System

Lymphatic vessels drain fluid from the body, filter it through lymph nodes, and return it to the circulatory system. A summary of lymphatic drainage sites is presented in Table 3-3. The **right lymphatic duct** drains the right arm and right half of the head and neck, whereas the **thoracic duct** drains all other body parts. The fluid from the thoracic duct drains into the left subclavian vein, and that from the right lymphatic duct drains into the junction of the right subclavian and internal jugular veins.

### Peripheral Lymphoid Tissue

Collections of lymphocytes outside the spleen and lymph nodes that are at prime locations for antigen interaction are termed peripheral lymphoid tissue. Some examples of peripheral lymphoid tissue include:

- Gut-associated lymphoid tissue (GALT), which includes the tonsils, appendix, and Peyer patches (Figure 3-4) of the intestines.
- Mucosal-associated lymphoid tissue (MALT).
- Bronchial-associated lymphoid tissue (BALT).

**TABLE 3-3.    Lymphatic Drainage Sites**

| LYMPH NODE CLUSTER | AREA OF BODY DRAINED |
| --- | --- |
| Cervical | Head and neck |
| Hilar | Lungs |
| Mediastinal | Trachea and esophagus |
| Axillary | Upper limb, breast, skin above umbilicus |
| Celiac | Liver, stomach, spleen, pancreas, upper duodenum |
| Superior mesenteric | Lower duodenum, jejunum, ileum, colon to splenic flexure |
| Inferior mesenteric | Colon from splenic flexure to upper rectum |
| Internal iliac | Lower rectum to anal canal (above pectinate line), bladder, vagina (middle third), cervix, prostate |
| Para-aortic | Testes, ovaries, kidneys, uterus |
| Superficial inguinal | Anal canal (below pectinate line), skin below umbilicus (except popliteal area), scrotum, vulva |
| Popliteal | Dorsolateral foot, posterior calf |

Right lymphatic duct drains right side of body above diaphragm.
Thoracic duct drains everything else into junction of left subclavian and internal jugular veins.

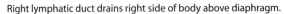

Modified with permission from Le T, et al. *First Aid for the USMLE Step 1: 2017.* New York: McGraw-Hill, 2017.

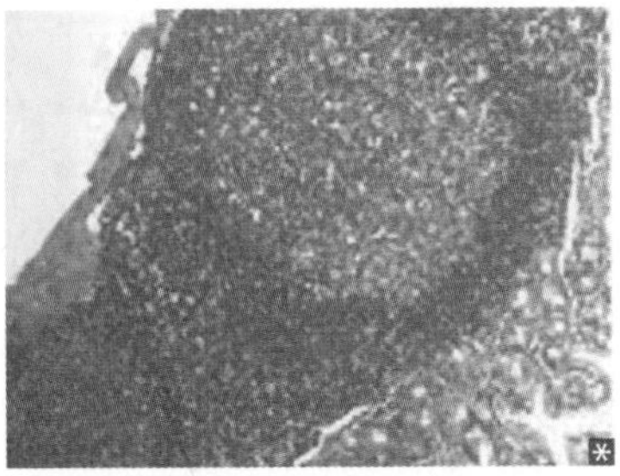

**FIGURE 3-4.    Peyer patches.**

## CELLS AND MOLECULES OF THE IMMUNE SYSTEM

### Innate Immunity

### Phagocytic Cells

Phagocytic cells engulf pathogens and debris and include:

- **Neutrophils** (Figure 3-5) are myeloid cells present in acute inflammatory responses. These cells contain multilobed (3–5 lobes) nuclei and abundant cytoplasmic myeloperoxidase granules for killing pathogens. Engulfed microbes trigger an oxidative burst that creates reactive oxygen species that are lethal to pathogens.
- **Macrophages** (Figure 3-6) are differentiated myeloid cells present in both pathologic and normal physiologic responses. These cells are large, amorphous, and have high phagocytic capacity and a longer life span than neutrophils. Macrophages are derived from monocytes that leave the bloodstream and differentiate in response to cytokines.
- **Dendritic cells** (Figure 3-7) are differentiated myeloid cells that engulf antigen in the epithelia of the skin, gastrointestinal, and respiratory tracts. Before antigen exposure, they can be identified by long, fingerlike processes of cytoplasm. After taking up antigen and becoming activated, they travel to lymph nodes where they present antigen to T cells.

### Antigen-Presenting Cells

APCs process engulf pathogens and express the resulting antigens to other immune cells. Some examples of APCs include:

- Dendritic cells
- Macrophages
- B cells

Following phagocytosis of extracellular pathogens, APCs digest the pathogen into peptides within phagolysosomes. The peptides are loaded on to a major histocompatibility complex (MHC) II molecule within an endosome, which fuses with the cell membrane so the MHC II–antigen complex may be presented to T cells.

### Natural Killer Cells

Natural killer (NK) cells contain lytic granules that attack and kill virus-infected or cancerous cells. Unlike lymphocytes, NK cells lack specific antigen receptors. Binding of the antibody constant region to NK cell surface receptors also triggers the release of lytic granules in a process known as **antibody-dependent cellular cytotoxicity (ADCC)**.

A summary of the cells of the innate immune system is provided in Table 3-4.

### The Complement System

The complement system comprises a cascade of proteins that result in the lysis of pathogenic cells, as shown in Figure 3-8 and Table 3-5. The complement cascade can be activated in three ways:

- The **classic pathway** is activated when C1 recognizes and binds the constant fragment of either IgG or IgM in an antigen-antibody complex.
- The **alternative pathway** is triggered when activated C3 or IgA antibodies recognize antigens on microbial surfaces. C3 recognizes nonspecific antigens, and IgA recognizes specific ones.
- The **lectin pathway** is activated when mannose-binding lectin, a serum protein, recognizes carbohydrate antigens on the surface of microorganisms such as encapsulated bacteria or viruses.

### CLINICAL CORRELATION

An oxidative burst is when the phagocyte nicotine adenine dinucleotide phosphate (NADPH) oxidase complex is activated, leading to the reactive oxygen species production. Patients with chronic granulomatous disease have a defect in NADPH oxidase and an increased susceptibility to catalase-positive organisms (eg, *staphylococcus aureus, pseudomonas, candida*).

### KEY FACT

In some instances, neutrophils may contain more lobes than usual, up to eight or nine. These hypersegmented neutrophils can be a sign of vitamin deficiencies, specifically $B_{12}$ and folate.

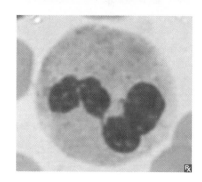

FIGURE 3-5.    **Neutrophils.**

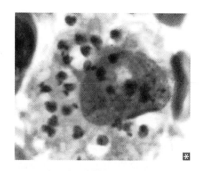

FIGURE 3-6.    **Macrophage.**

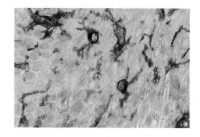

FIGURE 3-7.    **Dendritic cells.**

**TABLE 3-4.    Cells of the Innate Immune System**

| CATEGORY | CELL TYPES | FUNCTION | MECHANISMS |
|---|---|---|---|
| Phagocytes | Neutrophils, macrophages, dendritic cells | Engulf foreign particles | Phagocytosis |
| Antigen-presenting cells | Dendritic cells, macrophages, B cells | Present particles to T cells (ie, to adaptive immune system) | Complexing antigen with MHC II |
| Natural killer cells | Natural killer cells | Destroy virus-infected and tumor cells | Detect down-regulation of MHC I, antibody-dependent cellular cytoxicity |

MHC, major histocompatibility complex.

The three activation pathways converge on the generation of **C3 convertase,** an enzyme that remains associated with the pathogen surface to trigger cleavage of other complement proteins. C3 convertase breaks down C3 molecules to the enzymatically active **C3b** and the **anaphylatoxin** C3a, which mediates a local inflammatory response. C3b is also important in triggering phagocytosis of pathogens.

Binding of C3b to C3 convertase creates **C5 convertase,** which cleaves C5 into C5a (another anaphylatoxin) and C5b, which is inserted into the cell membrane of the pathogen. The binding of C6, C7, C8, and C9 to C5b follows, forming the **membrane attack complex (MAC),** which perforates the pathogen's cell membrane and causes major damage to the cell.

A summary of the functions of complement proteins is shown in Table 3-5.

As with the coagulation system, the formation of a few active enzymes can lead to rapid activation and amplification of the complement cascade. Therefore, regulatory proteins are important in maintaining control of the cascade.

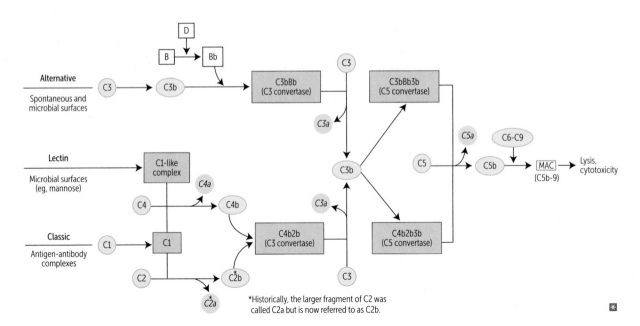

**FIGURE 3-8.    The complement system.** MAC, membrane attack complex.

**TABLE 3-5.** **Complement System Proteins**

| | FUNCTION | PATHWAYS INVOLVED | DEFICIENCY RESULTS |
|---|---|---|---|
| C1 | Recognize antigen-antibody complexes | C | |
| C2 | Part of C3 convertase | C, L | |
| C3a | Anaphylatoxin | C, A, L | Recurrent pyogenic infections (respiratory tract) |
| C3b | | C, A, L | |
| C4a | Anaphylatoxin | C, L | |
| C5a | Anaphylatoxin, neutrophil chemotaxis | C, A, L | |
| C5b, C6, C7, C8, C9 | Cytolysis (MAC) | C, A, L | Recurrent *Neisseria* infections (C6–C8) |

A, alternative pathway; C, classical pathway; L, lectin pathway; MAC, membrane attack complex.

Examples of this control are **C1 esterase inhibitor** and **decay-accelerating factor** (CD55), which disrupts the formation of C3.

In **paroxysmal nocturnal hemoglobinuria,** the protein that associates decay-accelerating factor (DAF) with the RBC membrane is abnormal, thus making the RBCs more susceptible to complement-induced lysis.

### Adaptive Immunity

Adaptive immunity can be divided into cell-mediated immunity and humoral immunity.

### T Cells

T cells are bone marrow derived, but mature in the thymus (T = thymus). They are involved in cell-mediated immunity and have two major responsibilities (Table 3-6).

- Helper T cells (Th): "Help" B cells produce antibodies and secrete cytokines that "help" other cells perform their functions. These cells are CD4 positive.
- Cytotoxic T cells (Tc): Directly kill infected or malignant cells. These cells are CD8 positive.

Within the thymus, T cells undergo differentiation to become mature CD4+ or CD8+ T cells. The mature T cells can also be divided into **helper T cells** ($T_H$) and **cytotoxic T cells** ($T_C$), as seen in Table 3-6. $T_H$ cells are CD4+ cells that "help" other immune cells perform their functions; they differentiate into $T_H1$ or $T_H2$ cells, depending on the cytokines found in their local environment. $T_C$ cells are CD8+ cells that kill target cells infected with viruses or intracellular bacteria. A summary of T-cell maturation is presented in Figure 3-9.

### B Cells

B lymphocytes are bone marrow–derived cells involved in **humoral immunity.** Their main function is to recognize extracellular pathogens and differentiate into **plasma cells** that produce antibodies to target pathogens for elimination from the body.

**TABLE 3-6.    Major Classes of T Cells**

| T CELL TYPE | CLUSTER DIFFERENTIATION (CD) MARKER | CYTOKINE INTERACTIONS | FUNCTION |
|---|---|---|---|
| $T_H1$ | CD4 | Activated by IL-12 and IFN-γ Inhibited by IL-4 and IL-10 | Activate macrophages and $T_C$ via IL-2 and IFN-γ |
| $T_H2$ | CD4 | Activated by IL-2 and IL-4 Inhibited by IFN-γ | Stimulate immunoglobulin production by B cells via IL-4 and IL-5 |
| $T_H17$ | CD4 | IL-6, TGF-β | Promote neutrophilic inflammation in response to extracellular bacteria and fungi |
| $T_C$ | CD8 | IL-2, IFN-γ | Kill cells infected with virus or intracellular bacteria |

IFN, interferon; IL, interleukin; TGF, transforming growth factor.

## Antibodies

Antibodies are proteins composed of two **heavy (H) chains** and two **light (L) chains.** Both heavy and light chains have a **constant ($C_H$ or $C_L$) region** that is identical for all antibodies of the same **isotype,** or class, as well as a **variable region ($V_H$ or $V_L$)** that has been designed by the B cell to specifically recognize an antigen. This general structure is shown in Figure 3-10.

Antibodies are composed of two antigen-binding fragments (**Fab**) and one constant fragment (**Fc**). The Fab fragments are each composed of one light chain and one N-terminal end of the heavy chain, which are normally attached to each other by disulfide bonds. The Fc fragment is composed of the two C-terminal ends of the heavy chains.

Antibodies have four major functions:

- **Opsonization:** The Fab portion of immunoglobulin, particularly IgG, binds to microbial surfaces. The other side of the antibody, the Fc portion, binds to cell surface receptors on the phagocytes, allowing phagocytosis.

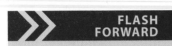

**FLASH FORWARD**

A systemic accumulation of immunoglobulin light chains (eg, in multiple myeloma) is responsible for Bence Jones proteinuria and amyloidosis.

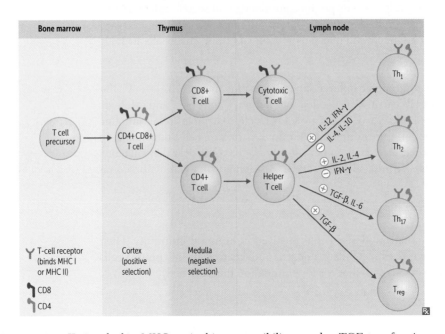

**FIGURE 3-9.    T-cell maturation.** IL, interleukin; MHC, major histocompatibility complex; TGF, transforming growth factor.

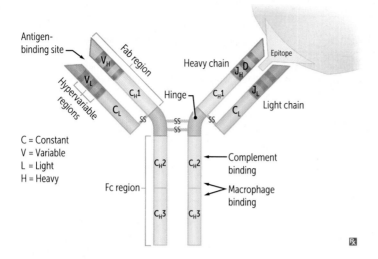

**FIGURE 3-10.    Antibody structure.**

- **Neutralization:** Binding to microbial surfaces can prevent adherence to and infection of host tissues. Furthermore, binding to antigens or inflammatory molecules can prevent an excessive immune response (eg, in passively administered anti–tumor necrosis factor [TNF]-α antibodies).
- **Complement activation:** Binding of IgG or IgM to antigens activates the complement system, leading to phagocytosis, anaphylaxis, and cytolysis.
- **ADCC:** Binding of antibodies to cell surface receptors on NK cells and eosinophils causes the release of cytotoxic granules.

Immunoglobulins with similar structures belong to the same class, or **isotype** ("same" type). There are five immunoglobulin isotypes, as determined by their heavy-chain constant regions. See Table 3-7 for a summary.

### Antibody Diversity

Although B cells contain a limited number of antibody-encoding genes, they can produce a diverse number of antibody molecules by four mechanisms:

- **Somatic recombination of VJ or VDJ genes:** Each B cell in an individual contains a given set of genes to transcribe and translate into antibody molecules. However, these genes have multiple exon segments in various regions (V and J regions for light chains and V, D, and J regions for heavy chains) that can be differentially spliced together. In this way, B cells can produce antibodies with different amino acid sequences, and thus different antigen specificities. This is also known as "combinatorial diversity."
- **Genetic recombination:** During VJ or VDJ recombination, various DNA segments are cut out of the genome. To repair the strand breaks, the enzyme **terminal deoxynucleotidyl transferase (TdT)** adds nucleotides to the sticky ends of the DNA strands.
- **Random combinations of heavy and light chains:** The differentially spliced heavy- and light-chain genes must then combine to form a functional antibody molecule.
- **Somatic hypermutation:** Once B cells have been activated by a helper T cell (following the binding of their B-cell receptor [BCR] to antigen), the variable regions of the immunoglobulin genes are subject to a high rate of random point mutations. At some point, these mutations result in an antibody that is more specific to the initial antigen than was the original antibody molecule; these B cells are selected to differentiate into plasma cells in a process known as **affinity maturation.**

**KEY FACT**

**Allotype:** Ig epitope that differs among members of the same species (polymorphism)
**Isotype:** Ig epitope common to a single class of Ig—determined by heavy chain (eg, IgG, IgA, etc)
**Idiotype:** Ig epitope determined by antigen-binding site (specific for given antigen)

**MNEMONIC**

**GAM**ma globulin is the most abundant antibody in human serum: Ig**G** > Ig**A** > Ig**M**

**TABLE 3-7.    Immunoglobulin Isotypes**

| | EXPRESSED BY | STRUCTURE | COMPLEMENT FIXATION | CROSSES PLACENTA | FUNCTION |
|---|---|---|---|---|---|
| **IgM** <br> J chain | Mature B cell (surface or secreted) | Monomer or pentamer (with J-chain) | Yes | No | Primary response |
| **IgD** | Mature B cell (surface) | Monomer | No | No | Functions as a B-cell receptor to help signal B-cell activation |
| **IgG** | Plasma cells (secreted; high concentration in serum) | Monomer | Yes | Yes | Important in secondary responses; opsonization and neutralization |
| **IgA** <br> J chain | Plasma cells (secreted) | Monomer or dimer (with J-chain) | No | No | Prevents pathogen attachment to mucous membranes; found in secretions |
| **IgE** | Plasma cells (secreted; low concentration in serum) | Monomer | No | No | Type I hypersensitivity (induces mast cell degranulation); parasite immunity |

## Cell Surface Proteins

In addition to their normal functions, cell surface proteins function as useful identifying markers of immune system components. Through flow cytometry, lymphocytes and other cells can be separated based on their cell surface components. This is useful when attempting to count the number of T or B lymphocytes in a patient or determining the level of differentiation of a population of cells (eg, when evaluating for immunodeficiency or lymphoid cancers).

## T-Cell Receptors

T-cell receptors (TCRs) are two-component cell surface receptors responsible for T-cell signaling on binding antigen. TCR components have both a constant region and a variable region that binds a particular antigen. Most TCRs have one α chain and one β chain (α:β TCR), but some are γ:δ.

TCRs interact with MHC molecules, as shown in Figure 3-11.

## B-Cell Receptors

A B cell binds a specific antigen with a BCR receptor, which then loads onto MHC II. The cell then migrates to the lymph node, where a T helper cell, specific to that same antigen, activates the B cell with appropriate co-simulation. The B cell then differentiates, undergoes isotype class switching, affinity maturation, and then becomes either a memory B cell or a plasma cell specific to a single isotype.

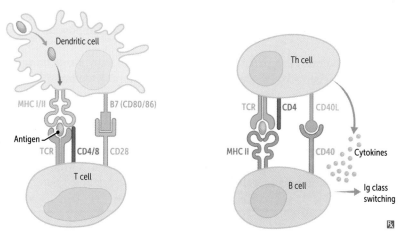

**FIGURE 3-11.    T- and B-cell activation.** MHC, major histocompatibility complex; TCR, T-cell receptor.

## Major Histocompatibility Complexes

Major histocompatibility complexes (MHCs) are surface proteins responsible for communication of T cells with other cells of the body. They are responsible for taking small protein sequences and presenting them extracellularly. This allows passing cells to identify what types of proteins are being made and degraded in that cell. The **human leukocyte antigen (HLA) genes** encode the MHC proteins. The characteristics of MHC I and II molecules are listed in Table 3-8.

MHCs are the most important molecules pertaining to organ and tissue transplantation. **HLA matching** allows for the determination of suitability of donor tissue for transplantation and the likelihood of rejection by the recipient. There are multiple types of tissue grafting:

- **Autografts:** Transfer of an individual's own tissue to another location. Skin autografts are used when transferring healthy skin to a burned or damaged location on the same individual.
- **Syngeneic grafts (isografts):** A transfer of tissue between genetically identical members of the same species, such as between identical twins.
- **Allografts (homografts):** Transfer of tissue between genetically different members of the same species. These grafts are commonly used for organ and tissue transplantation.

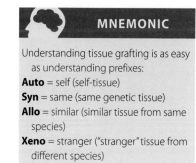

**MNEMONIC**

Understanding tissue grafting is as easy as understanding prefixes:
**Auto** = self (self-tissue)
**Syn** = same (same genetic tissue)
**Allo** = similar (similar tissue from same species)
**Xeno** = stranger ("stranger" tissue from different species)

**TABLE 3-8.    Characteristics of Major Histocompatibility Complexes (MHCs)**

|  | MHC I | MHC II |
| --- | --- | --- |
| Expressed by | All nucleated cells (except RBCs) | APCs |
| Present | Intracellular peptides (self- and viral peptides) | Extracellular peptides (engulfed pathogens) |
| Acquires peptide in | Rough ER (endogenous proteins) | Vesicles, after fusion with acidic endosomes (exogenous proteins) |
| Associated with | $\beta_2$–Microglobulin | Invariant chain (before transport to cell surface) |
| Encoded by | $\alpha$ Chain: HLA-A, -B, and -C genes | HLA-DR, -DP, and -DQ genes |
|  | $\beta$ Chain: Chromosome 15 ($\beta_2$– microglobulin) |  |
| Binds to | TCR and CD8 coreceptor | TCR and CD4 coreceptor |

APCs, antigen-presenting cells; ER, endoplasmic reticulum; HLA, human leukocyte antigen; TCR, T-cell receptor.

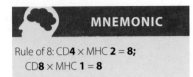

**MNEMONIC**

Rule of 8: CD**4** × MHC **2 = 8;**
CD**8** × MHC **1 = 8**

- **Xenografts (heterografts):** Transfer of tissue between different species. For example, some heart valve replacements are performed with modified porcine valves.

Even with meticulous HLA matching and proper drug therapy, tissue transplantation may not be fully accepted by the recipient. The body can undergo **transplant rejection** in a variety of ways, as presented in Table 3-9.

### Clusters of Differentiation

Clusters of differentiation (CDs) are surface protein complexes widely found on cells of the immune system. There are hundreds of known CDs, with a wide variety of functions. The most common and well-characterized CDs are presented here.

### T Cells

Mature T cells express different proteins that help identify them and the function they serve.

- Mature T cells express CD3 and either CD4 or CD8.
- CD4 on $T_H$ cells is a coreceptor for MHC II molecules on APCs and is also the receptor for HIV.
- CD8 on $T_C$ cells is a coreceptor for MHC I molecules on cells expressing abnormal intracellular peptides (typically virus-infected cells).
- T cells also express CD40 ligand, or CD40L, which is important in antibody isotype switching, and CD28, which is important in T-cell activation.

### B Cells

In addition to the BCR, B cells have a number of identifying receptors.

- CD19 and CD20 are markers for B lymphocytes.
- CD21 is also a B-cell marker, is involved in the complement pathway, and is the receptor for Epstein-Barr virus (EBV).
- B cells also express CD40, which binds CD40L of helper T cells. This interaction is a crucial costimulatory signal for B cells, stimulating differentiation and isotype switching.

A summary of the most common cell surface proteins is found in Table 3-10.

**TABLE 3-9.    Categories of Transplant Rejection**

| CATEGORY | FEATURES |
| --- | --- |
| Hyperacute | Occurs due the presence of preformed antidonor antibodies in the recipient (eg, ABO blood type antibodies). Seen within minutes of transplantation. |
| Acute | Occurs due to $T_C$ reaction with foreign MHCs and is reversible with immunosuppressants. Seen within weeks of transplantation. |
| Chronic | Occurs due to both direct CD8+ T-cell activation and antidonor antibody production, resulting in irreversible vascular fibrinoid necrosis. Seen within months to years of transplantation. |
| Graft-versus-host disease | Occurs in an irradiated immunocompromised host. Grafted immunocompetent T cells recognize the body as "foreign," causing widespread organ dysfunction. Common symptoms are rash, jaundice, and diarrhea. |

**TABLE 3-10.** **Summary of Cell Surface Proteins**

|  | CELL-SPECIFIC SURFACE PROTEINS | ADDITIONAL SURFACE PROTEINS |
|---|---|---|
| T cells | CD3, TCR | CD28 |
| Helper T cells | CD4 | CD40L |
| Cytotoxic T cells | CD8 | |
| B cells | IgM, CD19, CD20 | MHC II, B7, CD21, CD40 |
| Macrophages | — | MHC II, CD14, Fc receptors, C3b receptors |
| Natural killer cells | CD56 | CD16 |
| Nucleated cells | — | MHC I |

MHC, major histocompatibility complex; TCR, T-cell receptor.

## Cytokines

Cytokines are intercellular communication signals that are crucial in immune system function. Some important classes of cytokines include interleukins, chemokines, interferons (IFNs), and tumor necrosis factors (TFNs).

## Interleukins

A family of secreted proteins with a diversity of actions. The most common interleukins are summarized in Table 3-11.

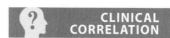

**CLINICAL CORRELATION**

Gram-negative bacteria carry an endotoxin lipopolysaccharide (LPS) that binds to and activates CD14, causing a large release of cytokines and vasodilators and potentially leading to sepsis or septic shock.

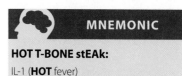

**MNEMONIC**

**HOT T-BONE stEAk:**

IL-1 (**HOT** fever)
IL-2 (**T** cells)
IL-3 (**BONE** marrow)
IL-4 (Ig**E**)
IL-5 (Ig**A**)

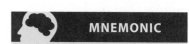

**MNEMONIC**

"Clean up on **aisle 8**": Neutrophils are recruited to clear infections by chemotactic factor **IL-8.**

**TABLE 3-11.** **Functions of Interleukins**

|  | SECRETED BY | ACTS UPON | RESULTS IN |
|---|---|---|---|
| IL-1 | Macrophages | T cells, B cells, neutrophils, fibroblasts, epithelial cells, hepatocytes | Growth, differentiation of cells; endogenous pyrogen; production of acute phase proteins |
| IL-2 | $T_H$ cells | $T_H$ and $T_C$ cells | Growth of cells |
| IL-3 | Activated T cells | Bone marrow stem cells | Growth and differentiation of cells |
| IL-4 | $T_H2$ cells | B cells | Growth of cells; class switching of IgE and IgG |
| IL-5 | $T_H2$ cells | B cells, eosinophils | Differentiation/activation of eosinophils; class switching of IgA |
| IL-6 | $T_H$ cells, macrophages | Hepatocytes, B cells | Production of acute phase proteins and immunoglobulins; endogenous pyrogen |
| IL-8 | Macrophages | Neutrophils | Chemotaxis |
| IL-10 | $T_H2$ cells | $T_H2$ and $T_H1$ cells | Turns off immune response; helps attenuate response to prevent autoimmunity |
| IL-12 | B cells, macrophages | NK and $T_H1$ cells | Activation of cells |
| IL-13 | $T_H2$ cells | Eosinophils | Activation of eosinophils |

IL, interleukin; NK, natural killer cell.

## Interferons

IFNs are secreted proteins from virus-infected cells that promote the transition of local cells to an antiviral state. IFNs bind to IFN receptors on the target cell surface, signaling the uninfected cell to degrade viral messenger ribonucleic acid (mRNA) and increase antigen presentation. IFNs also activate NK cells and stimulate them to kill infected cells. There are three types of IFNs:

- **IFN-α** and **IFN-β** signal cells to produce the enzyme ribonuclease L (RNase L), which degrades mRNA, resulting in a net decrease in protein synthesis and virus production.
- **IFN-γ** signals for increased expression of MHC I and MHC II, thus increasing antigen presentation in all cells that receive the signal. IFN-γ is also secreted by helper T cells to stimulate phagocytosis by macrophages.

### Tumor Necrosis Factors

TNF-α, a protein secreted by macrophages and T cells, is a key mediator of the inflammatory response during infection and autoimmune disease (Figure 3-12).

### Immune System Interactions

### T-Cell Activation

Naïve T cells are not activated until they receive stimulation from a specific APC called a dendritic cell. The TCR binds antigen presented on the MHC molecule of the APC (the **primary signal**). A **secondary (costimulatory) signal** is also required for T-cell activation; one example is the binding of the B7 surface glycoprotein of the APC to CD28 on the T cell. These two interactions result in clonal expansion of the T cell. A summary of this process is shown in Figure 3-13.

### Isotype Switching

Naïve (mature but inactive) B cells express IgM on their surface but do not secrete antibody until activation and **isotype switching** occur. Once IgM binds antigen, antigenic peptides are presented via MHC II. The binding of MHC II to the TCR and CD4 of $T_H$ cells, along with the binding of the appropriate costimulatory molecules (CD40 on the B cell and CD40L on the T cell), triggers the T cell to produce cytokines. These cytokines induce isotype switching. This results in the production of various immunoglobulin isotypes via changes in the constant region of heavy-chain genes. It also

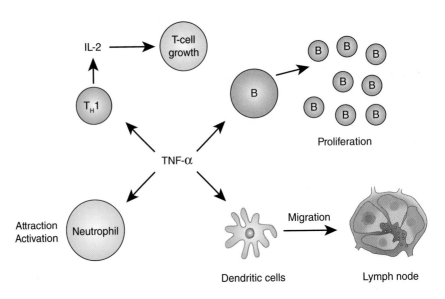

**FIGURE 3-12.** **Functions of tumor necrosis factor (TNF)-α.**

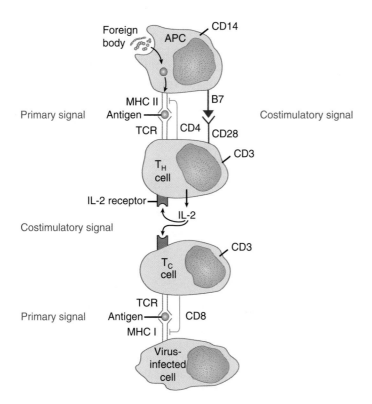

**FIGURE 3-13.** **T-cell activation.** Two signals are required for T-cell activation: Signal 1 (primary signal) and Signal 2 (costimulatory signal). Helper T-cell ($T_H$) activation: (1) Foreign body is phagocytosed by antigen-presenting cells (APC); (2) Foreign antigen is presented on major histocompatability complex (MCH) II and recognized by T-cell receptor (TCR) on $T_H$ cell (Signal 1); (3) "Costimulatory signal" is given by interaction of B7 and CD28 (Signal 2); (4) $T_H$ cell activated to produce cytokines. Cytotoxic T-cell ($T_C$) activation: (1) Endogenously synthesized (viral or self) proteins are presented on MHC I and recognized by TCR on $T_C$ cell (Signal 1), (2) Interleukin 2 (IL-2) from $T_H$ cell activates $T_C$ cell to kill virus-infected cell (Signal 2).

bridges the immune response to the memory stages, in which certain B cells will have the capability of producing specific immunoglobulins for years.

## Summary

Immune cells and the molecules they express or secrete are significantly interconnected to form a coordinated, efficient immune response to pathogens. These interactions are summarized in Figure 3-14.

## ANERGY AND TOLERANCE

Because T- and B-cell specificity is determined by random recombination events to create a large repertoire of antigen receptors, some developing immune cells react with self-antigen. These cells must be removed by one of the mechanisms discussed below to prevent autoimmune disease.

### T Cells

### Clonal Selection

T cells undergo both positive and negative selection during development (Figure 3-15). **Positive selection** occurs in the cortex of the thymus when T cells bind self-MHC. Positive selection ensures that T cells that do not recognize self-MHC do not survive in the periphery. **Negative selection** occurs next, in the thymic medulla, as T cells that

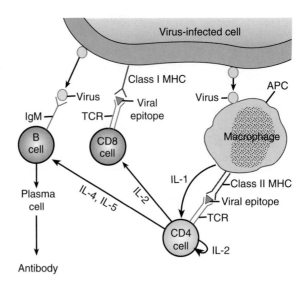

**FIGURE 3-14.** **Immune cell interactions.** APC, antigen-presenting cell; IL, interleukin; MHC, major histocompatibility complex; TCR, T-cell receptor.

react to self-antigens are deleted. T cells then proceed to the periphery. Clonal selection ensures that the mature T-cell population can react with foreign antigen (presented by MHC I and MHC II), but does not react with self-antigen. This is made possible by the autoimmune regulator (AIRE) protein, which allows the thymic epithelial cells to express a wide range of self-antigens that mimic organ-specific antigens.

### Peripheral Tolerance

Inevitably, some self-antigens are expressed at very low levels (or not at all) in the thymus, so that T cells reacting to these antigens do not undergo negative selection. These cells are released to the periphery (Figure 3-16), where they must be controlled through the following processes:

- **Clonal deletion:** A T cell that binds repeatedly (eg, because of a high concentration of self-antigen) undergoes programmed cell death.
- **Anergy:** Anergic T cells recognize self-antigen but remain inactive owing to a lack of the costimulatory molecules (CD80/CD86) required for activation of the T cell.
- **Active suppression:** Self-reactive T cells are kept nonfunctional when self-antigen is presented at low levels. The cells reacting at low levels differentiate into regulatory cells, which secrete regulatory cytokines to prevent other cells from reacting to that antigen. This is the most common mechanism for controlling peripheral T cells. Regulatory T cells (T suppressor cells) are recognized by their coexpression of both CD4 and CD25.
- **Ignorance:** Like any other T cell, if a self-reactive T cell never encounters its antigen, it will die from lack of stimulation.

### B Cells

#### Clonal Deletion

B cells that react with self-antigen can either be deleted or undergo receptor editing of the light chain during their development in the bone marrow. Receptor editing changes the antigen specificity of the cell with the goal of preventing recognition and binding to self-proteins. This receptor-editing event serves as the last chance for the autoreactive B cell to escape deletion. Failing this, the cell is deleted. This process is termed **negative selection.**

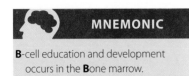

**MNEMONIC**

**B**-cell education and development occurs in the **B**one marrow.
**T**-cell maturation takes place in the **T**hymus.

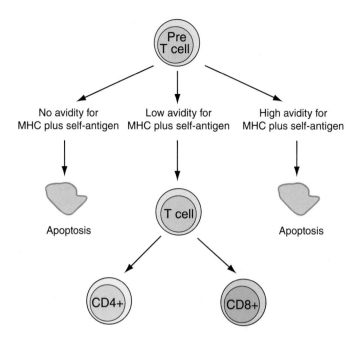

FIGURE 3-15.    **Central T-cell tolerance.** MHC, major histocompatibility complex.

## Anergy

Sometimes self-reactive B cells escape deletion and are accidentally released to the periphery. When these self-reactive cells encounter the antigen they recognize in the absence of costimulatory molecules, they are stimulated to become permanently **anergic.** Costimulatory molecules are activation signals expressed on APCs stimulated by the inflammatory response of the innate immune system (see Figure 3-17).

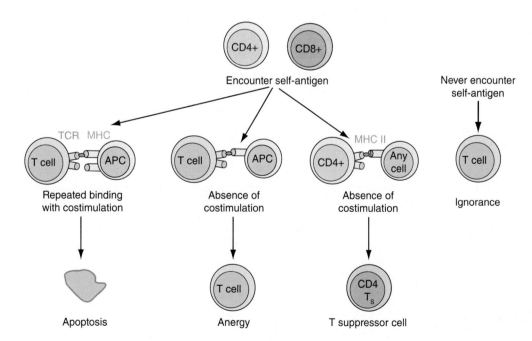

FIGURE 3-16.    **Peripheral T-cell tolerance.** APC, antigen-presenting cell; MHC, major histocompatibility complex; TCR, T-cell receptor.

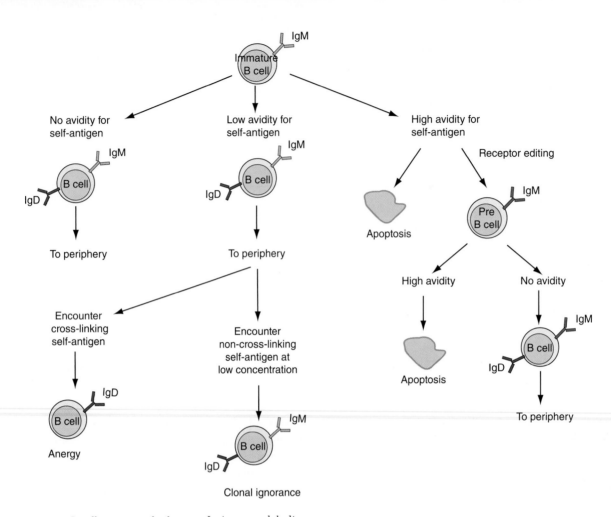

FIGURE 3-17. **B-cell anergy and tolerance.** Ig, immunoglobulin.

## Clonal Ignorance

Some B cells bind only weakly to self-antigen and so escape detection and deletion. These B cells are usually nonfunctional (since their binding is weak), but can become activated if the concentration of their antigen is unusually high.

Anergy and tolerance are very similar in T cells and B cells. Table 3-12 summarizes the key points related to each and allows for comparison between the two.

### IMMUNIZATIONS

An effective vaccine induces sustained, protective immunity in the recipient without causing illness. In general, an effective vaccine must provide several years of protection, although multiple doses (boosters) may be necessary. Effective vaccines stimulate the production of neutralizing antibodies or induce cell-mediated immunity. There are multiple types of vaccines:

- **Killed vaccines** contain inactivated whole organisms or viruses.
- **Live attenuated vaccines** contain live organisms or virus particles that have been altered to reduce pathogenicity.
- **Toxoid vaccines** contain inactivated toxins isolated from the microorganisms that produce them.
- **Recombinant vaccines** contain engineered protein components that can stimulate production of protective antibodies to a pathogen.

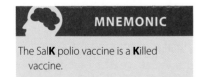

**MNEMONIC**

The Sal**K** polio vaccine is a **K**illed vaccine.

**TABLE 3-12.** **Summary of Anergy and Tolerance in B Cells and T Cells**

|  | REACTION TO ANTIGEN | LOCATION | OUTCOME | REACTIVATION? |
|---|---|---|---|---|
| **T cells** | | | | |
| Clonal selection | Normal signaling | Thymus | Positive and negative selection | —- |
| Clonal deletion | Strong and repeated reaction to self-antigen | Periphery | Cell death | No |
| Anergy | Normal recognition of self-antigen | Periphery | Cell nonfunctional, lack of costimulation | Yes |
| Active suppression | Low-frequency recognition of self-antigen | Periphery | Cell differentiates to a regulatory T cell | No |
| Ignorance | Never encounters self-antigen | Periphery | Cell death from lack of stimulation | No |
| **B cells** | | | | |
| Clonal deletion | Strong reaction to self-antigen | Bone marrow | Light-chain rearrangement or deletion | No |
| Anergy | Strong reaction to self-antigen | Periphery | Cell nonfunctional, lack of costimulation | No |
| Clonal ignorance | Weak reaction to self-antigen | Periphery | Cell nonfunctional, weak binding | Yes |

- **Conjugate vaccines** contain synthetic compounds designed to induce a stronger immune response than the original pathogen or compound. For example, carbohydrates are weakly antigenic, but when combined with a protein fragment, the resulting compound is better able to stimulate the production of protective antibodies.

Population-based vaccination schedules are important. Infants are on a specific vaccine schedule that allows them to gain immunity to protect themselves after the mother's passive immunity wears off. Another important group is pregnant women, who should not receive live vaccines, human papillomavirus (HPV) vaccines, or vaccines for the ToRCHeS (toxoplasmosis, other agents, rubella, cytomegalovirus, herpes simplex) infections. Important vaccines are listed in Table 3-13.

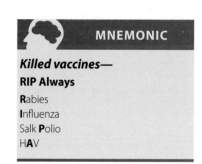

**MNEMONIC**

**Killed vaccines—**

**RIP Always**

**R**abies
**I**nfluenza
Salk **P**olio
H**A**V

## Pathology

### HYPERSENSITIVITY

There are four types of hypersensitivity, as seen in Table 3-14. Types I through III are antibody mediated, whereas type IV is mediated by T cells. The general effector mechanism of all four types is immune-mediated damage to otherwise normal, healthy tissue.

#### Type I: IgE-Mediated

Also called **immediate hypersensitivity,** the type I response can be **anaphylactic** (systemic) or **atopic** (local). After being sensitized to an antigen, the patient experiences an immune response to low concentrations of that same antigen. Free antigen cross-links IgE on presensitized mast cells and basophils, triggering immediate release of vasoactive amines (Figure 3-18). Genetic susceptibility plays a role in this reaction.

#### Pathogenesis

Figure 3-19 outlines the pathogenesis of type I hypersensitivity.

**MNEMONIC**

**For the types of hypersensitivity, remember—**

**ACID**

Type I: **A**topic and **A**naphylactic
Type II: **C**ytotoxic
Type III: **I**mmune Complex
Type IV: **D**elayed

**FLASH FORWARD**

Epinephrine is used to treat anaphylaxis because it rapidly constricts blood vessels.

**TABLE 3-13.    Common Vaccines**

| TYPE OF VACCINE | PREVENTS | PROTECTS FROM |
| --- | --- | --- |
| Killed | Polio[a] | Poliovirus |
| | Rabies | Rhabdovirus |
| | Influenza | An orthomyxovirus |
| | Hepatitis A | Hepatitis A virus (HAV) |
| | Cholera | *Vibrio cholerae* |
| Live attenuated | Measles[b] | A paramyxovirus |
| | Influenza (live attenuated influenza vaccine [LAIV]) (inhaled) | An orthomyxovirus |
| | Mumps[b] | A paramyxovirus |
| | Rubella[b] | A togavirus |
| | Polio[c] | Poliovirus |
| | Chickenpox | Varicella-zoster virus (VZV) |
| | Yellow fever | A flavivirus |
| | Smallpox | A poxvirus |
| | Pharyngitis, pneumonia | Adenovirus |
| | Tuberculosis (BCG)[d] | *Mycobacterium tuberculosis* |
| | Salmonellosis | *Salmonella typhi* |
| | Tularemia | *Francisella tularensis* |
| Toxoid | Diphtheria[e] | *Corynebacterium diphtheriae* |
| | Tetanus[e] | *Clostridium tetani* |
| | Whooping cough[e] | *Bordetella pertussis* |
| Recombinant | Hepatitis B | Hepatitis B virus (HBV) |
| | Cervical cancer | Human papillomavirus (HPV) |
| Conjugate | Meningitis | *Haemophilus influenzae* type b |
| | Meningitis | *Neisseria meningitidis* |
| | Pneumonia | *Streptococcus pneumoniae* |

[a]The Salk intramuscular polio vaccine (IPV) contains inactive poliovirus.

[b]The measles, mumps, and rubella vaccines are often combined (MMR).

[c]The Sabin oral polio vaccine (OPV) contains mutated poliovirus.

[d]The bacillus Calmette-Guérin (BCG) vaccine contains a different strain of the bacteria that causes tuberculosis. This vaccine is not used in the United States but is widely used in other countries.

[e]The diphtheria, tetanus, and pertussis vaccines are often combined (DTP or DTaP).

**TABLE 3-14.    Hypersensitivity**

|  | DESCRIPTION | TEST | HYPERSENSITIVITY DISORDERS | MNEMONIC |
|---|---|---|---|---|
| Type I | Anaphylactic and atopic IgE mediated | Skin test for specific IgE | Allergic and atopic disorders (eg, rhinitis, hay fever, eczema, hives, asthma) <br> Anaphylaxis (eg, bee sting, some food/drug allergies) | **1st** and fast |
| Type II | Cytotoxic IgM and IgG mediated | Direct and indirect Coombs tests | Acute hemolytic transfusion reactions <br> Autoimmune hemolytic anemia <br> Bullous pemphigoid <br> Erythroblastosis fetalis <br> Goodpasture syndrome <br> Graves disease <br> Guillain-Barré syndrome <br> Idiopathic thrombocytopenic purpura <br> Myasthenia gravis <br> Pemphigus vulgaris <br> Pernicious anemia <br> Rheumatic fever | Cy-**2**-toxic |
| Type III | Immune complex | Immunofluorescent staining | Arthus reaction <br> SLE <br> Polyarteritis nodosa <br> Poststreptococcal glomerulonephritis <br> Serum sickness | **3** things in an immune complex: antigen, antibody, complement |
| Type IV | Cell mediated (delayed type) | Patch test, PPD | Contact dermatitis (eg, poison ivy, nickel allergy) <br> Graft-versus-host disease <br> Multiple sclerosis | **4th** and last <br> **4 Ts** = **T** lymphocytes, **T**ransplant rejections, **T**B tests, **T**ouching (contact dermatitis) |

PPD, purified protein derivative (test for *Mycobacterium tuberculosis*); SLE, systemic lupus erythematosus.

Common manifestations include urticaria, allergic rhinitis, and asthma. All three are characterized by local effects, and patients generally have consistently high circulating levels of IgE.

**Urticaria,** or hives, is the mildest form of atopy. Histamine release causes vasodilation and a visible wheal and flare.

**Allergic rhinitis** and **asthma** result from inhalation of allergens. This can cause inflammation of either the nasal mucosa, leading to rhinitis, or the lower bronchi, resulting in bronchial constriction and air trapping (asthma).

**Anaphylaxis** is the most severe form of type I hypersensitivity. It occurs when vasoactive amines (ie, histamine) are released systemically. Widespread vasodilation and increased vessel permeability can result in hypotension and shock, accompanied by bronchoconstriction.

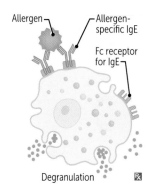

**FIGURE 3-18.    Type I hypersensitivity.** Free antigen cross-links IgE on mast cells and basophils, resulting in release of vasoactive amines.

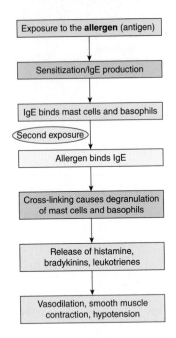

**FIGURE 3-19.    Pathogenesis of type I hypersensitivity.**

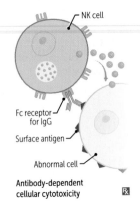

**FIGURE 3-20.    Type II hypersensitivity.** IgM and IgG bind to fixed antigen on the cell surface, resulting in cellular destruction.

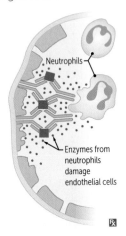

**FIGURE 3-21.    Type III hypersensitivity.** Antigen-antibody (IgG) complexes active complement, resulting in neutrophil attraction.

### Type II: Antibody-Mediated (Cytotoxic)

Antibody-mediated hypersensitivity occurs when antibodies are directed to fixed antigens on cell surfaces (Figure 3-20).

#### Pathogenesis

- Circulating antibody binds to an antigen on the pathogen.
- Complement is activated.
- Outcomes include:
    - Opsonization, followed by phagocytosis.
    - **ADCC.**
    - Cell death mediated by NK or T cells.
    - Immune response-mediated damage to healthy tissue.

Incompatible **blood transfusions** are a common example. The recipient has preformed antibodies to the donor's major RBC antigens, resulting in rapid destruction of the infused RBCs.

**Erythroblastosis fetalis** (hemolytic disease of the newborn) results from an Rh mismatch between mother and fetus. Rh– mothers exposed to fetal Rh+ blood (often during delivery) may make Rh antibodies. In subsequent pregnancies, anti-Rh IgG can cross the placenta and attack fetal Rh+ erythrocytes. Bilirubin, a byproduct of RBC destruction, can accumulate in the brain of the newborn, causing kernicterus. The mother is treated with anti-Rh IgG antibody (RhoGAM) at first delivery. RhoGAM binds fetal Rh+ erythrocytes, thus removing them from circulation before the mother's immune system can mount an anti-Rh response.

**Goodpasture syndrome** is caused by antibodies to the glomerular basement membrane (anti-GBM) and the alveolar basement membrane, which bind to type IV collagen. Antibodies form complexes in the kidneys and lungs, resulting in glomerulonephritis and pulmonary hemorrhage.

### Type III: Immune Complex-Mediated

Soluble antigen-antibody complexes form when antigen is abundant. Complex deposition in tissues causes type III hypersensitivity (Figure 3-21).

#### Pathogenesis

- Clearance of infections creates antigen-antibody complexes.
- Normally, the complexes aggregate into clusters that activate the complement system, which triggers an inflammatory response to clear the infection.
- Certain smaller complexes escape detection and are deposited in membranes and the walls of blood vessels. They accumulate on the endothelium and synovium of joints, leading to:
    - Complement activation resulting in tissue inflammation, which manifests as vasculitis (endothelium) or arthritis (synovium).
    - Chemotaxis of neutrophils that cause significant tissue damage or arthritis.

**Systemic lupus erythematosus (SLE)** is associated with antibodies to self-proteins known as antinuclear antibodies (**ANAs**). Kidney disease is a major consequence of SLE because the immune complexes are deposited in the glomerulus and cause inflammation and tissue damage.

**Serum sickness** occurs when serum or antibodies, such as horse antivenom for a snakebite victim, are administered to a patient. Approximately 1 week (5–10 days) following the treatment, antibodies are formed to the foreign proteins, leading to lymphadenopathy and systemic inflammatory symptoms such as fever, arthralgias, proteinuria, and urticarial plaques.

The **Arthus reaction** is a local swelling at the site of intradermal injection of an antigen to which the patient has been immunized. Antigen-antibody complexes form in the skin. The reaction occurs quickly and can be cleared within 24 hours. It is now most often seen at the site of desensitization allergy shots.

### Type IV: Cell-Mediated (Delayed Type)

T cells are primed as effector cells specific to intracellular antigens or aberrant cells (foreign or mutated) (Figure 3-22).

#### Pathogenesis

- Exposure to antigen or infection causes production of memory immune cells, among them effector T cells.
- On repeated exposure, effector T cells proliferate and activate a macrophage response to clear the infection (Figure 3-23). This process generally takes 1–2 days.

The **tuberculin skin test** uses hypersensitivity to determine whether a person has been previously exposed to *Mycobacterium tuberculosis*. Tuberculin purified protein derivative (**PPD**) is injected in the skin. If a T cell has been previously sensitized to the PPD antigen, its proliferation results in erythematous induration at the site of injection. It is important to note that with certain T-cell immunodeficiencies (ie, HIV), induration may not be seen despite previous exposure.

**Contact dermatitis** results from a similar reaction, except that the T cells are sensitized to topical antigens from poison ivy. These reactions generally involve both CD4+ and CD8+ T cells and can be as widespread as the area of contact. Exposure to a large volume of antigen increases the magnitude of the immune response, which consequently can cause severe local tissue damage, and in some cases, systemic responses.

### IMMUNODEFICIENCY

#### B-Cell Deficiencies

##### X-Linked (Bruton) Agammaglobulinemia

An X-linked recessive defect in Bruton tyrosine kinase (Btk), which functions in B-cell differentiation, maturation, and signaling. B cells fail to develop normally past the pre-B-cell stage, resulting in low levels of all classes of immunoglobulins after 6 months of age.

**FLASH FORWARD**

The most common cause of death in SLE is diffuse proliferative glomerulonephritis (DPGN).

**KEY FACT**

Most serum sickness is now caused by drugs (not serum) acting as haptens. Serum sickness is more common than Arthus reaction.

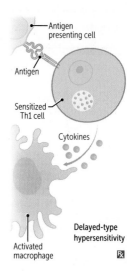

**FIGURE 3-22.** **Type IV hypersensitivity.** Sensitized T cells encounter antigens and release cytokines, resulting in macrophage activation.

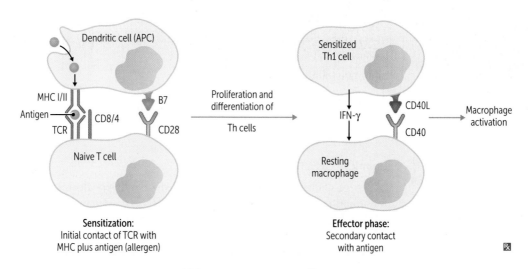

**FIGURE 3-23.** **Delayed-type hypersensitivity.** APC, antigen-presenting cell; IFN-γ, interferon gamma; TCR, T-cell receptor; Th, T helper cell.

### Presentation

Recurrent extracellular pyogenic and enterovirus infections.

### Diagnosis

B cells are absent on peripheral smear, immunoglobulin levels are low to undetectable, and the patient lacks tonsils. Lymph node biopsy showing lack of germinal centers is confirmatory.

### Treatment

Intravenous immunoglobulin (IVIG) from adult donors.

## Dysgammaglobulinemia (Selective Immunoglobulin Deficiency)

Lack of any immunoglobulin class due to defective B-cell class switching or activation. IgA deficiency is the most common primary immunodeficiency, affecting as many as 1 in 600 people. Affected individuals have decreased mucosal immunity and potentially increased susceptibility to autoimmune disease.

### Presentation

Often asymptomatic and diagnosed incidentally in patients with chronic lung disease. Common associated conditions include milk allergy, diarrhea, and chronic sinus infections.

### Diagnosis

Decreased serum titers of IgA, with normal IgG and IgM levels.

### Treatment

Antibiotics are given to symptomatic patients to help clear infections.

## Common Variable Immunodeficiency

B-cell differentiation defect that can be acquired at 20–30 years of age.

### Presentation

Affected individuals have an increased risk of autoimmune disease, bronchiectasis, lymphoma, and sinopulmonary infections.

### Diagnosis

Decreased plasma cells and immunoglobulins.

### Treatment

Immune globulin replacement.

See Table 3-15 for a summary of B-cell-related immunodeficiencies.

### T-Cell Deficiencies

## Thymic Aplasia (DiGeorge Syndrome)

DiGeorge syndrome is characterized by the triad of hypocalcemia (tetany), conotruncal abnormalities, and T-cell deficiency. The defect is caused by defective formation of the third and fourth pharyngeal pouches early in gestation. Thymic aplasia is associated with 22q11 chromosomal microdeletions. The syndrome results in a nondeveloping thymus and a lack of parathyroid glands, which cause T-cell and calcium deficiencies, respectively.

**TABLE 3-15.** Summary of B-Cell Immunodeficiency Syndromes

|  | DEFECT | PRESENTATION |
|---|---|---|
| X-linked (**B**ruton) agammaglobulinemia | Loss of Btk tyrosine kinase leads to complete absence of B cells | Recurrent bacterial and enteroviral infections after 6 months of age |
| Dysgammaglobulinemia (Selective immunoglobulin deficiency) | Defective class switching leads to decrease of immunoglobulin, most commonly Ig**A** | Sinopulmonary infections, GI infections, autoimmune disease, atopy, anaphylaxis |
| Common variable immunodeficiency (CVID) | Defect in B cell differentiation | Sinopulmonary infections, increased risk of autoimmune disease |

Btk, Bruton tyrosine kinase; GI, gastrointestinal; IgA, immunoglobulin A.

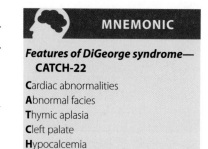

**MNEMONIC**

*Features of DiGeorge syndrome—* CATCH-22
**C**ardiac abnormalities
**A**bnormal facies
**T**hymic aplasia
**C**left palate
**H**ypocalcemia
Chromosome **22**q11

### Presentation

Neonatal tetany and recurrent opportunistic viral and fungal infections. Infants often also show facial abnormalities (velocardiofacial syndrome [VCFS]), or cardiac malformations (tetralogy of Fallot, truncus arteriosus), or both.

### Diagnosis

Patients generally present with **cyanosis** or **tetany** due to cardiac disease or hypocalcemia, respectively. Fluorescent in situ hybridization can be used to detect the 22q11 chromosomal deletion. Chest radiographs show absent or greatly reduced thymic shadow. Low to undetectable circulating T cells are seen, as well as low circulating levels of immunoglobulin (due to lack of B-cell activation by T cells), parathyroid hormone (PTH), and $Ca^{2+}$.

### Treatment

If the patient possesses any fragments of thymus, immunomodulatory agents can be given to stimulate thymic growth. If not, fetal thymic transplantation can be performed if the patient remains symptomatic.

### IL-12 Receptor Deficiency

An autosomal recessive disorder that is characterized by decreased T-cell differentiation, resulting in a diminished Th1 response.

### Presentation

Disseminated mycobacterial and fungal infections. May present after BCG vaccine.

### Diagnosis

Decreased levels of IFN-γ.

### Autosomal Dominant Hyper-IgE Syndrome (Job Syndrome)

Deficiency of Th17 cells due to *STAT3* mutation. Affected individuals have impaired recruitment of neutrophils to sites of infection.

### Presentation

Coarse facies, staphylococcal abscesses without inflammation, retained primary teeth, and eczema.

### Diagnosis

Increased levels of IgE and decreased levels of IFN-γ.

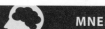

**MNEMONIC**

The features of **hyper-IgE (Job) syndrome** can be remembered by the mnemonic **FATED:**
**F**acies (coarse)
**A**bscesses (staphylococcal)
**T**eeth (retain primary teeth)
Ig**E** elevated
**D**ermatologic problems (eczema)

**QUESTION 1**

A 35-year-old woman presents with rapidly progressive symmetric ascending muscle weakness. Weakness began in the feet and migrated toward the trunk. She has just recovered from a GI infection. What is the most likely diagnosis? What type of hypersensitivity disorder is this syndrome?

**QUESTION 2**

A 55-year-old HIV-positive man is found to have bilateral ground-glass opacities on x-ray of his chest (CXR). Silver stain of lung tissue shows disk-shaped yeast. What is the most likely diagnosis? At what CD4+ T-cell count should HIV patients begin prophylaxis?

### Chronic Mucocutaneous Candidiasis

A selective lack of T-cell reactivity to *Candida* species.

#### Presentation

Recurrent *Candida albicans* infections on skin and mucosal areas.

#### Diagnosis

Laboratory studies show normal levels and functioning of both B and T cells. Diagnosis is made on highly specific T-cell challenge, which shows an absent T-cell response to *Candida* antigens.

#### Treatment

Antimycotic agents can aid the patient in clearing the infection, but avoidance of potential sources of infection is more effective.

### Acquired Immunodeficiency Syndrome

AIDS is the sequela of infection with HIV, which directly infects and kills CD4+ helper T cells. This immunosuppression manifests as a loss of cell-mediated immunity and can lead to opportunistic infections (Table 3-16) and malignancies. HIV and AIDS are discussed in greater detail in Chapter 4 (Microbiology).

#### Presentation

General wasting and constitutional symptoms (fever, weight loss, etc). Affected individuals also have increased occurrence of opportunistic infections and rare malignancies, such as the viral-mediated Kaposi sarcoma.

#### Diagnosis

HIV seropositivity is initially determined by enzyme-linked immunosorbent assay (**ELISA**) (highly sensitive) and then confirmed with Western blot (highly specific). A low peripheral blood CD4+ T-cell count is an indicator that an HIV-positive patient is progressing to AIDS.

#### Treatment

Control viral replication with highly active antiretroviral therapy (**HAART**) including reverse-transcriptase inhibitors or protease inhibitors (or both). Treat infections with appropriate antibiotics. Broad-spectrum antibiotics are often given prophylactically to decrease the occurrence of opportunistic infections.

See Table 3-17 for a summary of T-cell–related immunodeficiencies.

### Combined Deficiencies

### Severe Combined Immunodeficiency

A class of inherited disorders that leads to malfunctioning of both B and T cells. Enzyme deficiencies in **adenosine deaminase (ADA)** or purine nucleotide phosphorylase can cause accumulation of toxic metabolites in the purine degradation pathways of lymphocytes. **X-linked severe combined immunodeficiency (SCID)** is the most common and results from a defect in the **common gamma chain (IL-2R),** which is shared by many cytokine receptors. In the absence of treatment, death occurs within 1 year of birth.

#### Presentation

Failure to thrive, diarrhea, thrush, and chronic infections (of all types) in an infant with low lymphocyte counts.

**KEY FACT**

Trimethoprim-sulfamethoxazole (TMP-SMX) is administered to HIV patients as prophylaxis against *Pneumocystis jirovecii* infection (CD4+ count < 200 cells/mm$^3$). Azithromycin is administered for prophylaxis against *Mycobacterium avium* complex infection (CD4+ count < 50 cells/mm$^3$).

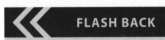

**FLASH BACK**

Adenosine deaminase deficiency causes a build up of adenosine triphosphate (ATP) and deoxyadenosine triphosphate (dATP). Feedback inhibition of ribonucleotide reductase prevents DNA synthesis.

**ANSWER 1**

The patient is demonstrating symptoms of Guillain-Barré syndrome (acute inflammatory demyelinating polyradiculopathy). This is a type II hypersensitivity disorder.

**ANSWER 2**

The most likely diagnosis is Pneumocystis pneumonia from a *Pneumocystis jirovecii* infection. Start prophylaxis (TMP-SMX) when CD4+ T cell count drops to < 200 cells/mm$^3$ in HIV patients.

**TABLE 3-16.** **Common Opportunistic Infections in Untreated AIDS Patients**

| | PATHOGEN | PRESENTATION | FINDINGS | CD4 COUNT |
|---|---|---|---|---|
| **Protozoa** | *Cryptosporidium* spp | Chronic, watery diarrhea | Acid-fast oocysts in stool | < 500 cells/mm$^3$ |
| | *T gondii* | Brain abscesses | Multiple ring-enhancing lesions on MRI | < 200 cells/mm3 |
| **Fungi** | *A fumigatus* | Hemoptysis, pleuritic pain | Cavitation or infiltrates on chest imaging | < 100 cells/mm$^3$ |
| | *C albicans* | Oral thrush | Scrapable white plaque, pseudohyphae on microscopy | < 500 cells/mm$^3$ |
| | *C neoformans* | Meningitis | Thickly encapsulated yeast on India ink stain | < 100 cells/mm$^3$ |
| | *H capsulatum* | Fever, weight loss, fatigue, cough, dyspnea, nausea, vomiting, diarrhea | Oval yeast cells within macrophages | < 100 cells/mm$^3$ |
| | *P jirovecii* | *Pneumocystis* pneumonia | "Ground-glass" opacities on CXR | < 200 cells/mm$^3$ |
| **Bacteria** | *B henselae* | Bacillary angiomatosis | Biopsy with neutrophilic inflammation | < 500 cells/mm$^3$ |
| | *L monocytogenes* | Meningitis | | |
| | *M avium-intracellulare, M avium* complex | Nonspecific systemic symptoms (fever, night sweats, weight loss) or focal lymphadenitis | | < 100 cells/mm$^3$ |
| | *M tuberculosis* | Tuberculosis symptoms (fever, night sweats, weight loss, nonproductive or productive cough, hemoptysis) | | |
| | *N asteroides* | Pulmonary infections | | |
| **Viruses** | Cytomegalovirus | Retinitis, esophagitis, colitis, pneumonitis, encephalitis | Linear ulcers on endoscopy, cotton-wool spots on fundoscopy / Biopsy reveals cells with intranuclear (owl eye) inclusion bodies | < 100 cells/mm$^3$ |
| | Epstein-Barr virus | Oral hairy leukoplakia | Unscrapable white plaque on lateral tongue | < 500 cells/mm$^3$ |
| | | B-cell lymphoma (eg, non-Hodgkin lymphoma, CNS lymphoma) | CNS lymphoma—ring enhancing, may be solitary (vs *Toxoplasma*) | < 100 cells/mm$^3$ |
| | HHV-8 | Kaposi sarcoma | Biopsy with lymphocytic inflammation | < 500 cells/mm$^3$ |
| | HIV | Dementia | | < 200 cells/mm$^3$ |
| | HPV | Squamous cell carcinoma, commonly of anus (men who have sex with men) or cervix (women) | | < 500 cells/mm$^3$ |
| | JC virus (reactivation) | Progressive multifocal leukoencephalopathy | Nonenhancing areas of demyelination on MRI | < 200 cells/mm$^3$ |
| | Varicella zoster virus | Shingles | | |

CXR, chest X-ray; HHV-8, human herpesvirus 8; HIV, human immunodeficiency virus; HPV, human papillomavirus; JC, John Cunningham (a human polyomavirus).

**TABLE 3-17.** **Summary of T-Cell Immunodeficiency Syndromes**

| | DEFECT | PRESENTATION |
|---|---|---|
| Thymic aplasia (DiGeorge syndrome) | Defective formation of 3rd and 4th pharyngeal pouches. 22q11 deletion | Cyanosis and/or tetany and absence of thymic shadow on CXR |
| IL-12 receptor deficiency | Decreased Th1 response (autosomal recessive) | Disseminated mycobacterial infections |
| Autosomal dominant hyper-IgE syndrome (Job syndrome) | Impaired recruitment of neutrophils to infection sites | Coarse facies, cold staph abscesses, retained primary teeth, elevated IgE, eczema |
| Chronic mucocutaneous candidiasis | T-cell dysfunction | Recurrent *Candida* infections |
| AIDS | HIV-induced depletion of CD4+ T cells | Opportunistic infections (see Table 3-16) |

CXR, x-ray of the chest; IgE, immunoglobulin E; IL, interleukin; staph, staphylococcal.

### Diagnosis

Flow cytometry indicating lack of lymphocytes, CXR showing absence of thymic shadow, and lymph node biopsy indicating germinal centers. More specific diagnosis is made by gene mutation analysis.

### Treatment

Bone marrow transplantation, prophylactic antibiotics. There are also several experimental gene therapy treatments for SCID that utilize viral-mediated delivery of the defective gene to bone marrow cells.

## Wiskott-Aldrich Syndrome

An X-linked defect occurs in Wiskott-Aldrich syndrome protein (WASP), causing cellular defects in the actin cytoskeleton. This affects all hematopoietic cells, especially platelets and T cells. T cells lose the ability to stimulate B cells in response to capsular polysaccharides present on some bacteria. Without treatment, most patients do not live beyond adolescence.

### Presentation

Pyogenic infections, bleeding diathesis, and eczema. Affected individuals also have an increased incidence of autoimmune disorders and lymphoma.

### Diagnosis

Low to normal levels of IgG and IgM, with elevated levels of IgE and IgA, abnormally small platelets on peripheral smear.

### Treatment

Bone marrow transplantation.

## Hyper-IgM Syndrome

This syndrome is caused by an X-linked defect in T-cell CD40-ligand. The CD40-CD40 ligand interaction is required for full activation of B cells as well as antibody class switching.

### Presentation

Recurrent bacterial infections. Opportunistic infection with *Pneumocystis*, *Cryptosporidium*, or cytomegalovirus (CMV). Individuals may also have increased susceptibility to autoimmune disorders or lymphoma.

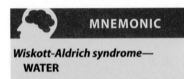

**MNEMONIC**

***Wiskott-Aldrich syndrome—*
WATER**

**W**iskott-**A**ldrich: **T**hrombocytopenic purpura, **E**czema, **R**ecurrent infections

### Diagnosis

Serum antibody titers reveal increased IgM and decreased IgA, IgG, and IgE.

### Treatment

Bone marrow transplantation. If no donor, immune function is augmented with IVIG and the administration of appropriate antibiotics to treat infections.

## Ataxia-Telangiectasia

Ataxia-telangiectasia is an autosomal recessive defect in the ataxia-telangiectasia mutated (ATM) protein that leads to insufficient cellular responses to DNA damage, including failure to repair double strand breaks. Lymphocytes are targeted because of high rates of proliferation and the need to rapidly divide. It is associated with IgA deficiency and malignancies. Most patients die of infections, cancer, or advanced neurodegenerative disease in their mid-20s.

### Presentation

Cerebellar ataxia and oculocutaneous telangiectasias in early childhood; increased susceptibility to mucosal infections.

### Diagnosis

Genetic defects on both alleles of *ATM* and clinical presentation, including lymphopenia, cerebellar atrophy, and increased α-fetoprotein (AFP). Serum antibody titers reveal decreased IgA, IgG, and IgE.

### Treatment

Antibiotics for infection.

See Table 3-18 for a summary of the combined immunodeficiencies.

## Phagocyte Deficiencies

The major phagocyte deficiency syndromes are summarized in Table 3-19.

## Leukocyte Adhesion Deficiency Syndrome (Type 1)

This syndrome occurs due to an autosomal recessive mutation in the lymphocyte function-associated antigen 1 (LFA-1) integrin (CD18) protein on phagocytes, which is responsible for phagocyte binding to endothelium. This prevents phagocytic infiltration at the site of infection or injury.

**TABLE 3-18. Summary of Combined Immunodeficiency Syndromes**

| | DEFECT | PRESENTATION |
|---|---|---|
| Severe combined immunodeficiency (SCID) | IL-2R gamma chain defect (X-linked), adenosine deaminase deficiency (autosomal recessive) | Failure to thrive, chronic diarrhea, recurrent infections, absent thymic shadow |
| Wiskott-Aldrich syndrome | X-linked defect in *WASP* gene | Pyogenic infections, bleeding diathesis, eczema |
| Hyper-IgM syndrome | X-linked defect in T-cell CD40 ligand | Early pyogenic infections |
| Ataxia-telangiectasia | Defects in *ATM* gene involved in DNA repair | Ataxia, spider angiomas, IgA deficiency |

IgA, immunoglobulin A; IgM, immunoglobulin M; IL, interleukin.

### Presentation

Increased frequency of bacterial infections in the first year of life with an absence of pus and impaired wound healing. Often preceded by delayed separation of the umbilical cord (> 30 days).

### Diagnosis

Leukocytosis, flow cytometric analysis of integrins, or phagocyte functional studies.

### Treatment

Bone marrow transplantation is the only treatment with documented benefit. Other options include prophylactic administration of antibiotics and regular leukocyte transfusions.

## Chronic Granulomatous Disease

Chronic granulomatous disease (CGD) is caused by a defective reduced nicotinamide adenine dinucleotide phosphate (NADPH) oxidase system (mutation in any of the four enzymes). It impairs the production of reactive oxygen intermediates required for the killing of phagocytosed pathogens. As a result, phagocytes can internalize bacteria but are unable to kill certain classes. This malfunction causes accumulations of immune cells in granulomas, which form at the site of infection.

### Presentation

Severe infections with catalase-positive bacteria (eg, *Staphylococcus aureus, Escherichia coli, Aspergillus*) or fungal infections, especially of the skin; hepatosplenomegaly; and lymphadenopathy.

### Diagnosis

Abnormal dihydrorhodamine (flow cytometry) test and negative nitroblue tetrazolium dye reduction test. The specific defect is determined by genetic testing.

### Treatment

Bone marrow transplantation can be curative. IFN-γ and prophylactic antibiotics are the current standard of care.

## Chédiak-Higashi Syndrome

This autosomal recessive mutation in lysosomal trafficking regulator (LYST) causes a failure of vesicle fusion in neutrophils (impaired phagosome-lysosome fusion), platelets, and melanocytes, among others.

### Presentation

Recurrent infections (especially *Streptococcus* and *Staphylococcus*), hair with a silvery metallic sheen, diffuse hypopigmentation of the skin with occasional acral (ears, nose) hyperpigmentation, prolonged bleeding times, and widespread lymphoproliferation. Peripheral neuropathy may also be seen.

### Diagnosis

Microscopic analysis of peripheral blood shows large granules in leukocytic cells (Figure 3-24).

### Treatment

Bone marrow transplantation ameliorates all symptoms except peripheral neuropathy. See Table 3-19 for a summary of phagocyte immunodeficiencies.

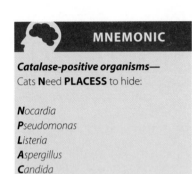

**MNEMONIC**

***Catalase-positive organisms—***
Cats **N**eed **PLACESS** to hide:

**N**ocardia
**P**seudomonas
**L**isteria
**A**spergillus
**C**andida
**E** coli
**S** aureus
**S**erratia

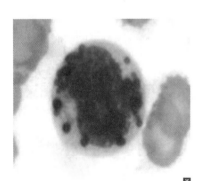

**FIGURE 3-24.** **Granulocytes in Chédiak-Higashi syndrome.** Granulocytes with giant granules are a hallmark of Chédiak-Higashi syndrome.

**TABLE 3-19.** **Summary of Major Phagocyte Deficiency Syndromes**

|  | DEFECT | PRESENTATION | TREATMENT |
|---|---|---|---|
| Leukocyte adhesion deficiency (type 1) | Autosomal recessive defect in LFA-1 | Recurrent pyogenic infections, delayed wound healing, absence of pus | Bone marrow transplantation |
| Chronic granulomatous disease | Mutation in any of 4 NADPH oxidase enzymes | Catalase + bacterial infections | |
| Chédiak-Higashi disease | Autosomal recessive mutation in LYST | Recurrent infections, partial albinism | |

LFA-1, lymphocyte function-associated antigen 1; LYST, lysosomal trafficking regulator; NADPH, reduced nicotinamide adenine dinucleotide phosphate.

## AUTOANTIBODIES AND ASSOCIATIONS

Although autoimmune disease is discussed in detail in the Pathology section, it is important to note key autoantibody associations, as found in Table 3-20.

## HLA ASSOCIATIONS

HLA associations are important when considering familial inheritance of disease or disease susceptibility. Table 3-21 lists important HLA-linked disorders.

## GENERAL AUTOIMMUNE PATHOLOGY

Under ordinary circumstances, the body is able to distinguish between its own normal cells and abnormal cells, or in other words, self and nonself. Immature B cells that strongly react to self-antigens in the bone marrow are either destroyed or undergo alteration of receptor specificity. Mature B lymphocytes encounter high concentrations of self-antigens in the peripheral lymphoid tissues, learn to recognize these antigens and do not mount immune responses against them. If these natural mechanisms of immunologic tolerance to self fail, then autoimmune pathology may develop. This development can be influenced by a number of factors, including genetics and infections.

Genes may predispose individuals to particular autoimmune diseases. **HLA genes** are an important type of gene frequently associated with autoimmunity. Individuals who inherit certain HLA alleles are at an increased risk of developing certain autoimmune diseases. However, autoimmune diseases are not *caused* by HLA alleles, and the majority of patients with a particular disease allele never develop that disease. The exact mechanism of autoimmunity is frequently unknown, but it has been hypothesized that particular HLA alleles may be inefficient at displaying self-antigens or may fail to stimulate T-cell regulation. Non-HLA genes may also be associated with particular autoimmune diseases.

**Infections** may activate self-reactive lymphocytes, leading to an autoimmune response, via the following mechanisms: (a) Infections may induce local immune responses and promote the survival of self-reactive T lymphocytes, (b) infections may injure tissues and release self-antigens that are normally isolated from the immune system, or (c) infectious organisms may produce peptides that are similar to self-antigens and trigger an autoimmune response via cross-reactivity (**molecular mimicry**).

**MNEMONIC**

***Antibodies that cross the placenta—***
**TAP D3**

Anti–**T**hyroid stimulating hormone (TSH)
Anti–**A**cetylcholine (ACh), Anti–**P**latelet
Anti–**D**esmoglein-**3**

**MNEMONIC**

Causes of a **false-positive Venereal Disease Research Laboratory (VDRL) test** for syphilis can be summed up by the mnemonic **VDRL:**

**V**iruses, **D**rugs, **R**heumatic fever, **L**upus and **L**eprosy

**TABLE 3-20.** **Autoantibodies and Their Associations**

| ANTIBODY | DISEASE |
| --- | --- |
| Anti-ACh receptor | Myasthenia gravis |
| Anti-basement membrane | Goodpasture syndrome |
| Anticardiolipin, lupus anticoagulant | SLE, antiphospholipid syndrome |
| Anticentromere | Limited scleroderma (CREST syndrome) |
| Antidesmin | Crohn disease |
| Anti-desmosome (anti-desmoglein) | Pemphigus vulgaris |
| Anti-dsDNA, anti-Smith | SLE |
| Anti-glutamic acid decarboxylase (GAD-65) | Type 1 diabetes mellitus |
| Antihemidesmosome | Bullous pemphigoid |
| Anti-histone | Drug-induced lupus |
| Anti-Jo-1, anti-SRP, anti-Mi-2 | Polymyositis, dermatomyositis |
| Antimicrosomal, antithyroglobulin | Hashimoto thyroiditis |
| Antimitochondrial | 1° biliary cirrhosis |
| Antimyelin | Multiple sclerosis |
| Antinuclear antibodies | SLE, nonspecific |
| Antiparietal cell, anti-intrinsic factor | Pernicious anemia |
| Antiplatelet | Thrombocytopenic purpura |
| Anti-RBC | Autoimmune hemolytic anemia |
| Anti-Scl-70 (anti-DNA topoisomerase I) | Scleroderma (diffuse) |
| Anti-smooth muscle | Autoimmune hepatitis |
| Anti-SSA, anti-SSB (anti-Ro, anti-La) | Sjögren syndrome |
| Anti-TSH receptor | Graves disease |
| Anti-U1 RNP | Mixed connective tissue disease |
| IgA anti-endomysial, IgA anti-tissue transglutaminase, antigliadin | Celiac disease |
| MPO-ANCA/p-ANCA | Microscopic polyangiitis, eosinophilic granulomatosis with polyangiitis (Churg-Strauss syndrome) |
| PR3-ANCA/c-ANCA | Granulomatosis with polyangiitis (Wegener) |
| Rheumatoid factor (IgM antibody that targets IgG Fc region), anti-CCP (more specific) | Rheumatoid arthritis |

ACh, acetylcholine; ANCA, antineutrophil cytoplasmic antibody; CCP, complement control protein; RNP, ribonucleoprotein; SLE, systemic lupus erythematosus; SRP, signal recognition protein; SSA/SSB, Sjögren syndrome-related antigen A/B; TSH, thyroid-stimulating hormone.

**TABLE 3-21.    HLA Subtypes Associated with Diseases**

| HLA TYPE | ASSOCIATED DISEASE | MNEMONIC |
|---|---|---|
| A1 | Graves disease, dermatitis herpetiformis | |
| A3 | Hemochromatosis | |
| B8 | Graves disease, celiac disease, autoimmune hepatitis, primary sclerosing cholangitis, dermatitis herpetiformis | |
| B27 | **P**soriatic arthritis, **A**nkylosing spondylitis, arthritis of **I**nflammatory bowel disease, **R**eactive arthritis (formerly Reiter syndrome) | **PAIR**. Also known as seronegative arthropathies |
| DQ2/ DQ8 | Celiac disease | |
| DR2 | Multiple sclerosis, hay fever, SLE, Goodpasture syndrome | |
| DR3 | Diabetes mellitus type 1, SLE, Graves disease, Hashimoto thyroiditis | |
| DR4 | **Rheu**matoid arthritis, diabetes mellitus type 1 | There are **4** walls in a "rheum" (room) |
| DR5 | Pernicious anemia (vitamin B deficiency), Hashimoto thyroiditis | |
| DR7 | Steroid-responsive nephrotic syndrome | |
| DR8 | Primary biliary cirrhosis | |

SLE, systemic lupus erythematosus.

## SYSTEMIC AUTOIMMUNE DISEASES

### Systemic Lupus Erythematosus

SLE is a chronic inflammatory autoimmune disorder characterized by immunologic abnormalities, such as the presence of **ANAs**. ANAs are polyclonal IgG, IgM, and IgA autoantibodies that are reactive with antigens in the cell nucleus. They are not organ-specific and are not cytotoxic to intact, viable cells. However, they are deposited as immune complexes, thus triggering inflammatory changes and tissue damage. ANAs are found in the serum of patients with SLE, but they may also be seen with other autoimmune disorders, such as rheumatoid arthritis (RA) and systemic sclerosis. Ninety percent of patients with SLE are females between the ages of 14 and 45. The disease is most common and severe in black females.

### Presentation

Many manifestations of SLE are possible. Symptoms often wax and wane over time. Rash, joint pain, and fever are the most common complaints. The arthritis associated with SLE is symmetrical and affects the small joints of the hands, feet, wrists, knees, and elbows. Other common findings in this disease can include:

- **Malar rash,** butterfly-shaped erythematous patches or plaques on the cheeks, as shown in Figure 3-25.
- **Discoid rash,** erythematous plaques with overlying hyperkeratosis and scale, often leading to atrophic scarring.
- **Nephritis** (occurring in one-half of all patients), which can lead to nephritic syndrome (DPGN) or nephrotic syndrome (membranous glomerulonephritis), renal failure, and death. As the renal disease progresses, a "wire loop" pattern, characteristic of DPGN and caused by the thickening of the capillaries, can be seen on biopsy.

**KEY FACT**

Lupus nephritis is a type III hypersensitivity disorder. Immune complexes consist of soluble antigen, antibody, and complement.

**KEY FACT**

The presence of antiphospholipid antibodies in patients with SLE may result in false-positive results on syphilis tests (rapid plasma reagin [RPR] and VDRL).

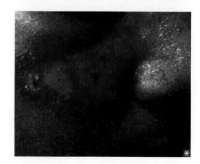

**FIGURE 3-25.    Malar rash.** Butterfly-shaped rash in young woman with systemic lupus erythematosus.

- **Hematologic abnormalities,** such as anemia (due to both chronic disease and circulating anti-RBC antibodies), thrombocytopenia (due to antiplatelet antibodies), and recurrent thromboses (particularly in association with antiphospholipid syndrome).
- **Cardiac manifestations,** such as pericarditis, myocarditis, valvulitis, or characteristic vegetations affecting both sides of cardiac valves (**Libman-Sacks endocarditis**).
- **Neurologic disturbances,** such as strokes and seizures.
- **Pulmonary abnormalities,** such as fibrosis and pulmonary hypertension.
- **Mucositis,** with ulcers in the nose and mouth.
- **Photosensitivity,** a rash that develops after exposure to sunlight.

### Diagnosis

- Diagnostic criteria for SLE include a history of at least four of the findings summarized by the mnemonic **I'M DAMN SHARP.**
- Laboratory tests may be useful for confirming the diagnosis. ANA is over 95% *sensitive* for SLE, but not very specific. Antibodies to double-stranded DNA (**anti-dsDNA**) are very *specific* and are associated with a poor prognosis. Anti-Smith (**anti-Sm**) antibodies, directed against spliceosomal small nuclear ribonucleoprotein (snRNP) particles, are also very specific for SLE, but not prognostic. **Antihistone** antibodies can be seen in certain cases of drug-induced lupus. Immune complex formation can lead to complement deficiency, including decreased C3, C4, and CH50.

### Treatment

The treatment for lupus depends on its manifestations. Nonsteroidal anti-inflammatory drugs (NSAIDs) are the typical treatment for arthritis, and sunscreen can be used for photosensitivity. **Systemic steroids** are often given if there is major organ involvement, but chronic use carries a risk of avascular necrosis, osteoporosis, diabetes, and ocular disease. Hydroxychloroquine is used for skin disease and arthritis. The cytotoxic agent cyclophosphamide and the antimetabolites mycophenolate mofetil and azathioprine are particularly useful for treating lupus nephritis.

### Prognosis

SLE is an unpredictable disease, and outcomes vary drastically. It is typical for patients to experience a series of relapses and remissions, although symptom-free periods may last for years. Prognosis is improved with early detection and treatment for kidney disease. Death can occur secondary to renal failure, cardiovascular disease, infection, or other complications.

### Scleroderma (Systemic Sclerosis)

A generalized rheumatologic disorder of connective tissue, systemic sclerosis is characterized by degenerative and inflammatory changes leading to fibrosis and collagen deposition. The disease is more common in women (75% female) and typically manifests between the ages of 30 and 50 years. The overall cause is unknown, but several pathogenic mechanisms have been proposed, including endothelial cell injury, fibroblast activation, and immunologic derangement. T cells sensitized to collagen and other skin antigens infiltrate the skin of patients with systemic sclerosis.

### Presentation

Skin involvement is almost universal in patients with systemic sclerosis. Skin may be edematous or indurated early in the disease, but progresses to sclerosis with hair loss, decreased sweating, and loss of the ability to make a skin fold. This gives the skin a characteristic tight and shiny appearance. Pitting of the fingertips is also observed (Figure 3-26). Other common manifestations of the disease include the following:

- **Raynaud phenomenon,** episodic attacks of vasospasm, which cause tingling and color change in the digits, progressing from white to blue to red (Figure 3-27). This phenomenon can be precipitated by cold temperature, emotional upset, and cigarette smoking.
- **Telangiectasias,** punctate macular lesions representing dilated small vessels just beneath the dermis. These can be seen on the face, palms, and digits (Figure 3-28).

In the GI tract, systemic sclerosis can manifest with dilation and impaired motility of the lower esophagus, atony of the small bowel with bacterial overgrowth and malabsorption, or dilation of the large intestine with formation of pseudodiverticula. In the lungs, pulmonary interstitial fibrosis and pulmonary hypertension can occur. Patients with rapidly progressive disease may experience the sudden onset of malignant hypertension leading to acute renal failure.

There are multiple subtypes of systemic sclerosis, with differing manifestations and prognoses.

- **Diffuse systemic sclerosis** is characterized by widespread skin involvement, rapid progression, and early visceral involvement. Skin changes appear rapidly following the development of Raynaud phenomenon. This subtype of systemic sclerosis is associated with anti-DNA topoisomerase I antibodies (formerly anti-Scl-70).
- Limited systemic sclerosis, or **CREST syndrome,** is associated with a more benign clinical course characterized by **calcinosis, Raynaud phenomenon, esophageal dysmotility, sclerodactyly,** and **telangiectasia.** Skin changes typically appear years after Raynaud phenomenon and are often limited to the face and distal extremities. This subtype of systemic sclerosis is associated with anticentromere antibodies.
- **Localized scleroderma,** or morphea, is confined to the skin, with no visceral involvement.

### Diagnosis

History and physical evaluation are typically the basis for a diagnosis of scleroderma. Serologic testing for anti-DNA topoisomerase I or anticentromere antibodies can be used to support the diagnosis but not exclude it. ANAs are present in about 95% of patients. Skin biopsy specimen demonstrating atrophy and thinning of the epidermis, fibrosis, focal collections of lymphocytes in the deep dermis, and loss of dermal appendages such as hair follicles and sweat glands can be helpful in some cases.

### Treatment

There are no Food and Drug Administration (FDA)–approved treatments for systemic sclerosis. D-Penicillamine may be used to treat the skin manifestations. Severe Raynaud phenomenon may be treated with calcium channel blockers. Angiotensin-converting enzyme (ACE) inhibitors are used to treat hypertension and prevent progression to renal crisis. Cyclophosphamide may be used for fulminant presentations or in cases of active alveolitis.

### Prognosis

Diffuse systemic sclerosis is a serious disease with a 10-year survival rate of about 20%. Prognosis is improving with increased use of ACE inhibitors to prevent renal crisis, which was formerly the leading cause of death. Pulmonary involvement is now the primary cause of mortality.

CREST syndrome is a more benign disease with a 10-year survival rate of > 70%.

### Sjögren Syndrome

A chronic autoimmune disorder, Sjögren syndrome is characterized by lymphocytic infiltration of the exocrine glands (Figure 3-29). It is the second most common rheu-

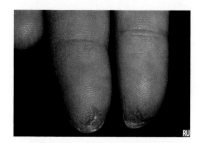

**FIGURE 3-26. Fingertip pitting.** A clinical manifestation of systemic sclerosis (scleroderma).

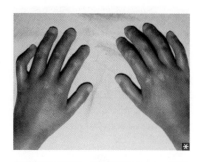

**FIGURE 3-27. Systemic sclerosis.** Hands of a patient with juvenile systemic sclerosis. Skin is shiny and shows a light reddish discoloration over knuckles.

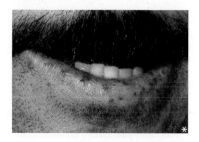

**FIGURE 3-28. Telangiectasias on the lips.** Tight lips are also characteristic.

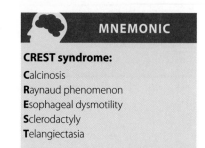

**MNEMONIC**

**CREST syndrome:**

**C**alcinosis
**R**aynaud phenomenon
**E**sophageal dysmotility
**S**clerodactyly
**T**elangiectasia

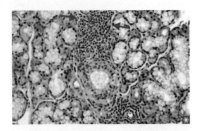

**FIGURE 3-29. Sjögren syndrome.** Destruction of exocrine glands by lymphocytic infiltrates.

**KEY FACT**

The classic triad of findings in Sjögren syndrome is xerophthalmia, xerostomia, and arthritis. The combination of xerostomia and xerophthalmia is known as the **sicca complex.**

**KEY FACT**

The **seronegative spondyloarthropathies** are a group of related inflammatory joint diseases associated with HLA-B27. These include the **PAIR** diseases:
- **P**soriatic arthritis
- **A**nkylosing spondylitis
- **I**nflammatory bowel disease with enteropathic arthritis
- **R**eactive arthritis
Serologic testing for RF is typically negative in these diseases.

**MNEMONIC**

**Reactive arthritis:**

Can't see (conjunctivitis)
Can't pee (urethritis)
Can't bend my knee (arthritis)

matologic disorder (after RA), and it predominantly affects females 40–60 years old. It can occur either as a primary disease or secondary to other autoimmune disorders, such as RA and SLE. The pathogenesis of the disease involves circulating autoantibodies that cause activated T and B cells to accumulate around blood vessels and ducts, particularly in the salivary and lacrimal glands. These autoantibodies target the **muscarinic ACh receptor,** chronic stimulation of which ultimately causes parenchymal tissue to lose the ability to produce fluid (eg, saliva and tears). As the disease progresses, it may affect other major organ systems and can rarely evolve into malignant lymphoma.

### Presentation

The hallmark symptoms of Sjögren syndrome are dry mouth (**xerostomia**) and dry eyes (**xerophthalmia**). This combination of symptoms can lead to difficulty chewing, dysphagia, dental caries, periodontal disease, keratoconjunctivitis, impairment in vision, and corneal ulcerations. Parotid gland enlargement is common. Other symptoms can include arthralgias, myalgias, Raynaud phenomenon, and nonthrombocytopenic purpura.

### Diagnosis

Both ANA and rheumatoid factor (RF) are usually present. **Anti-Ro (SS-A)** and **anti-La (SS-B)** are associated with earlier onset, longer duration, and more extraglandular manifestations. Salivary gland biopsy reveals a **lymphocytic infiltrate.**

### Treatment

Treatment of Sjögren syndrome focuses on relieving symptoms and includes artificial tears, lozenges, and oral hygiene.

### Prognosis

Primary Sjögren syndrome generally has a good prognosis unless significant extraglandular manifestations develop. The prognosis for secondary disease depends on the primary autoimmune disorder. Patients have a small risk of developing lymphoma.

### Reactive Arthritis

Reactive arthritis is an autoimmune disease characterized by urethritis, conjunctivitis, arthritis, and mucocutaneous lesions. Also known by its older name, Reiter syndrome, this disease occurs in two forms. The **postvenereal** (endemic) form is triggered following urethritis or cervicitis, usually caused by *Chlamydia trachomatis* or *Mycoplasma pneumoniae.* The **postdysenteric** (epidemic) form is triggered following infectious diarrhea, usually due to *Shigella flexneri, Salmonella,* or *Yersinia,* or *Campylobacter.* The postvenereal form occurs almost exclusively in males, whereas the postdysenteric form affects both sexes equally. HLA-B27 is present in 80% of patients.

### Presentation

Symptoms generally appear 1–3 weeks after the inciting episode of urethritis/cervicitis or diarrhea. **Urethritis** ultimately occurs regardless of the inciting infection. **Arthritis** mainly affects the lower extremities and is asymmetrical. **Conjunctivitis** is usually accompanied by mucopurulent discharge, lid edema, and anterior uveitis. **Mucocutaneous lesions** can include painless superficial ulcers of the palate and buccal mucosa, painless ulcers on the penis (balanitis circinata), and a hyperkeratotic rash affecting the soles, palms, scrotum, trunk, and scalp (keratoderma blennorrhagica).

### Diagnosis

History and physical evaluation are sufficient to make the diagnosis of reactive arthritis. Aspirates of joint fluid are usually sterile, and examination of biopsy specimen of the rash is indistinguishable from that for psoriasis.

## Treatment

NSAIDs are the mainstay of treatment for joint symptoms. Sulfasalazine is an alternative for patients who have a contraindication to or do not experience relief from NSAIDs.

## Prognosis

The disease is usually self-limited, lasting between 2 and 6 months. Symptoms recur in about 50% of patients, but permanent joint damage is uncommon.

## Sarcoidosis

Sarcoidosis is a multisystemic disorder characterized by an exaggerated cellular immune response to an unknown antigen, leading to the formation of **noncaseating, "naked" granulomas** in affected tissues. It is most common in black females between the ages of 20 and 40.

## Presentation

Sarcoidosis is characterized by immune-mediated, widespread noncaseating granulomas (Figure 3-30A). It can occur in any organ system, but most commonly affects the lungs and lymph nodes. It is asymptomatic in about 50% of patients and is often diagnosed incidentally after radiographic imaging for other reasons. Bilateral hilar adenopathy or coarse reticular opacities are often observed on CXR (Figure 3-30B) and CT (Figure 3-30C). **Dyspnea** is the most common complaint. Additional clinical findings include erythema nodosum, Bell palsy, uveitis, and hypercalcemia (due to increased 1-α-hydroxylase–mediated vitamin D activation in macrophages). Patients may also present with vague constitutional symptoms, such as fever, malaise, weight loss, and fatigue.

## Diagnosis

Chest radiography is an important tool in differentiating sarcoidosis from other granulomatous diseases involving the lungs, as described in Table 3-22. Definitive diagnosis is made by biopsy, often requiring 5–10 samples from the lung parenchyma. Epithelioid granulomas contain microscopic Schaumann and astroid bodies. Histologic characteristics of sarcoidosis in comparison with other granulomatous diseases are described in Table 3-23.

## Treatment

Steroids are the mainstay of therapy for patients with symptomatic sarcoidosis, although exact regimens vary drastically according to the location and severity of the disease.

## Prognosis

Most cases of sarcoidosis resolve spontaneously, usually over a period of about 2–5 years. One-third of cases persist for longer than 5 years, and 5% result in death. Pulmonary fibrosis and extrapulmonary manifestations such as chronic iritis, lupus pernio (violaceous plaques on the face [nose, ears, cheeks] or digits), and tracheal involvement are associated with a less favorable prognosis.

**TABLE 3-22. Differentiating Granulomatous Diseases by Chest Film**

| | SARCOIDOSIS | TUBERCULOSIS | HYPERSENSITIVITY PNEUMONITIS |
|---|---|---|---|
| Hilar adenopathy | Bilateral | Unilateral | Absent |
| Parenchymal infiltrate | Lower/middle fields | Localized or miliary | Diffuse |
| Cavity formation | Rare | Common | Rare |
| Pleural effusion | Unusual | Common | Absent |

**MNEMONIC**

The major features of sarcoidosis can be remembered with the mnemonic **A GRUELING D**isease:

**A**CE levels increased
**G**ranulomas
**R**heumatoid arthritis
**U**veitis
**E**rythema nodosum
**L**ymphadenopathy (bilateral, hilar)
**I**nterstitial fibrosis
**N**oncaseating granulomas
**G**ammaglobulinemia
Vitamin **D** levels increased

**KEY FACT**

Sarcoidosis is associated with restrictive lung disease (interstitial fibrosis).

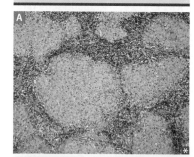
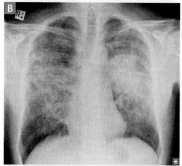
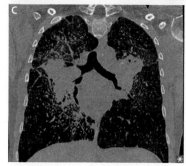

**FIGURE 3-30. Clinical findings associated with sarcoidosis.** **A** Noncaseating granulomas. **B** Chest x-ray showing bilateral adenopathy and coarse reticular opacities. **C** CT showing hilar and mediastinal adenopathy.

**TABLE 3-23.    Differentiating Granulomatous Diseases by Histology**

|  | SARCOIDOSIS | TUBERCULOSIS | HYPERSENSITIVITY PNEUMONITIS |
|---|---|---|---|
| Caseation | Absent | Present | Rare |
| Necrosis | Rare | Present | Rare |
| Inclusions | Present (70%) | Rare | Rare |
| Eosinophils | Present | Minimal | Prominent |
| Bronchiolitis | Rare | Rare | Present |

## OTHER AUTOIMMUNE DISEASES

Autoimmune diseases associated with specific organ systems are covered in greater detail elsewhere, but autoantibody targets and clinical features are summarized in Table 3-24.

**TABLE 3-24.    Autoantibody Targets and Clinical Features of Autoimmune Diseases**

| DISEASE | AUTOANTIBODY TARGET(S) | CLINICAL FEATURES |
|---|---|---|
| **Systemic Autoimmune Diseases** | | |
| Systemic lupus erythematosus (SLE) | Cell nucleus (ANA), double-stranded DNA, Smith, histone (drug-induced lupus) | Arthritis, malar rash, nephritis, serositis, photosensitivity |
| Antiphospholipid syndrome | Cardiolipin, lupus anticoagulant | Thrombosis, spontaneous abortion, elevated aPTT |
| CREST syndrome | Centromere | **C**alcinosis, **R**aynaud phenomenon, **e**sophageal dysmotility, **s**clerodactyly, **t**elangiectasias |
| Mixed connective tissue disease | U1-RNP (ribonucleoprotein) | Overlapping SLE, polymyositis, and scleroderma symptoms |
| Sjögren syndrome | Ro/SSA, La/SSB | Xerostomia, xerophthalmia, arthritis, parotid enlargement |
| Reactive arthritis | Unknown | Urethritis, conjunctivitis, arthritis, mucocutaneous lesions |
| Sarcoidosis | Unknown | Dyspnea, constitutional symptoms, bilateral hilar adenopathy on chest film |
| **Diseases of the Vascular System** | | |
| Vasculitis (multiple) | Neutrophil cytoplasm components (eg, c-ANCA, p-ANCA) | Hemoptysis (lung involvement), hematuria and proteinuria (renal involvement), palpable purpura (skin involvement) |
| **Diseases of the Endocrine System** | | |
| Diabetes mellitus type 1 | Pancreatic islet cells, insulin | Thirst, polyuria, hyperglycemia, retinopathy, nephropathy, neuropathy, ketoacidosis |
| Graves disease | Thyroid-stimulating hormone receptor, thyroid peroxidase | Hyperthyroidism, proptosis, pretibial myxedema |
| Hashimoto thyroiditis | Thyroid peroxidase, thyroglobulin, microsomal | Hypothyroidism with episodes of hyperthyroidism |

*(continues)*

**TABLE 3-24.** **Autoantibody Targets and Clinical Features of Autoimmune Diseases** *(continued)*

| DISEASE | AUTOANTIBODY TARGET(S) | CLINICAL FEATURES |
|---|---|---|
| **Diseases of the Gastrointestinal System** | | |
| Celiac disease (nontropical sprue) | Tissue transglutaminase, gliadin, endomysium | Ingestion of gluten causes diarrhea, steatorrhea, nausea, vomiting |
| Primary biliary cirrhosis | Mitochondria | Pruritus, jaundice, hepatomegaly, xanthelasma, transaminitis, hypercholesterolemia |
| Primary sclerosing cholangitis | Neutrophil cytoplasm components (p-ANCA) | Pruritus, jaundice, hepatomegaly, "beading" of bile ducts on ERCP |
| Autoimmune hepatitis | Smooth muscle, liver-kidney microsome | Jaundice, ascites, spider angiomata, esophageal varices, transaminitis |
| **Diseases of the Blood** | | |
| Autoimmune hemolytic anemia | Red blood cells | Pallor, fatigue |
| Pernicious anemia | Parietal cells, intrinsic factor | Cobalamin (vitamin $B_{12}$) deficiency, megaloblastic anemia, atrophic glossitis, neuropathic pain and paresthesias, myelopathy |
| Idiopathic thrombocytopenic purpura | Platelet membrane glycoproteins (eg, glycoprotein IIb/IIIa) | Petechiae, ecchymoses, epistaxis, easy bruisability |
| Heparin-induced thrombocytopenia | Heparin-bound platelet factor 4 (PF4) | Thrombosis and thrombocytopenia |
| **Diseases of the Musculoskeletal System** | | |
| Rheumatoid arthritis | Fc portion of IgG (rheumatoid factor), cyclic citrullinated peptide (specific) | Symmetrical arthritis, swan-neck and boutonnière deformities, morning stiffness |
| **Diseases of the Skin** | | |
| Pemphigus vulgaris | Desmoglein-3 and desmoglein-1 | Oropharyngeal erosions, flaccid cutaneous vesicles and bullae |
| Pemphigus foliaceus | Desmoglein-1 | Crusts and occasionally, delicate flaccid cutaneous vesicles and bullae |
| Epidermolysis bullosa acquisita | Type VII collagen (anchoring fibrils) | Tense vesicles and bullae leading to erosions on extensor surfaces of hands, elbows, knees, and ankles |
| Bullous pemphigoid | Hemidesmosome, BPAg1, BPAg2 (type XVII collagen) | Intensely pruritic urticarial patches followed by tense vesicles, bullae on the trunk and extremities |
| Dermatitis herpetiformis | Epidermal transglutaminase-3 | Pruritic vesicles and crusts on elbows, knees, and buttocks (associated with celiac disease) |
| **Diseases of the Nervous System** | | |
| Myasthenia gravis | Postsynaptic nicotinic acetylcholine receptors | Facial muscle weakness that spreads to the trunk and limbs. Can also be limited to the ocular muscles (ocular myasthenia gravis) |
| Lambert-Eaton myasthenic syndrome | Voltage-gated calcium channels on the presynaptic motor nerve terminal | Proximal muscle weakness of the lower extremities, autonomic dysfunction (dry mouth, constipation, pupillary constriction, sweating) |
| Multiple sclerosis | Myelin | Fatigue, paresthesias, tremor, optic neuritis |
| Autoimmune inner ear disease | Various inner ear antigens | Bilateral sensorineural hearing loss |

*(continues)*

**TABLE 3-24.**    **Autoantibody Targets and Clinical Features of Autoimmune Diseases** *(continued)*

| DISEASE | AUTOANTIBODY TARGET(S) | CLINICAL FEATURES |
|---|---|---|
| **Diseases of the Renal System** | | |
| Goodpasture syndrome | Glomerular basement membrane, pulmonary basement membrane | Oliguria, nephritic syndrome, pulmonary hemorrhage |

ANA, antinuclear antibody; aPTT, activated partial thromboplastin time; BPA, bullous pemphigoid antigen; c-ANCA, cytoplasmic antineutrophil cytoplasmic antibody; ERCP, endoscopic retrograde cholangiopancreatography; IgG, immunoglobulin G; p-ANCA, perinuclear antineutrophil cytoplasmic antibody; SSA/SSB, Sjögren syndrome-related antigen A/B.

# Microbiology

# Bacteriology

## BACTERIAL STRUCTURES

Bacteria are prokaryotic organisms and exhibit several structural components.

### Cytoplasmic Structures

Eukaryotes and prokaryotes differ in their cytoplasmic structures (Table 4-1). Bacteria carry the following intracellular components:

- **Bacterial chromosome:** Circular, double-stranded, and contained within the nucleoid.
- **Plasmids:** Smaller extrachromosomal DNA, often containing important genes, such as those that confer resistance to antibiotics.
- **Bacterial ribosome:** Consists of 30S and 50S subunits that form the 70s ribosome, and these are coupled in bacterial transcription and translation.

### Bacterial Cell Walls

With the exception of **Mycoplasma,** which has **no cell walls,** the cell walls of bacteria are composed of layers of **peptidoglycan** that surround their cytoplasmic membranes. Important functions of the cell wall include:

- Resisting osmotic stress.
- Serving as a primer for its own synthesis, which is necessary for cell division.
- Defining the shape of the bacteria; **coccus, bacillus** (*Staphylococcus, Vibrio*), **spirillum** (spirochete).
- Providing some protection from innate immune responses in humans.

The organization of the cell wall differs among gram-positive and gram-negative organisms (Figure 4-1, and Table 4-2) as follows:

- **Gram-positive bacteria:** Thick cell wall, composed of many layers of **peptidoglycan.** The linkage between one layer of peptidoglycan and another (via the third and fourth amino acids of glucosamine pentapeptide) is further extended by a pentaglycine bridge, whereas gram-negative bacteria link their pentapeptide chains directly. Without peptidoglycan, the bacteria would lyse due to the differential in osmotic pressure across the cytoplasmic membrane. Gram-positive bacteria also have **teichoic** and

**KEY FACT**

Because bacterial ribosomes and RNA polymerases differ from those in humans, they are ideal targets for antibiotics.

**KEY FACT**

*Mycoplasma* do not have cell walls and therefore cannot be seen with Gram stain.

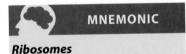

**MNEMONIC**

**Ribosomes**

**E**ukaryotes begin with an **E**ven number
Pr**O**karyotes begin with an **O**dd number.

**TABLE 4-1. Eukaryotic Versus Prokaryotic Cytoplasmic Structures**

| CYTOPLASMIC STRUCTURES | EUKARYOTE | PROKARYOTE |
| --- | --- | --- |
| Nucleus | Nuclear membrane present | Nuclear membrane absent |
| Chromosomes | Linear, diploid DNA | Circular, haploid DNA |
| Ribosome | 80S (60S + 40S) | 70S (50S + 30S) |
| Cell membrane | Contains sterols | No sterols[a] |
| Mitochondria | Present | Absent |
| Golgi bodies | Present | Absent |
| Endoplasmic reticulum | Present | Absent |
| Respiration | Via mitochondria | Via cell membrane |

[a]Mycoplasmas are an exception, as they incorporate sterols.

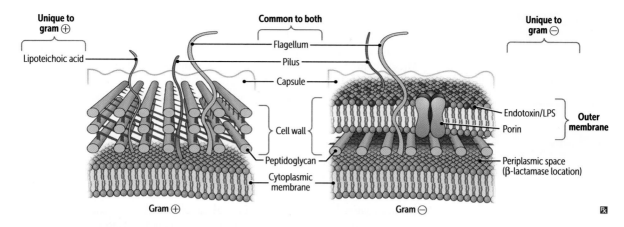

**FIGURE 4-1.** Key differences between Gram-positive and Gram-negative bacterial cell walls.

**lipoteichoic acids** within their cell walls. These copolymers vary between species and provide distinguishing qualities that allow further classification within a species (serotypes). Teichoic acids also promote bacterial interactions with human cell receptors, and initiating host immune responses.

■ **Gram-negative bacteria:** Consist of both a **peptidoglycan layer,** making up only 5–10% of the cell wall, and **an outer membrane.**

The peptidoglycan cell wall is synthesized mainly through the action of two enzymes: **transglycosylase** and **transpeptidase,** which catalyze formation of glycosidic and peptide bonds respectively, to cross-link peptidoglycan monomers.

### External Bacterial Structures

There are several external bacterial structures of interest (Figure 4-1):

■ **Bacterial capsules** are usually composed of **polysaccharide glycocalyx,** with the exception of *Bacillus anthracis* (specifically containing D-glutamate). It is an important virulence factor that help to resist opsonization and phagocytosis.

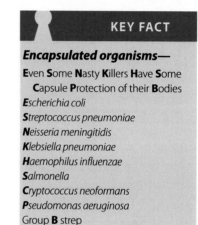

**KEY FACT**

*Encapsulated organisms—*
**E**ven **S**ome **N**asty **K**illers **H**ave **S**ome **C**apsule **P**rotection of their **B**odies
*Escherichia coli*
*Streptococcus pneumoniae*
*Neisseria meningitidis*
*Klebsiella pneumoniae*
*Haemophilus influenzae*
*Salmonella*
*Cryptococcus neoformans*
*Pseudomonas aeruginosa*
Group **B** strep

**TABLE 4-2.** Gram-Positive and Gram-Negative Bacterial Membrane Structures

| GRAM-POSITIVE | | GRAM-NEGATIVE | |
| --- | --- | --- | --- |
| STRUCTURE | CHEMICAL CONSTITUENTS | STRUCTURE | CHEMICAL CONSTITUENTS |
| Peptidoglycan | Chains of GlcNAc and MurNAc peptide bridges cross-linked by pentaglycine chains | Peptidoglycan | Thinner compared to gram-positive bacteria, with direct peptide bridging and no pentaglycine chains |
| Teichoic acid | Glycerol phosphate or polyribitol phosphate cross-linked to peptidoglycan | Periplasmic space | Enzymes involved in transport, degradation, and synthesis |
| Lipoteichoic acid | Lipid-linked teichoic acid | Outer membrane | Fatty acids and phospholipids |
| | | Lipopolysaccharide (LPS) | Core polysaccharide, O antigen, lipid A |
| Proteins | Porins, transport proteins | Proteins | Porins, lipoprotein, transport proteins |
| Plasma membrane | Phospholipids, proteins, and enzymes involved in generation of energy, membrane potential and transport | Plasma membrane | Same as gram-positive bacteria |
| Capsule | Disaccharides, trisaccharides, and polypeptides | Capsule | Polysaccharides and polypeptides |

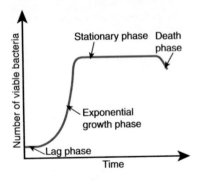

**FIGURE 4-2. Bacterial growth curve.** Depicted are lag phase, exponential growth phase, and stationary phase.

- **Biofilms** are bacterial communities embedded in a matrix that form on a surface that can protect bacteria from antibiotics and host immune defenses.
- **Flagella** are **coiled protein subunits (flagellin)** anchored in bacterial membranes. They provide bacterial motility and express **antigenic (H antigen)** and **strain determinants** useful for serotyping bacteria.
- **Fimbriae** are hair-like structures on the outside of bacteria, composed of repeating subunits of the protein **pilin.** Fimbriae often promote **adherence** to other bacteria or to host cells.
- **Periplasmic space:** Area between the cytoplasmic membrane and the outer membrane. Contains enzymes necessary for metabolism and **virulence factors,** such as proteases, phosphatases, lipases, nucleases, collagenases, hyaluronidases, and β-lactamases.
- Gram-negative bacteria contain **lipopolysaccharide (LPS-endotoxin),** which allow for serotyping gram-negative bacteria. LPS is a potent activator of immune cells and stimulates release of major pyrogenic substances such as **interleukin-1 (IL-1), IL-6,** and **tumor necrosis factor (TNF),** the major **cytokine responsible for shock.**

## BACTERIAL GROWTH AND METABOLISM

### Bacterial Growth and Death

Bacteria need a source of carbon and nitrogen, water, and various ions for growth. Bacteria must also obtain or synthesize the **amino acids, carbohydrates,** and **lipids** necessary for building proteins, structures, and membranes. A cascade of regulatory events then initiates **DNA synthesis,** which then runs to completion.

Bacterial growth occurs in **four phases** (Figure 4-2):

- **Lag phase:** Gathering of necessary growth requirements. No divisions occur during this phase.
- **Log phase** (or exponential growth phase): Growth and cell division begin. The doubling time varies among different strains and conditions.
- **Stationary phase:** Depicts the point at which bacteria run out of metabolites, and toxic products begin to accumulate. The same number of bacteria multiply and die, leading to plateau. This is the phase in which sporulation occurs.
- **Decline phase:** Death of bacterial cells after stationary phase.

Bacterial growth is assessed in three ways: Viable cell counts, optical density, and metabolic products.

- **Viable cell counts** (colony-forming units per milliliter [CFU/mL]).
- **Optical density** (spectrophotometry).
- **Indirect measurement** of bacterial numbers by detection of metabolic by-products ($CO_2$).

Bacterial growth is controlled by subjecting bacterial populations to heat, antimicrobial chemicals, and antibiotics (see following discussion).

**Key mechanisms** of bacterial growth control include (Table 4-3):

- Alteration of membrane permeability.
- Denaturation of proteins.
- Interference with DNA replication—alkylating agents.
- Oxidation.

### Bacterial Metabolism

**Essential elements** necessary for bacterial metabolism include carbon, hydrogen, nitrogen, sulfur, phosphorus, potassium, magnesium, calcium, iron, sodium, chloride, and $O_2$.

**TABLE 4-3.** Methods of Controlling Bacterial Growth

| METHOD | EFFICACY, MECHANISM | SPECTRUM |
|---|---|---|
| **Heat** | | |
| Steam autoclave 121°C for 15 min | High, damages cell membranes, protein denaturant | All bacterial growth phases, viruses, fungi. **Spores can only be destroyed by autoclaving** |
| Boiling | High, damages cell membranes, protein denaturant | Most growth phases, some spores, viruses, fungi |
| Pasteurization | Intermediate, damages cell membranes, protein denaturant | All bacterial growth phases, some viruses, fungi |
| Dry heat | High, damages cell membranes, protein denaturant | All bacterial growth phases, viruses, fungi |
| **Chemical** | | |
| Ethylene oxide gas | Sterilizing, alkylating agent | All bacterial growth phases, viruses, fungi |
| Sodium hypochlorite (bleach) | High, oxidizing agent | Bacteria, viruses, fungi |
| Alcohol | Intermediate, damages cell membranes, protein denaturant | All bacterial growth phases, some viruses, fungi |
| Hydrogen peroxide | High, damages cell membranes, oxidizing agent | All bacterial growth phases, viruses, fungi |
| Chlorine | High, oxidizing agent | All bacterial growth phases, viruses, fungi |
| Iodine compounds | Intermediate, iodination, oxidation | All bacterial growth phases, viruses, fungi |
| Phenolics, phenol, hexachlorophene, chlorhexidine | Intermediate, damages cell membranes | All bacterial growth phases, some viruses, fungi |
| Glutaraldehyde | High, alkylating agent | All bacterial growth phases, viruses |
| Formaldehyde | High, alkylating agent | All bacterial growth phases, viruses, fungi |
| Quaternary ammonium compounds | Low, damages cell membranes, cations | All bacterial growth phases, viruses, fungi |
| **Radiation** | | |
| Ultraviolet | High, DNA damage and protein crosslinking | All bacterial growth phases, viruses, fungi |
| Ionizing | High, DNA damage and protein crosslinking | All bacterial growth phases, viruses, fungi |
| **Physical** | | |
| Filtration | High, size exclusion | All bacterial growth phases, fungi, some viruses |

Bacteria requiring $O_2$ can be divided into four groups:

- **Obligate (or strict) anaerobes:** Cannot grow in the presence of $O_2$.
- **Facultative anaerobes:** Can grow either in the presence or absence of $O_2$.
- **Obligate (or strict) aerobes:** Require molecular $O_2$.
- **Microaerophilic:** Require very low levels of $O_2$ for growth.

A **carbon source** is required by all bacteria. Genera can be differentiated based on the type of carbon they metabolize (ie, **lactose, glucose,** and **galactose**).

Bacteria can produce energy via aerobic respiration, anaerobic respiration, or fermentation.

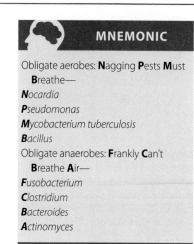

**MNEMONIC**

Obligate aerobes: **N**agging **P**ests **M**ust **B**reathe—
**N**ocardia
**P**seudomonas
**M**ycobacterium tuberculosis
**B**acillus
Obligate anaerobes: **F**rankly **C**an't **B**reathe **A**ir—
**F**usobacterium
**C**lostridium
**B**acteroides
**A**ctinomyces

■ **Aerobic respiration:** Completely converts glucose into $CO_2$ and $H_2O$ and forms adenosine triphosphate (ATP) through **substrate level** and **oxidative phosphorylation.**

■ **Anaerobic respiration:** ATP is also formed through substrate level phosphorylation; however, other high-energy molecules such as $SO_4^{2-}$ and $NO_3^-$ are used as the terminal electron acceptors rather than $O_2$. Anaerobic respiration produces slightly less ATP than aerobic respiration, but is more efficient than fermentation.

■ **Fermentation:** In the absence of $O_2$ and following substrate level phosphorylation, certain bacteria are able to ferment pyruvic acid. The **end products** of this process are two- and three-carbon compounds. These organic molecules act in lieu of $O_2$ as **electron acceptors** to **recycle** the **reduced form of nicotinamide adenine dinucleotide (NADH)** to **nicotinamide adenine dinucleotide (NAD).**

The end products of fermentation can also be used to distinguish particular bacteria.

### Bacterial Genetics

The bacterial **genome** consists of the single **haploid chromosome** of the bacteria in addition to extrachromosomal genetic elements (**plasmids** and **bacteriophages**). These elements may be independent of the bacterial chromosome and, in most cases, can be transmitted from one cell to another.

Exchange of genetic material between bacterial cells can occur via three mechanisms (Figure 4-3):

■ **Conjugation: One-way transfer of DNA** from a donor cell to a recipient cell through the sex pilus. The $F^+$ plasmid contains genes necessary for the pilus and conjugation.

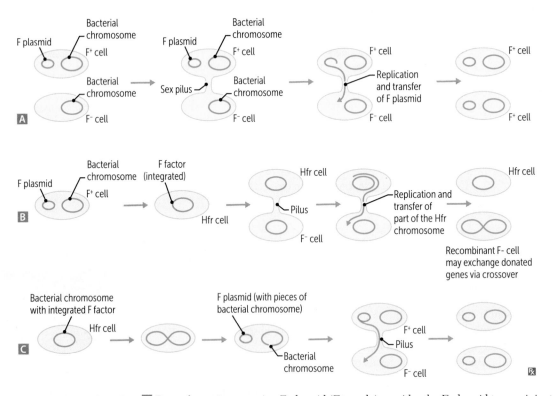

**FIGURE 4-3.** **Bacterial conjugation.** **A** Donor bacterium carrying F plasmid ($F^+$, male) provides the F plasmid to a recipient bacterium ($F^-$, female) via a sex pilus. **B** The F plasmid can integrate into chromosomal DNA leading to a cell in a high-frequency recombination (Hfr) state. Conjugation with an $F^-$ recipient cell can lead to transfer of a replicated DNA strand that includes a part or all of the integrated F plasmid. Once in the $F^-$ recipient, the strand can integrate into chromosomal DNA, giving rise to a recombinant $F^-$ cell. **C** The F plasmid may be excised back out from the Hfr cell's chromosome, generating the F prime plasmid. This plasmid carries pieces of chromosomal DNA due to imprecise excision. Like the F plasmid, the F prime plasmid can be transferred via a sex pilus to an $F^-$ recipient.

Conjugation typically occurs between members of the same species or related species. Recipient bacteria transform into donors following completion of conjugation.

- Donor bacteria carry an episomal F plasmid (F+ male), while recipients do not (F− female). The F plasmid carries the genes necessary for the pilus and the initiation of conjugation.
- In the case of F+ and F− (F+ × F−) conjugation, the episomal F+ plasmid is first replicated, and a copy is transferred to the F− recipient via the pilus, resulting in two F+ bacteria. Only the episome is transferred without sharing of any chromosomal DNA.
- The F+ plasmid can occasionally integrate directly into the F+ bacteria's chromosomal DNA, converting the bacterium into a high-frequency recombination (Hfr) state. Conjugation (**Hfr × F−**) can result in transfer of not only the F+ sequence, but also of small pieces of the donor's chromosomal DNA.
- Integrated F+ plasmids can be excised back out into an episome, and small errors in the excision can carry along pieces of flanking chromosomal DNA. The resulting plasmid is an F prime (F′) plasmid, and conjugation (F′ × F−) will also result in sharing of both plasmid and chromosomal DNA, similar to Hfr × F−.
- **Transformation:** Bacteria take up **fragments of naked DNA** and **incorporate** them into their genomes if the recipient chromosome is sufficiently **homologous** for **recombination** to occur. Certain species of bacteria such as *H influenzae, S pneumoniae, Bacillus* species, and *Neisseria* species are capable of taking up exogenous DNA.
- **Transduction:** Genetic transfer mediated by bacteria-targeting viruses (**bacteriophages**). This is a very efficient way for bacteria to pass genetic information such as antibiotic resistance. There are two forms of transduction:
  - Generalized: A "packaging" event. **Lytic** phage infects bacterium, leading to cleavage of bacterial DNA and synthesis of viral proteins. Parts of bacterial chromosomal DNA may become packaged in viral capsid. Phage infects another bacterium, transferring these genes.
  - Specialized: An "excision" event. **Lysogenic** phage infects bacterium; viral DNA is incorporated into bacterial chromosome. When phage DNA is excised, flanking bacterial genes may be excised with it. DNA is packaged into phage viral capsid and can infect another bacterium.

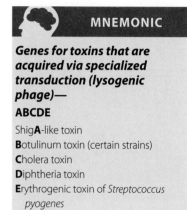

## Bacterial Defenses—Pathogenic Factors

Bacteria have multiple defensive **virulence factors** that protect them from the human immune system while also enabling them to enter the host and promote disease. A few of these factors include capsules (explained previously), the sporulation process, toxins, proteases, hemolysins, coagulase, and catalase (Table 4-4).

## Spore

The spore is a dehydrated, multicelled structure that allows bacteria to survive when nutrients are limited. The spores are composed of:

- Inner membrane
- Two peptidoglycan layers
- Outer protein coat

The complete copy of the bacterium's chromosome, as well as the essential proteins and ribosomes necessary for germination, are confined within the spore. A spore can survive for decades, protecting bacterial DNA from heat, radiation, enzymes, and chemical agents (eg, most disinfectants).

**TABLE 4-4.** **Defensive Virulence Factors**

| DEFENSE MECHANISMS | SPECIES OF BACTERIA |
| --- | --- |
| Spores | *Clostridium tetani, Clostridium botulinum,* or *Clostridium difficile, Bacillus anthracis* |
| IgA proteases | *Streptococcus pneumoniae, Neisseria meningitidis, Neisseria gonorrhoeae, Haemophilus influenzae* |
| Cellular invasion | *Rickettsia* and *Chlamydia, Salmonella, Shigella, Brucella, Mycobacterium, Listeria, Francisella, Legionella, Yersinia* |
| Hemolysis | *Streptococcus pneumoniae, Streptococcus pyogenes, Streptococcus agalactiae, Staphylococcus aureus, Listeria monocytogenes, Enterococcus* |
| Catalase | *Staphylococcus, Micrococcus, Listeria* |
| Coagulase | *Staphylococcus aureus* |
| Toxins | *Streptococcus pyogenes, Staphylococcus aureus, Clostridium diphtheriae, Pseudomonas aeruginosa, Shigella dysenteriae, Escherichia coli, Vibrio cholerae, Bordetella pertussis, Clostridium difficile, Clostridium perfringens, Clostridium tetani, Clostridium botulinum* |

## IgA Proteases

*Streptococcus pneumoniae, N meningitidis, Neisseria gonorrhoeae,* and *H influenzae* carry IgA proteases. These proteases cleave IgA, which is found on mucosal surfaces and functions as a first line of defense against pathogens. Cleavage by the proteases prevents opsonization of these bacteria, thus allowing bacteria to enter unnoticed by the host's immune system.

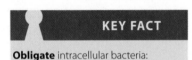

**KEY FACT**

**Obligate** intracellular bacteria: *Rickettsia* and *Chlamydia*.
**Facultative** intracellular bacteria: *Salmonella, Shigella, Brucella, Mycobacterium, Listeria, Francisella, Legionella,* and *Yersinia.*

## Cellular Invasion

Some bacteria are able to live and replicate intracellularly to avoid the host's immune system. There are obligate intracellular (strictly intracellular only) and facultative intracellular (capable of existing either intracellularly or extracellularly) bacteria.

## Hemolysis

Hemolysis is the breakdown of red blood cells in culture by hemolysins. Hemolysis is useful in categorizing types of streptococci. **Three types** of hemolysis are identified (Figure 4-4):

- α-**Hemolysis** results in greenish darkening of the blood agar. The green color change of the agar is caused by peroxide produced by the bacteria, not hemolysin, and therefore α-hemolysis is often referred to as **partial hemolysis** (*S pneumoniae*) (Figure 4-5).
- β-**Hemolysis** results in complete clearing of the blood agar (complete hemolysis by hemolysin) (*S pyogenes*) (Figure 4-5).
- γ-**Hemolysis** designates no hemolysis (no change to the color of the blood agar) (*Enterococcus*).

## Catalases

Catalases are enzymes that catabolize hydrogen peroxide ($H_2O_2$) into water and $O_2$. The presence or absence of catalase can be used to categorize gram-positive cocci.

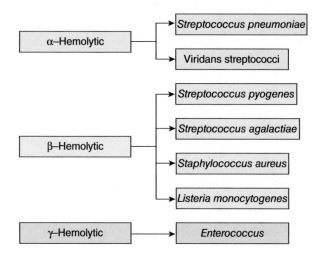

**FIGURE 4-4.** **Types of hemolysis.** Note that many other organisms besides enterococci are nonhemolytic, whereas enterococci can also be β, α, or γ.

## Coagulases

These enzymes are used to **distinguish** *S aureus* (the most common species of staphylococci found in humans that produces the enzyme coagulase) from other forms of staphylococci. In common usage, the latter are referred to as coagulase-negative staphylococci (CoNS).

## Toxins

Three major types of toxins exist: endotoxin, exotoxin, and enterotoxin.

- **Endotoxin,** or lipopolysaccharide (**LPS**), is found in the outer cell membrane of gram-negative bacteria and can cause fever and shock.
- **Exotoxins** are **polypeptides** secreted by bacteria that cause harm to the host by altering cellular structure or function. Exotoxins are very potent and a very low dose may be lethal to the host.
- **Enterotoxins** are toxins that act on the gut.

Toxins have a wide range of function (Table 4-5).

**KEY FACT**

In plasma, coagulase binds to serum factor and coverts fibrinogen to fibrin, forming a clot.

**KEY FACT**

Superantigens:
- *S pyogenes:* Scarlet fever toxin
- *S aureus:* Toxic shock syndrome toxin

**CLINICAL CORRELATION**

Toxins that ↑ cAMP (eg, cholera toxin) lead to ↑ chloride secretion in the gut, followed by $H_2O$ efflux, leading to secretory diarrhea.
Toxins that ↑ cGMP (eg, heat-stable enterotoxin) ↓ NaCl resorption (and hence, $H_2O$ resorption) in the gut, leading to diarrhea.

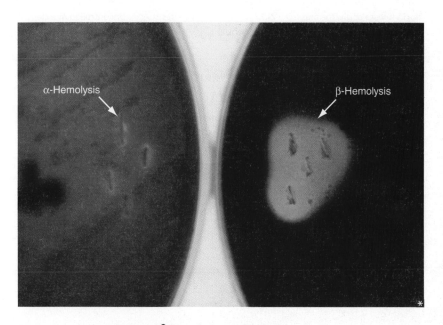

**FIGURE 4-5.** **α-Hemolysis and β-hemolysis on blood agar.**

**TABLE 4-5.** **Bacterial Toxicity in Brief**

| MICROORGANISM | TOXIN TYPE | MECHANISM | MOLECULAR RESULT | CLINICAL RESULT |
|---|---|---|---|---|
| *Corynebacterium diphtheriae* | Diphtheria toxin | Inactivates EF-2 via ADP–ribosyltransferases | Inhibits protein synthesis | Upper respiratory tract infection. Sore throat Low fever |
| *Pseudomonas aeruginosa* | Exotoxin A | Inactivates EF-2 via ADP–ribosyltransferases | Inhibits protein synthesis | UTIs and many nosocomial infections (eg, HCAP) |
| *Escherichia coli* | Heat-labile (LT) enterotoxin (ETEC) | Activates adenylate cyclase via ADP ribosylation of *Gs* | Activates second-messenger pathway ↑ cAMP (**Labile** like the **Air**) | Secretory diarrhea |
| | Heat-stable (ST) enterotoxin (ETEC) | Activates guanylate cyclase | Activates second-messenger pathway ↑ cGMP (**Stable** like the **G**round) | Secretory diarrhea |
| | Shiga-like toxin, (eg, EHEC strain *O157:H7*) | Binds to Gb3 receptor on glomerular epithelial cells and is endocytosed; inactivates ribosomes via RNA *N*-glycosidase | Inhibits protein synthesis | Abdominal pain, fever. Bloody, mucoid, WBCs in stools. Reactive arthritis (formerly Reiter symptoms) Swelling and fibrin deposits in glomerulus |
| *Shigella dysenteriae* | Shiga toxin | Inactivate ribosome via RNA *N*-glycosidase by binding 60S ribosome | Inhibits protein synthesis | Bloody and inflammatory diarrhea |
| *Vibrio cholerae* | Cholera toxin | Activates adenylate cyclase via ADP ribosylation of *Gs* | Activates second-messenger pathway ↑ cAMP | Hypersecretory diarrhea with great loss of fluid and electrolytes |
| | Heat-labile (LT) enterotoxin | | | |
| *Bordetella pertussis* | Pertussis toxin | Activates adenylate cyclase via ADP ribosylation of *Gi* | Activates second-messenger pathway ↑ cAMP | ↑ Secretion in upper respiratory tract Other tissue effects |
| *Clostridium tetani* | Tetanospasmin | Blocks release of glycine and GABA from inhibitory neurons | Zinc-dependent proteases cleave SNARE | Uncontrolled muscle spasms Spastic paralysis |
| *Clostridium botulinum* | Botulinum toxin (A, B, E) | Blocks release of acetylcholine at neuromuscular junctions | Zinc-dependent proteases cleave SNARE | Flaccid paralysis |
| *Bacillus anthracis* | Edema factor (EF), lethal factor (LF), and protective antigen (PA) | Calmodulin-dependent calcium activation | Activates second-messenger pathway ↑ cAMP | Edema, lethal |

ADP, adenosine diphosphate; cAMP, cyclic adenosine monophosphate; cGMP, cyclic guanosine monophosphate; EF-2, elongation factor 2; *Gs,* G protein, S polypeptide; *Gi,* G protein, I polypeptide; SNARE, soluble NSF (*N*-ethylmaleimide-sensitive factor) attachment protein receptors; UTI, urinary tract infection.

## MICROBIOLOGIC STAINS

The microscopic examination and subsequent identification of microorganisms are greatly aided by the use of differential stains, which generate artificial contrast so the organism can be visualized.

Bacteria can be seen microscopically via:

- **Direct examination:** Performed by suspending bacteria in liquid (sometimes called a **wet mount**). This is useful for detecting motility, for distinguishing larger organisms (eg, yeasts and parasites) from bacteria, and for visualizing *Treponema pallidum*, using darkfield microscopy.
- **Acid-fast stains** include **Ziehl-Neelsen, Kinyoun,** and **auramine-rhodamine.** They are used to stain the bacteria only if pretreated with acid-alkali solutions because the bacteria resist decolorization. Acid-fast staining is particularly useful in identifying **mycobacteria.** However, other acid-fast organisms include *Nocardia, Rhodococcus, Cryptosporidium, Isospora,* and *Cyclospora.*
- **Fluorescent stains** include acridine orange, auramine-rhodamine, calcofluor, and direct/indirect fluorescent antibody stains.
- **Fluorescent antibody staining** is based on the recognition of pathogens by staining with fluorescently labeled antibodies specific for the pathogens.

### Gram Stain

Gram stain is the best-known and most widely used differential stain for bacteria (Table 4-6; depicting respective staining patterns of different bacterial species) because it permits identification of the bacteria based on the chemical and physical properties of their cell walls. This method is fast and reliable when rapid diagnosis is needed. It is usually performed on bodily fluids (eg, cerebrospinal fluid [CSF] for meningitis or synovial fluid for septic arthritis).

In a Gram stain preparation, gram-positive bacteria appear dark blue to **purple,** and gram-negative bacteria are **red.** The procedure includes:

1. Application of a sample to a glass slide and fixation under a flame.
2. Application of the primary stain—crystal violet (CV).
3. Application of iodine to bind and "set" the dye.
4. Washing away of unbound CV from gram-negative organisms during decolorization.
5. Counterstaining of gram-negative organisms with the red dye safranin.

The mechanism of staining is based on the following properties or interactions:

- CV penetrates the cell wall and membrane of both gram-positive and gram-negative cells.
- **Iodine** interacts with CV and forms complexes of CV and iodine within the inner and outer layers of the bacterial cells.
- **Decolorizer** disintegrates the lipids of the cell membranes; thus gram-negative cells lose their outer membrane, exposing the peptidoglycan layer, whereas gram-positive cells dehydrate following treatment with ethanol.
- Decolorization washes out the CV–iodine complexes and outer membrane from gram-negative cells.

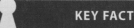

**KEY FACT**

Botulinum toxin ↑ flaccid paralysis. Tetanus toxin ↑ spastic paralysis.

**KEY FACT**

The waxy coat of mycobacteria resists acid, thus making them **acid-fast.** They stain red with the acid-fast stain.

**KEY FACT**

Bacteria that **are not visualized on Gram stain** are:
- *Treponema*
- *Rickettsia*
- *Mycobacteria*
- *Mycoplasma*
- *Legionella*
- *Chlamydia*

**FLASH FORWARD**

**β-Lactam** antibiotics target the enzymes—penicillin-binding protein (PBPs)—responsible for cross-linking amino acids in peptidoglycan. Eukaryotes (like us) possess neither peptidoglycan nor PBPs and thus are intrinsically "resistant" to these antibiotics.

**TABLE 4-6. Gram-Staining Patterns of Various Bacterial Species**

| STAIN | GRAM-POSITIVE | GRAM-NEGATIVE |
|---|---|---|
| **Bacteria** | *Staphylococcus, Streptococcus, Clostridium, Listeria, Bacillus, Corynebacterium* | *Neisseria, H influenzae, Pasteurella, Brucella, B pertussis, Klebsiella, E coli, Enterobacter, Citrobacter, Serratia, Shigella, Salmonella, Proteus, Pseudomonas* |

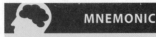

**MNEMONIC**

Gram-**p**ositive bacteria stain **purple;** gram-**n**egative bacteria do **not.**

**MNEMONIC**

Gram-**ne**gative bacteria are the only ones containing **en**dotoxin.

**FLASH FORWARD**

Don't forget the important nonmicrobiologic tissue–based stains: **Congo red** for **amyloid; Sudan black** for **fat droplets; periodic acid–Schiff** for **glycogen,** and **trichrome** for **tissue collagen.**

- CV–iodine complexes remain "trapped" within the gram-positive cells' thick peptidoglycan.
- Following decolorization:
  - **Gram-positive** bacteria remain (stain) **purple.**
  - **Gram-negative** bacteria **lose** their **purple** color.

### Intracellular Microorganisms

*Rickettsia* spp (*Coxiella*), *Ehrlichia* spp, and *Chlamydia* spp are all small, obligate intracellular parasites that live in the cytosol of infected cells. They stain poorly with Gram stain, but share membrane characteristics with gram-negative organisms. Microscopy is generally not useful in the diagnosis of diseases caused by these organisms. *Listeria monocytogenes*, a gram-positive rod that is primarily intracellular, also does not take up CV and is usually visualized on clinical specimens via a silver stain.

The limitations of Gram staining (due to differences in composition of various microorganisms) are bypassed by using other staining methods (Table 4-7).

### Other Microbiologic Stains and Microscopic Techniques

For most common bacteria, a Gram stain can help in making an accurate diagnosis. However, in certain cases, such as the identification of nonstainable organisms, fungi, and parasites, other techniques must be used (Tables 4-8 and 4-9).

## BACTERIAL CULTURE

Growing bacteria on agar plates can aid identification. For example, bacteria with polysaccharide capsules generally have "wet" or **mucoid**-appearing colonies. Some bacteria also produce visibly pigmented colonies on agar:

- *P aeruginosa* produces a fluorescing blue-green pigment.
- *S aureus* produces a **gold** pigment (think of **Au**reus, the abbreviation for gold on the periodic table).
- *S marcescens* produces a red pigment. (Think: maraschino red cherries.)

Generally, bacteria from clinical specimens are first grown on an agar-based, permissive, nonselective medium, with an additional nutrient source (either hydrolyzed soy protein or sheep's blood). Isolated colonies from these agar plates can then be aseptically selected and used for further laboratory diagnosis.

- **Selective media** are supplemented with antibiotics or other substances that **prevent the growth** of certain contaminating bacteria.
- **Differential media** contain **indicators** that provide further biochemical information about the microorganisms.

**TABLE 4-7. Gram Stain Limitations**

| BACTERIA | PREFERRED STAINING METHOD |
| --- | --- |
| *Treponema* | Darkfield microscopy and fluorescent antibody staining |
| *Rickettsia* | Immunofluorescent and immunoperoxidase staining |
| *Mycobacterium* | Acid-fast |
| *Mycoplasma* | Do not stain |
| *Legionella pneumophila* | Silver stain |
| *Chlamydia* | Immunofluorescent staining |

**TABLE 4-8.** Microscopy Techniques and Stains Used in Microbiology

|  | ORGANISMS | RATIONALE |
|---|---|---|
| Darkfield microscopy | Spirochetes | Thin organisms are more easily identified by this technique |
| KOH (potassium hydroxide) preparation | Fungi | Bacteria are killed in this strong alkali solution, leaving fungi behind (which are stable in alkali solution) |
| India ink | *Cryptococcus* in CSF specimens | Cryptococcal polysaccharide capsule scatters ink, rendering it bright against dark background<br>(However, latex agglutination test to detect polysaccharide capsular antigen is preferred for identification of *Cryptococcus*) |
| Wright/Giemsa | *Borrelia recurrentis*<br>Blood parasites (*Plasmodium* spp, *Trypanosoma* spp and *Babesia microti*)<br>*Chlamydia* and *Rickettsia* | A routine stain for peripheral blood |
| Silver (methenamine silver) | Fungi<br>*Listeria monocytogenes*<br>*Pneumocystis jirovecii* | Tissue stain for fungus; is also used to detect certain poorly Gram-staining organisms. Technically difficult |
| Acid-fast (Ziehl-Neelsen or carbol-fuchsin) | *Mycobacterium*<br>*Nocardia*<br>Some protozoa | High lipid content of cell wall prevents stain from being washed out by acid alcohol decolorizer |
| Iron hematoxylin and trichrome | Protozoa |  |
| Fecal wet mount (ova and parasites) | Protozoa, helminth eggs | Large size, can be easily visualized |

CSF, cerebrospinal fluid.

## MacConkey Agar

- Selective and differential medium.
- Inhibits the growth of gram-positive bacteria.
- Also differentiates whether a microorganism can use lactose as a nutrient source.
- Lactose utilizers form red colonies (vs white colonies in lactose nonfermenters).
- Used to distinguish among different enteric bacteria.

**TABLE 4-9.** Specialized Media for Microbial Growth

| ORGANISM | MEDIUM |
|---|---|
| All bacteria | Blood agar |
| Gram-negatives, lactose fermenters | MacConkey agar |
| Gram-negatives, lactose fermenters | EMB (eosin-methylene blue) agar |
| *H influenzae* | Chocolate agar |
| *Neisseria* | Thayer-Martin (VCN) agar |
| *B pertussis* | Bordet-Gengou medium |
| *Corynebacterium diphtheriae* | Tellurite agar |
| Group D streptococci | Bile esculin agar |

VCN, vancomycin, colistin, nystatin.

### Eosin-Methylene Blue Agar

- Like MacConkey's, eosin-methylene blue (EMB) agar inhibits gram-positive bacterial growth and allows assay of lactose as a sugar source.
- Lactose utilizers form dark-green, metallic-appearing colonies.

### Chocolate Agar

- *Haemophilus* spp are pathogens that are highly fastidious in their growth requirements and require enriched medium to survive in vitro.
- **X factor** (hemin) and **V factor** (NAD) are required. *Haemophilus* can also be grown in media with *S aureus*, which lyses RBCs and provides *Haemophilus* with the factors it needs to grow.
- Present in sheep's blood agar, but gentle heating (or "chocolatizing") is required to remove V factor inhibitors.

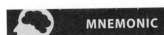

**MNEMONIC**

Say **HI** (*H influenzae*) to the townsfolk on your way to the **five and dime** (**V** and **X**) to buy some **chocolate.**

### Thayer-Martin (VCN) Agar

Like *Haemophilus*, *Neisseria* spp are highly fastidious microbes and require X and V factors for growth in the laboratory. Thayer-Martin (VCN) agar is a selective medium made of **chocolate agar supplemented with vancomycin, colistin,** and **nystatin (VCN).** It is used for the isolation of N *gonorrhoeae* from mucosal surfaces. The three powerful antimicrobial agents suppress growth of other commensal organisms present in vaginal, rectal, and pharyngeal specimens.

### Bordet-Gengou Medium

*Bordetella pertussis* is a highly fastidious respiratory pathogen that is difficult to grow under typical laboratory conditions. Specimen collection must be performed with a calcium alginate swab (sterile cotton is toxic to the microbe), and freshly prepared special medium (charcoal and horse blood) is required for growth.

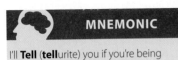

**MNEMONIC**

I'll **Tell** (**tell**urite) you if you're being **Corny** (**Coryne**bacterium).

### Tellurite Agars

Various selective media (potassium tellurite agar, cysteine tellurite agar) are used to isolate *Corynebacterium diphtheriae* from the respiratory tracts of affected individuals. Positive colonies are characteristically black on these agar plates.

### Bile Esculin Agar

This selective medium is used to differentiate group D streptococci (including *Enterococcus* spp) from other streptococci, which are unable to grow in the presence of bile salts.

**GRAM-POSITIVE COCCI**

Gram positive bacteria is identified in Figure 4-6. Microbes from the genera *Streptococcus* and *Staphylococcus* make up the bulk of clinically relevant gram-positive cocci (Figure 4-6) are responsible for diseases affecting diverse organ systems. Streptococci and staphylococci can be easily differentiated based on microscopic morphology; staphylococci appear in clusters ("bunches of grapes"), whereas streptococci are seen in pairs (**diplococci**) or chains (Figure 4-7). In addition, the **catalase** test easily discerns between the two genera; staphylococci are catalase-positive, and streptococci are catalase-negative.

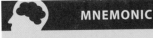

**MNEMONIC**

Stre**P**to**C**occi are seen in **P**airs and **C**hains.
**STAPH**ylococci are in clusters, like the **staff** of the hospital.

### *Streptococcus* and *Enterococcus*

The catalase-negative, gram-positive cocci (*Streptococcus* and the closely related *Enterococcus*, from now on referred to together as streptococci for simplicity) are a diverse group of coccoid organisms. Many medically important streptococci were first classified serologically by their **Lancefield group antigen,** a polymorphic immunogen located on the C carbohydrate component of the cell wall. Today, only three medically important

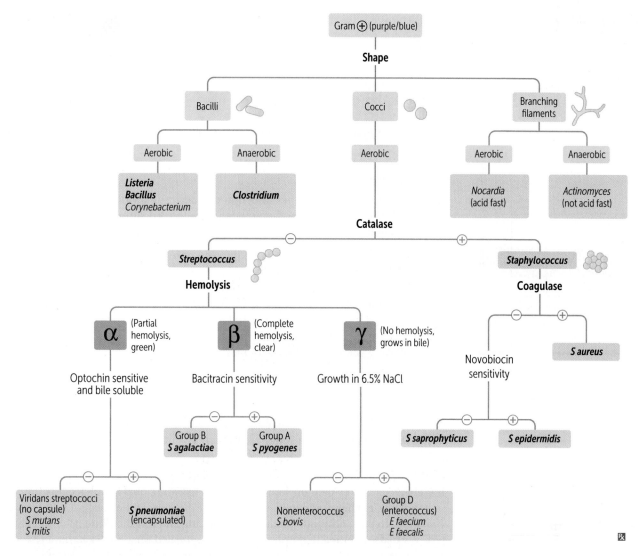

**FIGURE 4-6.    Gram-positive laboratory algorithm.** Important tests are in **bold**. Important pathogens are in ***bold italics***. Note: *Enterococcus* is either α- or γ-hemolytic.

groups of streptococci are known by their Lancefield antigens. Streptococci can be differentiated from one another on the basis of hemolysis patterns on blood agar.

***Streptococcus pyogenes*** (Lancefield Group A)

Characteristics

- **Pyogenic,** as the name suggests, meaning a pus-producing organism.
- 1- to 2-μm spherical coccus found in chains (Figure 4-7).
- β-hemolytic.
- Catalase-negative.
- Bacitracin-susceptible.
- Colonizes the upper respiratory mucosa (especially the oropharynx). Asymptomatic carriage in healthy individuals is common.

Pathogenesis

*S pyogenes* has a number of important virulence factors.

- **M protein** is a part of the cell wall that inhibits complement activation, preventing opsonization. Antibodies produced by the immune system that are directed against M protein can cause rheumatic fever. Specific antibodies produced by the immune system (type 2 hypersensitivity) are directed against the M protein.

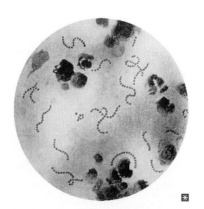

**FIGURE 4-7.    Photomicrograph of *Streptococcus pyogenes* in long chains.**

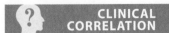
- **Streptolysin S** and **streptolysin O** are hemolytic enzymes responsible for the characteristic β-hemolytic pattern in vitro.
- **Pyrogenic exotoxins** are superantigens capable of causing the characteristic rash of scarlet fever as well as the multiple-organ system failure seen in streptococcal toxic shock syndrome.
- **Streptokinases** mediate the spread of infection through infected tissues.

Spread by respiratory droplets, so crowded conditions (eg, day-care facilities) facilitate person-to-person transmission.

### Clinical Symptoms

Clinical sequelae of *S pyogenes* infection can be easily divided into diseases caused by toxic effects of the bacteria themselves (often termed **suppurative** infections) and diseases caused by activation of the host immune system.

- Due to toxic effects of bacteria (eg, invasion or released toxins):
  - Skin and soft tissue infection
  - Streptococcal pharyngitis (strep throat)
  - Toxic shock syndrome (discussed under *S aureus* infections)
- Due to host immune system (eg, production of cross-reacting antibodies):
  - Rheumatic fever
  - Poststreptococcal glomerulonephritis

### Streptococcal Pharyngitis

Strep throat is a common streptococcal infection that involves the pharynx and possibly the tonsils and larynx. It is spread by direct contact with an infected individual and occurs more frequently in crowded areas, such as schools and the military.

### Clinical Symptoms

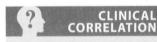
It is characterized by pain on swallowing, high fever, regional lymphadenopathy, and, most notably, erythema and frank white exudate on the palatine tonsils. Distinguishing viral from streptococcal sore throat can be difficult, and throat culture or a "rapid Strep test" is usually required. Complications from untreated pharyngitis include retropharyngeal and parapharyngeal abscesses, as well as immunologic sequelae (described later).

A variant of streptococcal pharyngitis, caused by strains containing a lysogenized pyrogenic exotoxin, is **scarlet fever.** Following the sore throat, a sandpaper-like rash appears on the chest and spreads centrifugally (outward), sparing the palms, soles, and face.

### Treatment

Penicillin V is the antibiotic of choice. Erythromycin or clindamycin is used for those with penicillin allergies.

### Skin and Soft Tissue Infections

#### Clinical Symptoms

Several distinct syndromes are caused by *Streptococcus* infection of epidermal, dermal, or fascial components.

- **Impetigo** is a common childhood skin infection of the upper epidermis by *S pyogenes* or *S aureus*. It is characterized by perioral vesicular/blistered lesions that eventually develop a honey-colored crust (Figure 4-8).
- **Erysipelas** and **cellulitis** are both acute infections of the skin characterized by erythema, edema, warmth, and systemic symptoms; cellulitis also involves deeper sub-

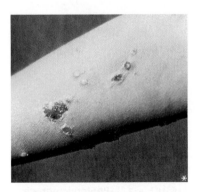

**FIGURE 4-8. Impetigo.**
These lesions on the forearm are *Streptococcal* impetigo.

cutaneous/dermal tissues. Both can be caused by other organisms as well (*S aureus* in immunocompetent individuals).

- **Necrotizing fasciitis** (or "flesh-eating bacteria") is a rapidly progressive infection of deep subcutaneous tissues. Symptoms include purple-blue **bullae** on the overlying skin following a cellulitis-like picture; overt gangrene, systemic symptoms, and multiorgan failure soon follow.

## Rheumatic Fever

### Pathogenesis

Rheumatic fever is caused by cross-reaction of antibodies raised against the *Streptococcus* bacteria with antigens in the heart, causing an initial **pancarditis.** Further cardiac damage in the form of valvular disease may occur many years later.

### Clinical Symptoms

In addition to symptoms of valvular cardiac disease, joint, cutaneous, and neurologic involvement is common.

Prevention of rheumatic fever is effectively accomplished by the early diagnosis and treatment of streptococcal pharyngitis with antibiotics, thus preventing the synthesis of the responsible antistreptococcal antibodies.

Those affected by rheumatic fever can have recurrences with subsequent streptococcal infections, and may be placed on long-term prophylactic antibiotics. Prophylaxis may be lifelong for patients who suffered rheumatic carditis.

## Poststreptococcal Glomerulonephritis

Renal sequelae of streptococcal infection can occur following either pharyngitis or skin or soft tissue infection. **Immune complexes** (antigen-antibody complexes) arising from streptococcal infection are deposited in the basement membrane of the glomerulus.

### Clinical Symptoms

The immune complex deposition causes typical glomerulonephritic symptoms of hematuria, hypertension, gross proteinuria, and facial edema all secondary to glomerular inflammation. Prognosis is generally good in the pediatric population.

### Treatment

*S pyogenes* is penicillin-sensitive. Patients with rheumatic fever may require lifelong prophylactic antibiotics because the fevers can often recur. Glomerulonephritis is usually treated with supportive care because immunosuppressive therapy to eliminate the immune complex deposition is ineffective.

### *Streptococcus agalactiae* (Lancefield Group B Streptococcus)

### Characteristics

*Streptococcus agalactiae*, a common cause of neonatal infection, is indistinguishable from *S pyogenes* by microscopy and is also characterized by β-hemolysis on blood agar.

- Unlike *S pyogenes*, *S agalactiae* is resistant to the antibiotic bacitracin.
- Approximately 10–30% of pregnant women are asymptomatically colonized with this organism.

### Pathogenesis

Transmission can occur transplacentally in utero or during delivery.

**KEY FACT**

Rheumatic fever follows untreated streptococcal pharyngitis, **not** streptococcal skin or soft tissue infection!

**MNEMONIC**

The **J♥NES** cr**ITERIA** are used to formally diagnose rheumatic fever.
**Required criterion**—documented evidence of recent group A streptococcal infection.

**Major criteria:**
**J**oint pains (migratory arthritis)
**♥** (carditis)
**N**odules (subcutaneous)
**E**rythema marginatum (spreading circular rash with red edges)
**S**ydenham chorea

**Minor criteria:**
**I**nflammatory cells (leukocytosis)
**T**emperature (fever)
**E**SR (erythrocyte sedimentation rate) or CRP (C-reactive protein) ↑
**R**heumatic fever (history of rheumatic disease)
**I**ncreased PR interval
**A**rthralgias
Two major criteria, or one major and two minor criteria are required for diagnosis.

**KEY FACT**

*S pyogenes* is always sensitive to penicillin. Penicillin resistance has never been detected in isolates, and transformation of pyogenes is notoriously difficult.

### Clinical Symptoms

*Streptococcus agalactiae* most commonly causes bacteremia without clear source, skin and soft tissue infections, and urinary tract infections. It is a relatively common cause of UTI in pregnant women. Other group B streptococcal (GBS) infections of adults are uncommon and generally occur in immunocompromised individuals.

Given the high rate of asymptomatic carriage in pregnant females, it is no surprise that *S agalactiae* is the most common cause of **neonatal septicemia** (sepsis) and meningitis. GBS can also cause **pneumonia in neonates.**

### Treatment

Like S *pyogenes*, GBS is also **penicillin-sensitive,** although higher concentrations are required for treatment. To prevent neonatal disease, current recommendations call for **screening** of pregnant women at 35–37 weeks' gestational age for GBS colonization via vaginal swab and culture. Women with positive cultures and those at high risk for intrapartum infection are given penicillin G (or ampicillin) during delivery.

### Viridans Streptococci

#### Characteristics

The viridans group of *Streptococcus* consists of several **nongroupable** (ie, not classified according to the Lancefield classification) streptococci that are α-hemolytic on blood agar. ("Viridis" is Latin for "green" to describe the green α-hemolysis.)

### Pathogenesis

Although viridans streptococci are commensals of the oropharynx and nasopharynx and are ordinarily nonpathogenic, they can cause disease, given the right opportunity.

### Clinical Symptoms

There are several members of the viridans streptococci group:

- *S mutans*, which is responsible for dental caries.
- *S interemdius*, which can be found in abscesses.
- *S sanguis*, which causes subacute bacterial endocarditis (SBE).

SBE is an indolent infection affecting previously damaged (ie, secondary to rheumatic fever or congenital bicuspid aortic valve) cardiac valves. Transient bacteremia is caused by dental procedures, and bacteria settle on the damaged valves. Associated symptoms include fevers, night sweats, fatigue, and new-onset murmurs.

### Treatment

Like the other streptococci, the viridans group are susceptible to penicillins. Resolution of SBE can require long-term use of parenteral antibiotics (penicillin or ceftriaxone and aminoglycoside, or vancomycin).

### Enterococcus and Other Group D Streptococci

#### Characteristics

The genus *Enterococcus*, members of which possess the group D Lancefield antigen, are distinguished from nonenterococcal group D streptococci by their growth under harsh conditions, namely 6.5% sodium chloride and 40% bile salts. Mostly γ-hemolytic, although hemolysis patterns can vary.

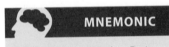

### Clinical Symptoms

Two species of enterococci, *Enterococcus faecalis* and *Enterococcus faecium*, are clinically relevant.

- Responsible for disease in immunocompromised patients and up to 10% of all infections in hospitalized patients. Patients on extended courses of broad-spectrum antibiotics are also at risk.
- UTIs in catheterized patients, postsurgical peritonitis, and SBE are the most common clinical entities caused by these microorganisms.

Of note, *Streptococcus bovis* is an uncommon cause of endocarditis. It is associated with gastrointestinal (GI) malignancy for an unknown reason; all patients with documented *S bovis* infections should receive a complete workup for GI malignancies.

### Pathogenesis

Enterococcal infections occur after genitourinary (GU)/GI procedures. Though enterococci do not produce potent toxins, they possess virulence factors that allow evasion of the immune system, like the enterococcal surface protein (Esp).

### Treatment

In the past, therapy for enterococcal infections has been the synergistic combination of ampicillin and an aminoglycoside. In the 1990s, rising resistance prompted the use of vancomycin to treat resistant strains. Unfortunately, resistance to vancomycin is rising (up to 20% of *E faecium* isolates), and novel antibiotic therapy has been required to treat these **vancomycin-resistant enterococci** (VRE) infections.

- Linezolid and daptomycin have activity against VRE; linezolid is bacteriostatic and has significant side effects.
- Antibiotics such as nitrofurantoin are another option for the treatment of VRE UTIs.

### *Streptococcus pneumoniae*
### Characteristics

The nontypable *S pneumoniae*, commonly known as pneumococcus, is one of the most clinically important gram-positive cocci. Microscopically, pneumococci are commonly seen as "lancet-shaped" organisms in pairs (diplococci). Hemolysis patterns on blood agar vary, but usually α-hemolysis is seen.

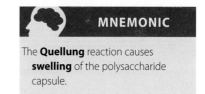

**MNEMONIC**

The **Quellung** reaction causes **swelling** of the polysaccharide capsule.

Identification of the pneumococcus is facilitated by several individualized assays.

- The **Quellung** reaction can identify pneumococci in a clinically derived sample such as sputum; the polysaccharide capsule is microscopically visualized by the addition of anticapsular antibodies, which cause the capsule to swell.
- Colonies of *S pneumoniae* are differentiated from other α-hemolytic streptococci (eg, viridans streptococci and enterococci) on agar plates by means of optochin susceptibility (*S pneumoniae* is susceptible, while viridans streptococci are resistant) and by adding bile to the culture medium. (*S pneumoniae* fail to grow in bile.)

### Pathogenesis

Virulence of pneumococcus is mainly mediated by the presence of a polysaccharide capsule, which inhibits phagocytosis.

Transmission of *S pneumoniae* is through airborne droplets; asymptomatic carriage is common. Disease is caused by oropharyngeal infection with a noncolonizing serotype. The microorganism then spreads from the oropharynx via respiratory mucosa to the paranasal sinuses, the lower respiratory tract, or the meninges.

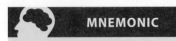

**MNEMONIC**

**Streptococcus pneumoniae *is the most common cause of—***
**MOPS**
**M**eningitis
**O**titis media
**P**neumonia
**S**inusitis

### Clinical Symptoms

- Pneumococcus is the most common cause of bacterial **pneumonia** in adults. A lobar pattern is seen on chest film, and high fevers with shaking and chills are common. Frank blood and diplococci may be found in an induced sputum sample.
- *S pneumoniae* is also the number one cause of **meningitis** in adults.
- Pneumococcal **sinusitis** in adults and **otitis media** in children are commonly seen.
- Pneumococcus can also cause **sepsis**, often preceded by meningitis. Individuals with **asplenia** (including functional asplenia seen in sickle cell disease) are also at increased risk for pneumococcal bacteremia and sepsis.

### Treatment

Penicillin was once the mainstay of treatment for pneumococcal infection. However, rapidly increasing resistance has forced the use of alternative therapies in certain areas with intermediate or high rates of resistance. **Ceftriaxone** or **vancomycin** (or a combination of the two) is used in these cases.

A 13-valent pneumococcal conjugate vaccine is recommended for all infants younger than 2 years. Adults at high risk—including immunocompromised, asplenic, and elderly individuals as well as some transplant recipients—should receive a **23-valent polysaccharide vaccine** to protect against pneumonia and invasive disease.

### *Staphylococcus*

Staphylococci make up the other major medically relevant group of gram-positive cocci. Like streptococci, they are colonizers of body surfaces and commonly cause skin and soft tissue substructure infections. Fortunately, they are easily differentiated from streptococci based on microscopy and the laboratory test for the **catalase** enzyme (using hydrogen peroxide as a substrate, Table 4-10). Staphylococci assume the form of purple clusters (called a "bunch of grapes") when Gram-stained.

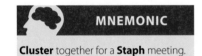

**MNEMONIC**

**Cluster** together for a **Staph** meeting.

Three common and medically relevant species of *Staphylococcus* are *S aureus*, *S epidermidis*, and *S saprophyticus*.

#### *Staphylococcus aureus*

### Characteristics

Because of its propensity for colonization and high degree of virulence, *S aureus* is a cause of both community-acquired and nosocomial morbidity and mortality. Like other staphylococci, on microscopic examination, it looks like purple clusters (Figure 4-9). Large β-hemolytic mucoid colonies that produce a **gold pigment** are seen when the organism is grown on blood agar.

*S aureus* is unique among the staphylococci in that it contains the enzyme **coagulase.** Other species of *Staphylococcus* do not have this enzyme and are thus often referred to in laboratory reports as "coagulase-negative *Staphylococcus.*"

*S aureus* is a part of the normal flora of human skin, and transient colonization of moist skin folds and the nasopharyngeal cavity is common. It also survives for long periods of

**TABLE 4-10.** ***Staphylococcus* Compared With *Streptococcus***

|  | STAPHYLOCOCCUS | STREPTOCOCCUS |
|---|---|---|
| **Microscopy** | Clusters | Pairs and chains |
| **Catalase test** | Positive | Negative |
| **Penicillin-sensitive** | Rarely (except *S saprophyticus*) | Commonly |

time on dry surfaces. Transmission is either via shedding of microbes or contaminated **fomites,** inanimate objects that serve as vectors for microbial transmission. The rate of hospital-acquired methicillin-resistant *S aureus* (MRSA) infections is almost certainly due to transmission via fomites.

### Pathogenesis

Like *S pyogenes, S aureus* features a number of different virulence factors that can be divided into several groups. Not all strains carry all virulence factors.

Immune modulators:

- **Protein A:** Specifically binds the $F_c$ component of immunoglobulin, preventing immune-mediated destruction via **opsonization.**
- **Coagulase:** An enzyme that builds an insoluble fibrin capsule that surrounds the microorganism, thus preventing immune cell access.
- **Hemolysins** (also known as cytotoxins) α, β, γ, and δ: Directly toxic to hematopoietic cells.
- **Leukocidin:** A toxin specific for white blood cells.
- **Catalase:** Prevents toxic action of neutrophil-derived hydrogen peroxide.
- **Penicillinase:** A secreted form of β-lactamase, can inactivate penicillin and derivatives.

Factors permitting penetration through tissues:

- **Hyaluronidase:** Hydrolyzes hyaluronic acid present in connective tissue.
- **Fibrinolysin** (also known as **staphylokinase**):Dissolves fibrin clots.
- **Lipases:** Break down lipids to allow for survival and spread in fat-rich areas of the body, such as in the sebaceous glands.

Secreted toxins:

- **Exfoliatin:** Causes the exfoliation of the skin, causing staphylococcal scalded skin syndrome (SSSS).
- **Enterotoxins** (heat-stable): Cause vomiting and diarrhea.
- **Toxic shock syndrome toxin (TSST-1):** A **superantigen** that cross-links the major histocompatability complex (MHC) class II molecules on antigen-presenting cells, causing a massive nonspecific T-cell response, leading to toxic shock syndrome.

### Clinical Symptoms

*S aureus* is capable of invading almost any organ. Both toxin-mediated (sterile) and invasive diseases are common (Table 4-11).

### Staphylococcal Scalded Skin Syndrome

SSSS is a relatively common disease of infants that presents with perioral exfoliation of the middle layer of the epidermis followed by the diffuse formation of blisters containing

### FLASH FORWARD

The development of multidrug (or methicillin)-resistant *S aureus* (MRSA) has complicated the treatment of *S aureus* infections. Drugs such as vancomycin are now needed to treat such infections.

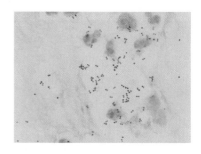

**FIGURE 4-9.** *Staphylococcus aureus.* Clusters of gram-positive cocci.

### KEY FACT

**Superantigens** are substances that can cause a massive, **nonspecific** overstimulation of the immune system by chemically cross-linking the MHC class II molecules on antigen-presenting cells.

**TABLE 4-11.** **Spectrum of Staphylococcal Disease**

| EXOTOXIN-MEDIATED | INVASIVE |
| --- | --- |
| Staphylococcal scalded skin syndrome (SSSS) | Skin and soft tissue infections |
| Food poisoning | Endocarditis |
| Toxic shock syndrome | Pneumonia and empyema |
| | Osteomyelitis |
| | Septic arthritis |

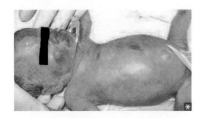

**FIGURE 4-10. Staphylococcal scalded skin syndrome.** Red skin lesions with epidermal peeling on the face and body.

**KEY FACT**

*Staphylococcus aureus* preformed enterotoxin is the only cause of food poisoning whose onset occurs acutely (within 4 hours).

**CLINICAL CORRELATION**

Usually there is a diffuse red rash involving the trunk and systemic hypotension due to widespread histamine release.

**KEY FACT**

Most cases of IE occur on **left-sided** valves and have a poor prognosis due to brain emboli; IV drug users get **right-sided** IE, which has a much better prognosis.

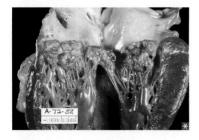

**FIGURE 4-11. Infective endocarditis.** Note the large, friable-appearing vegetations on the valves.

sterile fluid (Figure 4-10). Unless there is bacterial superinfection, the disease resolves within approximately one week without further sequelae; morbidity and mortality rates are low.

### Gastroenteritis

*S aureus*–induced gastroenteritis is common and notable for its rapid onset (within 4–6 hours after ingestion of tainted food), due to preformed heat-stable enterotoxin produced by the bacteria. Symptoms include abrupt and copious vomiting and nonbloody diarrhea. The bacteria are spread via food that is prepared by someone with a skin infection or by asymptomatic nasal carriage. Common culprit food items are salads made with tainted mayonnaise, processed meats, custard, and nondairy creamers. The illness generally runs a short (< 24 hours) and uncomplicated course, and antibiotics are unnecessary.

### Toxic Shock Syndrome

Tampons left in place for too long can become a nidus for infection and is a common cause of toxic shock syndrome. But toxic shock syndrome can also occur in wounds with draining fluid collections. *S aureus* microbes multiply in the nutrient-rich menstrual or wound fluid and secrete TSST-1, which causes a systemic inflammatory response due to the nonspecific activation of T cells. Symptoms include abrupt onset of fever and hypotension, and multiple organ dysfunction are seen; a desquamating rash of the palms and soles is typical as well. Treatment includes blood pressure support and empiric antibiosis with vancomycin and clindamycin, which also serves to suppress protein synthesis of TSST-1.

### Skin and Soft Tissue Infections

#### Characteristics

Like group A *Streptococcus*, *S aureus* can also cause various **skin and soft tissue infections,** such as cellulitis and impetigo. The following skin substructure infections are more commonly caused by *S aureus*:

- **Folliculitis** is an infection of the base of the hair follicle. Patients present with a small, raised, erythematous bump. This infection can occur anywhere on the skin, but is most common in areas with abundant hair.
- A **furuncle** is a conglomeration of several adjacent inflamed follicles. It presents as a large, painful nodule.
- **Carbuncles** are coalesced furuncles that often extend into the dermis. They can cause systemic symptoms such as fever as well as staphylococcal bacteremia.
- **Staphylococcal wound infections** are common because they are commensals that normally live on the skin.

#### Treatment

Appropriate antibiotic therapy can be administered either systemically or locally via topical creams or ointments.

### Infective Endocarditis

Infective endocarditis (IE) of undamaged (native) valves is commonly caused by *S aureus* migrating from infected surgical wounds or contaminated intravenous (IV) catheters. Unlike SBE, acute IE is characterized by a rapid onset of high fever with rigors, myalgias, and possibly a right-sided regurgitation murmur. Large infective vegetations, which can break off and cause septic pulmonary emboli, can be seen on the affected valves (Figure 4-11).

### Pneumonia

Staphylococcal **pneumonia** is rare in the community but is a common cause of nosocomial pneumonia, especially in the elderly following infection with influenza. Characterized by the rapid onset of fever and chills and a nonspecific radiographic pattern. **Cavitations** in the lung tissue are seen on gross dissection. Infected parapneumonic effusions (known as **empyema**) are also common. Certain strains can cause an even more severe variant known as **necrotizing** pneumonia, characterized by massive hemoptysis and septic shock.

## Osteomyelitis

Osteomyelitis is characterized by a deep-seated infection of the bone. This disease is seeded hematogenously from distant sites (usually cutaneous staphylococcal infections) or from contiguous, overlying skin infections (eg, diabetic foot ulcers). The symptoms are localized pain and fever, and further hematogenous spread is common. Plain radiographs or MRI are used to screen for distant disease. Several weeks to months of appropriate antibiotic therapy usually results in a complete cure.

## Septic Arthritis

### Characteristics

*S aureus* is the most common cause of **septic arthritis** seen in pediatric and elderly age groups (*N gonorrhoeae* is the most common cause among sexually active individuals).

### Pathogenesis

Disease can be caused by local introduction of the organism by synovial puncture via needle or via hematogenous spread from distant foci of infection.

### Clinical Symptoms

Classic symptoms include an erythematous, swollen joint with decreased range of motion; the key laboratory finding from **arthrocentesis** (joint aspiration) is an elevated neutrophil count.

### Treatment

Prompt treatment with antibiotics is generally effective; drainage may be required.

Since most *S aureus* isolates carry a penicillinase enzyme, first-generation penicillins are not used for antibiotic therapy.

**Methicillin-sensitive *S aureus*** (MSSA) make up approximately 70% of *S aureus* strains and are appropriately treated with semisynthetic, second-generation penicillins such as nafcillin, oxacillin, and dicloxacillin, which are not broken down by penicillinase. First-generation cephalosporins are also highly efficacious. Note that methicillin is no longer used clinically because of nephrotoxicity.

Unfortunately, methicillin-resistant strains of *S aureus* (MRSA) have developed in the past half-century. MRSA contain an altered penicillin-binding protein (PBP) that does not bind β-lactams well, rendering them resistant to the semisynthetic penicillins. Previously, these strains were found only in settings where broad-spectrum antibiotics were commonly used. However, community-acquired MRSA is seen increasingly, especially in skin and skin substructure infections. **Vancomycin** is the cornerstone of MRSA therapy. However, clindamycin and trimethoprim-sulfamethoxazole (TMP-SMX) may also be used.

### Coagulase-Negative *Staphylococcus*

### Characteristics

*S epidermidis* and *S saprophyticus* are commonly isolated *Staphylococcus* species. Both appear as gram-positive cocci in small clusters and are catalase-positive, but do not contain the coagulase enzyme. Of note, *S epidermidis* is sensitive to the antibiotic **novobiocin,** whereas *S saprophyticus* is resistant.

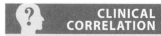

**CLINICAL CORRELATION**

*S aureus* is the most common cause of osteomyelitis overall, but in certain patient populations other bacteria are more common (eg, *Salmonella typhi* in sickle cell disease, and *P aeruginosa* in diabetic foot ulcer).

**KEY FACT**

*S epidermidis* is one of the most frequently isolated organisms from blood cultures in hospitals. This is usually due to contamination rather than true *S epidermidis* bacteremia.

### Pathogenesis

*S epidermidis* is a constituent of normal skin flora. In healthy individuals, this species is not a major cause of disease. However, its unique polysaccharide capsule allows the organism to adhere to various surfaces with ease (eg, medical equipment), which can lead to opportunistic infections.

### Clinical Symptoms

Infections of mechanical prostheses (eg, prosthetic joints, mechanical heart valves), as well as indwelling catheters, are common. These infections demonstrate an indolent course with slow development of systemic symptoms.

*S saprophyticus* is the second most common cause of community-acquired UTIs in sexually active women (*E coli* being the most common). Symptoms are typical and include dysuria, pyuria, and bacteruria.

### Treatment

Over 50% of *S epidermidis* isolates are methicillin-resistant and thus require vancomycin or alternative treatment. *S saprophyticus* responds to typical empiric treatment for UTIs with TMP-SMX, fluoroquinolones, and others.

## GRAM-POSITIVE RODS

Gram-positive rods fall into two general categories: the spore-forming—or **sporulating**—rods and the non–spore-forming rods. The anaerobic *Clostridium* spp and the aerobic *Bacillus* spp form **endospores** under conditions of metabolic stress. *L monocytogenes*, *Corynebacterium diphtheriae*, and the actinomycetes (*Actinomyces* spp and *Nocardia* spp) make up the heterogeneous group of nonsporulating gram-positive rods.

### Sporulating Gram-Positive Rods

The medically important gram-positive rods in this category are universally soil microbes, and the endospore they produce is thought to be an evolutionary adaptation to dehydration. Pathogenically, these microorganisms cause disease by secreting powerful exotoxins. Invasive disease is not characteristic and, since the toxins are usually preformed, antibiotics are of limited efficacy in treatment of disease.

#### *Clostridium botulinum*

##### Characteristics

*Clostridium botulinum* is a gram-positive, sporulating rod that is anaerobic, thus growing only in specially designed anaerobic environments. It produces a highly virulent exotoxin that leads to **flaccid muscular paralysis.**

##### Pathogenesis

The botulinum exotoxin most commonly enters the body via ingestion of endospores, and is a **heat-labile A-B neurotoxin** that inhibits the release of acetylcholine (ACh) at neuromuscular junctions, leading to flaccid paralysis. There are seven serotypes, A–G; however, the serotypes that most commonly cause disease are **A, B,** and **E.** People never develop natural immunity to botulism toxin because of its extreme toxicity; even amounts too small to initiate an immune response can be fatal if untreated. Botulinum toxin is a potential biologic weapon and is listed as a CDC category A **bioterrorism agent.**

##### Clinical Symptoms

There are three clinical presentations of botulinum toxicity.

- **Food-borne botulism** occurs 1–2 days after eating tainted canned or preserved goods.

### FLASH BACK

*Botulinum exotoxin* targets the synaptosomal-associated protein 25 (SNAP25) fusion protein, preventing neurotransmitter-filled vesicles from fusing to the membrane and releasing ACh.

- Once ingested, the exotoxin is absorbed through the gut and travels in the blood to nerve synapses.
- Patients complain of blurred or double vision, difficulty speaking or swallowing, droopy eyes or muscle weakness, and GI symptoms. The paralytic effects progress in a descending fashion (from head to toe).
- Patients need to be treated immediately because the toxin may compromise respiratory muscles. Treatment includes antitoxin and respiratory support.
- **Infant botulism** results when babies ingest spores found in household dust or **honey.**
  - The spores germinate in the gut and produce the exotoxin, which is absorbed into the blood. Toxin can be detected in stool sample.
  - Symptoms include constipation, limpness, loss of head control, dysphagia, weak feeding, and weak crying. This disease is sometimes referred to as **floppy baby syndrome** because of the severe loss of muscle tone and control.
  - Treatment includes respiratory support and human-derived polyvalent antitoxin (serotypes A, B, and E). A human-derived antitoxin rather than the equine-derived antitoxin is given to prevent any risk of type III hypersensitivity reaction.
  - Prognosis is good, even without the use of humanized antitoxin.
- **Wound botulism** occurs from trauma and germination of spores at the wound site.
  - Botulinum toxin is produced in vivo and disseminated throughout the body. Symptoms are the same as those for food-borne botulism, without GI symptoms.
  - Patients are treated with respiratory support, equine-derived polyvalent antitoxin, and antibiotics to eradicate the bacteria.

### Treatment

**Antitoxin** is the cornerstone of treatment for all varieties of botulism. Antitoxin is a fraction of serum (usually equine) obtained from an animal that has been inoculated with the toxin. This serum contains polyclonal antibodies that can neutralize the botulinum toxin.

### *Clostridium tetani*

### Characteristics

Like other *Clostridium* species, this anaerobic gram-positive rod produces spores that are generally found in the soil.

### Pathogenesis

The spores are inoculated into puncture wounds (eg, stepping on a rusty nail), which provide an ideal environment for germination. The bacteria produce **tetanus toxin,** also known as tetanospasmin, a neurotoxin that binds peripheral nerve terminals and travels intra-axonally from the site of entry to the CNS. It binds ganglioside receptors at the presynaptic inhibitory nerve ending, selectively cleaves synaptobrevin, a protein component of the synaptic vesicle, and **prevents the release of the inhibitory neurotransmitters** (γ-aminobutyric acid [GABA] and glycine). Without inhibitory signals, excitatory neurons are unopposed, causing sustained muscle contraction or **tetany.**

### Clinical Symptoms

Patients with tetanus present with severe, unopposed muscle contractions. Often, this is most evident in the muscles of the jaw, producing the characteristic **risus sardonicus** (strange grin), or lockjaw.

### Treatment

Treatment of active tetanus infection is accomplished with antibiotics (usually metronidazole), antitetanus immune globulin, an immediate tetanus booster, extensive debridement, and muscle relaxants. Rapid response is critical to prevent death secondary to respiratory complications. Benzodiazepines and supportive care (mechanical ventilation) may be provided to allow breathing until the effects of the toxin wears off.

**KEY FACT**

**Never feed babies honey!** Their immature GI tracts do not have the normal flora that prevent spores from germinating.

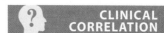

**CLINICAL CORRELATION**

Antitoxin of any variety given to a human can produce **serum sickness** because of the foreign protein antigens present in animal-derived sera. This is an example of type III hypersensitivity.

The major modality for control and prevention of tetanus is the **tetanus toxoid** vaccine. This is a formalin-inactivated toxin that is first injected as part of the **DTaP** (diphtheria-tetanus-acellular pertussis) vaccine. Since immunity is fleeting, booster shots are given every 10 years.

### Clostridium perfringens

#### Characteristics

This anaerobic, spore-forming soil bacterium is the only non-motile member of the *Clostridium* species.

#### Pathogenesis

Traumatic implantation of the spores into muscle tissue (ie, by a puncture wound) causes germination and the release of the **α toxin,** a lecithinase that can necrotize tissue and destroy blood and vascular cells. Other toxins are released as well, some of which are capable of catalyzing a **fermentation reaction,** causing the release of intra-parenchymal **gas.**

#### Clinical Symptoms

The most serious infection caused by *Clostridium perfringens* is **gas gangrene,** also known as **clostridial myonecrosis.** This infection is characterized by **tissue crepitus** (the palpable and audible presence of air or gas) and rapid, widespread necrosis of muscular tissue with rapidly ensuing death. Other soft tissue infections with significantly less severe presentations, and gastroenteritis (watery diarrhea), are also possible sequelae.

#### Treatment

Treatment of gas gangrene involves debridement, high-dose penicillin, and hyperbaric $O_2$ (to provide a toxic atmosphere for the anaerobic clostridia). Mortality is unfortunately still high in the most severe infections.

### Clostridium difficile

#### Characteristics

*C difficile* is another anaerobic, spore-forming organism that causes **colitis** (the severe variant is known as **pseudomembranous colitis**), which is common among hospitalized patients, especially those on broad-spectrum antibiotics.

#### Pathogenesis

*Clostridium difficile* is a normal component of the intestinal flora of some people (and is easily spread to others via its hardy spores). Because of its relative antibiotic resistance, it has the tendency to proliferate in the colon during treatment with broad-spectrum antibiotics, thus outcompeting the susceptible normal enteric flora. At this point, the organism produces **enterotoxin** and **cytotoxin,** which cause the characteristic secretory diarrhea.

#### Clinical Symptoms

Clinically, patients with colitis present with an acute episode of watery diarrhea and abdominal cramping. In severe cases, a **pseudomembrane** composed of sloughed inflammatory cells, fibrin, and mucus is seen overlying intact colonic mucosa (Figure 4-12). Extreme cases can progress to **toxic megacolon,** which can require surgical intervention.

#### Treatment

Appropriate treatment is discontinuation of broad-spectrum antibiotics and treatment with **oral vancomycin,** or intravenous metronidazole.

**KEY FACT**

Clindamycin, fluoroquinolones, and broad spectrum β-lactams are most often associated with *C difficile* colitis, although all antibiotics are capable of causing this side effect.

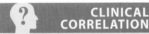

**CLINICAL CORRELATION**

Despite claims to the contrary, *C difficile* colitis cannot be diagnosed based on the smell of the offending stool alone. One or both toxins must be isolated from stool specimens.

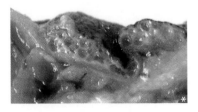

**FIGURE 4-12.**
**Pseudomembranous colitis.**

*Bacillus anthracis*

### Characteristics

This spore-forming facultative anaerobe is the causative agent of **anthrax.** It is a non-motile gram-positive rod that primarily infects herbivores or lives in the soil as a resilient spore. Transmission to humans is usually via traumatic implantation or inhalation of spores from infected animals or, more recently, via inhalation of intentionally placed spores.

### Pathogenesis

Spores are transmitted via inhalation or contact through an open wound. The organism possesses a unique, immunogenic capsule composed of a poly-D-glutamate polypeptide that prevents phagocytosis. **Protective antigen** allows entry of other toxins into cells, and **edema toxin** activates adenylate cyclase, causing osmotic cell swelling. The **lethal factor** is a cytotoxic protein that causes inflammation, macrophage activation, and cell death.

### Clinical Symptoms

There are three categories of clinical anthrax, which correspond completely with the route of contact with the pathogen or its spores.

- **Cutaneous anthrax** occurs through skin contact with *B anthracis* spores. A characteristic papule progresses to vesiculation/ulceration and subsequently to a **black eschar** with central necrosis at the original site of inoculation (Figure 4-13). While the lesion is painless, painful regional lymphadenopathy and systemic disease can develop.
- **Pulmonary (inhalational) anthrax** occurs when spores are inhaled, either from animals (**woolsorter's disease**) or in cases of bioterrorism. Nonspecific symptoms such as fever, headache, cough, malaise, and chest pain are the usual initial manifestations. Untreated, this will lead to **massively enlarged mediastinal lymph nodes,** pulmonary hemorrhage, meningeal symptoms, and often (50%) death.
- **Gastrointestinal anthrax** is caused by ingestion of live spores; it is highly lethal but rare.

### Treatment

Ciprofloxacin is the agent of choice, although several alternatives are available. Immediate antibiotic treatment as soon as the diagnosis is suspected is the key to preventing fatality. Prevention is focused on **animal vaccination;** a human vaccine is available but has major side effects and is given only to at-risk populations.

*Bacillus cereus*

### Characteristics

*Bacillus cereus* is another motile, spore-forming gram-positive rod, but its virulence is much lower than that of *B anthracis*.

### Pathogenesis

The spores are ubiquitously found in nature and are typically ingested in food sources. **Reheated fried rice** is a common source.

### Clinical Symptoms

Two forms of GI disease are possible: An **emetic** form manifesting as rapid-onset vomiting and diarrhea, and a **diarrheal** form characterized by watery, secretory diarrhea.

### Treatment

Both forms typically resolve without sequelae, and antibiotic treatment is not indicated.

**KEY FACT**

The only organism with a polypeptide capsule (poly-D-glutamate) is *B anthracis*. All other known capsules are composed of polysaccharides.

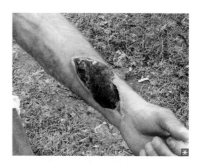

**FIGURE 4-13.** **Cutaneous anthrax on a forearm.**

## Nonsporulating Gram-Positive Rods

### Listeria monocytogenes

#### Characteristics

*Listeria* is an uncommon human pathogen responsible for important diseases affecting neonates. It is a short gram-positive rod that exhibits **tumbling motility** at room temperature and is easily grown on agar, **even at cold temperatures.** Like many opportunistic pathogens, it is ubiquitous in nature and can be found in animals, soil, and even as an asymptomatic colonizer of the human GI tract. When a source is identified, it is often a refrigerated, contaminated food product such as soft cheese, cabbage, or milk.

#### Pathogenesis

Infection is often precipitated by ingestion and subsequent transmucosal uptake by cells of the GI tract. Unpasteurized dairy products and spoiled deli meats are common sources. Transplacental transmission in utero and vaginal transmission during birth are also possible. *L monocytogenes* is also a facultative intracellular organism, enabling it to evade clearance by phagocytosis. Patients with compromised cell-mediated immunity are at a higher risk due to the intracellular nature of infection.

#### Clinical Symptoms

Neonatal listeriosis can take on two forms. **Early-onset disease** (also known as **granulomatosis infantiseptica**) occurs as a result of transplacental transmission and is characterized by late miscarriage or birth complicated by sepsis, multiorgan abscesses, and disseminated granulomas. The mortality rate is extremely high. **Late-onset disease** typically is transmitted during childbirth and manifests as meningitis or meningoencephalitis occurring 2–3 weeks later. Therefore, pregnant women are advised to avoid eating soft cheeses and unpasteurized dairy products.

Adult listeriosis manifests variably depending on the demographic: pregnant women may develop amnionitis or septicemia or experience spontaneous abortion; immunocompromised patients can develop meningitis; and healthy individuals develop mild gastroenteritis.

#### Treatment

*Listeria monocytogenes* is intrinsically resistant to cephalosporins, and the mainstays of treatment are IV penicillin or ampicillin, often combined with gentamicin for synergy.

### Corynebacterium diphtheriae

#### Characteristics

These important **comma-shaped** bacteria are the cause of **diphtheria.** They are small, pleomorphic, irregular-staining gram-positive rods that are observed to contain **metachromatic** (red or blue) **granules** when stained with methylene blue (Figure 4-14). They can grow on most media, but **tellurite-containing medium** is often used to selectively isolate the organism from pharyngeal swab specimens.

Because of an extensive childhood vaccination campaign, *C diphtheriae* has become rare in the developed world, but cases are still relatively common in impoverished urban areas worldwide.

#### Pathogenesis

Transmission is via respiratory droplets from unvaccinated individuals or asymptomatic vaccinated carriers. The main virulence factor is **diphtheria toxin,** an exotoxin that is encoded on a lysogenic bacteriophage virus called a **β-phage.** Not all bacteria express the toxin, since expression relies on prior infection of the bacterium by a bacteriophage. The toxin is a classic A-B toxin: component B allows entry of the A subunit into the

---

**KEY FACT**

Always include intravenous ampicillin for meningitis in neonates and immunocompromised patients.

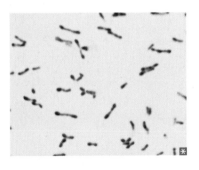

**FIGURE 4-14.** *Corynebacterium diphtheriae.* This photomicrograph depicts numerous gram-positive asporogenous, rod-shaped, *Corynebacterium diphtheriae* bacteria.

cells. The A subunit in this case is an adenosine triphosphate (ADP)–ribosyltransferase enzyme that **inactivates elongation factor (EF-2)** via ADP-ribosylation, thereby inhibiting protein synthesis.

### Clinical Symptoms

Diphtheria manifests as an **exudative pharyngitis** causing dysphagia (pain on swallowing), fever, and malaise following an incubation period of less than 1 week. As the disease progresses, a thick **pseudomembrane** (made up of fibrin, dead cells, bacteria, and leukocytes) forms on the posterior oropharynx and tonsils. This membrane is **gray** and tightly adherent and **cannot be scraped off** without causing bleeding of the underlying tissue. After another week, this membrane spontaneously dislodges, although complications can arise from airway compromise caused by the membrane. Other features of the disease include cervical lymphadenopathy and edema, resulting in the characteristic **bull-neck** appearance. Cardiac and lower respiratory complications are rare but potentially fatal.

Diagnosis of diphtheria is usually clinical, but clinical specimens are generally tested for pathogenicity using the **Elek test,** an in vitro assay that tests for the production of exotoxin.

### Treatment

Treatment of active diphtheria is the early administration of **diphtheria antitoxin** and appropriate antibiotic therapy (penicillin or erythromycin).

Prevention has been largely successful in the United States, owing to routine childhood immunization with nontoxic **diphtheria toxoid** as part of the DTaP vaccine series.

### Gram-Positive Branching Organisms

These gram-positive rods typically live in soil and have unique, fungus-like microscopic morphology with branching and hyphal forms. There is a staggering number of these organisms, many of which cause rare opportunistic or pulmonary infections. Two of them are particularly important and are discussed here.

#### *Actinomyces israelii*

### Characteristics

Unlike *Nocardia*, *A israelii* is an **anaerobic** actinomycete that is **not acid-fast.** It is a constituent of the normal mouth flora of some humans that may lead to opportunistic infection.

### Pathogenesis

Because *A israelii* is not normally virulent, a break in integrity of the mucous membrane through trauma or oral surgery is necessary for infection.

### Clinical Symptoms

Typically causes slowly developing oral and facial abscesses with an underlying yellow color due to the presence of so-called **sulfur granules.** These granules are actually massive collections of *Actinomyces* organisms. Sinus tract drainage of these abscesses to the skin surface is common. Other potential sites for actinomycosis are the brain, chest cavity, and abdominopelvic region. Mycetomas are also possible.

### Treatment

Surgical incision and drainage coupled with penicillin or ampicillin.

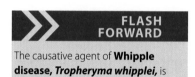

**FLASH FORWARD**

The causative agent of **Whipple disease, *Tropheryma whipplei,*** is also an actinomycete.

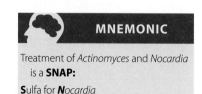

**MNEMONIC**

Treatment of *Actinomyces* and *Nocardia* is a **SNAP:**

**S**ulfa for **N**ocardia
**A**ctinomyces needs **P**enicillin

*Nocardia*

### Characteristics

*Nocardia* is strictly aerobic. It can be differentiated from *A israelii* as it is **partially acid-fast** on carbol-fuchsin stain.

### Pathogenesis

*Nocardia* is opportunistic, with the majority of infected patients being immunocompromised. During its filamentous growth phase, the organism is resistant to phagocytosis. The most common route of transmission is via inhalation, as the organism can adhere to dust particles. Ingestion of contaminated food, as well as direct inoculation into the skin via trauma, can also occur.

### Clinical Symptoms

*Nocardia* causes indolent bronchopulmonary infections, especially in individuals with **decreased T-cell immunity.** Cavitary pulmonary lesions as well as hematogenous spread to the skin and CNS are common. Primary cutaneous lesions such as cellulitis, subcutaneous abscesses, and **mycetomas** can develop as well. Mycetomas are chronic, destructive cutaneous lesions caused by actinomycetes that generally feature sinus tracts communicating with the epidermal surface, painless edema, and subcutaneous abscesses.

### Treatment

Treatment is with sulfonamides or TMP-SMX.

## GRAM-NEGATIVE COCCI

For an algorithm that identifies gram-negative bacteria, see Figure 4-15.

### *Neisseria*

The only two medically important gram-negative cocci are *N meningitidis* or **meningococcus,** which causes meningitis and sepsis; and *N gonorrhoeae* or **gonococcus,** which causes gonorrhea, disseminated gonococcal disease, and ophthalmia neonatorum. All *Neisseria* are small, aerobic, gram-negative cocci typically seen on microscopy as coffee-bean-like **diplococci** or in clumps (Figure 4-16). Both are oxidase-positive (in contrast to the oxidase-negative Enterobacteriaceae).

### *Neisseria meningitidis*

#### Characteristics

Meningococcus is the organism responsible for most cases of bacterial meningitis in adolescents and certain at-risk populations (military trainees, dormitory residents). In addition, it can cause debilitating sepsis known as **meningococcemia.** The microorganism is transmitted by respiratory droplets and can be a normal constituent of the oropharyngeal flora.

#### Pathogenesis

Except for the meningococcal capsule, *N meningitidis* and *N gonorrhoeae* share the same virulence factors:

- **Por proteins:** Form outer membrane pores that allow passage of nutrients and waste materials and, in some cases, prevent complement-dependent killing of the bacteria.
- **Opa proteins:** Involved in surface adhesion.
- **Lipooligosaccharide (LOS):** A variant of gram-negative endotoxin (LPS) that does not possess the O-polysaccharide moiety present in LPS but still possesses endotoxin-like cytotoxic capabilities.
- **IgA proteases:** Cleave the immunoglobulin IgA into its inactive constituents to evade mucosal adaptive immunity.

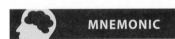

**MNEMONIC**

*N* go**NO**rrhoeae—
**NO** capsule, **NO** maltose, and **NO** vaccine.

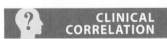

**CLINICAL CORRELATION**

**Complement-mediated cytolysis** is required for the immune system to clear a meningococcus infection. Repeated meningococcal infections in a child should prompt a search for hereditary terminal (C5–C9, components of the MAC) complement deficiency.

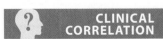

**CLINICAL CORRELATION**

While *N gonorrhoeae* exhibits antigenic variation of its pili, *Salmonella* exhibits antigenic variation of its flagella. This antigenic variation prohibits vaccine development against these bugs.

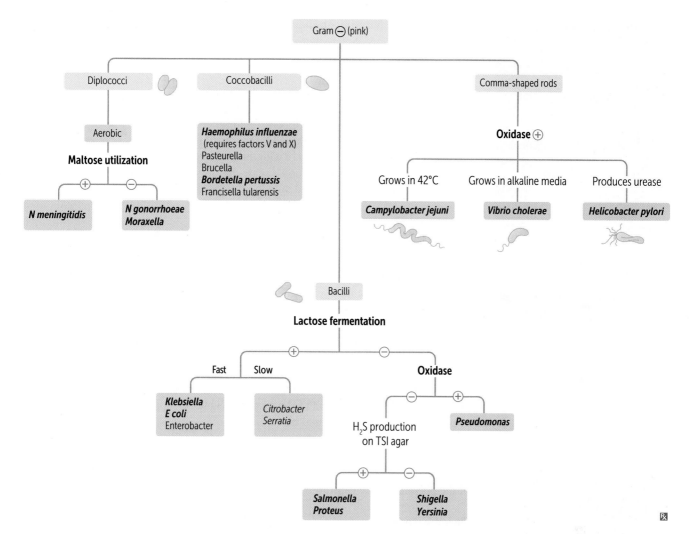

FIGURE 4-15.    **Gram-negative laboratory algorithm.** Important tests are in **bold**. Important pathogens are in ***bold italics***.

- **Siderophores:** Allow collection of iron from human iron-binding proteins (transferrin).
- **Antiphagocytic polysaccharide capsule:** The basis of subclassification of N *meningitidis* into its serogroups. Serogroups A, B, C, Y, and W-135 are responsible for most infections. The capsule is immunogenic and is used to synthesize the meningococcal vaccine.

### Clinical Symptoms

Once inside the nasopharynx, N *meningitidis* leads to local symptoms, including dysphagia and fever. From there, it can easily spread to other subepithelial tissues to cause more significant disease.

**Meningococcemia** is a life-threatening meningococcal sepsis that results in severe multiorgan disease accompanied by small-vessel thrombosis and disseminated intravascular coagulation (DIC). As a result, a characteristic **petechial** or **purpuric rash** is often seen on the trunk and lower extremities (Figure 4-17). Fulminant meningococcemia can result in septic shock and bilateral **hemorrhagic destruction of the adrenal glands**, known as **Waterhouse-Friderichsen syndrome.**

**Meningococcal meningitis** results from infection of the meninges. Typical symptoms include an abrupt onset of fever, chills, stiff neck, headache, and vomiting. Meningeal signs are often present as well. Mortality rate is approximately 10% in appropriately treated patients, and long-term neurological complications are rare.

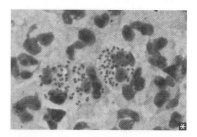

FIGURE 4-16.    ***Neisseria gonorrhoeae.*** Microorganisms are arranged in side-by-side pairs and small clumps.

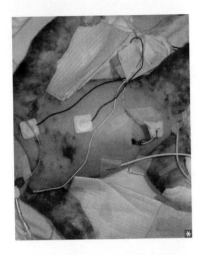

**FIGURE 4-17.**   **Purpura fulminans.**

Meningococcus is an uncommon cause of pneumonia and is usually observed with signs and symptoms of pharyngitis.

### Treatment

*N meningitidis* is almost universally sensitive to penicillin. However, due to poor oral bioavailability of penicillin, treatments are given parenterally in cases of severe meningococcal infection. **Rifampin** can be used for chemoprophylaxis of close contacts of affected individuals. Currently, the American Academy of Pediatrics recommends vaccinating all adolescents at age 11–12 with the meningococcal conjugate vaccine, which covers four of the five most common disease-causing serogroups. (There is a serogroup B vaccine, but it is recommended only for at-risk groups like those who are asplenic.)

#### *Neisseria gonorrhoeae*

### Characteristics

Like N meningitidis, N gonorrhoeae is an aerobic gram-negative coccus that is responsible for serious infections in humans. It possesses the same virulence factors as N meningitidis except that it lacks a polysaccharide capsule. It is responsible for the sexually transmitted infection **gonorrhea** as well as a disseminated variant. Passage through an infected vaginal canal during parturition can result in purulent gonococcal infection of the eye, termed **ophthalmia neonatorum.** Transmission is otherwise via unprotected sexual contact.

Attempts to isolate gonococcus from clinical samples (eg, urethral swabs) are usually performed on **Thayer-Martin (VCN) medium,** which is supplemented with antibiotics to prevent overgrowth of normal genital flora.

### Pathogenesis

All virulence factors are the same as those of N meningitidis, except there is an absence of the polysaccharide capsule.

### Clinical Symptoms

In men, uncomplicated genital gonorrhea presents as acute, purulent urethritis accompanied by dysuria and discharge (Figure 4-18). Infected women may experience abdominal pain, vaginal discharge, and dysuria, but the infection is often asymptomatic.

A complication of untreated disease in women is ascending genital tract infection, termed **pelvic inflammatory disease (PID),** in which the infection spreads to the uterus and ovaries. Symptoms are protean and include abdominal pain, cervical motion tenderness, dysuria, fever, nausea, and vomiting. Serious sequelae of PID include **tubo-ovarian abscess, infertility,** and increased probability of **ectopic pregnancy.**

**Gonococcal pharyngitis** is an uncommon cause of sore throat, caused by orogenital contact.

**Disseminated gonococcal infection** via hematogenous spread is also possible following local gonococcal infection. This is often manifested as acute, painful, asymmetrical migratory polyarthralgia, frequently seen in a clinical triad with **tenosynovitis** (inflammation of the tendon capsule, often on the dorsum of the hand) and a painless, nonpruritic **rash.** Acute suppurative **septic arthritis** with swollen, painful knees, wrists, and ankles is also seen in disseminated infection.

**Gonococcal ophthalmia neonatorum** manifests as an acute purulent conjunctivitis several days after birth. All newborns in the United States routinely receive intraocular antibiotics as prophylaxis against ocular gonococcal and chlamydial infections.

## Treatment

Resistance rates to penicillin and tetracycline are high, and resistance to the previous first-line therapy of fluoroquinolones is on the rise. Therefore, first-line therapy is usually a **third-generation cephalosporin,** such as intramuscular ceftriaxone. Prior infections do not confer immunity, so efforts at disease prevention are currently focused on barrier methods of contraception.

## GRAM-NEGATIVE RODS

The gram-negative rods are numerous and have been grouped according to the major site of disease in this book to allow for easier learning by categorization (Table 4-12).

### Gram-Negative Rods Causing Respiratory and Mucosal Infections

These organisms all appear as small, gram-negative "coccoid" rods when viewed under the microscope and are sometimes described as "coccobacillary" for this reason. The zoonotic bacteria *Brucella* spp and *Pasteurella multocida* are also coccobacillary.

### *Haemophilus influenzae*

#### Characteristics

Formerly a major cause of severe childhood respiratory disease, the highly virulent *H influenzae* serotype b (Hib) is now under better control due to remarkable successes in vaccination.

- *H influenzae* culture can be grown on blood agar supplemented with factors V and X. Chocolate agar, composed of lysed blood cells, is also suitable for culture.
- *H influenzae* appear as small, gram-negative, nonmotile coccobacillary organisms.
- Both encapsulated and nonencapsulated (nontypable) strains exist.
- Encapsulated strains have been characterized as **serotypes a through f.**
- In the prevaccination era, **serotype b** (also known as **Hib**) was responsible for over 95% of invasive pediatric disease.
- Most *H influenzae* disease is now caused by serotypes c, f, and nontypable strains (which can only cause local disease).

Children younger than 3 years old are uniquely susceptible to infection with encapsulated serotypes of *H influenzae* because specific adaptive immune response to polysaccharide antigens is deficient in young children. Infants younger than 6 months have relative protection due to maternal antibodies passed transplacentally and via breast milk. Immunocompromised, nonvaccinated, and asplenic patients are also at risk.

#### Pathogenesis

Nontypable *H influenzae* contributes to normal bacterial flora of the nasopharyngeal mucosa from an early age, and endogenous infection from these sites is responsible for

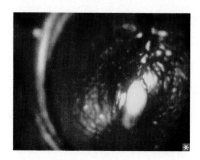

**FIGURE 4-18.   Urethral discharge secondary to gonorrhea.** Frank purulent discharge is a common feature, especially in infected men.

### CLINICAL CORRELATION

Empiric antibiotic therapy for genital gonorrhea should always include coverage for coinfection with **C trachomatis.** For this reason, **azithromycin** or **doxycycline** is usually added to standard single-dose intramuscular **ceftriaxone** for gonorrhea.

### KEY FACT

*H influenzae* does **not cause influenza,** although it is an important cause of postinfluenza pneumonia.

**TABLE 4-12.   Gram-Negative Rods**

| RESPIRATORY/MUCOSAL PATHOGENS | ENTERIC PATHOGENS | ZOONOTIC PATHOGENS |
| --- | --- | --- |
| *Haemophilus influenzae* | Enterobacteriaceae family | *Yersinia pestis* |
| *Haemophilus ducreyi* | *Vibrio* spp | *Francisella tularensis* |
| *Gardnerella vaginalis* | *Pseudomonas aeruginosa* | *Brucella* spp |
| *Bordetella pertussis* | *Bacteroides fragilis* | *Pasteurella multocida* |
| *Legionella pneumophila* | *Campylobacter* | *Bartonella henselae* |

most localized disease (otitis media, sinusitis, pneumonia). Transmission is by respiratory droplets.

Like all gram-negative organisms, *H influenzae* possesses endotoxin, which is responsible for many of its deleterious effects. Other virulence factors include pili and nonpilus adhesins, which mediate attachment, and the antiphagocytic polysaccharide capsule in encapsulated strains.

### Clinical Symptoms

*H influenzae* is responsible for a number of respiratory diseases with varying degrees of severity.

- **Epiglottitis** is perhaps the most memorable of the clinical entities caused by *H influenzae*. It is uncommon now because it is **caused only by Hib.** Affected children are 2–4 years old and present sitting bolt upright with copious drooling, stridor, sore throat, fever, and dyspnea. Rapid airway obstruction leading to death can occur, and **laryngoscopy in the operating room** that shows a cherry-red epiglottis is required for definitive diagnosis.
- **Meningitis** also only results from infection with serotype b. Formerly, it was the major causative organism of meningitis in infants 6 months to 3 years old. Since children at this age do not commonly present with the typical meningitic symptom of stiff neck, the diagnosis is suspected based on nonspecific signs such as fever, poor feeding, vomiting, and irritability. Mortality is low, but residual neurologic deficits are common.
- Upper and lower respiratory tract disease (**otitis media** in children, and **pneumonia, conjunctivitis,** and **sinusitis** in anyone) are common manifestations of endogenous *H influenzae* infection caused by colonization with nontypable strains. The organism is among the top two causative agents of otitis media and sinusitis (*S pneumoniae* is the other); pneumonia usually occurs only in previously damaged lungs (smokers and patients recovering from influenza or viral pneumonia, for example).

### Treatment

Minor respiratory tract infections generally respond to treatment with ampicillin or amoxicillin, although resistance rates are increasing (currently approximately 15%). Other options are azithromycin or cephalosporin. Meningitis requires prompt therapy with CNS-penetrant third-generation cephalosporins (ceftriaxone or cefotaxime).

Chemoprophylaxis of susceptible close contacts is required and rifampin is the drug of choice. More important, immunization of all children with the univalent conjugate vaccine against the *H influenzae* serotype b polysaccharide capsule is recommended. Three doses are generally given before 6 months of age.

*Haemophilus ducreyi*

### Characteristics

Gram-negative, anaerobic coccobacillus that is common in developing countries but rare in the United States.

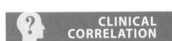

### Pathogenesis

*Haemophilus ducreyi* is mainly spread sexually to genital areas, and the resulting ulceration is an important cofactor for HIV transmission.

### Clinical Symptoms

The causative organism of **chancroid,** a sexually transmitted infection. Patients have a tender perineal nodule that eventually ulcerates (Figure 4-19) and is associated with inguinal lymphadenopathy. The differential diagnosis of this condition is important (Table 4-13).

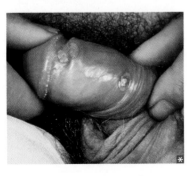

**FIGURE 4-19.** **Infection from** *Haemophilus ducreyi* **resulting in an enlarging chancroid.**

**TABLE 4-13. Differential Diagnosis of Genital Ulceration**

| | CHANCROID (*HAEMOPHILUS DUCREYI*) | CHANCRE (SYPHILIS) | GENITAL HERPES (HSV-2) | LYMPHOGRANULOMA VENEREUM (*CHLAMYDIA* L1-3) |
|---|---|---|---|---|
| Number of ulcers | Single | Single, rolled edges | Multiple, vesicular | Single |
| Ulcer painful? | Pain**ful** | Pain**less** | Pain**ful** | Pain**less** |
| Regional lymphadenopathy | Unilateral, painful, suppurative | Bilateral, painless, nonsuppurative | None, but systemic symptoms present | Pain**ful**, suppurative; appear after ulcer disappears |

## Treatment

Treatment is with erythromycin. The major complication is increased rate of transmission of other sexually transmitted diseases through the open sore.

### Gardnerella vaginalis

## Characteristics

*Gardnerella vaginalis* is a gram-variable coccobacillary rod organism that has been isolated from the vaginal mucosa of both asymptomatic women and those with **bacterial vaginosis (BV)**.

## Clinical Symptoms

BV is a polymicrobial colonization of the vagina with G *vaginalis* in addition to a number of anaerobic bacteria. Clinically, it is characterized by intense pruritus, dysuria, and a characteristic **fishy odor** of the copious, frothy secretions when treated with potassium hydroxide (KOH) preparation. **Clue cells**, which are vaginal epithelial cells covered with coccobacillary bacteria, are seen on wet mount of the discharge (Figure 4-20).

## Treatment

Treatment is with metronidazole to cover both G *vaginalis* and anaerobes.

### Bordetella pertussis

## Characteristics

Like *H influenzae* serotype b, *B pertussis* is a former major cause of pediatric morbidity and mortality that has been largely controlled by an effective vaccination program. It is responsible for **whooping cough.**

- *B pertussis* is an extremely small, coccobacillary, gram-negative rod.
- It is highly sensitive to drying, so care must be taken when collecting and transporting patient samples.
- The microbe has fastidious nutritional requirements, so specialized media (Bordet-Gengou or Regan-Lowe agars) are required for growth.
- Only 50% of all clinically diagnosed patients have positive cultures.

## Pathogenesis

*B pertussis* is highly infective via the nasopharyngeal/respiratory route and infects only humans. Although it is traditionally considered a pediatric disease, whooping cough is now seen in older individuals as well, a phenomenon thought to be secondary to decreased protective effects of childhood vaccination.

*B pertussis* has a number of virulence factors that contribute to its toxicity. **Filamentous hemagglutinin** and **pertactin** are proteins that mediate specific adhesion to ciliated respiratory epithelial cells. **Tracheal cytotoxin** destroys respiratory epithelium directly and may be responsible for the characteristic violent cough. **Pertussis toxin** is a two-part (A-B) exotoxin in which the B component binds the respiratory epithelial cell, allowing

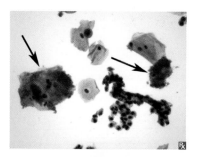

**FIGURE 4-20. Clue cells of bacterial vaginosis.** The image shows the organisms coating squamous cells, forming a purple, velvety coat.

entry of the A component. The A component then constitutively inactivates the inhibitory G protein G$\alpha_i$, causing increased cAMP levels and therefore increased respiratory secretions. The **adenylate cyclase toxin** also increases cAMP levels to the same effect.

### Clinical Symptoms

**Pertussis,** or whooping cough, is characterized by four stages with relatively distinct clinical features.

- The asymptomatic **incubation** period is 7–10 days.
- The **catarrhal stage** lasts about 10 days. This stage is characterized by typical upper respiratory infection symptoms such as sneezing, low fever, and rhinorrhea. Despite its nonspecific symptoms, this stage harbors the period of maximum infectivity.
- The **paroxysmal stage** then lasts for 2 weeks to 1 month and is characterized by the "whoops" of whooping cough. Patients have periodic paroxysms consisting of repetitive nonproductive coughing followed by an inspiratory "whoop"; this then cycles and is often terminated only by posttussive emesis or exhaustion. Hypoxemia and cyanosis are also seen.
- Finally, the **convalescent stage** lasts for approximately 1 month and is characterized by the gradual reduction in intensity and frequency of paroxysms.

### Treatment

Macrolide antibiotic therapy is effective only when given during the incubation or catarrhal stages of the disease. Other treatment is generally supportive in nature and is focused on maintenance of a patent airway. Household contacts of patients with pertussis undergo chemoprophylaxis with 14 days of erythromycin.

The acellular pertussis vaccine—which has replaced the complication-prone whole-cell pertussis vaccine—is a key component of the DTaP recommended for all infants. Five total doses are given. TdaP (tetanus-acellular pertussis) is a booster vaccine to reimmunize adolescent and adult individuals who have probable waning immunity from their childhood DTaP series.

*Legionella pneumophila*

### Characteristics

*Legionella pneumophila* is a motile, pleomorphic, gram-negative rod that is facultatively intracellular. The organism is poorly visualized on Gram stain; therefore, silver or fluorescent antibodies are used. Culture is possible on **buffered charcoal yeast extract agar** supplemented with **cysteine and iron,** but diagnosis is usually made using urine serology.

### Pathogenesis

Transmission is usually via inhalation of infectious aerosols. Once engulfed, the organism multiplies inside the phagosomes of alveolar macrophages following phagocytosis, specifically inhibiting lysosome fusion so that it is not destroyed.

### Clinical Symptoms

The mild form of legionellosis is an influenza-like illness called **Pontiac fever.** It is characterized by epidemic outbreaks with a high attack rate, as well as a clinical syndrome of fever, chills, and myalgias with resolution in about 1 week without treatment. Legionnaires disease is a severe community-acquired pneumonia that generally affects elderly persons with underlying lung disease. Clinical presentation includes a nonproductive cough, high fevers, headache, confusion, and watery diarrhea, with a rapid deterioration often leading to death if antibiotic therapy is not promptly started.

### Treatment

The mainstay of treatment is fluoroquinolones; penicillins are not effective because of the presence of β-lactamase.

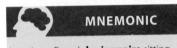

**MNEMONIC**

Imagine a French **legionnaire** sitting around a campfire **(charcoal)** with an **iron** dagger—he is no sissy **(cysteine).**

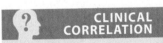

**CLINICAL CORRELATION**

Patients with a more severe presentation of pneumonia, associated with confusion, diarrhea, and hyponatremia, may be infected with legionella instead of other, more common, bugs.

### Enteric Gram-Negative Rods

Many enteric microbes constitute the normal flora of the GI tract. Pathogenic enteric microbes infect the lumen of the lower alimentary canal and can produce syndromes along **two** clinical spectra: diarrheal disease and systemic disease.

Four taxonomic families of enteric organisms are important in medicine:

1. **Enterobacteriaceae:** A large family consisting of organisms such as *Shigella dysenteriae*, *E coli*, *Salmonella enterica*, and *K pneumoniae*. Other notable members of the family include *Yersinia enterocolitica*, *Proteus mirabilis*, *Enterobacter cloacae*, and *S marcescens*.
2. **Vibrionaceae:** Notable organisms are *Vibrio cholerae*, *Campylobacter jejuni*, and *Helicobacter pylori*.
3. **Pseudomonadaceae:** *P aeruginosa*, commonly seen in hospitalized patients.
4. **Bacteroidaceae:** *Bacteroides fragilis*, an anaerobe that can cause gastrointestinal infections.

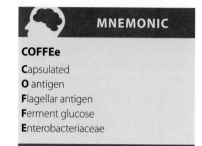

**MNEMONIC**

**COFFEe**
**C**apsulated
**O** antigen
**F**lagellar antigen
**F**erment glucose
**E**nterobacteriaceae

### Enterobacteriaceae

- **All** are oxidase-negative, facultative anaerobes.
- The **lactose fermentation test** (often accomplished on the selective and differential eosin-methylene blue (EMB) or MacConkey agar) and the ability to **produce hydrogen sulfide (H₂S) gas** are two biochemical tests that help characterize and differentiate members of the Enterobacteriaceae family.
- If motile, flagella are usually peritrichous (ie, numerous flagella projecting in many directions).

All Enterobacteriaceae have **O, K,** and **H** antigens, which differ between genera and species and are used to serologically classify clinical isolates. The heat-stable **O antigen** is the outermost polysaccharide layer of the LPS (endotoxin) component of the cell wall. The heat-labile **K antigen** refers to the polysaccharide capsule if present, and the heat-labile **H antigen** is a flagellar protein that may be present.

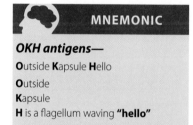

**MNEMONIC**

**OKH antigens—**
**O**utside **K**apsule **H**ello
**O**utside
**K**apsule
**H** is a flagellum waving **"hello"**

#### *Shigella* Species

#### Characteristics

- **Nonmotile,** gram-negative rod-shaped organisms that do **not ferment lactose** but are able to produce **H₂S gas.**
- The four species that make up the genus *Shigella* are **highly virulent** enteric bacteria responsible for many cases of GI disease, especially in pediatric populations and in areas with potentially substandard hygiene (eg, day-care centers).
- Humans are the only host of *Shigella*; in contrast to many other Enterobacteriaceae, there is **no animal reservoir.**

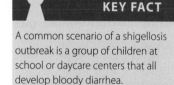

**KEY FACT**

A common scenario of a shigellosis outbreak is a group of children at school or daycare centers that all develop bloody diarrhea.

#### Pathogenesis

Transmission is from person to person via the fecal-oral route, and as few as 10 organisms may cause symptomatic infection. *Shigella* species cause **invasive** gastroenteritis by attaching to and invading immune cells located in Peyer patches. Much of *Shigella's* virulence can be ascribed to the presence of the highly virulent exotoxin called **Shiga toxin.** Shiga toxin is a typical A-B toxin in which the B subunit binds to enterocytes, allowing the A unit to penetrate the cells and cause cell death.

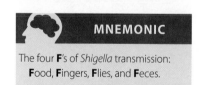

**MNEMONIC**

The four **F**'s of *Shigella* transmission:
**F**ood, **F**ingers, **F**lies, and **F**eces.

#### Clinical Symptoms

The invasive diarrhea caused by *Shigella* species is called **shigellosis** and is characterized by **bloody stools** with pus, fever, and abdominal pain occurring 1–3 days after ingestion of the organism. Initially, diarrhea is often watery. **S *dysenteriae*** specifically produces the Shiga toxin and can cause a more severe form of the disease termed **bacterial dysentery;** this species is also occasionally associated with the **hemolytic-uremic syndrome.**

### Treatment

First-line treatment is azithromycin or fluoroquinolones. Ampicillin and TMP-SMX have widespread resistance. Other treatments are supportive in nature.

### *Salmonella* Species

#### Characteristics

- *Salmonella* species are **motile**, gram-negative rods that, like *Shigella*, produce **$H_2S$ gas,** and do **not ferment lactose.**
- Like *Shigella*, the main route of *Salmonella* invasion is via the M cells of the Peyer patches of the intestine, which may result in hematogenous spread. *S typhi* can **reside in macrophage vesicles**, allowing it to be carried to extraintestinal sites to cause typhoid fever.
- Unlike infection with *Shigella*, *Salmonella* is normally acquired by eating **contaminated** food products such as **chicken, egg, or dairy** products.
- Several species exist due to antigenic variation, but the most important distinction is between *Salmonella typhi* (the causative agent of typhoid fever) and the other species.
    - *S typhi* is the only *Salmonella* species that does **not** produce $H_2S$. Also, *S typhi* can cause **typhoid fever** because it expresses **Vi antigen** on its polysaccharide capsule.
    - Unlike other *Salmonella* subspecies, *S typhi* is propagated by a **human host** (fecal-oral route), often from asymptomatic carriers that harbor the organism in their gallbladders.

#### Clinical Symptoms

**Four** different clinical symptoms can result from *Salmonella* infection: gastroenteritis, bacteremia/sepsis, typhoid fever, and an asymptomatic carrier state.

- *Salmonella* **gastroenteritis** is the most common form of salmonellosis. It manifests as an invasive diarrhea characterized by nausea, frequent stools ranging from watery to slightly bloody with mucus, and abdominal pain. Antibiotic therapy does not shorten the course of the disease.
- *Salmonella* **sepsis** is uncommon and has a higher incidence in immunocompromised, pediatric, or elderly patients. Asplenic individuals have difficulty clearing the organism due to its polysaccharide capsule, so hematogenous spread to various end organs (bone, joints, heart) is possible in these individuals. Sickle cell patients are at risk of hematogenous spread to bone causing **osteomyelitis.**
- **Typhoid fever** (also known as enteric fever) results from *S typhi* invasion of enterocytes and subsequent intracellular residence in circulating macrophages. It is characterized by the onset of fever, headache, and abdominal pain, and can be mistaken for appendicitis. Symptoms occur 1–3 weeks after exposure. Clinical signs include splenomegaly and occasionally a transient rash (termed **rose spots**) on the abdomen of the patient (Figure 4-21).
- **Asymptomatic carriers** of *S typhi* constitutively excrete the organism in stool due to colonization of the gallbladder but are completely asymptomatic. This represents the source and reservoir of salmonellosis.

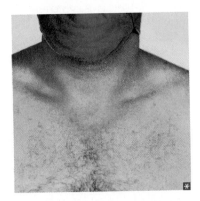

**FIGURE 4-21.** **Rose spots of typhoid fever.** These pathognomonic spots appear transiently on light-skinned individuals.

### Treatment

Ciprofloxacin and ceftriaxone, among other agents, are appropriate treatments for disseminated disease or typhoid fever. Treatment of asymptomatic carriers is strongly suggested as a public health measure and may require surgical excision of the gallbladder. A vaccine for *S typhi* is available but is only routinely given to individuals traveling to endemic areas.

*Escherichia coli*

Characteristics

*E coli* is associated with many diseases affecting different organ systems.

- *E coli* is a **motile,** gram-negative, medium-sized rod.
- It is a **lactose fermenter,** thus appearing purple on MacConkey agar.
- *E coli* does **not** produce $H_2S$ gas.
- It is the most common gram-negative rod in the digestive tract.

Clinical Symptoms

Diseases caused by *E coli* are numerous and varied.

- *E coli* **infectious diarrhea** is a major cause of infant mortality worldwide, usually due to dehydration. Several variants of diarrheal illness caused by *E coli* have been characterized in humans. They differ from each other based on affected populations, clinical presentation, pathogenic factors, and severity (Table 4-14).
- The **hemolytic-uremic syndrome (HUS)** is one of the most feared complications of enterohemorrhagic *E coli* (EHEC) infection in children. Approximately 5–10% of infected children younger than 10 years develop the clinical **triad of renal failure, hemolytic anemia,** and **thrombocytopenia,** in addition to bloody diarrhea.
- *E coli* is the **number one cause of UTIs.** Strains of *E coli* possess **P1 pilus-bound** adhesion factors, allowing them to attach to the urethral wall and ascend the urinary tract, causing **bacterial cystitis.** This is characterized by dysuria and increased urinary frequency. A common complication of cystitis is **pyelonephritis** or ascending infection of the kidney parenchyma; this complication is commonly associated with **fever, flank pain,** and **vomiting.**
- *E coli* is the second most common cause of **neonatal meningitis.**
- Gram-negative sepsis is most commonly caused by *E coli*. It primarily affects debilitated, hospitalized patients, especially following instrumentation or intra-abdominal surgery. Septic shock is the most common cause of death in this group, presumably caused by the endotoxin component of the cell wall.

**TABLE 4-14.   Diarrhea Caused by *Escherichia coli***

| VARIANT | EPIDEMIOLOGY | PRESENTATION | PATHOGENESIS | SEVERITY |
|---|---|---|---|---|
| ETEC | Affects travelers (traveler's diarrhea) and infants in developing countries. Found in contaminated water. | Copious, watery, non-bloody diarrhea and abdominal cramping. | Cholera-like heat-labile toxin (LT) overactivates adenylate cyclase to ↑ cAMP, leading to ↑ Cl– secretion and $H_2O$ efflux in the gut, while the heat-stable toxin (ST) overactivates guanylate cyclase to ↑ cGMP, leading to ↓ resorption of NaCl and $H_2O$ in the gut. | Can be fatal in infants without proper hydration. |
| EPEC | Affects infants in developing countries. | Watery diarrhea. | Microcolony formation on the surface of intestinal epithelium with subsequent loss of microvilli, leading to ↓ absorption. | Mild to moderate. |
| EIEC | Rare in developed countries; uncommon worldwide. | Bloody diarrhea with pus, fever, and abdominal pain. | Shares virulence factors with *Shigella* (but not Shiga toxin) and can invade enterocytes directly, causing an inflammatory reaction and colitis. | Usually mild, but can progress to dysentery. |
| EHEC (strain O157:H7) | Most common pathogenic strain. Found in ground beef and unpasteurized milk. | Hemorrhagic colitis: abdominal pain, bloody diarrhea, but no fever. Can cause HUS. | Expresses Shiga-like toxin, inhibiting protein synthesis leading to enterocyte death. | Usually self-limiting, but HUS can be fatal. |

EHEC, enterohemorrhagic *E coli*; EIEC, enteroinvasive *E coli*; EPEC, enteropathogenic *E coli*; ETEC, enterotoxigenic *E coli*; HUS, hemolytic-uremic syndrome; LT, heat-labile toxin; ST, heat-stable enterotoxin.

### Treatment

Antibiotics are often **not** indicated in diarrheal infections. Antibiotic choice is dictated by susceptibility testing in the case of disseminated or serious disease. UTIs are usually treated empirically with TMP-SMX, and fluoroquinolones.

### Klebsiella pneumoniae

#### Characteristics

*Klebsiella* is an encapsulated, indole-negative, lactose-fermenting member of the Enterobacteriaceae family. The colonies look very mucoid due to the presence of abundant polysaccharide capsules.

#### Pathogenesis

Diabetic and immunocompromised patients, as well as patients with increased aspiration of oral secretions (eg, alcoholics), are at greater risk for opportunistic infections with *K pneumoniae*. Nosocomial infections are common among patients on ventilators (pneumonia) and those with indwelling plastic devices like intravenous or urinary catheters.

#### Clinical Symptoms

*Klebsiella*-induced pneumonia is characterized by bloody, **currant-jelly** sputum. The pneumonia is **lobar,** severe, often **necrotizing,** and **cavitating.** It can also cause gram-negative sepsis.

#### Treatment

Various isolates of *Klebsiella* have different susceptibilities, which include fluoroquinolones, cephalosporins, and carbapenems. Due to widespread use of broad-spectrum antibiotics, carbapenem-resistant *Klebsiella* strains are on the rise.

### Proteus mirabilis

#### Characteristics

This organism is characterized by its extreme **motility** (which causes a **swarming** phenotype on agar), and its ability to chemically split urea into two molecules of ammonia via its **urease** enzyme.

#### Pathogenesis

Infection of the urinary tract ascends from the periurethral area into the bladder. The adhesive fimbriae and flagella *P mirabilis* allow it to ascend against the flow of urine. After colonization, *P mirabilis* further climbs the ureters and can initiate infection of the renal pelvis.

#### Clinical Symptoms

*P mirabilis* is a common cause of UTI for patients with indwelling bladder catheters and structural or functional abnormalities of the kidney and urinary tract. In these cases, urinalysis confirms the bacterial diagnosis owing to the **alkaline pH of the urine.**

#### Treatment

*P mirabilis* responds to cephalosporins and penicillins.

### Yersinia enterocolitica

#### Characteristics

This bacterium is a zoonotic pathogen, infecting mostly farm animals and pets.

#### Pathogenesis

It is spread through pet feces (eg, from puppies), contaminated milk, or pork.

**MNEMONIC**

**Remember the 4 A's of KlebsiellA—**

**A**spiration pneumonia
**A**bscess in lungs and liver
**A**lcoholics
di**A**betics

**KEY FACT**

*Proteus* infections are associated with struvite stones/staghorn calculi because they are urease positive. Ureases digest urea ammonia thereby increasing the pH of urine. This facilitates the precipitation of phosphate and magnesium to form struvite ($NH_4MgPO_4 \cdot 6H_2O$) kidney stones. These can form a nidus for recurrent infection.

### Clinical Symptoms

*Y enterocolitica* causes an **invasive gastroenteritis** associated with fever, abdominal pain, and diarrhea (sometimes bloody). It can also spread to the **mesenteric lymph nodes** and produce symptoms of abdominal pain that closely mimic appendicitis (pseudoappendicitis).

### Treatment

First-line treatment includes aminoglycosides and TMP-SMX.

### *Citrobacter, Enterobacter, Morganella, Serratia, Edwardsiella,* and *Providencia*

Certain other Enterobacteriaceae **rarely infect immunocompetent patients** and are included here for completeness. *Enterobacter* infections are known for **broad antibiotic resistance.** *S marcescens* infections are usually nosocomially acquired. *S marcescens* culture produces characteristic **bright-red** colonies on agar.

### Vibrionaceae

- Important members of the family are *V cholerae, C jejuni,* and *H pylori.*
- *Vibrio* species are **curved, motile, oxidase-positive** gram-negative rods with a **single polar flagellum.**
- Three medically relevant members of the *Vibrio* genus exist. The well-known *V cholerae* produces the profuse watery diarrhea of cholera. *Vibrio parahaemolyticus* and *V vulnificus* are both acquired by eating **contaminated shellfish** and cause self-limiting gastroenteritis and wound infections, respectively.

### *Vibrio cholerae*

### Characteristics

*V cholerae* is a major cause of infant mortality worldwide due to the effects of its **exotoxin.** It is a comma-shaped gram-negative rod that has no specific culture requirements (Figure 4-22).

*V cholerae* is generally found in developing or impoverished countries in standing or brackish water contaminated by human feces. The organism can easily multiply and contaminate drinking water, causing epidemics and pandemics. The "**El Tor**" biotype of serogroup O1 was responsible for the most recent worldwide pandemic in the latter half of the previous century. Person-to-person transmission is rare, and inhabitants of endemic areas are often immune.

### Pathogenesis

The **cholera toxin,** also known as choleragen, is an A-B exotoxin that is secreted upon binding of the cholera bacteria to enterocytes. Once the A subunit gains entry into the cell, it causes constitutive activation of the G protein, $G_{\alpha s}$, which results in the **buildup of cAMP** in a manner similar to the action of pertussis toxin. Because of this cAMP accumulation, sodium and chloride ions are actively extruded into the colon lumen and reabsorption is inhibited.

### Clinical Symptoms

Affected individuals are rapidly afflicted with "**rice-water stools**" named for their appearance. Massive fluid diarrhea due to osmotic pull of secreted sodium chloride occurs, with **isotonic** fluid losses potentially up to 20 L/day. Electrolyte imbalances (hypokalemia, metabolic acidosis) and hypovolemic shock can occur and lead to death if affected persons are untreated.

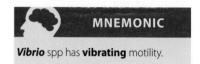

**MNEMONIC**

*Vibrio* spp has **vibrating** motility.

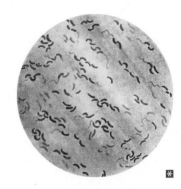

**FIGURE 4-22.** *Vibrio cholerae.* This Gram stain depicts flagellated *Vibrio comma* bacteria, a strain of *Vibrio cholerae.*

### Treatment

The cornerstone of therapy for cholera is fluid replacement; the use of inexpensive **oral rehydration therapy** in developing countries has saved countless lives. Antibiotic therapy with doxycycline or TMP-SMX can shorten the course of the disease.

#### *Campylobacter jejuni*

### Characteristics

- Similar to *V cholerae*, *C jejuni* is a small, curved (comma-shaped), motile gram-negative rod with a polar flagellum.
- Culture conditions require special nutrients contained in **Campy agar,** as well as a **microaerophilic** atmosphere (3–15% $O_2$) and a temperature of **42°C** for growth.
- Acquisition of the organism is from contaminated food and water; undercooked chicken and unpasteurized milk are common sources. Transmission can also occur from domestic animals to humans via a fecal-oral route.
- Although usually not stressed in microbiology textbooks, *Campylobacter* is the single **most common cause of invasive diarrhea.** Over two million incident cases of *C jejuni* infection occur in the United States each year.

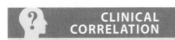

**CLINICAL CORRELATION**

*C jejuni* **infection** has been shown to be associated with the development of **Guillain-Barré syndrome** and **reactive arthritis** resulting from cross-reactivity of antibodies directed against the bacteria.

### Pathogenesis

As indicated by its species name, *C jejuni* causes an invasive diarrhea with tissue invasion largely in the **distal small bowel.** Pathologic specimens show ulceration, crypt abscesses, and acute inflammation.

### Clinical Symptoms

Like other invasive infectious diarrheas, *C jejuni* enteritis is characterized by **bloody diarrhea,** fever, malaise, and abdominal pain. The disease is self-limited. Complications are rare and include sepsis, spontaneous abortion, and Guillain-Barré syndrome.

### Treatment

Routine regional enteritis of *C jejuni* infection usually responds to fluid replacement and does not require antibiotic therapy. More serious infections require azithromycin.

#### *Helicobacter pylori*

### Characteristics

*H pylori* is an important cause of gastroduodenal pathology.

- Diagnosis is usually made by:
    - Examination of endoscopic biopsy specimens
    - Testing for serum antibodies against *H pylori*
    - Performing the highly specific **urease breath test**
    - Applying immunoassay detection of *H pylori* antigen in stool
- It is a corkscrew-shaped, highly motile, gram-negative rod that grows best under microaerophilic conditions.
- Although it shares many characteristics with *C jejuni*, *H pylori* does **not** grow at 42°C.

**KEY FACT**

*H pylori* infection is associated with increased risk of gastric adenocarcinoma and gastric lymphoma.

### Pathogenesis

It possesses a **urease** enzyme capable of splitting urea into alkaline ammonia, which allows it to survive in the highly acidic gastric microenvironment.

### Clinical Symptoms

It is found in biopsy specimens of **duodenal ulcers** and **chronic gastritis,** but without evidence of tissue invasion.

## Treatment

**Triple therapy** (either bismuth-metronidazole-tetracycline/amoxicillin or metronidazole-omeprazole-clarithromycin) eradicates the organism and prevents recurrence of ulcer and gastritis.

## Pseudomonaceae

### Characteristics

*P aeruginosa* and related organisms constitute a group of microbes that are **opportunistic pathogens** of humans; that is, they mainly infect immunocompromised patients. These **strictly aerobic**, gram-negative rods **do not ferment lactose** and are differentiated from the nonfermentative Enterobacteriaceae (*Shigella*, *Salmonella*, and others) by the fact that they are **oxidase-positive.** *P aeruginosa* is by far the most common and important of these organisms; the others that make up this group are listed only for completeness: *Burkholderia* spp, *Stenotrophomonas maltophilia*, and *Acinetobacter* spp.

### *Pseudomonas aeruginosa*

### Characteristics

*Pseudomonas* can be easily identified in a microbiology lab because of its characteristic odor and color. Cultures of this organism (as well as infected surface wounds) have a **bluish green tint** due to the production of the **water-soluble** pigments **pyocyanin** and **fluorescein.** In addition, the bacteria produce a sweet (some people liken it to **grapes**) odor.

*Pseudomonas* is a **soil** contaminant and is commonly found in **moist** environments, especially within hospitals in respiratory ventilators. The organism is **resistant** to many antibiotics and disinfectants, and is primarily transmitted from contaminated surfaces.

### Pathogenesis

*Pseudomonas* features a number of virulence factors, but does not possess significant invasive ability in healthy hosts. Infection targets hospitalized, immunocompromised patients.

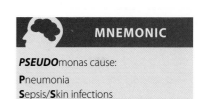

**MNEMONIC**

**PSEUDO**monas cause:

**P**neumonia
**S**epsis/**S**kin infections
**E**ndocarditis/**E**xternal otitis
**U**TI/corneal **U**lcers
**D**iabetic infections
**O**steomyelitis

- **Exotoxin A** serves as an inhibitor to EF-2, effectively disrupting protein synthesis in mammalian cells.
- **Endotoxin** (LPS) is a major player in pseudomonal sepsis.
- Some strains have an antiphagocytic polysaccharide **capsule.**
- The organism has connective tissue hydrolases, including **elastases** and an **alkaline protease,** allowing facile spread through infected tissues.

### Clinical Symptoms

In immunocompromised patients, *Pseudomonas* infection can lead to various outcomes (Table 4-15).

### Treatment

*Pseudomonas* can acquire **resistance** to many commonly used antibiotics, including antipseudomonal penicillins or cephalosporins (eg, piperacillin/tazobactam or cefepime), and fluoroquinolones. Aminoglycosides are used to treat life-threatening infections and those caused by drug-resistant strains of bacteria.

Prevention of pseudomonal infection is achieved through appropriate use of broad-spectrum antibiotics.

**TABLE 4-15.    Diseases Caused by *Pseudomonas aeruginosa***

| DISEASE | SUSCEPTIBLE POPULATION(S) | CLINICAL SYNDROME |
|---|---|---|
| Pneumonia | CF patients | Almost all CF patients are **colonized** with *Pseudomonas,* and exacerbations of the underlying disease are often associated with a necrotizing, destructive pseudomonal pneumonia. In CF patients, *Pseudomonas* forms **mucoid biofilms** that inhibit phagocytosis and decrease antibiotic penetration, thus establishing pseudomonal colonization of the CF patient's lungs. |
|  | Patients who had prior therapy with broad-spectrum antibiotics, or respiratory instrumentation | Diffuse, bilateral necrotizing pneumonia with high mortality rate. |
| UTI | Urinary instrumentation, broad-spectrum antibiotics | Typical UTI symptoms of dysuria, pyuria, and urgency. |
| Osteomyelitis | Diabetics | *Pseudomonas* is often the causative agent of infected **diabetic** foot ulcers, though *Staphylococcus aureus* is the most common cause. |
|  | Children after puncture trauma | Through-and-through **puncture** into the foot can lead to the introduction of *Pseudomonas* from the moist shoe environment into the wound. |
| Malignant OE | Diabetics | Typical OE is characterized by **pain on ear traction** and sometimes discharge; malignant OE is a severe and potentially fatal complication characterized by spread into the mastoid, with resultant destruction of bone and cranial nerves. |
| Wound infections | Patients with burns | The moist environment of the burn surface is an ideal breeding ground for *Pseudomonas.* One of the most feared complications of topical burns is gram-negative sepsis. |
| Hot tub folliculitis | Anyone | Inflammation of hair follicles with characteristic rash after immersion in warm, contaminated water. |
| Sepsis | Patients with neutropenia, diabetes, extensive burns, leukemia | Extremely high mortality rate for gram-negative sepsis. |
| Corneal ulcers | Contact lens wearers | Usually occurs after incidental trauma to the eye; can rapidly progress if untreated. |
| Ecthyma gangrenosum | Immunocompromised patients | First presents as a painless macule that grows to a hemorrhagic bulla. Eventually, the lesion ruptures, forming a gangrenous ulcer with grey-black eschar surrounded by an erythematous halo. Dermal necrosis occurs as a result of vascular thrombosis secondary to bacterial growth in the vessel wall. |

CF, cystic fibrosis; OE, otitis externa; UTI, urinary tract infection.

### Bacteroidiaceae

Although the anaerobic Bacteroidiaceae family has several medically relevant members, the most important is *B fragilis*, commonly implicated in visceral abscesses. Other members of the family include organisms causing periodontal disease and aspiration pneumonia such as *Bacteroides* spp, *Fusobacterium* spp, and *Porphyromonas* spp. In general, **anaerobic infections tend to be polymicrobial,** with a number of different organisms responsible for pathology.

Culturing obligate anaerobic bacteria presents a special problem; specific culture media as well as an $O_2$-free atmosphere are required. Treatment of these infections must include clindamycin, metronidazole, or other antibiotics with activity against anaerobes.

*Bacteroides fragilis*

### Characteristics

This **obligate anaerobe** is a gram-negative organism that lives within the alimentary and female reproductive tracts.

### Pathogenesis

As *B fragilis* is naturally present in the gut and reproductive tracts. Disruption in these barriers (eg, surgery, septic abortion, PID, intestinal rupture) is required for the organism to seed the intraperitoneal cavity and form abscesses.

### Clinical Symptoms

Fever and localized pain are the presenting symptoms of *B fragilis* abscesses, and systemic hematogenous spread can result.

### Treatment

Antibiotics that target anaerobes (eg, clindamycin and metronidazole) are popular choices for the treatment of bacteroides.

## Zoonotic Gram-Negative Bacteria

Zoonotic infections are acquired from reservoirs principally existing in animals: humans are usually accidental hosts. Transmission usually occurs by direct contact with the animal in question.

*Yersinia pestis*

### Characteristics

*Yersinia pestis* is the causative organism of the **plague,** the "Black Death" that decimated the population of Europe during the 1300s. As a gram-negative, lactose-fermenting rod, it is related to the enteric pathogen *Y enterocolitica* but produces a markedly different clinical syndrome. It is a facultatively intracellular organism and is disseminated throughout the body by macrophages following phagocytosis.

The natural reservoirs of *Y pestis* are **rats** in the urban setting and other wild rodents, especially prairie dogs, in rural areas. Transmission is accomplished either by the bite of an infected rodent or by a secondary vector such as a flea. Currently, very few cases are reported in the United States, with most cases restricted to the American Southwest.

### Pathogenesis

*Y pestis* possesses an antiphagocytic **protein** capsule (called **F1**) as well as the **V** and **W** antigens, of unknown function. These antigens allow the organisms to reside in the phagosomes of macrophages without destroying them. Very few organisms are required for infection to occur.

### Clinical Symptoms

Two syndromes are associated with *Y pestis* infection: **bubonic plague** and **pneumonic plague.**

- **Bubonic plague** occurs after direct contact with an infected rodent or flea and is characterized by the presence of **buboes**—erythematous, painful, and swollen inguinal or axillary lymph nodes that become indurated about 1 week after exposure (Figure 4-23). High fever and cutaneous hemorrhage follow, and bacteremia and multiorgan involvement are inevitable without treatment. The mortality rate is approximately 75% if untreated.

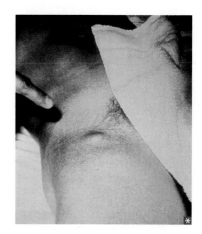

**FIGURE 4-23. Bubonic plague.** Note the swollen inguinal lymph node or bubo.

- **Pneumonic plague** has an incubation period of only 3 days after which the micro-organism can be aerosolized and spread. Constitutional and respiratory symptoms predominate, and the mortality rate is even higher (90% if untreated) than that for bubonic plague.

### Treatment

Appropriate treatment for plague involves the administration of an aminoglycoside: streptomycin (given intramuscularly) or gentamicin. Rodent control and vaccination of at-risk populations can help control the spread of this disease.

#### Francisella tularensis

### Characteristics

*Francisella tularensis* is another rare zoonotic bacterium, which is the causative agent of **tularemia.** It is an extremely small gram-negative coccobacillus that, like Y *pestis,* is a facultative intracellular bacterium that spreads from the point of entry into the body via macrophage phagosomes. It is fastidious to culture and requires either "chocolate" or buffered charcoal yeast extract agar and an extended period for growth in the lab.

The animal reservoirs for *F tularensis* are wild rodents, especially **rabbits.** In the United States, tularemia is seen mostly in the Central Plains states, although most states have reported cases. The species is **highly virulent;** only a few organisms are required to produce infection.

### Pathogenesis

Humans are usually infected either by contact with a domestic animal that has killed an infected rodent or by a tick bite. *F tularensis* has an antiphagocytic polysaccharide capsule, which protects against opsonization. It is resistant to intracellular killing in the phagosomes of macrophages.

### Clinical Symptoms

Tularemia can manifest as a variety of different syndromes.

- The **ulceroglandular** variant is the most common form. Lesions resemble bubo formation at the site of initial infection except that the skin surface ulcerates as well; the bacteria can spread from there to the blood.
- **Pneumonic** tularemia results from contact with aerosolized bacteria and can lead to a bilateral pneumonia.
- **Oculoglandular** tularemia affects the eye and cervical lymph nodes.
- **Typhoidal** tularemia has GI and systemic symptoms.

### Treatment

Streptomycin and gentamicin are standard therapies for tularemia. Tick prophylaxis (light-colored clothing, insect repellents, and long sleeves) and avoidance of known reservoirs of infection serve to decrease the incidence of disease in endemic areas.

#### Brucella

### Characteristics

*Brucella* species (*B melitensis, B abortus, B suis,* and *B canis*) are facultatively intracellular, small, nonmotile, encapsulated gram-negative organisms that infect mammals such as **cows, goats,** and **pigs.** Spread to humans is usually through contact with infected meat, aborted placentas, or unpasteurized milk products. Brucellosis is rare in the United States owing to cattle immunization and milk pasteurization.

### Clinical Symptoms

Brucellosis generally manifests with nonspecific symptoms; one common finding is an intermittent fever (**undulant fever**). Progressive involvement of the gastrointestinal or respiratory tracts or skeleton is possible.

### Treatment

A combination of doxycycline and rifampin is used to eradicate the organism.

#### *Pasteurella multocida*

### Characteristics

*Pasteurella* is a nonmotile, encapsulated gram-negative organism distantly related to *Haemophilus,* which asymptomatically colonizes the mouths of dogs and especially **cats.**

### Pathogenesis

Infection occurs following a bite or scratch from an infected cat or dog.

### Clinical Symptoms

Localized wound infection, cellulitis, and lymphadenopathy.

### Treatment

Doxycycline or penicillin as well as appropriate wound care.

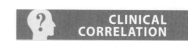

**CLINICAL CORRELATION**

Because of the risk of *Pasteurella* (and other) infections, animal (and human) bite wounds are generally **not** closed with sutures.

#### *Bartonella henselae*

### Characteristics

*Bartonella* species are **aerobic** gram-negative rods that are poorly characterized to date. They are found in a number of animal reservoirs, often with insects as intermediate vectors. The most clinically important member of the genus is *B henselae,* the causative agent of **cat-scratch fever.** *B quintana* causes **trench fever,** a 5-day illness frequently seen during World War I, characterized by fever and bone pain.

### Pathogenesis

*B henselae* can be spread after being scratched by a cat that is parasitized by infected fleas. When cats scratch themselves, the infected flea excrement is embedded into their claws. *B quintana* has no known animal reservoir; transmission occurs via the bite of a human body louse.

### Clinical Symptoms

Cat-scratch fever is a lymphadenitis occurring mainly in children. Lymph nodes near the site of infection become enlarged and painful, and chronic low-grade fevers may develop.

### Treatment

The infection is self-limited.

## GRAM-INDETERMINATE BACTERIA

Several other groups of medically important bacteria do not Gram stain. These bacteria include *Mycobacteria, Mycoplasma, Chlamydia,* and *Rickettsia.*

#### *Mycobacterium*

Mycobacteria are small, nonmotile, **aerobic** rods with a complex cell wall that differs from those of both gram-positive and gram-negative organisms. The cell walls of mycobacteria possess complex lipids called **mycocides—mycolic acid** residues on the most external surface—and various additional membrane proteins and cross-linkages of the peptidoglycan layer. This cell wall structure causes mycobacteria to stain positive with **acid-fast stains (Ziehl-Neelsen stain)**, as described previously. It also acts as a virulence factor, resulting in resistance to common antimicrobial agents, such as β-lactam and cephalosporin antibiotics.

Many pathogenic mycobacteria are either **very slow-growing** or unable to be grown in bacterial cultures. The three most important members of the genus are *M tuberculosis*, the causative agent of **TB**, *M leprae*, which causes **Hansen disease** (formerly known as leprosy), and *M avium–intracellulare* (MAC or MAI), an opportunistic pathogen that causes disseminated infection in immunodeficient persons.

### *Mycobacterium tuberculosis*

#### Characteristics

*M tuberculosis* infection is a life-threatening chronic condition affecting individuals in both impoverished and developed countries.

- *M tuberculosis* is a small, acid-fast, obligate aerobe that resides inside macrophages and can establish lifelong infection.
- It is found worldwide—primarily in Southeast Asia, Africa, and Eastern Europe—and is spread by infectious aerosols from person to person (without animal reservoirs).
- One-third of the world's population carries some form of infection, but because of efficacious treatment regimens and strict reporting of cases, disease burden in the United States has been steadily decreasing.
- Risk factors for TB (in the United States) include:
  - Incarceration
  - Immunodeficiency—especially untreated HIV infection
  - Homelessness
  - Travel to endemic areas
  - Exposure to individuals with known active TB
  - Drug and alcohol abuse
  - Employment in a health care setting

#### Pathogenesis

Primary *M tuberculosis* infection usually begins when infectious particles are inhaled and phagocytosed by alveolar macrophages. Once inside, the microbe evades lysosomes by **inhibiting lysosomal fusion;** however, a chronic inflammatory response is produced. This inflammatory response damages tissue parenchyma, especially the lungs, resulting in the soft, deliquescent **caseous granulomas** composed of infected macrophages and debris. Eventual control of the infection is achieved with **cell-mediated** ($T_H1$-based) immunity, but viable *M tuberculosis* bacteria continue to exist within the granulomas and can **reactivate** when host immune function is depressed. **Virulent** strains can form microscopic "serpentine **cords**" (hence, the term *cord factor* to describe virulence) in which the bacilli are arranged in parallel chains.

#### Clinical Symptoms

The first infection, termed **primary tuberculosis,** usually results in an asymptomatic lung infection (Figure 4-24). Primary infection is generally established in **central (perihilar) lung fields** (Figure 4-25). The characteristic finding on chest radiograph is a **Ghon complex,** which consists of **enlarged perihilar lymph nodes adjacent to a calcified granuloma.** Occurs in the elderly, pediatric, or immunosuppressed populations.

- **Latent tuberculosis** is an asymptomatic state in which the bacteria lie dormant inside caseous granulomas.
- **Reactivation (secondary) tuberculosis** occurs when the host undergoes a decrease in immune function, allowing escape of the organisms from the granuloma (Figure

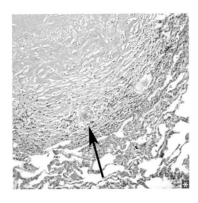

**FIGURE 4-24. Caseating granuloma from lung parenchyma infected with *Mycoplasma tuberculosis*.**

4-26). Most commonly, the **apices of the lungs** are affected because of the microbe's predilection for areas of high $O_2$ concentration (Figure 4-25).

- Symptoms include **fever, night sweats, weight loss,** and **hemoptysis.**
- Without treatment, the bacteria and resultant inflammatory response slowly erode the lung parenchyma.
- TB can also reactivated in a number of **extrapulmonary organs:** The CNS (causing lymphocytic meningitis), vertebra (causing compression fractures and referred to as **Pott disease**), kidneys, lymphoreticular system, and GI tract.
- **Miliary TB** occurs when tubercular bacteremia causes distal seeding. This is seen mainly in immunosuppressed populations and has a high mortality rate. The radiographic and pathologic presentations of this disease are remarkable.

Diagnosis of active TB is usually clinical and radiographic, but the **purified protein derivative (PPD)** skin test provides a measure of whether individuals can mount a cell-mediated response to *M tuberculosis*. Purified protein particles from killed bacteria are injected intradermally; a few days later, the area of induration (hard, raised bump; not the area of redness) is measured. Positive tests correlate with active, latent, or resolved infection; unfortunately, false-positive results are common (due to cross-reactivity in recipients of the bacillus Calmette-Guérin [BCG] vaccine) and false-negative (due to anergy in immunosuppressed patients). Another test uses interferon-γ (IFN-γ) release as a marker for latent TB by measuring the amount of IFN-γ released when WBCs are exposed to mycobacterial antigens.

### Treatment

The mainstay of treatment for active TB is **prolonged multidrug therapy** to prevent the onset of resistance.

- Generally, a four-drug regimen consisting of isoniazid (INH), ethambutol, pyrazinamide, and rifampin for 2 months followed by INH/rifampin for 4–6 more months

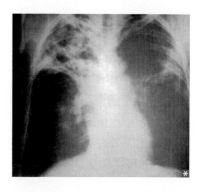

**FIGURE 4-25.** **An anteroposterior x-ray of advanced bilateral pulmonary tuberculosis.** This x-ray of the chest reveals the presence of bilateral pulmonary infiltrate, and "caving formation" present in the right apical region. The diagnosis is advanced tuberculosis.

---

**KEY FACT**

The PPD test will be positive if patient has current infection or past exposure. For high-risk populations (eg, IV drug users, HIV+, immunocompromised) an erythematous induration, ≥ 10 mm is considered a positive result, whereas for the general population at low risk, ≥ 15 mm is considered positive. False positives can occur with BCG vaccination. (To avoid cross-reactivity, the interferon-γ release assay is preferred over PPD.) The PPD test will be negative if there is no infection, or if the patient is anergic (on steroids, malnourished, immunocompromised), or in cases of sarcoidosis.

---

**CLINICAL CORRELATION**

Worldwide, TB is the major infectious cause of **adrenal insufficiency (Addison disease).** Other infections that can cause adrenal insufficiency include HIV and chronic fungal infections such as histoplasmosis.

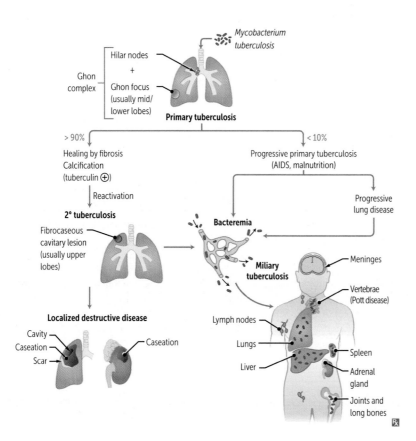

**FIGURE 4-26.** **Primary and secondary tuberculosis.**

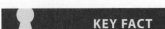

### KEY FACT

Treatment of *M tuberculosis* will always involve two or more agents because resistance develops quickly.

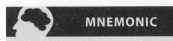

### MNEMONIC

**Treatment for TB—**

TB is **RIPE** for treatment:

**R**ifampin
**I**NH
**P**yrazinamide
**E**thambutol

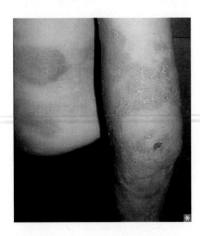

**FIGURE 4-27. Lepromatous leprosy.** Elbow after two weeks of multi-drug therapy.

is used, although alternative combinations are required if resistance or drug intolerance develops.

■ Chemoprophylaxis for exposure to active TB or a positive PPD test without symptoms is generally 9 months of INH. The BCG vaccine is given in some endemic countries to prevent primary infection. It prevents major sequelae of TB (disseminated or miliary) without actually preventing spread.

### *Mycobacterium leprae*

#### Characteristics

*M leprae* is an acid-fast, aerobic rod that causes the disfiguring disease known as **leprosy,** or **Hansen disease.** Humans and armadillos are the only known hosts. The disease is spread through contact with infected lesions. Better control of Hansen disease has caused a 90% reduction in its incidence since 1985. *M leprae* **cannot** be grown in culture.

#### Pathogenesis

*M leprae* has a predilection for **cool** surfaces, and therefore most of its pathogenic features occur in superficial tissues such as the **skin** and the **peripheral nerves.**

#### Clinical Symptoms

**Two** clinical forms of leprosy are known: **Tuberculoid leprosy** and **lepromatous leprosy** (Figure 4-27). They develop based on differential responses of the immune system to the bacteria (Table 4-16).

#### Treatment

Therapy for the tuberculoid variant involves the antibiotics **dapsone** and **rifampin** for 6 months. Longer therapy of 12 months and the addition of clofazimine are required for the lepromatous variant.

### Atypical Mycobacteria

#### Characteristics

The atypical mycobacteria such as *M avium-intracellulare, M kansasii, M scrofulaceum,* and so on, tend to cause disease in specific populations. Atypical bacteria are grouped according to speed of growth in media as well as pigmentation.

*M avium-intracellulare* (MAI) (also known as *M avium* complex, or **MAC**) is a ubiquitous atypical mycobacterium present in **soil and water.**

**TABLE 4-16. Pathogenesis and Clinical Features of Lepromatous and Tuberculoid Leprosy**

| FEATURE | LEPROMATOUS LEPROSY | TUBERCULOID LEPROSY |
|---|---|---|
| Immunopathogenesis | Failed cell-mediated (T$_H$1) immunity; primarily ineffective humoral response | Successful cell-mediated immunity; lesions contained |
| Skin lesions | Many nodular growths with tissue compromise; stocking-and-glove peripheral neuropathy but no anesthesia around lesions; skin thickening | Few, hypopigmented macules; complete sensory loss in/around lesions; presence of granulomas and vigorous chronic inflammatory response |
| Organism presence in skin lesions | Always, innumerable | Few to none |
| Infectivity of skin lesions | Highly | Minimal |
| Prognosis | Poor; can lead to death, if untreated | Can be self-limiting |

### Pathogenesis

The atypical mycobacteria are not readily transmitted from person to person, and are instead considered opportunistic organisms.

### Clinical Symptoms

Rarely, *M avium-intracellulare* can cause pulmonary infections or lymphadenitis in immunocompetent individuals. Pulmonary infections are typically **nodular** and **bronchiectatic.** More importantly, MAC is a major cause of chronic disseminated disease in **patients with active AIDS.** This infection generally afflicts patients who have CD4+ T-cell counts below 10/mm³. The disease manifests as an overwhelming, disseminated infection in virtually all tissues. Patients present with cough, diarrhea, osteomyelitis, anemia, and wasting.

### Treatment

Multidrug resistance is common. Susceptible AIDS patients are routinely treated **prophylactically** for MAI with **macrolide** antibiotics (usually azithromycin).

Other atypical mycobacteria include:

- *M kansasii*, which is a **rare** cause of a syndrome clinically **identical** to pulmonary TB.
- *Mycobacterium scrofulaceum* is the causal agent of the pediatric disease **scrofula,** a chronic cervical lymphadenitis.
- *M marinum* inhabits standing water and can cause ulceration and granulomas at sites of open wounds.

## *Mycoplasma*

Mycoplasma are the smallest free-living bacteria in nature. They are so small that they were originally thought to be viruses. They are unique in that they **do not possess cell walls,** therefore drugs that inhibit cell wall synthesis (penicillins, cephalosporins and vancomycin) are ineffective against mycoplasma. Mycoplasma also have a plasma membrane reinforced with **cholesterol,** a sterol usually found in eukaryotic cells. Mycoplasma can be grown (very slowly) on artificial media in the lab but have complex nutritional requirements. They assume a **fried-egg** appearance after a few weeks of culture. The most important of the species is *Mycoplasma pneumoniae*, which causes atypical pneumonia. *Ureaplasma urealyticum* can cause nongonococcal urethritis (like *C trachomatis*).

### *Mycoplasma pneumoniae*

### Characteristics

*M pnemoniae's* plasma membrane is fortified with sterols for stability, and is antigenic. Human anti-*Mycoplasma* cell membrane antibodies **cross-react** with erythrocyte antigens and agglutinate RBCs but **only at low temperatures (4°C but not 37°C).** Thus, the **cold agglutinin test** is a simple (but nonspecific) test for an anti-*Mycoplasma* immune response that can be performed at the bedside.

### Pathogenesis

The plasma membrane of *M pneumoniae* contains the P1 protein, which is capable of binding specifically to respiratory epithelia.

Clinical Symptoms

*M pneumoniae* is a common cause of **atypical pneumonia** in young adults and manifests as gradual-onset, persistent low fever with a hacking, nonproductive cough and associated pharyngitis and malaise. Chest radiograph usually reveals patchy bilateral infiltrates that appear much worse than the clinical picture.

Treatment

Macrolides, or third-generation fluoroquinolones, such as levofloxacin.

### Chlamydiae and Rickettsiae

Chlamydiae and rickettsiae are tiny organisms. They are **obligate intracellular,** meaning that they are unable to live outside eukaryotic cells because they do not produce their own ATP. They stain gram-negative and possess a modified gram-negative cell wall, but the organisms are so small that they are invisible under conventional microscopy.

*Chlamydia* spp cause a variety of **respiratory and mucosal diseases** because of their **tropism to ciliated columnar epithelial cells,** whereas *Rickettsia* spp (and the closely related pathogens *Coxiella* and *Ehrlichia*) tend to cause **fever and rash syndromes** owing to a **predilection for endothelium.** Diseases caused by these organisms are also commonly treated with tetracyclines, macrolides, or (rarely) chloramphenicol.

#### *Chlamydia* Species

*Chlamydia* spp are distinguished from all other bacteria because of their **unique replicative cycle.** The infectious particle is the **elementary body (EB),** which is structurally similar to a spore in that much of its exterior peptidoglycan is cross-linked, protecting it from the elements. This peptidoglycan does **not** possess **muramic acid** and is not susceptible to disruption by penicillin antibiotics.

Once the EB form is taken up by the host cell, the cross-linkages are lost, and it transforms into a noninfectious **reticulate body** (RB, also known as an **initial body**). In this form, the microbe is metabolically active and amplifies its DNA, RNA, and protein production, **using host ATP.** These RBs are visible under microscopy as **cytoplasmic inclusions.** The intracellular RBs then differentiate into EBs, which are extruded from the host cell to start the cycle again.

The three medically important members of the *Chlamydia* genus are *C trachomatis,* which causes optic, genital tract, and neonatal pulmonary infections, and *C pneumoniae* and *C psittaci,* both of which cause atypical pneumonia.

The EB of *C trachomatis* is capable of infecting only certain types of cells—generally columnar or transitional epithelium, depending on the **serologic variant** of the organism. Different serovars have different epidemiologic and disease patterns (Table 4-17).

#### *Rickettsia* Species and Related Organisms

Like *Chlamydia, Rickettsia* and the closely related organisms *Coxiella burnetii, Orientia tsutsugamushi,* and *Ehrlichia chaffeensis* are tiny obligate intracellular organisms with structures similar to gram-negative rods. As with *Chlamydia* infections, treatment is almost always with doxycycline, or with chloramphenicol in children. However, these organisms differ from *Chlamydia* spp in several ways:

■ Unlike *Chlamydia* infections, which affect only humans, these organisms generally have **arthropod vectors (tick, mite, and louse)** (except for *Coxiella*).

**TABLE 4-17.** *Chlamydia trachomatis* **serotypes**

| SEROLOGIC VARIANT | CLINICAL SYMPTOMS | MNEMONIC/NOTES |
|---|---|---|
| Types A, B, and C | Chronic infection, cause blindness due to follicular conjunctivitis in Africa | **ABC** = **A**frica, **B**lindness, **C**hronic infection |
| Types D–K | Urethritis/PID, ectopic pregnancy, neonatal pneumonia (staccato cough) with eosinophilia, neonatal conjunctivitis | D–K = everything else Neonatal disease can be acquired during passage through infected birth canal |
| Types L1, L2, and L3 | Lymphogranuloma venereum—small, painless ulcers on genitals → swollen, painful inguinal lymph nodes that ulcerate (buboes). Treat with doxycycline | |

Reproduced with permission from Le T, et al. *First Aid for the USMLE Step 1 2017*. New York, NY: McGraw-Hill Education, 2017.

- Reproduction is by **binary fission.**
- Intracellular localization is within the **cytoplasm** and **nucleus.**
- Disease symptoms usually consist of headache, fever, and rash, resulting from the **vasculitis** secondary to the replication of the rickettsiae inside endothelial cells (Table 4-18).

**TABLE 4-18.   Rickettsial Diseases**

| ORGANISM/DISEASE | AFFECTED LOCATIONS | VECTOR/RESERVOIR | CLINICAL SYMPTOMS | RASH |
|---|---|---|---|---|
| *R rickettsii*: Rocky Mountain spotted fever | Southeastern and south central United States | "Hard" *Dermacentor* ticks | High fever, chills, headache, and myalgias | Macular, centripetal spread (extremities to trunk) and palms/soles |
| *R akari*: Rickettsial pox | Rare in United States | Mites that live on field mice | Fever, chills, headache; mild | Vesicular, generalized |
| *R prowazekii*: Epidemic typhus | Latin America, Africa in areas of poor hygiene | *Pediculus* body louse | Fever, chills, myalgias, headache, arthralgias, mental status changes | Petechial or macular, centrifugal spread (trunk to extremities) |
| *R typhi*: Endemic typhus | Warm areas | Fleas that live on rodents | Gradual onset of fever, chills, myalgias, nausea | Maculopapular, restricted to chest/abdomen |
| *O tsutsugamushi*: Scrub typhus | Asia, Pacific islands | Larvae (chiggers) of mites | High fever, headache, myalgias | Maculopapular, centrifugal spread |
| *C burnetii*: Q fever | Worldwide | Endospore inhalation | Headache, high fever, chills, myalgias, atypical pneumonia | None |
| *E chaffeensis*: Ehrlichiosis | Southern United States, Asia | *Amblyomma* ticks | Headache, fever, chills, myalgias; GI symptoms; leukopenia | Macular, centripetal spread |

GI, gastrointestinal.

## SPIROCHETES

Spirochetes are spiral-shaped bacteria with an **internal flagellum**:

- Technically gram-negative (ie, contain endotoxin), but not well visualized with light microscopy. Can be visualized with **darkfield** or fluorescent microscopy.
- Three clinically important genera: *Borrelia*, *Treponema*, and *Leptospira* (Table 4-19).
- Treated with β-lactams.

### TREPONEMA

The *Treponema* genus consists of **venereal** treponema (*T pallidum*, subspecies *pallidum* (simply referred to as *T pallidum*) as well as **nonvenereal** treponema that cause various infections such as **yaws, pinta,** and **bejel.**

### Treponema pallidum (Syphilis)

#### Characteristics

- *T pallidum* is a microaerophilic, extracellular spirochete with an internal flagellum between the outer membrane and cell wall.
- Humans are the only host.

#### Diagnosis

Diagnosis of *T pallidum* is based on clinical presentation, **darkfield** microscopy (cannot be grown in culture), and, most reliably, serology. Serological tests for diagnosing *T pallidum* include:

- *T pallidum* enzyme-linked immunosorbent assay (ELISA, TP IgG).
- **VDRL** (Venereal Disease Research Laboratories, for only CSF) or **RPR** (rapid plasma reagin):
  - Testing is based on a **nontreponemal** antibody (reagin) that reacts with cow heart cardiolipin-lecithin in vitro.

**TABLE 4-19.    Summary of Spirochete Diseases**

| PATHOGEN | GENERAL | TRANSMISSION | DIAGNOSIS | INFECTION | TREATMENT |
|----------|---------|--------------|-----------|-----------|-----------|
| *Treponema pallidum* (syphilis) | Microaerophilic, extracellular | Skin-skin contact Transplacental (**TO**RCH) | Serology: VDRL, then FTA-Abs | *Primary:* Painless chancre *Secondary:* Condylomata lata, palm and sole rash *Tertiary:* Aortitis, gummas, Argyl-Robertson pupil, tabes dorsalis | Penicillin G |
| *Borrelia burgdorferi* (Lyme disease) | Common vector-borne disease Microaerophilic, intracellular | Deer tick (*Ixodes scapularis*) | Clinical, serology | *Stage 1:* Erythema migrans, flulike symptoms *Stage 2:* Bell palsy, AV block *Stage 3:* Chronic arthritis, encephalopathy | Doxycycline |
| *Borrelia recurrentis* | Antigenic variation | *Pediculus humanus corporis* (human body louse) | Blood samples during fever | Sudden onset of fever, etc Spontaneous resolution and relapse | Tetracycline, penicillin |
| *Leptospira interrogans* | Aerobic | Animal urine | Microscopy | *Initial:* Flulike symptoms, photophobia *Later:* Liver damage with jaundice, renal failure | Penicillin G; doxycycline for prophylaxis |

AV, atrioventricular; FTA-Abs, fluorescent treponemal antibody absorption; TORCH, Toxoplasmosis; Other infections (syphilis, parvovirus B19, hepatitis B virus, HIV, varicella-zoster virus), Rubella, Cytomegalovirus, Herpes simplex virus; VDRL, Venereal Disease Research Laboratory.

- Screening tests: **High sensitivity,** low specificity.
- Turn positive 1 week after infection.
- False-positive in systemic lupus erythematosus (SLE), Epstein-Barr virus (EBV) infection, leprosy, hepatitis B (HBV) infection, and many others.
- **Fluorescent treponemal antibody absorption (FTA-Abs):**
  - Tests for **antitreponemal** antibody.
  - **Confirmatory** test—used to follow up positive VDRL/RPR.
  - Highly sensitive and **highly specific.**
  - Expensive.

### Pathogenesis

- Transmitted through sexual contact, contact with open chancre, or transplacentally.
- Outer membrane carries endotoxin-like lipids.
- Spirochetes penetrate mucous membranes, leading to bacteremia and seeding of organs throughout the body.

### Clinical Symptoms

There are **three** clinical stages of syphilis:

- **Primary syphilis** (following a 3- to 6-week incubation period).
  - A single **painless,** indurated ulcer with smooth margins **(chancre)** at **site of inoculation,** that heals within 3–6 weeks (Figure 4-28).
  - Early spread to regional lymph nodes and early bacteremia.
  - Self-limited primary stage, but **highly contagious.**
- **Secondary syphilis** (1–3 months later; rarely coexists with primary syphilis):
  - Manifests with flulike symptoms and a maculopapular rash on **palms, soles,** and mucous membranes.
  - May include condylomata lata (**highly infectious** wartlike lesions on perianal skin).
  - May cause infection in any organ or part of body (eg, hepatitis, arthritis, meningitis, etc).
  - Relapsing and remitting course, with cyclic symptoms and episodes of latency.
- **Tertiary syphilis** (decades later):
  - **Aortitis**—aortic insufficiency, ascending aortic aneurysm.
  - Neurosyphilis—**tabes dorsalis** (posterior column disease); **Argyll Robertson pupil** (accommodates but does not react to light), psychosis, and meningitis.
  - **Gummas**—soft granulomas of bone, skin, viscera (Figure 4-29).

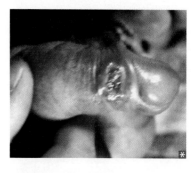

**MNEMONIC**

**Gram-indeterminate organisms—**

**S**ome **E**rrant **R**ascals **M**ay **M**icroscopically **L**ack **C**olor

**S**pirochetes
*Ehrlichia*
*Rickettsia*
*Mycobacterium*
*Mycoplasma*
*Listeria*
*Chlamydia*

**FIGURE 4-28. Chancre of primary syphilis.**

**FLASH FORWARD**

Tabes dorsalis occurs late and is characterized by demyelination of the posterior columns and dorsal roots. Corresponding symptoms include:
- Ataxia and wide-based gait (particularly in the dark or with eyes closed).
- Paresthesias and anesthesias (loss of proprioception and vibration sense).
- "Shooting" pains in lower extremities, loss of deep tendon reflexes and joint damage (Charcot joints)

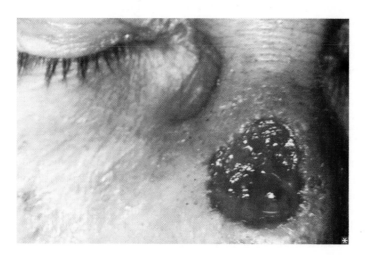

**FIGURE 4-29.** **Gumma of nose due to a long-standing tertiary syphilitic *Treponema pallidum* infection.**

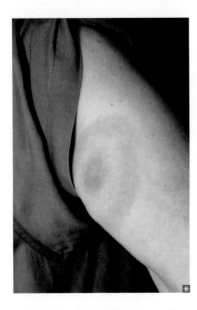

**FIGURE 4-30. Pathognomonic erythematous rash (erythema chronicum migrans).** Rash in the pattern of a bull's-eye of stage 1 Lyme disease.

## Treatment

- Benzathine penicillin G is used for primary and secondary syphilis as well as for prophylaxis to contacts. Aqueous penicillin G is used to treat neurosyphilis (due to poor CNS penetration of benzathine penicillin).
- Complication of treatment due to lysis of treponeme = Jarisch-Herxheimer reaction (fevers, chills, myalgias).
- No vaccine.
- Reinfection can occur as immunity to previous syphilis infection is incomplete.

Dependent on stage of infection and affected organs. Early syphilis and neurosyphilis tend to resolve well; however, aortitis may result in permanent structural defects.

### Nonvenereal Treponemal Infections

- Nonvenereal treponemal infections (yaws, pinta, and bejel) generally occur in **hot, humid areas** such as sub-Saharan Africa, the Middle East, Southeast Asia, Central and South America, and sometimes Mexico.
- **All** cause **cutaneous** disease sometimes, with internal organ involvement.
- Unlike syphilis, nonvenereal treponemal infections are **not** transmitted sexually and do **not** cause congenital disease. These infections are transmitted by direct person-to-person contact.
- Like syphilis, the causative spirochetes **cannot** be grown in culture. Importantly, nonvenereal treponemal infections yield **positive** VDRL/RPR and FTA-Abs test results.
- **All** treponemal infections are treated with penicillin G.

## BORRELIA

Generally, microbes of the *Borrelia* genus are more loosely coiled than treponemes and are **arthropod-borne** (not sexually or transplacentally transmitted).

### *Borrelia burgdorferi* (Lyme Disease)

#### Characteristics

*Borrelia burgdorferi* is the most common tick-borne agent in the United States. Reservoirs include the white-tailed deer and the white-footed mouse, and patients may be coinfected with *Ehrlichia* or *Babesia*.

#### Pathogenesis

- Transmission is via the bite of *Ixodes scapularis* (deer or black-legged tick); successful transmission requires the tick to feed for more than 24 hours.
- *B burgdorferi* is capable of changing its surface protein profile to escape the host immune response, known as **antigenic variation.**
- Invades skin and spreads hematogenously; leads to immune complex deposition.
- Can access immunoprivileged sites such as CNS, tendons, and synoviae.

#### Clinical Symptoms

There are **three** clinical stages of Lyme disease:

1. **Primary (early):** Erythema chronicum migrans (EVM) (spreading, **red target lesion,** Figure 4-30) and constitutional symptoms—fever, chills, fatigue, headache, myalgias or arthralgias.
2. **Secondary,** disseminated phase (days to weeks after infection):
   - Bell palsy (CN VII), aseptic meningitis, peripheral neuropathy.
   - Atrioventricular (AV) block, carditis.
   - Multiple erythema chronicum migrans (ECM) (secondary lesions).
   - Migratory myalgias, transient arthritis.
   - Other: Fever, stiff neck, headache, limb numbness or pain, malaise, fatigue.

3. **Tertiary,** late (months to years after infection):
   - Chronic polyarthritis.
   - Neurologic impairment, fatigue.
   - Acrodermatitis chronicum atrophicans (skin atrophy).

### Diagnosis

Often clinical, based on history of tick bite with characteristic erythema chronicum migrans. Serology may also be tested, although many false-negatives result, owing to antigenic variation and intracellular location. **Skin biopsy** can also be performed and result is positive if motile spirochetes are visible under darkfield microscopy. Other diagnostic tests include **PCR** and **culture** (modified Kelly medium).

### Treatment

**Doxycycline (oral)** for primary-stage Lyme disease and **ceftriaxone (IV)** for later-stage disease.

### *Borrelia recurrentis* (Relapsing Fever)

### Characteristics

*Borrelia recurrentis* can be diagnosed from a blood sample and looking for serum antibodies, or via darkfield microscopy with a Giemsa stain.

### Pathogenesis

*B recurrentis* is most commonly transmitted through the bite of the human body louse. Like *B burgdorferi*, *B recurrentis* is also capable of antigenic variation. Proliferation in the bloodstream can stimulate a subsequent immune response.

### Clinical Symptoms

- Inoculation: Transmitted by **human body louse.**
- Bacteremia presents with onset of shaking chills, fever, myalgias, headache, delirium, cough, lethargy, hepatosplenomegaly.
- Spontaneous resolution and recurrence (less severe) due to antigenic variation and recurrent septicemia.

### Treatment

Penicillin or tetracycline. Treatment may cause Jarisch-Herxheimer reaction via lysis of bacteria and release of antigens.

### *Leptospira interrogans* (Leptospirosis, Icterohemorrhagic Fever)

### Characteristics

- *Leptospira interrogans* is an aerobic spirochete with hooked ends and two periplasmic flagella (Figure 4-31).
- Diagnosis is achieved via microscopy (spirochetes in blood, CSF, or urine), as well as serology.

### Pathogenesis

Transmission is fecal-oral through **animal urine** (variety of wild and domesticated animals, especially rodents, dogs, fish, and birds). Most common modes of transmission: puddle stomping, recreation in contaminated water, working in sewers (rat urine).

*L interrogans* is also capable of antigenic variation due to its variable LPS structure.

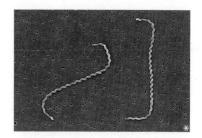

**FIGURE 4-31.   Scanning electron micrograph of *Leptospira interrogans*.**

### Clinical Symptoms

Leptospirosis presents with flulike symptoms and photophobia. Mild infection, known as anicteric leptospirosis, can lead to aseptic meningitis. Severe infection, known as **Weil**

**disease**, presents with hemorrhagic vasculitis that can lead to kidney damage (renal failure) and hepatitis (jaundice). Although the mortality rate is high in Weil disease, prognosis is generally good for mild cases.

### Treatment

Penicillin G for treatment, doxycycline for prophylaxis.

# Mycology

## FUNGI

### General Characteristics

- Nonmotile eukaryotes with a chitinous cell wall that take the form of yeasts, hyphal molds, or dimorphic fungi.
- Cause an array of diseases including skin, lung, opportunistic, and systemic infections.
  - Fungi can cause **endemic** infections as well as **localized** infections (ie, **superficial, cutaneous,** or **subcutaneous**). Some fungi are **opportunistic** pathogens that cause disease in immunocompromised hosts.
- Grow on **Sabouraud** agar, which is selective for fungi due to its low pH, which inhibits growth of most bacteria.
- Cell **membrane** contains **ergosterol** and cell **wall** is composed of **chitin.**

### Morphology

Fungi exist in **two** forms: yeast and molds. Many fungi can be found in either life form, depending on the **temperature** at which they are growing (Figure 4-32 and Table 4-20).

### Endemic Mycoses

- **Inhaled** particles primarily cause pulmonary infections but can disseminate through the bloodstream, producing endemic symptoms involving multiple organs.
- Pathogens include *Histoplasma, Blastomyces, Coccidioides,* and *Paracoccidioides,* all of which:
  - Are dimorphic fungi (existing in two forms) and can be treated with **fluconazole** (or itraconazole) for local infections, amphotericin B for endemic infections.
  - Can be diagnosed with sputum cytology, sputum cultures on blood agar, special media, and peripheral blood cultures (*Histoplasma* in particular).
  - Can induce **granuloma formation** that may calcify over time (similar to TB).
- Endemic fungal infections are **not** transmittable from person to person (in contrast with TB).

#### *Histoplasma capsulatum*

##### Characteristics

- Found in the Mississippi and Ohio River Valleys; transmitted by inhalation of **bird** and **bat droppings.**
- At 20°C, grows as hyphae with macronidia and micronidia.
- At 37°C, found as yeast inside macrophages in the body (Figure 4-33).

##### Pathogenesis

- Reservoir: **Soil, bird,** and **bat droppings** contain spores.
- Transmission: Spores are inhaled from dust.
- Macrophages phagocytose spores and carry them systemically.

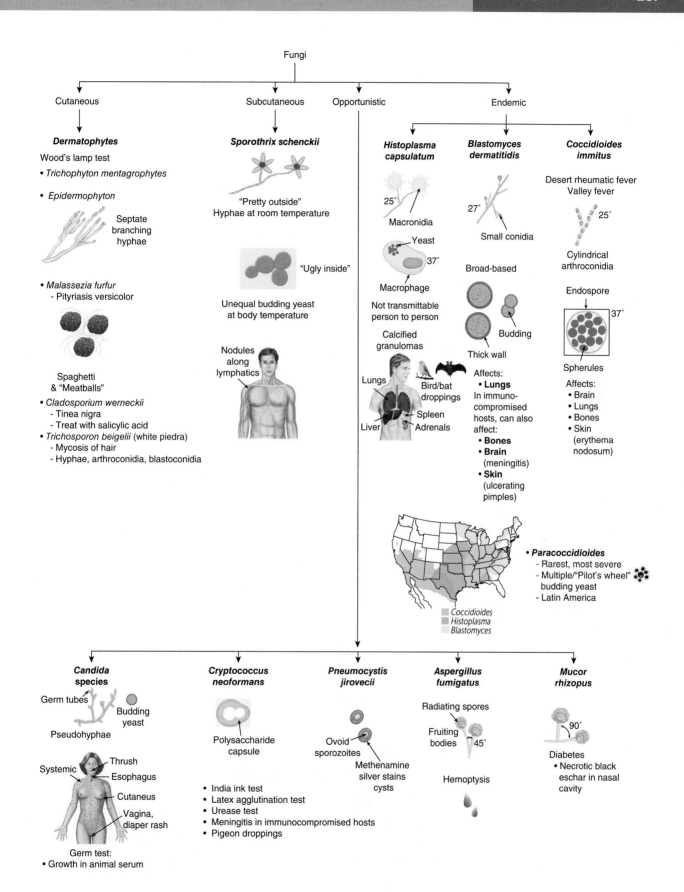

**FIGURE 4-32.** **Classification of fungi.** Fungi with histologies shown and clinical symptoms depicted by diagrams.

**TABLE 4-20.    Fungi Morphology**

|  | YEAST | MOLDS |
|---|---|---|
| Cellularity | Unicellular | Multicellular |
| Form | Budding cells | Hyphae (long filamentous tubular cells) |
| Other forms | **Pseudohyphae** (long chains of cells formed by incomplete budding) | **Septate** hyphae—membranes separate cells <br> **Aseptate** hyphae—no membranes between cells, multinucleated cells |

- Budding yeast forms **inside** macrophages, causing local infections throughout the body.

### Clinical Symptoms

- Asymptomatic in immunocompetent patients.
- Systemic infection in immunocompromised patients.
- Calcified granulomas in infected tissues.
- Pneumonitis that appears similar to miliary TB.
- Infection may involve liver, spleen, and adrenal glands in immunocompromised patients.

### Diagnosis

- Dimorphic yeast.
- Granulomas.
- Small budding cells within macrophages on biopsy.
- Calcified lung lesions that may become **cavitary** in chronic progressive form.

### Treatment

- Cell-mediated immunity required.
- Itraconazole for moderate infection.
- Amphotericin B for severe infection.

*Blastomyces dermatitidis*

### Characteristics

- Found in the Ohio and St. Lawrence River Valleys.
- **Rarest** of all endemic mycoses.
- At 20°C, found as hyphae with small conidia.
- At 37°C, found as budding yeast with broad base in tissue or in culture (Figure 4-34).

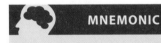

**MNEMONIC**

**BBB**

**B**lastomyces are found as **B**udding yeast with a **B**road **B**ase.

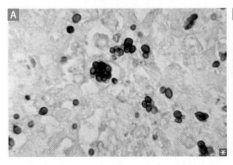
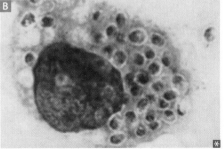

**FIGURE 4-33.    *Histoplasma* morphologies.** A Tissue form, and B intracellular form.

## Pathogenesis

- Reservoir: **Soil** and **rotten wood** contain spores.
- Transmission: Inhaled spores.
- Spores form yeast in the body, causing local infections.
- Yeast spreads systemically over time and causes granulomas throughout the body (lungs, bones, and skin).

## Clinical Symptoms

- Ulcerating pimples or verrucous skin lesions
- Pneumonitis, night sweats, weight loss
- Meningitis
- Arthritis
- Does **not** reactivate

## Diagnosis

- Dimorphic yeast
- Thick-walled spores
- Lung lesions do **not** calcify
- Granulomas

## Treatment

- Cell-mediated immunity required.
- Itraconazole for moderate infection or meningeal involvement.
- Amphotericin B for severe infection without meningeal involvement.

## Prognosis

Fair; **most severe** of endemic mycoses.

### *Coccidioides immitis*

## Characteristics

- Found in the southwestern United States, Mexico, and South America; known as "desert rheumatic fever" or "valley fever."
- At 20°C (room temperature), grows as cylindrical arthroconidia.
- At 37°C (in tissue), grows as endospores in spherules (Figure 4-35).

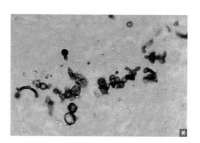

**FIGURE 4-34.    *Blastomyces* morphology.**

**KEY FACT**

Remember **B dermatitidis** is the only endemic fungus commonly seen in the U.S. that causes ulcerating pimples.

**KEY FACT**

Systemic infection with **B dermatitidis** often occurs in the absence of lung disease.

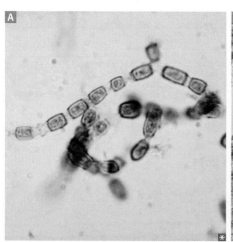 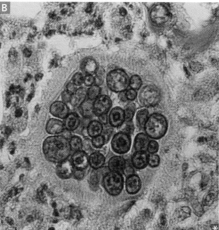

**FIGURE 4-35.    *Coccidioides* morphologies.** **A** Tissue form (arthroconidia) and **B** spore form (spherule filled with endospores).

### Pathogenesis

- Reservoir: **Soil.**
- Transmission: Airborne. Inhaled arthroconidia become endospores in body.

### Clinical Symptoms

- Majority of infections are subclinical.
- Most common clinical presentation: Mild pneumonia, cough, fever, with possible hemoptysis.
- Erythema nodosum
- Pneumonitis
- CNS involvement
- Arthritis
- Dissemination to bone and skin
- AIDS patients: Meningitis, mucocutaneous lesions
- Pregnancy: Severe dissemination in third trimester

### Diagnosis

- Dimorphic yeast (no hyphae).
- Thick-walled spores.
- Granulomas.
- Biopsy specimen shows **endospores inside spherules,** all inside giant cells (Figure 4-35).

### Treatment

- **Cell-mediated immunity** is required.
- Itraconazole for mild infections.
- Amphotericin B for severe infections without CNS involvement.
- Fluconazole for CNS involvement (good CNS penetration).

### Prognosis

Fair, but may be fatal for elderly patients, and the immunocompromised are at risk for developing complications.

### *Paracoccidioides brasiliensis*

### Characteristics

- Found in **Latin America.**
- Appears as multiple budding yeasts often described as **"spokes of a wheel,"** or **"pilot's wheel"** (Figure 4-36).
- Affected population: 90% **male.**

### Pathogenesis

- Reservoir: Spores found in **soil.**
- Transmission: Inhalation of spores.

### Clinical Symptoms

Symptoms are similar to those of *Blastomyces.*

### Diagnosis

Dimorphic yeast.

### Treatment

- Itraconazole
- Sulfamethoxazole/trimethoprim (Bactrim)
- Amphotericin B

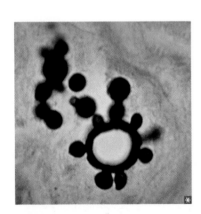

**FIGURE 4-36.**
***Paracoccidioides*—"pilot's wheel."**

Prognosis

Good.

## Cutaneous Mycoses

Dermatophytes

### Characteristics (Figure 4-37)

- Includes three main types of fungi that infect the skin: *Trichophyton*, *Microsporum*, and *Epidermophyton*.
- Septate branching hyphae with arthroconidia and cross-walls.

### Pathogenesis

- Reservoir: **Soil, animals, humans.**
- Transmission: Spread by contact with infected individuals or animals.
- Colonize **keratinized** epithelium (dead, horny layer) in warm, moist areas.
- Infection spreads centrifugally with curvy worm-like borders ("ringworm").
- Fungal antigens are released from the hyphae and may induce **delayed-type hypersensitivity** reaction (dermatophytoses: inflammation, itching, scaly skin, pustules).
- Fungal antigens may diffuse systemically and cause dermaphytid reactions: Hypersensitivity responses (vesicles) at distant sites such as fingers.

### Clinical Symptoms

- Head and scalp (**tinea capitis** [Figure 4-38A]).
- Body infection (**tinea corporis**): Ring lesion ("ringworm") on skin that appears to spread centrifugally (Figure 4-38B).
- Athlete's foot (**tinea pedis** [Figure 4-38C]).
- Jock itch (**tinea cruris**).
- Onychomycoses (tinea unguium): Nail infection, discoloration of nails.

### Diagnosis

- Scrapings of infected skin are placed in KOH preparation, which destroys nonfungal cells and allows visualization of fungal hyphae.
- Wood's lamp (**UV** light) detects *Microsporum*.

### Treatment

- Topical antifungal creams for skin infections (imidazole).
- Oral antifungals for hair follicle and nail infections.

### Prognosis

Good, but relapse is common.

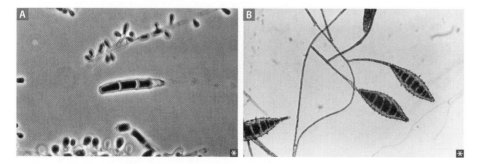

**FIGURE 4-37.   Dermatophytes.** A Macroconidia budding from multiseptate conidiophores and B spindle-shaped macroconidia of *Microsporum*.

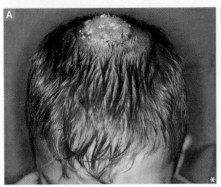
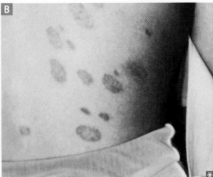
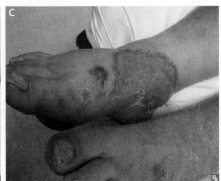

FIGURE 4-38.    **Tineas.** A Tinea capitis; B tinea corporis; and C tinea pedis with onychomycosis (tinea unguium).

### *Malassezia furfur*

#### Characteristics

**Natural flora** of skin.

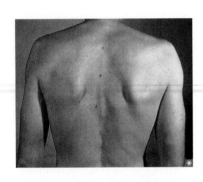

FIGURE 4-39.    **Hypopigmented, patchy rash of tinea versicolor.**

#### Pathogenesis

- Reservoir: Animals, humans, soil.
- Transmission: Contact.

#### Clinical Symptoms

Pityriasis (tinea) versicolor: **Pale** spots on the skin, often on the back, chest, and neck (Figure 4-39).

#### Diagnosis

- KOH prep.
- Spherical yeast.
- "Spaghetti and meatballs" appearance (Figure 4-40).

#### Treatment

Topical antifungals: Imidazole.

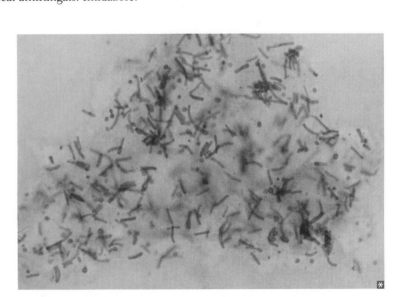

FIGURE 4-40.    ***Malassezia furfur.*** Spaghetti and meatballs appearance, shown on Gram stain.

Prognosis

Good.

## Opportunistic Fungal Infections

Opportunistic fungi include *Candida, Aspergillus, Cryptococcus, Mucor, Pneumocystis,* and many others. These fungi cause symptoms almost exclusively in immunocompromised hosts. However, candidal disease can occur after prolonged **antibiotic** use or contamination of **indwelling catheters** in immunocompetent hosts.

### *Candida albicans*

#### Characteristics

- **Natural flora** of skin.
- Appear as budding yeast with **pseudohyphae** in tissue biopsy (Figure 4-41).
- Causes mucosal and systemic infections in compromised hosts, and device-related infections in otherwise normal hosts.

#### Pathogenesis

- Reservoir: GI flora and normal skin flora in moist areas such as underneath breasts or in skin folds.
- Growth: Forms "**germ tubes**" (Figure 4-42) at 37°C and pseudohyphae when invading tissue. Grows rapidly if not controlled.
- **Antibiotic use,** immunocompromise, and cancer increase risk of infection.

#### Clinical Symptoms

- In immunocompetent hosts:
    - Oral **thrush**
    - **Vulvovaginitis** ("yeast infection")
    - **Diaper rash**
- In immunocompromised hosts:
    - **Esophagitis**
    - Skin infection
    - Disseminated systemic infection and septicemia
- Endocarditis in **IV drug users.**

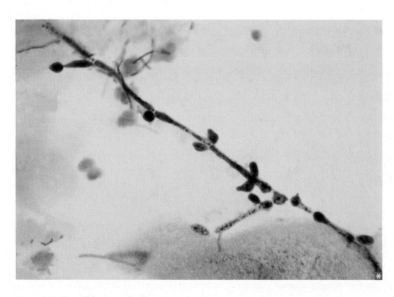

**FIGURE 4-41.** *Candida* **morphology.**

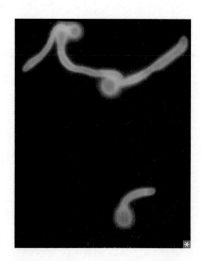

**FIGURE 4-42.** *Candida.* Germ tube morphology.

### Diagnosis

- **Silver** stain.
- **KOH** stain for pseudohyphae, budding yeast.
- **Germ tube test**—grow in animal serum.

### Treatment

- Nystatin/fluconazole for mucosal infection.
- Fluconazole, other azoles, echinocandins, or amphotericin B for systemic infections; echinocandins are emerging as first-line therapy.
- Other *Candida* species cause similar disease to *C albicans* but are more likely to be azole-resistant.

### Prognosis

Good, but *Candida* infections cause serious morbidity and some mortality in immunocompromised hosts.

### *Cryptococcus neoformans*

#### Characteristics

- Appears as budding yeast (Figure 4-43).
- Has **thick polysaccharide capsule.**
- Mostly affects patients with AIDS or other defects in cell-mediated immunity.

#### Pathogenesis

- Reservoir: Bird (especially **pigeon**) droppings.
- Transmission: Inhaled yeast from droppings results in lung infection (often asymptomatic).
- Spreads hematogenously to CNS, causing meningitis, abscess formation, and increased intracranial pressure.
- Affects people with poor T-cell–mediated immunity.

#### Clinical Syndromes

- Meningitis
- Pneumonia
- Fungemia

#### Diagnosis

- **Latex agglutination test** for capsular antigen in blood or CSF.
- Ring-enhancing brain abscesses.

#### Treatment

- Amphotericin B plus flucytosine for meningitis.
- Fluconazole for lifetime suppression in AIDS patients, along with restoration of immune function with antiretroviral therapy.

#### Prognosis

Fair.

### *Pneumocystis jirovecii* (formerly known as *Pneumocystis carinii*)

#### Characteristics

- Appears as dark **ovoid sporozoites within cysts** on **silver stain** (Figure 4-44).
- Frequently affects AIDS patients.
- May also affect severely malnourished children and patients on long-term high-dose steroid therapy.

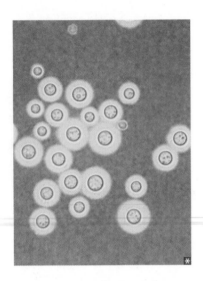

**FIGURE 4-43.** *Cryptococcus* **morphology.** Budding yeast in India ink preparation.

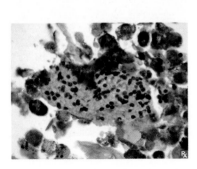

**FIGURE 4-44.** *Pneumocystis jirovecii* **in tissue with silver stain.**

## Pathogenesis

- Transmission: Cyst is inhaled by most people in childhood, leading to an asymptomatic or mild pneumonia, then to a latent infection in the lungs.
- In immunocompromised hosts: Reactivation, uncontrolled growth, and an inflammatory response can lead to pneumonia.

## Clinical Symptoms

- Pneumonitis.
- Classically may cause **pneumothorax.**

## Diagnosis

**Silver stain** (from lung biopsy or lavage) showing cysts containing **dark oval bodies** (Figure 4-44), other stains, or DFA testing.

## Treatment

- Sulfamethoxazole/trimethoprim (Bactrim)—single strength, atovaquone, pentamidine, or dapsone for prophylaxis.
- Sulfamethoxazole/trimethoprim (Bactrim)—double strength, or pentamidine for treatment.
- Corticosteroids may be given in addition to antipneumocystis regimens to reduce inflammation during treatment initialization.

## Prognosis

Fair.

### Microsporidia

## Clinical Symptoms

Causes self-limiting watery diarrhea in immunocompetent persons, but can result in massive, chronic watery diarrhea in immunocompromised patients (eg, AIDS patients).

## Diagnosis

Fecal sample reveals gram-positive and acid-fast spores.

## Treatment

- Supportive for the immunocompetent.
- Albendazole for the immunocompromised.

### Aspergillus fumigatus

## Characteristics

- Found in many environmental reservoirs; most people are constantly exposed to spores.
- **Septate** hyphae **branching at a 45-degree angle in tissue** (Figure 4-46).

**CLINICAL CORRELATION**

Classic clinical presentation of *Pneumocystis carinii* pneumonia (PCP): Severe hypoxia with ground glass on x-ray (Figure 4-45) in severely immunocompromised patient; treatment includes steroids.

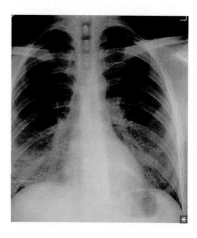

**FIGURE 4-45.** **Classic clinical presentation of *Pneumocystis jirovecii* pneumonia.**

**KEY FACT**

*Pneumocystis jirovecii* pneumonia is still called **PCP** (*Pneumocystis carinii* **p**neumonia) in the medical community. In AIDS patients, PCP **prophylaxis** is initiated when the CD4 count is < **200.**

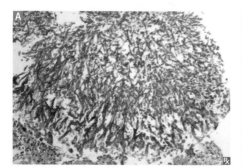
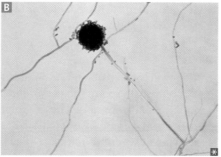

**FIGURE 4-46.** ***Aspergillus* morphology.** **A** 45-degree angle branching septate hyphae in a fruiting body. **B** Conidial head with spores.

- Fruiting bodies borne on stalks.
- Primarily affects **neutropenic** patients.

### Pathogenesis

- Reservoir: Mold grows on **decaying vegetation.**
- Transmission: Spores are inhaled.
- May stimulate IgE response, leading to bronchospasm and **allergic bronchopulmonary aspergillosis (ABPA)**, especially in patients with asthma or CF.
- May be deposited in lung cavity to form aspergillus ball (aspergilloma or fungus ball), especially after a previous TB infection.
- May invade lung tissue and enter bloodstream in the immunocompromised host. Can occlude blood vessels, leading to pulmonary **infarction.**
- Can produce aflatoxins, carcinogenic toxins associated with hepatocellular carcinoma.

### Clinical Syndromes

- Various lung diseases, including fungus ball, acute and chronic pneumonitis, and disseminated systemic disease.
- *Aspergillus* can produce aflatoxins, which induce p53 mutations, and are associated with the development of hepatocellular carcinoma.
- Pneumonitis often with **hemoptysis;** severe illness with high mortality in persistently neutropenic patients.

### Diagnosis

- Tissue biopsy reveals branching hyphae (45-degree angle).
- Sputum culture shows fungal colonies with hyphae and, in mature colonies, fruiting bodies bearing conidia (asexual spores).
- **X-ray** may detect aspergilloma or progressive and necrotic pulmonary infiltrates. *Aspergillus* galactomannan test is used for monitoring and presumptive diagnosis of invasive aspergillosis.
- Overall, diagnosis is difficult; tissue biopsy may be required.

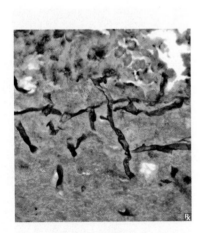

**FIGURE 4-47.** *Mucor and Rhizopus.*

### KEY FACT

*A fumigatus, Mucor,* and *Rhizopus* appear very similar in tissue biopsies, but *Aspergillus* branches at 45 degrees (acute) while *Mucor* and *Rhizopus* branch at 90 degrees. Also, *Aspergillus* has smaller septate (segmented) hyphae, but *Mucor* and *Rhizopus* hyphae are large and aseptate.

### Treatment

- ABPA: Corticosteroids, no antifungals needed.
- Aspergilloma: Surgery with antifungal therapy.
- Invasive aspergillosis: Voriconazole; if not tolerant or responding, can use echinocandin or amphotericin B.

### Prognosis

Depends on type of disease. For disseminated disease, prognosis is poor.

### *Mucor* and *Rhizopus*

### Characteristics

- **Aseptate** hyphae branch at **90-degree angle in tissue** (Figure 4-47).
- Afflicts patients with diabetes or other metabolic acidoses, neutropenia, or burns and other extensive wounds.

### Pathogenesis

- Reservoir: Spores ubiquitous in the environment.
- Transmission: Spores inhaled or inoculated.
- In immunocompromised hosts: Colonizes tissue and invades blood vessels, leading to necrosis (similar to aspergillosis).
- Can penetrate cribriform plate and infect brain, producing rhinocerebral or frontal lobe abscess and possible cavernous sinus thrombosis.

## Clinical Symptoms

- Nasal ulceration or necrosis (black eschar), painful periorbital or facial swelling, headache, and possible cranial nerve involvement.
- Invasive **rhinocerebral** infection, a medical and surgical emergency.
- Pneumonitis similar to *Aspergillus*.

## Diagnosis

- Tissue biopsy shows branching hyphae (branching at 90-degree angle) without septae.
- Shows a broad ribbon-like growth pattern. Culture insensitive even in cases where hyphae is seen in tissue.

## Treatment

- Control of diabetes
- Surgery for rhinocerebral infections
- Isavuconazole and Amphotericin B

## Prognosis

Poor.

### Subcutaneous Mycoses

*Sporothrix schenckii*

#### Characteristics (Figure 4-48)

- Found in soil.
- "Gardener's nodule": Often transmitted via prick of finger on **rose thorns.**
- At 20°C, appears as branching hyphae with rosette conidia (flower-shaped macroconidia).
- At 37°C, appears as elongated, unequally budding yeast.

#### Pathogenesis

- Subcutaneous infections affect skin and surrounding lymphatics.
- Reservoir: Spores in soil.
- Transmission: Spores enter skin through cuts and puncture wounds such as puncture by rose thorn.

#### Clinical Symptoms

Subcutaneous nodules form along lymphatics, usually in the upper extremity that was infected via break in the skin. Primary nodule becomes necrotic and ulcerates. Secondary nodules form along lymphatic tracts draining primary infection.

**QUESTION**

A patient with history of diabetes presents with polyuria, polydipsia, fever, and headache. What are the next steps in evaluating for possible mucormycosis?

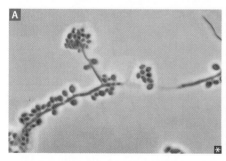 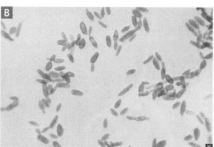 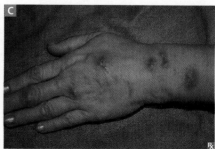

**FIGURE 4-48.** **Sporothrix schenckii morphologies and clinical presentation.** **A** Branching conidiophores and numerous conidia of the mold form. **B** Cigar-shaped budding yeast. **C** Ascending subcutaneous nodules.

### Diagnosis

- Culture at different temperatures reveals branched hyphae at 20°C and single cells (**cigar-shaped** budding yeast) at 37°C.
- Produces **black** pigment.
- Rosette conidia.
- Neutrophilic **microabscesses** in skin.

### Treatment

- Oral potassium iodide (mechanism unclear).
- Antifungals for extracutaneous involvement: Amphotericin B, itraconazole.

### Prognosis

Good.

## Parasitology

Medically important parasites comprise two groups: protozoa and helminths (worms). Relevant protozoa include *Plasmodium* (the malaria parasite) and organisms such as *Entamoeba* and *Giardia*. Notable helminths are the tapeworms and the pinworms, the soil-dwelling nematodes, and the flukes.

### PROTOZOA

Protozoa are **unicellular,** eukaryotic parasites. They can be classified into five groups based on sites of pathogenesis:

1. Intestinal protozoa: *Giardia, Entamoeba, Cryptosporidium, Cyclospora,* and *Cystoisospora.*
2. CNS protozoa: *Toxoplasma, Naegleria,* and *Trypanosoma brucei.*
3. Hematologic protozoa: *Plasmodium* and *Babesia.*
4. Visceral protozoa: *Trypanosoma cruzi* and *Leishmania.*
5. Sexually transmitted protozoa: *Trichomonas.*

### Intestinal Protozoa

#### Giardia lamblia

- Causes noninvasive gastrointestinal disease characterized by abdominal cramps, flatulence, and **foul smelling, "explosive" stools** with **steatorrhea.**
- Often seen in **campers** or **hikers** who drank from streams contaminated with *Giardia* cysts.
- Transmission between humans can be **fecal-oral** or **oral-anal.**
- Organism has characteristic "facelike" appearance (Figure 4-49). Diagnosis by antigen test is more sensitive than microscopy.
- Treatment: Metronidazole.

#### Entamoeba histolytica

- Infection may be **asymptomatic** or may cause **amebiasis,** amoebic dysentery (tenesmic diarrhea with blood and mucus), and visceral "anchovy paste" abscess, especially in the liver (Figure 4-50).
- Fecal-oral transmission.
- Exists in two life cycle stages: Cyst (infective stage) and trophozoite (invasive stage).
- Cyst has characteristic four nuclei, whereas trophozoite occasionally contains ingested RBCs (Figure 4-51). Antigen detection is more sensitive than microscopy for detection in stool. In patients with liver abscess, stool is often negative, therefore serology is useful.
- Treatment: Metronidazole.

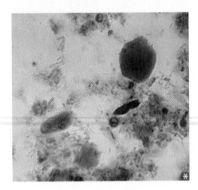

**FIGURE 4-49.** **Giardia lamblia cyst.**

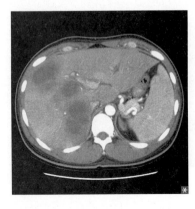

**FIGURE 4-50.** **Entamoeba histolytica.** CT of abdomen revealing multiple liver abscesses.

*Cryptosporidium, Cyclospora,* and *Cystoisospora*

- Cause self-limiting watery diarrhea in immunocompetent persons, but can result in massive, chronic watery diarrhea in immunocompromised patients (eg, AIDS patients).
- Fecal sample reveals:
  - *Cryptosporidium:* Modified acid-fast oocysts (Figure 4-52).
  - *Cyclospora:* Modified acid-fast oocysts.
  - *Cystoisospora:* Acid-fast oocysts.
- Treatment: Supportive for the immunocompetent. For the immunocompromised (eg, AIDS):
  - *Cryptosporidium:* Nitazoxanide.
  - *Cyclospora* and *Cystoisospora:* Bactrim (sulfamethoxazole/trimethoprim).

## CNS Protozoa

### *Toxoplasma gondii*

- Cause toxoplasmosis, which resembles mononucleosis in immunocompetent persons but can be severe (especially in AIDS patients), resulting in encephalitis with multifocal CNS lesions.
- Routes of infection: **Ingestion** of undercooked, **cyst-contaminated meat,** exposure to **oocysts** in **cat feces,** and **transplacental** transmission.
- Congenital disease (**T** in **TORCH** congenital disease mnemonic) is characterized by hydrocephalus, cerebral calcifications, and chorioretinitis.
- Diagnosis: by serology (IgM antibodies to toxoplasmosis antigen) for acute/congenital infection; IgG for exposure status in compromised hosts. Brain CT scan shows **ring-enhancing lesions** (Figure 4-53).
- **Treatment:** Pyrimethamine.

## Hematologic Protozoa

### *Plasmodium* Species

- Causes **malaria,** a mosquito-borne infection that affects 200–400 million people worldwide and kills about 650,000 people annually.
- Five species: *P falciparum, P vivax, P ovale, P malariae,* and the newly recognized *P knowlesi.*
- Vector: female *Anopheles* **mosquito.**
- Complex life cycle involving mosquito, human liver, and human erythrocytes.

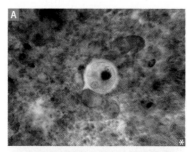

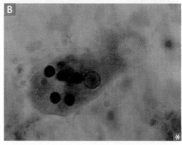

**FIGURE 4-51.** *Entamoeba histolytica* **stages.** A Cyst with two visible nuclei and chromatin body in its cytoplasm. B Trophozoite with single nucleus and multiple ingested red blood cells.

**? CLINICAL CORRELATION**

*Crypto* in AIDS patients
*Cryptosporidium* **p**arvum: **p**rotozoa, chronic watery diarrhea
*C* **n**eoformans: fu**n**gus, meningoencephalitis

**? CLINICAL CORRELATION**

Due to the risk of transplacental transmission, pregnant women are advised to **avoid cat-litter boxes** and **undercooked meat.**

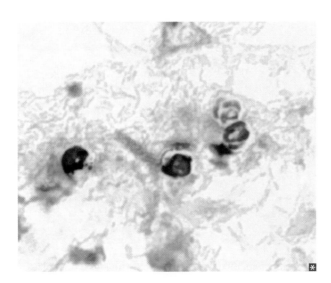

**FIGURE 4-52.** **Photomicrograph shows acid-fast *Cryptosporidium* spp oocysts.**

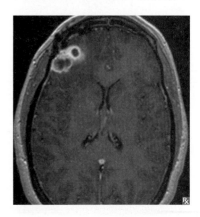

**FIGURE 4-53.** **CT of the head shows ring-enhancing lesions of *Toxoplasma gondii.***

- Malaria is characterized by **cyclical fever** with **hemolytic anemia** (parasites infect and rupture RBCs), **myalgias,** and sometimes **gastroenteritis and splenomegaly.**
- *P falciparum* malaria is a medical emergency that should usually be managed in an ICU setting; it's associated with brain, kidney, and lung complications as well as severe fevers and anemia and other complications.
- **Giemsa-stained** blood smear reveals **banana-shaped** gametocytes (*P falciparum* only), and **"ring" and developing trophozoite and schizont forms within RBCs** (Figure 4-54).
- Sickle cell gene likely has **protective** effect against malaria.
- **Treatment:** Quinines (chloroquine, primaquine, mefloquine), artemisinin, sulfadoxine-pyrimethamine.
- **Drug-resistance** to antimalarial medications is common. Primaquine is necessary to treat *P vivax* and *P ovale* infections.

### Babesia

- **Tick-borne** parasite that causes **malaria-like** illness in northeastern United States.
- Although *Babesia* infects RBCs and causes hemolytic anemia, it does **not** infect the liver like *Plasmodium.*
- Blood smear (Wright/Giemsa stain) reveals RBCs containing ring-form trophozoites, occasionally in a **"Maltese cross"** configuration (Figure 4-55).
- Asplenic (and other immunocompromised) patients are at risk for more severe infections, which can manifest with complications of acute respiratory distress syndrome (ARDS), DIC, and/or congestive heart failure (CHF).
- **Treatment:** Clindamycin and quinine.

## Visceral Protozoa

### Trypanosoma Species

- Includes *T brucei* and *T cruzi.*
- *T brucei* (*rhodesiense* and *gambiense*) transmitted by **tsetse fly,** causes **African sleeping sickness.**
- *T cruzi,* transmitted by the **reduviid (kissing) bug,** causes **Chagas disease.**
- **Chronic** manifestations of Chagas disease include **dilated cardiomyopathy, megaesophagus, megacolon,** and meningoencephalitis.
- **Treatment:** Complicated, toxic, and difficult; an specialist must be consulted.

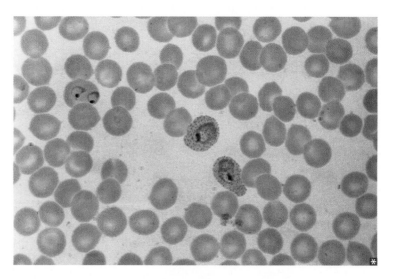

**FIGURE 4-54.** ***Plasmodium.*** Blood smear containing ring-form trophozoite and mature schizont.

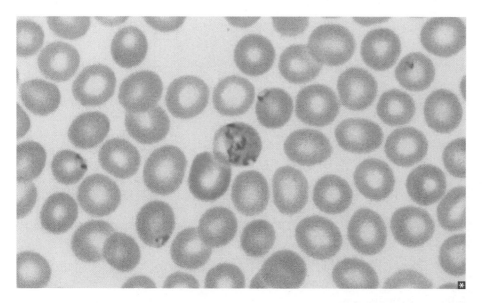

**FIGURE 4-55.** ***Babesia.*** Blood smear showing *Babesia* rings within erythrocytes.

### *Leishmania* Species

- Many species; the four most important are: *L donovani*, *L tropica*, *L mexicana*, and *L braziliensis*.
- Disease depends on species: ***L donovani*** causes visceral leishmaniasis, or "kala azar," resulting in fever, anemia, leukopenia and hepatosplenomegaly (Figure 4-56). Most of the other *Leishmania* species cause cutaneous or mucocutaneous disease
- Transmission: **Sand fly.**
- **Treatment:** Stibogluconate. Amphotericin in severe cases.

### Sexually Transmitted Protozoa

#### *Trichomonas vaginalis*

- **Sexually transmitted** urogenital infection.
- Infection (**vaginitis** in females) characterized by **greenish, foul-smelling,** watery and **itchy** discharge. Infected cervix has punctate hemorrhages ("strawberry cervix"). In pregnancy, associated with premature labor and delivery.
- Infected males are usually **asymptomatic** but may present with **urethritis** or **prostatitis**.
- **Wet mount** reveals motile organisms with four anterior flagella. Best diagnosed by molecular methods.
- Treatment: Metronidazole.

### Other Notable Protozoa

#### *Naegleria fowleri*

- An amoeba that causes **highly fatal, rapid-onset meningoencephalitis**.
- Humans are infected while **swimming** in contaminated **fresh waters**.
- **Treatment:** Amphotericin B and supportive care (almost always fatal).

## HELMINTHS

Helminths are multicellular parasites (worms) that are often associated with eosinophilia. Two general types of helminths are roundworms (nematodes) and flatworms (platyhelminths). Flatworms may be segmented (ie, cestodes, or tapeworms) or nonsegmented (ie, trematodes, or flukes) (Figure 4-57).

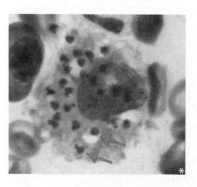

**FIGURE 4-56.** **Macrophage containing *Leishmania* amastigotes.**

---

**KEY FACT**

*Tricky "Trichs"*
*Trichomonas:* Protozoa → STD
*Trichinella:* Round worm → GI infection and skeletal muscle cysts
*Trichuris:* Round worm → GI infection and rectal prolapse

---

**Q    QUESTION**

A patient contracts malaria, is treated with chloroquine, and recovers. Three months later, he presents with a febrile illness similar to the malaria he had previously, and rings are found in his erythrocytes on peripheral blood smear. What are the most likely *Plasmodium* species indicated? What antimalarials should be considered? Before treatment, what additional test should be performed?

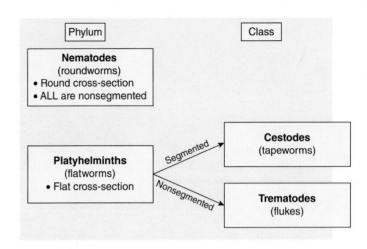

FIGURE 4-57.    **Helminth classification scheme.**

## Nematodes (Roundworms)

Nematodes are **nonsegmented** worms with a **circular** cross-section and complete digestive system. Table 4-21 contains a summary of nematodes.

### Intestinal Nematodes

*Enterobius vermicularis* (Pinworms)

#### Characteristics

Pinworms are small nematodes, about 1 cm long. Pinworm infection is the **most common helminthic infection in the United States.**

#### Pathogenesis

Transmission is **fecal-oral** via ingestion of eggs from contaminated surfaces or household dust. Eggs hatch in the digestive tract, where the larvae then mature and mate. Adult females migrate out through the anus and **lay eggs in perianal skin.**

#### Clinical Symptoms

Pinworms most often affect **children,** and the eggs cause **intense perianal itching.** Diagnosis is made using the **Scotch tape test,** in which a piece of tape is pressed against the perianal skin and then examined for eggs (Figure 4-58).

#### Treatment

Pyrantel pamoate, mebendazole, albendazole.

*Ascaris lumbricoides*

#### Characteristics

*Ascaris* is a large nematode that can grow up to 13 inches long. It is the **most common helminthic infection in the world** and is especially prevalent in tropical areas with poor sanitation.

#### Pathogenesis

Transmission is **fecal-oral** via ingestion of eggs from contaminated soil. Eggs hatch in the digestive tract, and larvae then penetrate the intestinal wall and enter the vasculature.

#### Clinical Symptoms

Ascariasis may be **asymptomatic** but may result in **pneumonia,** if large numbers of ova are ingested. Larvae can also mature into adult worms in the intestines, which may

ANSWER

*P ovale* and *P vivax.* Either add primaquine to a repeated chloroquine treatment or, if resistance is suspected, mefloquine + primaquine, or atovaquone/proguanil + primaquine. Before administering primaquine, test patient for glucose-6-phosphate dehydrogenase (G6PD) deficiency.

**TABLE 4-21.    Summary of Nematodes**

| MODE OF TRANSMISSION | WORM | SYMPTOMS | BUZZWORDS | LABORATORY DIAGNOSIS |
|---|---|---|---|---|
| **INTESTINAL NEMATODES** | | | | |
| Ingestion of eggs | *Enterobius vermicularis* (pinworm) | Anal pruritus | | Scotch tape test |
| | *Ascaris lumbricoides* | None, pneumonia, malnutrition, peritonitis | Bowel obstruction, bile obstruction | Eggs in stool |
| | *Trichuris trichiura* (whipworm) | None, diarrhea without pruritus | | |
| Larvae penetrate skin (usually feet) | *Strongyloides stercoralis* (threadworm) | None, pneumonitis, gastroenteritis | | Larvae in stool, string test |
| | *Ancylostoma duodenale* (Old World hookworm) | Pneumonitis, gastroenteritis, microcytic anemia | | Eggs in stool |
| | Cat or dog hookworm | Itching along worm's path | Cutaneous larva migrans | |
| | *Necator americanus* (New World hookworm) | Pneumonitis, gastroenteritis, microcytic anemia | | Eggs in stool |
| Ingestion of larvae | *Trichinella spiralis* (pork roundworm) | Diarrhea, myalgias, periorbital edema | Pork, wild game | |
| **TISSUE NEMATODES** | | | | |
| Arthropod bite | | | | |
| Blackfly | *Onchocerca volvulus* | River blindness, skin nodules, rash, hyperpigmentation | | |
| Deer fly | *Loa loa* (eye worm) | Blindness, swelling in skin | | |
| Mosquito | *Wuchereria bancrofti* | Elephantiasis, edema, fever, scaly skin | Enter bloodstream at night | |
| Ingestion of eggs | *Toxocara canis* (dog ascaris) | Hepatosplenomegaly, blindness | Visceral larva migrans | |
| Ingestion of larvae | *Dracunculus medinensis* (Guinea worm) | Painful subcutaneous nodules | Copepods | Roll out on a stick, surgery |

then migrate, penetrate, or obstruct the GI tract. As a result, *Ascari* infection may cause **malnutrition,** bowel obstruction, or biliary obstruction. Diagnosis is made by eggs in the stool (Figure 4-59) and **eosinophilia.**

Treatment

Pyrantel pamoate, mebendazole, albendazole.

*Strongyloides stercoralis* (Threadworm)

Pathogenesis

Larvae in contaminated soil are able to directly penetrate the skin, usually through the feet.

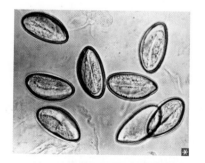

**FIGURE 4-58.    Eggs of *Enterobius vermicularis* mounted on tape.**

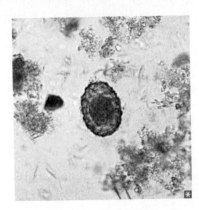

**FIGURE 4-59.** **Fertile egg of** *Ascaris lumbricoides.*

MNEMONIC

**ST**rongyloides is the only helminth whose larvae are **ST**rong enough to get into the **ST**ool.

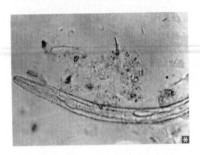

**FIGURE 4-60.** *Strongyloides stercoralis* **larva.**

MNEMONIC

Remember that both hookworms can cause **iron deficiency anemia:**
Dracula sucks blood from your **Nec**(ator).
*An*cylostoma forms an **an**astomosis with your gut.

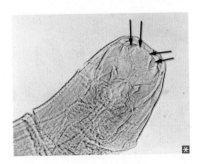

**FIGURE 4-61.** **Head of** *Ancylostoma duodenale* **worm with hooks in mouth (arrows).**

### Clinical Symptoms

Strongyloidiasis can be **asymptomatic.** However, **local itching** may occur at the site of entry, and larvae are transported through the vasculature to the lungs, where they may rarely cause **pneumonia.** From the lungs, they migrate up the trachea and into the pharynx where they are subsequently swallowed. Larvae can then mature and mate in the digestive tract. Females lay their eggs in the intestinal wall, which may cause abdominal pain and **diarrhea.** Once the eggs hatch, larvae may exit with feces or may penetrate the abdominal wall and reenter the bloodstream. In the latter case, larvae can then travel to the lungs and repeat the life cycle (**autoinfection**). Diagnosis is made by detection of eosinophilia and **larvae in the stool** (Figure 4-60). Serology is highly sensitive and specific and has replaced the "**string test,**" in which a patient swallows a long string that reaches the duodenum, after which larvae can then be pulled out via the string. Most immunocompetent patients with *Strongyloides* are asymptomatic, but steroid-treated and neutropenic patients can develop *Strongyloides* hyperinfection syndrome, in which large numbers of migrating larvae and adult worms can produce serious pneumonitis, gastroenteritis, and gram-negative sepsis.

### Treatment

Ivermectin, thiabendazole.

### *Ancylostoma duodenale* and *Necator americanus* (Old World and New World Hookworm)

### Characteristics

Both species of hookworms have characteristic "hooks" in their mouth that allow them to attach to the intestinal mucosa (Figure 4-61).

### Pathogenesis

Similar to *Strongyloides*, larvae in contaminated soil are able to directly penetrate the skin, usually through the feet.

### Clinical Symptoms

Similar to *Strongyloides*, **local itching** may occur at the site of entry. Larvae are then transported through the vasculature to the lungs, where they may rarely cause **pneumonia.** From the lungs, they migrate up the trachea and into the pharynx, where they are subsequently swallowed. Larvae then mature into adults in the GI tract. The adult form attaches to the intestinal mucosa using characteristic hooks. It then feeds off of the host's blood. Adults also mate in the intestines and release eggs into the stool.

- Initial symptoms may include abdominal pain and **diarrhea.**
- Over time, the host may develop a **hypochromic microcytic anemia.**
- Diagnosis is made by detection of eggs in the stool, along with **eosinophilia.**

### Treatment

Mebendazole, pyrantel pamoate. Treat anemia with iron and folic acid.

### Cat or Dog Hookworm

### Characteristics

Lacks the necessary collagenase to be able to penetrate the epidermal basement membrane in humans. The infection is especially prevalent in warm, humid climates and usually affects children.

### Pathogenesis

Larvae reside in soil contaminated with dog or cat feces. Similar to human hookworms, infection arises from direct skin contact, usually through the feet.

## Clinical Symptoms

Because the larvae cannot fully penetrate human skin, they are only able to migrate along the dermal-epidermal junction. Their path is marked by a serpiginous erythematous rash that is intensely pruritic. This is known as **cutaneous larva migrans** (Figure 4-62).

## Treatment

Infection is usually self-limited, and larvae usually die within several weeks.

### *Trichinella spiralis* (Pork Roundworm)

#### Characteristics

Most common cause of parasitic **myocarditis.**

#### Pathogenesis

Transmission occurs by ingestion of encysted larvae in **undercooked pork** or wild game. Larvae mature and mate in the human digestive tract and may subsequently penetrate the intestinal wall to enter the bloodstream. From the blood, larvae often migrate to skeletal **muscle.**

#### Clinical Symptoms

Symptoms of trichinellosis correlate with the worm's life cycle:

- Larvae in digestive tract: Nausea, vomiting, diarrhea.
- Migrating larvae in bloodstream: High fever, eosinophilia, periorbital edema, conjunctival and splinter hemorrhages, urticarial rash.
- Larvae occupation of muscle: Myalgias and calcified cysts.
- Infiltration of heart and brain: Myocarditis and encephalitis.

Diagnosis is confirmed via muscle biopsy or positive anti-*Trichinella* serology (or both). There are no eggs in the stool because the eggs hatch in the intestinal submucosa.

#### Treatment

Mebendazole, albendazole, and thiabendazole are effective for the intestinal stages of infection. Although there is no effective treatment for muscle cysts, **glucocorticoids** may be beneficial in cases of severe myositis or myocarditis.

### *Trichuris trichiura* (Whipworm)

#### Characteristics

Adult worms are typically 3–5 cm long, with a whiplike shape (narrow anterior, wide posterior).

#### Pathogenesis

Similar to pinworms, whipworm transmission is fecal-oral via ingestion of eggs. Eggs hatch in the digestive tract, where the larvae then mature and mate. Adult whipworms attach to the **superficial mucosa.**

#### Clinical Symptoms

Usually **asymptomatic,** but heavier worm burdens may result in malnutrition, abdominal pain, **bloody diarrhea,** tenesmus, and/or **rectal prolapse.** No anal pruritus. Diagnosis of whipworm is made by detection of eggs in the stool.

#### Treatment

Mebendazole, albendazole.

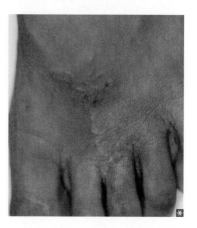

**FIGURE 4-62. Cutaneous larva migrans.** A serpiginous erythematous rash found on a patient's foot.

## Tissue Nematodes

### *Onchocerca volvulus* (River Blindness)

#### Characteristics

Arthropod-borne, endemic near rivers.

#### Pathogenesis

A bite from the **black fly** releases larvae into the **skin.** Larvae migrate through skin and mature into adults. Adults can mate and release microfilariae into subcutaneous tissues. To complete their life cycle, microfilariae are ingested via a second fly bite and then mature into larvae.

#### Clinical Symptoms

- Fibrosis can occur around adult worms, resulting in **subcutaneous nodules.**
- Migrating microfilariae result in an inflammatory response consisting of a thick, hyperpigmented, pruritic **rash.**
- If microfilariae reach the eye, local inflammation can also cause blindness (**river blindness**).
- Diagnosis can be made with a skin biopsy of a subcutaneous nodule or by detecting microfilariae in a skin-snip.

#### Treatment

Ivermectin is effective against microfilariae only. Subcutaneous nodules (ie, adult worms) must be surgically removed.

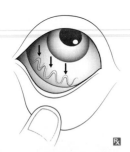

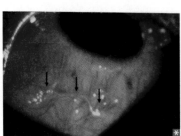

**FIGURE 4-63.** *Loa loa* **worm in subconjunctiva.**

### *Loa loa* (Eye Worm)

#### Characteristics

Arthropod-borne, similar to *Onchocerca.* Found in Africa.

#### Pathogenesis

A bite from the ***Chrysops*** **fly** releases larvae into the skin.

#### Clinical Symptoms

Infection is most often asymptomatic, but can lead to episodic swelling (Calabar swellings). Adult worms can sometimes be seen **migrating through the subconjunctiva** (Figure 4-63).

#### Treatment

Diethylcarbamazine.

### *Wuchereria bancrofti* and *Brugia malayi* (Elephantiasis)

#### Characteristics

Arthropod-borne, endemic in tropical areas. *Brugia malayi* is confined primarily to southern Asia.

#### Pathogenesis

A **mosquito** bite releases microfilariae into the **blood.**

#### Clinical Symptoms

Microfilariae reach the lymphatic system and mature into adults. Fibrosis around adult worms results in obstruction, leading to edema and scaly skin (**elephantiasis**), which usually involves the **genitalia** and **lower extremities** (Figure 4-64). Symptoms of elephantiasis can take 9 months to a year or more to develop after initial bites. Other signs and symptoms of infection may include fever, chills, lymphadenopathy, and eosinophilia. Diagnosis can be made by detecting microfilariae in the blood at **night.**

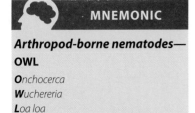

**MNEMONIC**

**Arthropod-borne nematodes— OWL**

**O**nchocerca
**W**uchereria
**L**oa loa

## Treatment

Diethylcarbamazine treats the parasite; however, doxycycline treats an obligate intracellular symbiont and has a high cure rate alone.

### *Toxocara canis* (Dog Ascaris)

#### Characteristics

*Toxocara canis* is similar to *A lumbricoides*, but can complete its life cycle only in dogs. Humans are dead-end hosts.

#### Pathogenesis

Transmission is fecal-oral via ingestion of eggs from soil contaminated with dog feces. Eggs hatch in the digestive tract, and larvae penetrate the intestinal wall and enter the vasculature.

#### Clinical Symptoms

Larvae can migrate to many different organs; therefore, this disease is known as **visceral** larva migrans. Common manifestations include **hepatosplenomegaly** and **blindness**. Diagnosis is made by presence of or detection of **epsinophilia** and anti-*Toxocara* **serology**.

#### Treatment

Infection is usually self-limited, but glucocorticoids may be helpful in severe cases.

### *Dracunculus medinensis* (Guinea Worm)

#### Characteristics

Larvae live in tiny aquatic crustaceans (called **copepods**).

#### Pathogenesis

Copepods are ingested in drinking water. *Dracunculus* larvae are then free to mature and mate in the human host.

#### Clinical Symptoms

Adult worms migrate to the **skin** to release their eggs back into the environment. They form painful subcutaneous nodules and can reach lengths up to 3 feet.

#### Treatment

Nodules can be removed surgically or by slowly pulling out the worm by rolling it on a stick (Figure 4-65). If the worm were to break during this process, **anaphylaxis** could result.

#### Prevention

Providing clean water, filtration for drinking water, case-finding and treatment, and treatment of reservoirs to eliminate copepod vectors have brought dracunculiasis to the brink of eradication.

### Cestodes (Tapeworms)

Cestodes are **segmented** flatworms, and **all** are transmitted by **ingestion.** In general, infected persons are treated with praziquantel (niclosamide, if praziquantel is unavailable) or albendazole (Table 4-22).

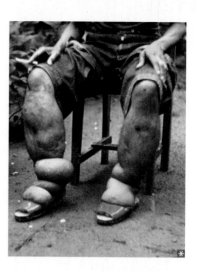

**FIGURE 4-64.** **Elephantiasis of the lower extremity.**

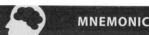

**MNEMONIC**

**Routes of nematode infection—**

- Ingested (You'll get sick if you **EATT** these.): **E**nterobius, **A**scaris, **T**oxocara, **T**richinella.
- Cutaneous (These get into your feet from the **SAN**d.): **S**trongyloides, **A**ncylostoma, **N**ecator.
- Bites (Lay **LOW** to avoid getting bitten.): **L**oa loa, **O**nchocerca volvulus, **W**uchereria bancrofti.

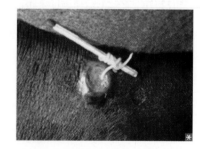

**FIGURE 4-65.** **Removing a *Dracunculus medinensis* worm from a patient's leg.**

**TABLE 4-22.** **Summary of Cestodes**

| MODE OF TRANSMISSION | TYPE OF INFECTION | WORM | SYMPTOMS | BUZZWORDS/ASSOCIATIONS | LAB FINDINGS |
|---|---|---|---|---|---|
| Ingestion of larvae | GI | *Taenia saginata* (**beef** tapeworm) | None, abdominal discomfort, malnutrition | Undercooked beef, proglottids | Eggs in stool |
| | GI | *Taenia solium* (**pork** tapeworm) | None, abdominal discomfort, malnutrition | Undercooked pork, proglottids | Eggs in stool |
| Ingestion of eggs | Tissue | *Taenia solium* (**pork** tapeworm) | Cysticercosis, seizures, blindness | Worm can be seen in vitreous humor! | Tissue cysts/ calcifications on x-ray |
| | GI | *Diphyllobothrium latum* (broad**fish** tapeworm) | None, B$_{12}$ deficiency, macrocytic anemia | Undercooked or pickled fish | Eggs in stool |
| | GI | *Echinococcus granulosus* (**dog** tapeworm) | Right upper quadrant pain, hepatomegaly, anaphylaxis | Liver cysts, hydatid cyst disease, sheep, dogs | Cysts on x-ray or CT |

*Taenia solium* (Pork Tapeworm)

Characteristics

Body plan similar to that of *Taenia saginata*. Ingestion of the *T solium* egg versus larva causes different diseases (Figure 4-66).

Pathogenesis

Ingesting the larval form through contaminated pork leads to infestation of intestines. The egg form is ingested through fecal contamination and hatches in the intestines. The larvae then penetrate the intestinal wall to enter the bloodstream and cause systemic infection.

Clinical Symptoms

Diagnosis rests on **cysticerci** on radiograph and serology; late in infection, after the organism has died, they may calcify.

Treatment

- GI infection: Praziquantel.
- Cysticercosis: Albendazole with prednisone.

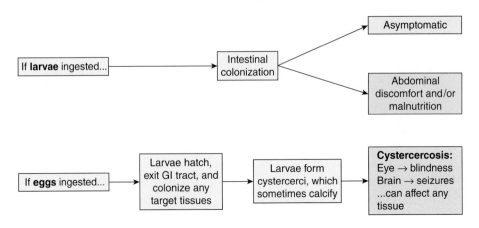

**FIGURE 4-66.** **Mechanisms of *Taenia solium* infection.**

*Taenia saginata* (Beef Tapeworm)

### Characteristics

Composed of scolex ("head") and proglottids (segmented "tail"). *Taenia saginata* can grow to several meters long.

### Pathogenesis

Adheres to mucosa via **scolex** and absorbs nutrients from host.

### Clinical Symptoms

- Ingestion of larvae in undercooked beef leads to infection that may be asymptomatic or may present with abdominal discomfort or malnutrition (or both).
- Diagnosis is by detection of proglottids or eggs in **stool.**

### Treatment

Treat with praziquantel.

*Diphyllobothrium latum* (Fish Tapeworm)

### Characteristics

Can grow to several meters long.

### Pathogenesis

Ingestion of infected undercooked or pickled freshwater fish results in intestinal colonization. May absorb nutrients and **outcompete host for vitamin B$_{12}$.**

### Clinical Symptoms

Diagnosis is based on finding eggs in **stool** (Figure 4-67). Infection is often asymptomatic, but can also cause **B$_{12}$ deficiency** with a megaloblastic, macrocytic anemia.

### Treatment

Praziquantel.

*Echinococcus granulosus* (Dog Tapeworm)

### Characteristics

Tapeworm stage does not infect humans; large tissue (usually liver) cysts.

### Pathogenesis

Ingestion of eggs from canine fecal contamination allows larvae to hatch in the GI tract. They can then penetrate the intestinal wall and migrate to target tissues, where they form **hydatid cysts.**

### Clinical Symptoms

- **Diagnosis** is based on plain film or CT visualization of cysts in tissue (Figure 4-68). Clinical manifestations of infection include **hydatid cyst disease,** which can affect the liver, lungs, and brain, resulting in organ **dysfunction.**
- **Ruptured cysts** can release high levels of antigen and may cause **anaphylaxis.**
- **Liver cysts** can present with **right upper quadrant pain** and **hepatomegaly.**

### Treatment

Albendazole followed by careful cyst aspiration.

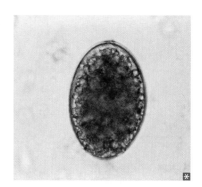

FIGURE 4-67. *Diphyllobothrium latum* **egg.**

 **KEY FACT**

Modes of transmission:
- Undercooked seafood: *Clonorchis sinensis, Paragonimus westermani, Diphyllobothrium latum*
- Undercooked beef: *Taenia saginata*
- Undercooked pork: *Taenia solium, Trichinella spiralis*
- Human feces: *Ascaris lumbricoides, Enterobius vermicularis, Trichuris trichiura*
- Dog feces: *Toxocara, Echinococcus*
- Drinking water: *Dracunculus*

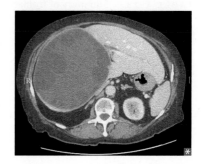

FIGURE 4-68. *Echinococcus granulosus.* CT of the abdomen showing a giant hydatid cyst in the liver of an infected patient.

### Trematodes (Flukes)

The trematode genera (flukes) consist of **nonsegmented** flatworms. Their life cycles are complex and involve **snails** as intermediate hosts. They are most often treated with **praziquantel** (Table 4-23).

#### Schistosomes (Blood Flukes)

#### Characteristics

- Male folds its body ventrally to hold female in **permanent copulation.**
- Eggs are highly **immunogenic,** resulting in chronic inflammation of tissues (Figure 4-69).
- Transmission: Larvae released into fresh water penetrate the skin, then enter the bloodstream to reach target tissues.
- Clinical manifestations of infection: Patient may be asymptomatic or may present with constitutional symptoms (Katayama fever) or early dermatitis with pruritus at the entry site (or both). Late manifestations are due to chronic inflammation of target tissue.
- Three species: *Schistosoma japonicum, S haematobium,* and *S mansoni.*
- Clinical manifestations: *S japonicum* and *S mansoni* can mature in the **portal circulation,** resulting in periportal fibrosis and portal hypertension. They can also affect the mesenteric circulation, resulting in intestinal polyps.
- *S haematobium:*
  - Clinical manifestations: *S haematobium* can mature in the blood vessels supplying the **bladder,** resulting in **hematuria,** dysuria, frequency, and urgency. Long-term infection is associated with **squamous cell carcinoma of the bladder,** presumably as a result of chronic inflammation. (Note that most primary bladder cancers are transitional cell carcinoma.)
  - Diagnosis: Eggs found in stool (all *Schistosoma*) and eggs in urine (*S haematobium*).

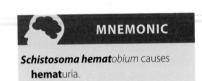

**MNEMONIC**

*Schistosoma hemat*obium causes **hemat**uria.

#### Treatment

**All** flukes are treated with praziquantel.

#### *Clonorchis sinensis* (Chinese Liver Flukes)

#### Characteristics

Endemic in Southeast Asia.

**TABLE 4-23.    Summary of Trematodes**

| MODE OF TRANSMISSION | TYPE OF INFECTION | WORM | SYMPTOMS | BUZZWORDS/ASSOCIATIONS | LAB FINDINGS |
|---|---|---|---|---|---|
| Larval penetration of skin | Tissue | *Schistosoma mansoni, Schistosoma japonicum* | Pruritus at entry sites, constitutional symptoms (Katayama fever) | **Portal hypertension,** intestinal polyps, snails | Eggs in stool |
| | Tissue | *Schistosoma haematobium* | Pruritus at entry sites, constitutional symptoms (Katayama fever), **hematuria** | **Squamous cell carcinoma of the bladder,** snails | Eggs in stool and urine |
| Ingestion of encysted larvae | GI | *Clonorchis sinensis* (Chinese liver fluke) | Biliary tree infection | Undercooked fish, **cholangiocarcinoma** | Eggs in stool |
| Ingestion of eggs | Lung | *Paragonimus westermani* | Hemoptysis, cough, fever | Shellfish (crab meat) | Eggs in stool and sputum |

## Pathogenesis

Encysted larvae are ingested in **raw or undercooked freshwater fish.** The larvae migrate through the GI tract and mature in the **biliary tree.**

## Clinical Symptoms

Diagnosis is by detection of eggs in stool. Manifestations range from asymptomatic to vague right upper quadrant pain, cholangitis, and/or biliary obstruction. Associated with **cholangiocarcinoma.**

## Treatment

**All** flukes are treated with praziquantel.

### *Paragonimus westermani* (Lung Fluke)

#### Characteristics

Endemic in Asia, Africa, and South America.

#### Pathogenesis

Ingestion of eggs from infected **shellfish.**

#### Clinical Symptoms

Diagnosis is via detection of eggs in sputum and stool. Clinical manifestations of infection include **hemoptysis,** cough, and fever.

#### Treatment

**All** flukes are treated with praziquantel.

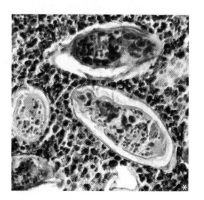

**FIGURE 4-69.** **Schistosoma haematobium.** Histopathology of bladder shows *Schistosoma haematobium* eggs with dense eosinophilic infiltrate.

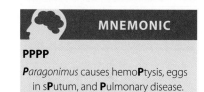

**MNEMONIC**

**PPPP**

*Paragonimus* causes hemo**P**tysis, eggs in s**P**utum, and **P**ulmonary disease.

# Virology

## BASIC STRUCTURE

### Virus Particles: Virions

Viruses are obligate intracellular pathogens and can only replicate inside an appropriate host cell. Because they lack their own machinery for self-replication and are not technically living cells, viral infectious particles are instead dubbed "virions." They are composed of a genome encased in a protein coat (**capsid**). Depending on the life cycle of the virus, the capsid may or may not be surrounded by a lipoprotein envelope (Figure 4-70).

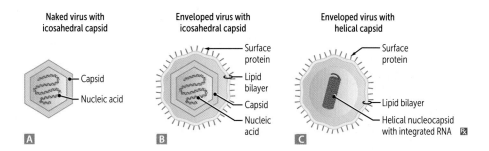

**FIGURE 4-70.** **Schematic diagram of the components of the complete virus particle (the virion).** A Naked virus with icosahedral capsid. B Enveloped virus with icosahedral capsid. C Enveloped virus with helical capsid.

Viral genome + Nucleocapsid ± Virus-encoded enzymes =
Nonenveloped (naked) virus

Viral genome + Nucleocapsid ± Virus-encoded enzymes +
Host membrane with virus-encoded glycoproteins = Enveloped virus

### Viral Classification

Viruses are primarily classified as follows:

- Type of genome (DNA or RNA, double-stranded (ds) or single-stranded (ss), positive-sense or negative-sense, circular or linear, and segmented or nonsegmented).
- Type of capsid (icosahedral, helical, or complex).
- Presence or absence of lipid envelope.

### Viral Genome

The viral genome is composed of a nucleic acid sequence made up of either DNA or RNA (but not both). There is great variation in genomic structure:

- ds or ss
- Segmented or nonsegmented
- Linear, circular, or partial circular

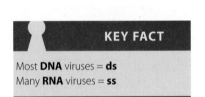

**KEY FACT**

Most **DNA** viruses = **ds**
Many **RNA** viruses = **ss**

A virus with a **ss genome** can be:

- **Positive-stranded (positive-sense) RNA:** Genome exhibits mRNA-like characteristics; thus, it can be directly translated by the host cell.
- **Negative-stranded (negative-sense) RNA:** The virus must first make a complementary copy of its genome before it can undergo translation. Negative-stranded viruses must carry their own enzymes, such as **RNA-dependent RNA polymerases,** to transcribe the complement strand after infecting a host cell.
- **Ambisense:** Genome contains both positive-stranded and negative-stranded nucleic acids. This arrangement requires two rounds of transcription to be carried out.

### Viral Ploidy

Traditionally, ploidy refers to the number of sets of chromosomes in a biological cell. When referring to viruses, ploidy refers to the number of copies of the viral genome contained in each virion. Nearly all viruses are haploid, meaning they have one copy of their DNA or RNA genome. Retroviruses are the exception—they are diploid, possessing two identical copies of their ssRNA genome.

### Capsid

The capsid forms an outer shell that holds and protects the viral genome and virus-encoded enzymes. It is composed of structural proteins called **capsomeres** that are uniquely determined by the viral genome and serve as antigenic stimuli for antibody production; that is, the molecular "tags" by the immune system identify viruses as foreign. The capsid can exhibit several **shapes:**

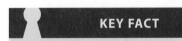

**KEY FACT**

Viral envelopes mediate attachment to the host cell and initiation of infection and also serve as antigenic stimuli for antibody production.

- **Icosahedral** (symmetrically sided polygon—polyhedron with 20 symmetrical triangular faces)
- **Helical**
- **Complex** (including a mix of polyhedral and helical shapes)

## ENVELOPED VERSUS NONENVELOPED VIRUSES

General characteristics of viral species that are human pathogens are depicted in Figure 4-71.

### Enveloped Viruses

Enveloped viruses are surrounded by a lipoprotein membrane acquired when the virus is nonlytically released from the host cell. **Virus-encoded glycoproteins present in the lipid membrane** are essential for attachment to the host cell and initiation of infection. The glycoproteins also serve as viral antigens and stimulate antibody production.

- **Most DNA** viruses acquire their envelopes from the host's plasma membrane as the virus exits the cell.
- **Exceptions** are **poxviruses,** because they replicate and acquire their envelope (through "Golgi wrapping") in the cytoplasm.

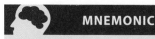

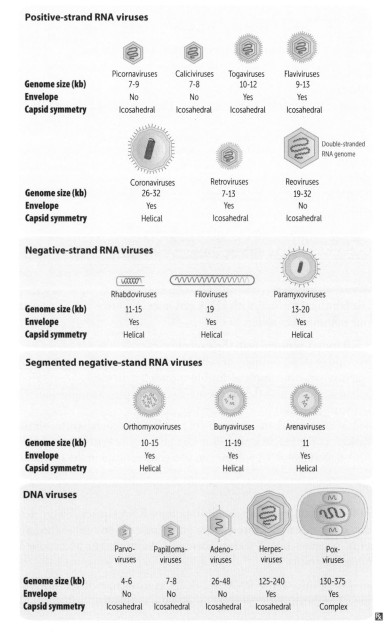

**FIGURE 4-71. Schematic diagram of the major virus families including species that infect humans.** The viruses are grouped by genome type and are drawn approximately to scale.

In addition to their primary function, viral glycoproteins also serve as **viral attachment proteins (VAPs)** that bind to host cell structures. Some examples are:

- Influenza **hemagglutinin (HA)**: Binds to exposed sialic acid to mediate viral entry.
- Influenza **neuraminidase (NA)**: Facilitates release of virion from host cell.
- **Fusion (F) proteins**: Facilitates fusion of virion and the host cell.

Viral envelopes provide an additional layer of metabolic and immunological protection for viruses and provide them with more options for invasion and long-term replication within infected cells but are vulnerable to environmental disruption. Because of acid-sensitivity, enveloped viruses are rarely GI pathogens.

### Nonenveloped Viruses

Nonenveloped viruses have no envelopes and are usually more stable than enveloped viruses because they are better equipped to withstand injury from the damaging agents mentioned earlier. Enteric viruses such as reoviruses and picornaviruses are transmitted via the **fecal-oral** route. Other viruses are transmitted via respiratory droplets and contact with fomites.

There are four families of **nonenveloped (naked) DNA** viruses:

- Parvoviridae
- Adenoviridae
- Papovaviridae (now classified into separate Papilloma and Polyoma families)

There are four families of **nonenveloped (naked) RNA** viruses:

- Astroviridae
- Reoviridae
- Picornaviridae
- Caliciviridae

## DNA VERSUS RNA VIRUSES

### DNA Viruses

There are **six families** of viruses **with DNA genomes** (Figure 4-72). These viruses share the following common characteristics:

1. **Double-stranded genome** with the exception of:
   - Parvoviridae (B19)—**single-stranded** DNA genome.
   - Hepadnavirus—**incomplete double-stranded** genome.
2. **Linear** viral genomes with the exception of papovaviruses (papilloma/polyoma) and hepadnavirus—**circular.**
3. **Icosahedral capsid** with the exception of poxviruses, which have a **complex** capsid.
4. **Replication** in the nucleus with the exception of poxviruses, which carry their own DNA-dependent RNA polymerase and can replicate in the cytoplasm.

### RNA Viruses

There are **14 major** families of medically important **RNA viruses** (Figure 4-73), which are generally categorized into **three** major groupings: positive-sense (positive-strand), negative-sense (negative-strand), and ambisense RNA viruses. The terms *sense* and *strand* are used interchangeably.

- Genomes of **positive-sense RNA** viruses act as messenger RNA (mRNA) and can be directly translated once the virus invades the host cell.

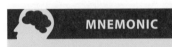

**MNEMONIC**

***Naked DNA viruses—***

A woman needs to be naked for a **PAP** smear.

**P**arvovirus
**A**denovirus
**P**apovavirus (**P**apilloma/**P**olyoma)

**MNEMONIC**

***Nonenveloped RNA viruses—***

**A** virus needs to be nonenveloped for **A PCR** reaction.

**A**strovirus
**P**icornavirus
**C**alicivirus
**R**eovirus

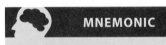

**MNEMONIC**

***For DNA viruses—***

Think **HHAPPPP**y

**H**erpes
**H**epadna
**A**deno
**P**apilloma
**P**olyoma
**P**arvo
**P**ox

**MNEMONIC**

All RNA viruses are single-stranded, except for the one that **RE**peats strands. **RE**ovirus = **RE**peat-o-virus.

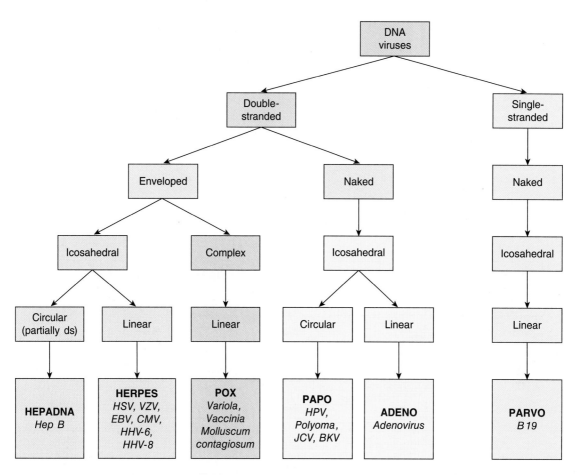

**FIGURE 4-72.** **Flowchart of DNA viruses.** Each family is categorized by the type of viral genome and capsid shape. Important examples of each viral family are highlighted.

- **Negative-sense RNA** viruses carry their own **RNA-dependent RNA polymerase** and make a positive-sense copy once the virus infects the host cell. The copy is then used as both a genomic template and as mRNA for protein synthesis.
- The genomes of **ambisense RNA** viruses have portions that are both positive- and negative-sense.
- **Segmented viral genomes** are seen mostly in human RNA viruses. After replication, these viral genomes are cleaved into two or more smaller, physically separate segments of nucleic acid. When the virion attaches to and infects another cell, these segments reassemble noncovalently, and join to form a complete genome.

Because of the great number and diversity of the RNA viruses, they have fewer shared characteristics than the DNA viruses. However, they do share a few **common traits** (Table 4-24):

- Single-stranded genome—except for reoviruses, which have a double-stranded RNA genome.
- Replicate in the cytoplasm—except for orthomyxoviruses and retroviruses, both of which replicate at least partially in the nucleus.

## PATHOGENESIS

### General Considerations

Several key properties influence viral **pathogenesis** (the interaction of viral and host factors that lead to production of disease):

**KEY FACT**

RNA viruses have the ability to produce great genetic diversity, which is generated by both **mutation** and **reassortment.**

**MNEMONIC**

**Viruses with segmented genomes—**
**BOAR**

**B**unyaviruses: 3 segments
**O**rthomyxoviruses: 8 segments
**A**renaviruses: 2 segments
**R**eoviruses: 10 or 11 segments

**MNEMONIC**

**All RNA viruses divide in the cytoplasm—**

**OR not**
**O**rthomyxovirus
**R**etrovirus

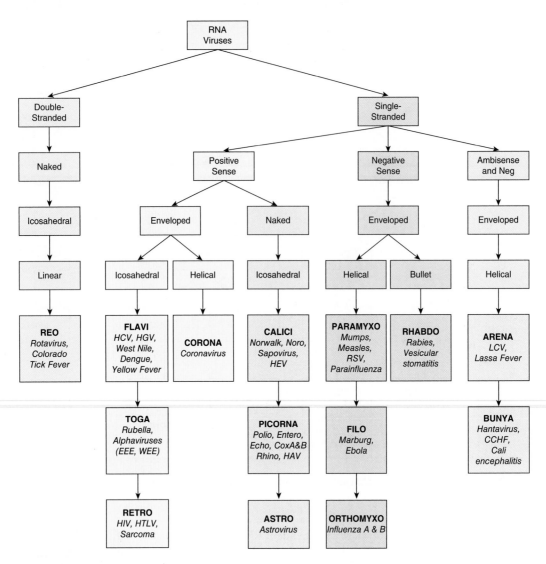

**FIGURE 4-73.** **Flowchart of RNA viruses.** Each family is categorized by the type of viral genome and capsid shape. Important examples of each viral family are highlighted.

■ **Virulence:** Ability of the virus to cause disease by avoiding or otherwise overcoming the host's defense mechanisms and by damaging host cells or causing them to malfunction.

■ **Cellular tropism:** The specificity of a virus for a given host cell or host tissue, determined by surface receptors and intracellular content within the host cell. Infection

**TABLE 4-24.** **Common Traits of RNA Viruses**

| TRAIT | SINGLE-STRANDED; REPLICATE IN CYTOPLASM, EXCEPT AS NOTED |
|---|---|
| Positive sense | Picornaviridae, Flaviviridae, Togaviridae, Calicivirus, Coronaviridae, Retroviridae |
| Negative sense | Paramyxoviridae, Filoviridae, Orthomyxoviridae, Rhabdoviridae |
| Ambisense | Arenaviridae, Bunyaviridae |
| Replicate in nucleus | Orthomyxoviridae, Retroviridae |
| Double-stranded genome | Reoviridae |

by a certain virus tends to affect a specific organ or group of organs (**target organs**), causing the typical symptoms for that particular virus.

- **Host range:** Range of cells (or species) that can become a host to a virus or bacteriophage; dictated by the presence or absence of specific receptors that enable active viral infection.

## Infection

To produce a disease, viruses must enter the host, interact with susceptible cells or tissues, replicate, and produce cell injury. Humans are infected with viruses by the same basic mechanisms that allow the spread of other microorganisms. Common **modes of transmission** include:

- Direct contact with bodily fluids or an infected source.
- Vertical transmission (transplacental—mother to child).
- Direct inoculation through injections or trauma; organ transplant.
- **Vectors,** such as insects and small rodents. Humans can become infected through bites of vector species or inhalation of viral particles from the vector's hair, fur, or bodily fluids.
  - **Arthropod-borne viruses—arboviruses:** Mainly belong to four families of viruses—Flaviviridae, Togaviridae, Bunyaviridae, and Reoviridae. The most common arthropod vectors are mosquitoes and ticks. Classic examples of arboviruses include dengue or "break-bone" fever and yellow fever (both flaviviruses).
  - **Rodent-borne viruses—roboviruses:** Belong to the Arenaviridae and Bunyaviridae families. These viruses are generally transmitted by rats and mice. Perhaps the most well known examples are lymphocytic choriomeningitis virus (LCMV), hantavirus, and Lassa fever, all arenaviruses.

**Reinfection:** Secondary infection that occurs after recovery from a previous infection and is caused by the same agent.

**Coinfection:** Concurrent infection of a host (single cell/tissue) by two or more viruses.

**Superinfection:** Process by which a host previously infected by one virus acquires coinfection with another virus at a later point in time (eg, HIV superinfection). Superinfection can also be caused by other microorganisms owing to the host's compromised immune system or the microorganisms' resistance to previous antibiotics (eg, *C difficile* infection after broad-spectrum antibiotic use).

## Replication

As obligate intracellular parasites, viruses must infect host cells in order to replicate. This process involves several sequential steps:

- **Attachment to host cell:** Binding of viruses to host cells is mediated through the interaction of viral surface proteins with specific and nonspecific host cell surfaces.
- **Penetration and entry:**
  - Most nonenveloped viruses enter host cells through **receptor-mediated endocytosis.**
  - **Viropexis:** Upon attachment to the host cell surface, hydrophobic (lipophilic) structures of certain naked viruses' capsid proteins are exposed, thus enabling them to directly penetrate the host cell.
  - **Enveloped viruses** enter host cells by **fusing** with the cell membrane, thus allowing the nucleocapsid or the viral genome to be delivered directly into the cytoplasm.
  - The fusion activity can be mediated by **VAPs,** fusion proteins, or other glycoproteins found in the viral membrane.
  - Optimal fusion pH is specific to each type of virus.

**KEY FACT**

The virulence level of a virus is variable and genetically determined by both virus and host.

**KEY FACT**

Cell tropism determines the target organ of each virus.

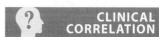

**CLINICAL CORRELATION**

**ARBO**virus = **AR**thropod-**BO**rne virus, including some members of **F**lavivirus, **T**ogavirus, and **B**unyavirus, ie, **F**ever **T**ransmitted by **B**ites.

**KEY FACT**

**Enveloped viruses** mediate host cell attachment through their glycoproteins **VAPs.**
**Nonenveloped viruses** use **capsid surface proteins** to attach to host cells (receptor-mediated endocytosis).

- If the optimal pH is neutral, the enveloped virus can fuse with the outer cell membrane.
- If the optimal pH is acidic, the virus must first be internalized by endocytosis and fuse with the endosomal membrane at low pH.
- **Uncoating of the virion:** Once a virus is internalized, the nucleocapsid must be brought to the site of replication and removed. Uncoating of a virion results in the loss of infectivity.

### Replication of DNA Viruses

DNA viruses (except for poxviruses) enter the nucleus and utilize the host cell's DNA-dependent RNA polymerase to transcribe its mRNA from the negative-strand template. There is a specific **temporal pattern of transcription:** immediate early, delayed early, and late mRNA transcripts.

Key steps in DNA virus replication (Figure 4-74A):

- mRNA transcripts undergo modification: Addition of a poly A tail and methylated cap takes place in the host cell's **nucleus.**
- Transcripts then are transported to the **cytoplasm** and translated on cytoplasmic polysomes.
- Newly synthesized proteins are then transported **back** to the nucleus, where the capsid is assembled and the viral genome and enzymes are packaged before the virus is released.

Genomic replication is performed by a **DNA-dependent DNA polymerase. HBV** is a **unique DNA virus** because the genome is partially double-stranded with single-stranded regions scattered throughout. Before it can be delivered to the nucleus and replicate, this virus must first generate a fully double-stranded genome. HBV carries an **RNA-dependent DNA polymerase** with reverse transcriptase properties that uses an RNA template to synthesize the DNA.

### Replication of RNA Viruses

Both replication and transcription of RNA viruses (except for orthomyxoviruses and retroviruses) occur **in the cytoplasm** (Figure 4-74B). This is possible because RNA viruses encode for their own **RNA-dependent DNA polymerases (replicases** and **transcriptases).**

Negative-sense RNA viruses carry these enzymes in their capsids. The genomes of positive-sense RNA viruses can serve as mRNA. Once inside the host cell, the genome can be directly translated to synthesize proteins (Table 4-25).

### Release of Newly Synthesized Viruses

The process of releasing newly synthesized viruses differs between nonenveloped and enveloped viruses:

- **Nonenveloped (naked) viruses** kill the host cell through cytolysis in order to be released; thus, they are unable to establish persistent productive infections because infected cells are lysed in the process.
- **Enveloped viruses** are released from infected host cells through a process referred to as "budding"; thus, the infected host cell survives and budding can lead to **cell senescence.** Budding involves synthesis of virally encoded glycoproteins within the host cell, which are temporarily anchored in the host cell's membrane. As the virus is released through the process of exocytosis, it is surrounded by the region of the cell membrane studded with glycoproteins, thus creating the viral envelope.

Once viruses are surrounded by the lipoprotein membrane and are released from the host cell, they are considered infective.

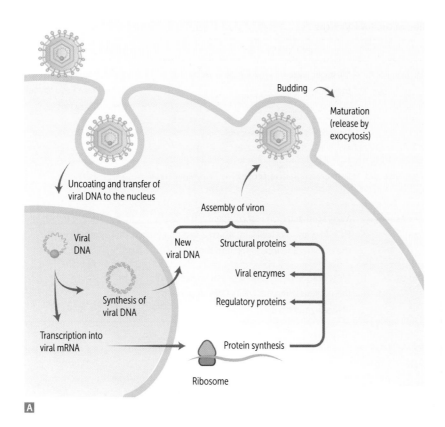

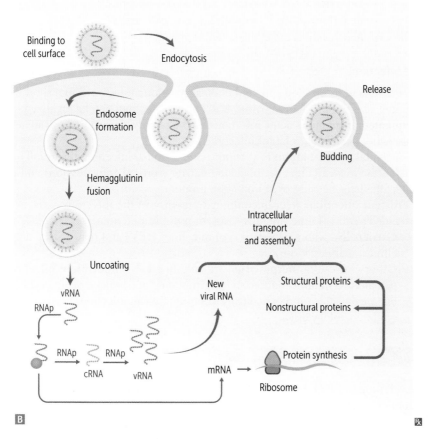

**FIGURE 4-74.** **Replicative cycles of DNA and RNA viruses.** The replicative cycles of DNA-encoded and RNA-encoded **B** viruses. mRNA, messenger RNA; vRNA, viral RNA; RNAp, RNA polymerase; cRNA, complementary RNA.

**TABLE 4-25.** Specifics of Genomic Replication of the RNA Viruses

| VIRUS | GENOME | REPLICATION PROCESS | ENZYMES |
|---|---|---|---|
| Negative-sense RNA viruses | Complementary to mRNA | Must generate positive-sense copy before translation | Carry RNA-dependent RNA polymerase used to make mRNA transcript |
| Positive-sense RNA viruses | Acts as mRNA transcript | Genome is directly translated | None |
| Ambisense RNA viruses | Some portions are positive-sense and others are negative-sense | Similar to negative-sense RNA virus replication | |
| Retroviruses | Positive-sense genome, but cannot be used as mRNA transcript | Must synthesize circular complementary DNA (cDNA) copy in cytoplasm, which is brought into the nucleus and integrated into the host's DNA | Carry reverse transcriptases that synthesize cDNA |
| Delta virus | Single-stranded RNA genome | Most unique replication process; replicates in the nucleus using host cell's DNA-dependent RNA polymerase II | None |

## CLINICAL CORRELATION

**HBV** can establish persistent productive infections; that is, infected cells produce virus by slowly spreading in a noncytolytic fashion, remaining morphologically intact over time.

## KEY FACT

Subclinical infections can stimulate an immune response and generate protective immunity from future or further infections.

## MNEMONIC

*Congenital infections—*
**TORCH**

**T**oxoplasmosis
**O**ther infections*
**R**ubella
**C**ytomegalovirus
**H**erpes simplex virus
*Other infections include syphilis, parvovirus B19, hepatitis B, virus, HIV, and varicella-zoster virus.

## KEY FACT

Persistent infection = recurring disease with cycles of symptomatic outbreaks and silent periods.

## Patterns of Infections

### Subclinical Infections

Subclinical infections are either asymptomatic or cause a less severe, nonspecific illness that may not be recognized or identified as the result of a specific virus.

- The virus inoculum is small, or only a few host cells are infected.
- The virus may reach its target tissue, but replication is curtailed.

### Acute Infections

- Acute infections develop apparent clinical symptomatology within a short period of time after the incubation period of the virus. Infections can be **localized** or **disseminated.** In addition, acute infections can be **rapidly cleared** or they can develop into either **persistent** or **latent** infections.
- **Congenital malformations** result from acute maternal infections that result in viremia. The virus can cross the placental barrier (**vertical transmission**) and easily infect the fetus because of its immature immune system.
- **Persistent infections** refer to continued presence of the infectious virus over an extended period of time (months, years, or possibly a lifetime).
  - **Carriers** live with a persistent viral infection (HBV) and may or may not have clinical manifestations.
  - Other viruses (eg, **herpesvirus**) are able to establish persistent infections in patients in a noninfectious form (no symptoms, viral antigen or viral cytopathology are detected) and periodically reactivate into an infectious form (full-blown symptomatology/disease).

## VIRAL GENETICS

Viral variations and alterations that lead to new strains can result from a number of different processes:

- Changes directly affecting the genome: **Genetic reassortment** (resulting in **genetic shift**) and **genetic drift** (resulting in **antigenic drift**).

- Strictly phenotypic changes that do not modify viral genomes: **Complementation, phenotypic mixing,** and **phenotypic masking.**

Many of these processes occur when a single cell is infected by multiple strains of a virus or by multiple viruses.

### Genetic Reassortment (Genetic Shift)

When two strains of a segmented virus infect the same cell, respective segments can intermingle in the cytoplasm during replication.

- As viral particles undergo assembly, the segmented genomes from the respective strains can trade segments during replication, thus creating a new (progeny) strain with a genome containing sequences from both (parental) strains.
    - Recombination can also occur between genes within the same segment. In general, the recombination frequency between genetic loci increases as the distance between the loci increases.
    - Changes in the **genome** resulting from genetic reassortment are referred to as **genetic shift.**
    - Genetic shift alters the antigenic properties of the affected viruses; hence, the term **antigenic shift** (Figure 4-75). This creates phenotypic variation; for example, novel surface proteins may allow viruses to infect previously resistant hosts, gain increased virulence, or allow immune escape (antigenic).
- Generated changes in the genome are drastic, yet may be positively selected, thus providing a source for major viral outbreaks, epidemics, or pandemics.
- A prototypic example of a virus with an ability to produce great genetic diversity via genetic reassortment is **influenza A** virus. This ability is secondary to its wide host range (Figure 4-76). Influenza B and C viruses do not exhibit antigenic shift because few related viruses exist in animals.

### Genetic (Antigenic) Drift

Genetic drift comprises the spontaneous mutations in viral genomes that create slight antigenic changes, which may or may not alter the virulence of the virus (Figure 4-75).

It is **most notable in RNA viruses,** especially in **HIV** and **orthomyxoviruses,** because their replication processes are error-prone.

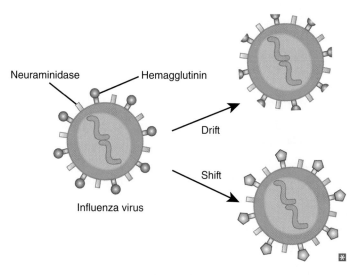

**FIGURE 4-75.    Antigenic shift and antigenic drift.** Antigenic shift generates viruses with entirely novel antigens (develops within a short period of time; source for epidemics/pandemics), whereas antigenic drift creates influenza viruses with moderately modified antigens (develops over years).

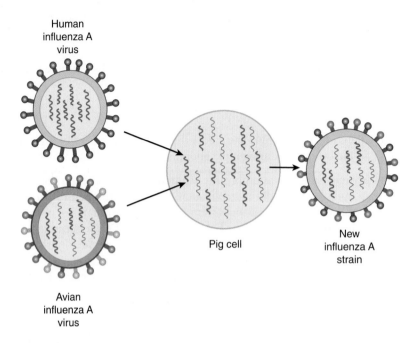

**FIGURE 4-76.** **New influenza A strain generated via genetic reassortment of human and avian strains of the virus.**

### Complementation

A defective mutant strain of a virus may be missing a gene encoding an enzyme or factor necessary for replication. Complementation refers to the **rescue** of such a mutant via **co-replication** with **another mutant** or cell line that expresses the missing protein (eg, hepatitis D depends on HBV, and its HBsAg envelope protein, in order to replicate).

- The newly established (**rescued**) genome, though still defective, is able to replicate and form progeny.
- The progeny derived from the original (**mutant**) genome still lack the same gene and are not able to replicate unless they, too, are rescued.

### Phenotypic Mixing

When two related, yet **antigenically distinct** viruses infect a **single host cell,** their proteins can mingle. Capsid proteins can merge during the assembly process, resulting in a capsid composed of a mixture of structural and surface proteins from both strains. The **genomes** remain **unchanged,** but the **capsids** are **hybrids** of the two strains, which may then alter the host range or develop resistance to antibody neutralization (Figure 4-77).

### Phenotypic Masking (Transcapsidation)

Similar to phenotypic mixing, phenotypic masking occurs when a **single** host cell is infected with **two related viral strains.**

- The genome of one strain is packaged in the capsid of the other.
- **Unlike** phenotypic mixing, the capsid is completely composed of proteins encoded by one strain.
- Phenotypic masking can occur with two completely different types of viruses and can result in what is called "**pseudotypes.**"

### Viral Vectors

With the use of recombinant DNA technology, viruses can be manipulated to serve as vectors, which deliver foreign genes into human cells. Viral vectors can be used to transfer DNA for gene therapy, as vaccines, and as killers that target specific tumor cells.

**KEY FACT**

The risk of reversion is one of the reasons why the killed (Salk) polio vaccine is preferentially used over the live, oral (Sabin) polio vaccine in the United States.

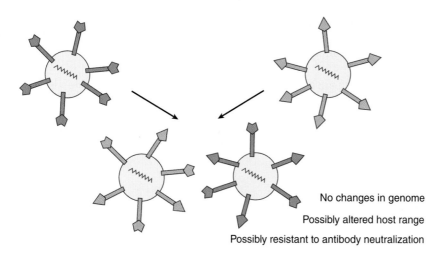

No changes in genome

Possibly altered host range

Possibly resistant to antibody neutralization

FIGURE 4-77. **Phenotypic mixing.**

**Defective viruses** are usually used as vectors because they cannot replicate, but they can infect and deliver genetic material into a targeted cell.

## VACCINES

Active immunization with virus vaccines exposes patients to a virus or its antigenic proteins, thus inducing an immune response that may protect from subsequent infection (protection immunity).

### Live Virus Vaccines

Live vaccines incorporate **attenuated** viral strains that are relatively nonvirulent. These viral vaccines are effective against enveloped viruses, which require a cell-mediated immune response to clear the infection.

- The **immune response** to a live virus vaccine mimics natural infection by generating $T_H1$ and $T_H2$ responses, thus stimulating both humoral and cell-mediated antibody immunity.
- **Routes of administration** can be parenteral, oral, or by inhalation to mimic the natural route of infection.
- **Immunity** derived from a live virus vaccine is long-lasting; thus, "boosters" are generally not needed. Notable exceptions include measles and chickenpox.

Immunization with a live virus vaccine carries a greater risk than vaccination using an inactivated virus. Live virus vaccines carry the **potential to revert** to a virulent form of the virus and may actually cause disease. Measles, mumps, and rubella (MMR) is the **only** live-attenuated vaccine that can be given to HIV-positive patients, although there is currently a move to allow them to receive others.

### Inactivated Vaccines

Inactivated vaccines contain either killed (inactivated) virus or viral subunits. Once an inactivated vaccine is injected into the patient, the body mounts a response to the immunogenic surface antigens found on the viral capsid or envelope.

- The **immune response:**
  - Predominantly a $T_H2$ (antibody) response, generating IgG that neutralizes and opsonizes the inactive virus.
  - Local secretory IgA response is not sufficient.
  - There is not a strong cell-mediated response.

**KEY FACT**

Pregnant women and other immunocompromised patients should not receive live virus vaccines.

**MNEMONIC**

*Live virus vaccines—*
**MMR PARVVY**

**M**easles
**M**umps
**R**ubella
**P**olio
**A**denovirus
**R**otavirus
**V**ariola
**V**ZV
**Y**ellow fever

**QUESTION**

A patient states that she received the influenza vaccine two years ago. Does she need to be re-vaccinated this year? What viral genetic process is at work?

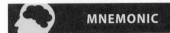
- **Routes of application:** Generally parenteral.
- **Immunity:** Not as long lasting as with live vaccines; **boosters** are usually required to maintain immunity.

Killed virus vaccines are generally very safe. However, they can stimulate a hypersensitivity reaction in some people.

Advantages and disadvantages of the respective types of vaccines are depicted in Table 4-26.

### Recombinant Vaccines

Recombinant vaccines utilize bacteria or yeast to generate a large amount of a single protein, which is then purified and injected into the patient. Two recombinant vaccines widely used in the clinical setting are:

- **HBV** vaccine (containing the viral envelope protein known as recombinant hepatitis B surface antigen [HBsAg]).
- **Human papillomavirus (HPV)** vaccine (2vHPV) protects against types 16 and 18, associated with cervical cancer; 4-valent HPV vaccine (4vHPV) protects against types 16, 18, as well as types 6 and 11, associated with genital warts; 9-valent vaccine (9vHPV) protects against types 6, 11, 16, 18, 31, 33, 45, 52, and 58.

### DIAGNOSTIC TESTS

Although the history and clinical signs and symptoms are often used to diagnose many viral illnesses, collected specimens can be used in the laboratory to confirm or to diagnose atypical or unusual cases. Most commonly used tests are described below.

- **Cytology** is a rapid detection method. Direct microscopic examination of collected specimens or monolayer cell culture samples is used to detect viruses.
- **Viral culture with examination for cytopathic effects (CPE):** Viruses can also be characterized and identified by the type of cells they infect, the rate of viral growth, and specific patterns of cellular changes caused by infection (Figure 4-78).
  - **Syncytia** (multinucleated giant cells) form when individual infected cells fuse together. They are often observed with **HSV, paramyxoviruses,** and **VZV.**
  - **Inclusion bodies** can also be seen in the cytoplasm or nucleus of infected cells.
- **Detection of viral genetic material:** Northern and Southern blot analyses, restriction endonuclease fragment lengths, **genetic probes,** and **PCR** can all be used to detect viral genetic material. This has become the most common approach to viral diagnosis in recent years.

**TABLE 4-26.** **Comparison of Advantages and Disadvantages of Live and Killed/Inactivated Vaccines**

|  | LIVE | KILLED/INACTIVATED |
|---|---|---|
| Immunity duration | Long-lasting | Short-term |
| Doses | Single | Multiple (boosters) |
| Antibody response | IgG, IgA | IgG |
| Cell-mediated response | Good | Poor |
| Side effects | Mild symptoms | Soreness around injection site |
| Temperature-sensitive | Yes | No |
| Reversion to virulence | Possible | Never |

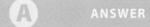

- **Detection of viral proteins:** Immunohistochemistry is used to detect and quantify viruses or their antigens in clinical specimens or culture samples. **Immunofluorescence, ELISA,** radioimmunoassay (**RIA**), and latex agglutination (**LA**) tests are commonly used methods.
- **Serologic tests:** Virus-specific antibodies may be detected, identified, and quantified in blood or serum samples.
  - **Seroconversion** indicates current infection and is determined by observing at least a fourfold increase in the antibody titer between serum collected during the acute and convalescent phases of an infection.
  - Virus-specific **IgM**—usually present during the first 2–3 weeks of a **primary infection.**
  - High titers of **IgG** are usually detected a few weeks after infection; they may be detected earlier in a **reinfection.**
  - In patients who experience frequent recurrence of disease, antibody titers tend to remain high.

## DNA VIRUSES

All viruses have a protein capsid. The capsid of all known DNA viruses is either icosahedral or complex. In addition to their capsid, some DNA viruses also have an outer phospholipid envelope. DNA viral genomes are either single-stranded or double-stranded and can be linear or circular (Table 4-27).

### Herpesvirus Family

#### General Characteristics

Herpesviruses are unique in that they are assembled in the nucleus and are the only viruses whose envelopes are derived from the **nuclear** membrane. Because they are assembled in the nucleus, infected cells can often be identified histologically by the presence of **intranuclear inclusion bodies** (see Figure 4-78). Infections may also become **latent.**

#### Herpes Simplex Virus 1 (HSV-1)

#### Characteristics

Common; prevalence ranges from 65–90% worldwide. HSV-1 is also the **most common cause of sporadic encephalitis** in the United States.

#### Pathogenesis

Transmitted by respiratory secretions or saliva. The virus invades mucous membranes and can cause a local infection. HSV may also invade nearby sensory nerve endings; it is then transported back to the cell body and becomes latent.

#### Clinical Symptoms

Most infections are **asymptomatic.** Initial symptoms may include vesicular ulcerating lesions of the mouth and gums (**gingivostomatitis**) or eye (**keratoconjunctivitis**). HSV can also infect the hand, causing a vesicular lesion called **herpetic whitlow** (Figure 4-79). HSV-1 may become latent in the **trigeminal** ganglia and can be reactivated under conditions of stress. Reactivation can result in recurring gingivostomatitis, keratoconjunctivitis, or **herpes labialis** (cold sores or fever blisters, Figure 4-79). Recurrent keratoconjunctivitis may lead to blindness. In some cases, the virus can be transported into the brain (via cranial nerves), where it characteristically infects the temporal lobe. Symptoms of **temporal lobe encephalitis** include fever, headache, neck stiffness, and **olfactory hallucinations.** Permanent neurologic damage or death may ensue. Diagnosis of HSV encephalitis can be made by **PCR** of the CSF. Diagnosis of cutaneous lesions can be made by PCR of the lesion or by direct fluorescent antibody (DFA) test, dem-

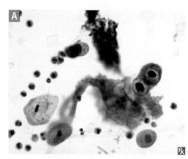
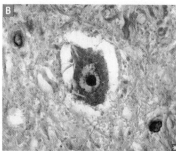
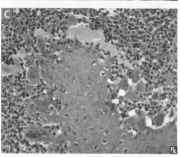

**FIGURE 4-78. Cytopathic effects of viruses.** A Urine sediment epithelial cells with "owl's eye" inclusions indicative of cytomegalovirus infection. B Negri body associated with rabies virus infection. C Multinucleated cells (syncytia) with intranuclear inclusions characteristic of HSV infection.

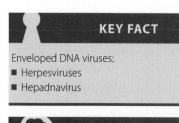

**KEY FACT**

Enveloped DNA viruses:
- Herpesviruses
- Hepadnavirus

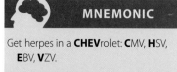

**MNEMONIC**

Get herpes in a **CHEV**rolet: **C**MV, **H**SV, **E**BV, **V**ZV.

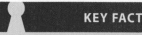

**KEY FACT**

HSV-1 above the waist; HSV-2 below. (However, the reverse may be true in up to one-third of cases.)

**TABLE 4-27.** **Summary of DNA Viruses**

| FAMILY | STRUCTURE | DISEASE | ROUTE OF TRANSMISSION | IMPORTANT FACTS |
|---|---|---|---|---|
| **Herpesviridae** | | | | |
| Herpes simplex virus (HSV) | dsDNA, enveloped, icosahedral, linear | Cold sores (usually HSV-1), genital herpes (usually HSV-2), encephalitis (often with characteristic necrosis of the temporal lobes) | Mucous membranes, breaks in skin, sex | Most commonly diagnosed cause of acute sporadic encephalitis in the US. |
| Varicella-zoster virus (VZV) | dsDNA, enveloped, icosahedral, linear | Chickenpox, shingles (herpes zoster), pneumonia | Airborne, close contact | Remains latent in sensory nerve ganglia throughout the body after infection. |
| Epstein-Barr virus (EBV) | dsDNA, enveloped, icosahedral, linear | Fever, pharyngitis, lymphadenopathy (heterophile-positive mononucleosis), encephalitis | Airborne, close contact, mucous membranes | Associated with malignancies, (eg, Burkitt lymphoma, Hodgkin lymphoma, nasopharyngeal carcinoma, oral hairy-cell leukoplakia), post-transplant lymphoproliferative disease. |
| Cytomegalovirus (CMV) | dsDNA, enveloped, icosahedral, linear | Fever, pharyngitis, lymphadenopathy (heterophile-negative mononucleosis), infection in immunocompromised individuals (particularly transplant recipients), congenital abnormalities (TORCH) | Close contact (perinatal, venereal), transfusion, transplacental, organ transplantation | One of the TORCH pathogens; causes teratogenic symptoms in fetus. |
| Human herpesvirus 6 (HHV-6) | dsDNA, enveloped, icosahedral, linear | Fever, rash, adenopathy (cause of roseola or sixth disease), hepatitis | Saliva | 90% of all humans infected by age 3, usually benign course. |
| Human herpesvirus 8 (HHV-8) | dsDNA, enveloped, icosahedral, linear | Primary infection asymptomatic; causes Kaposi sarcoma in AIDS patients | Sexual and body fluids | Causes purpuric, raised skin lesions of Kaposi sarcoma. |
| **Hepadnaviridae** | | | | |
| Hepatitis B (HBV) | Partially dsDNA, ssDNA gap, enveloped, icosahedral, circular | Infectious hepatitis | Blood, blood products, sexual activity, shared needles | Cause of primary hepatocellular carcinoma, cirrhosis, hepatitis. |
| **Adenoviridae** | | | | |
| Adenovirus | dsDNA, naked, icosahedral, linear | Pharyngitis/pneumonia, conjunctivitis, gastroenteritis, acute hemorrhagic cystitis (children) | Fecal-oral, aerosol, close contact | 51 known serotypes of human adenoviruses. |
| **Parvoviridae** | | | | |
| Parvovirus B19 | ssDNA, naked, icosahedral, linear | Erythema infectiosum (fifth disease), aplastic anemia, hydrops fetalis | Respiratory droplets, oral secretions, parenterally | The only parvovirus known to cause human disease. |

**TABLE 4-27.    Summary of DNA Viruses** *(continued)*

| FAMILY | STRUCTURE | DISEASE | ROUTE OF TRANSMISSION | IMPORTANT FACTS |
|---|---|---|---|---|
| **Papillomaviridae** | | | | |
| Human papillomavirus (HPV) | dsDNA, naked, icosahedral, circular | Cervical or vaginal intraepithelial neoplasia (CIN/VIN), cervical carcinoma and anogenital cancers (mostly types 16, 18, but others as well); genital warts/condylomata (types 6, 11) | Sex, contact | Highly restricted in tissue tropism and replicates only in epithelial cells. Many serotypes. |
| **Polyomaviridae** | | | | |
| Polyomavirus | dsDNA, naked, icosahedral, circular | Causes no disease in humans | Sex, contact | Causes no human malignancy. |
| JC virus | dsDNA, naked, icosahedral, circular | Progressive multifocal leukoencephalopathy (PML) | Sex, contact | Fatal disorder of CNS that can occur in immunodeficient patients. |
| BK virus | dsDNA, naked, icosahedral, circular | Hemorrhagic cystitis, ureteral stenosis, and urinary tract infections | Sex, contact | Oncogenic in animal models, not in humans. Important cause of renal disease and graft failure in transplant recipients. |
| **Poxviridae** | | | | |
| Variola | dsDNA, enveloped, complex, linear | Smallpox | Respiratory droplets or close contact | Lesions develop at the same pace; therefore are all at the same stage of development. Currently eradicated in the wild; high mortality in the pre-vaccine era. |
| Vaccinia | dsDNA, enveloped, complex, linear | Cowpox "milkmaid's blisters" | Contact | Used to make smallpox vaccine. |
| Molluscum contagiosum | dsDNA, enveloped, complex, linear | Small, spontaneously regressing, umbilicated, flesh-colored skin lesions | Contact | Common among wrestlers; patients with HIV. |

ds, double-stranded; ss, single-stranded; TORCH, toxoplasmosis, other (eg, syphilis), rubella, cytomegalovirus, herpes simplex.

onstration of multinucleate giant cells on a **Tzanck** smear of an opened skin vesicle, or by the presence of intranuclear Cowdry A inclusion bodies on skin **biopsy.**

### Treatment

Acyclovir to decrease the duration of active infection or prevent recurrence (not curative). Valacyclovir and famciclovir are also used and have increased bioavailability, allowing less frequent dosing. All three function by inhibiting viral DNA replication.

### Herpes Simplex Virus 2 (HSV-2)

### Characteristics

Less widespread than HSV-1, but still a common infection; approximately one in six adults between the ages of 14 and 49 are seropositive. HSV is one of the **TORCH** infections!

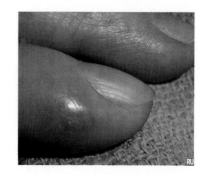

**FIGURE 4-79.    Herpetic whitlow.** Painful, grouped, confluent vesicles on an erythematous edematous base on the finger.

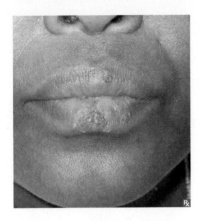

**FIGURE 4-80. Herpes labialis due to HSV-1 infection.** Connective tissue erosion of the lip with scalloped border and vesicles on an erythematous base.

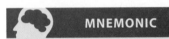

**MNEMONIC**

**Tzanck** goodness if you don't have herpes!

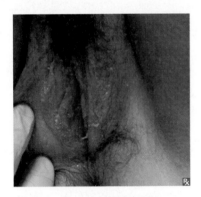

**FIGURE 4-81. Multiple genital lesions due to HSV-2 infection.**

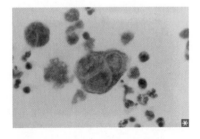

**FIGURE 4-82. Tzanck smear.** Multinucleated giant cell (Tzanck cell) from ulcerated penile tissue of a herpes infection.

### Pathogenesis

Transmitted by sexual contact or perinatally. Like HSV-1, HSV-2 invades mucous membranes and can cause a local infection (Figure 4-81). It may also invade nearby sensory nerve endings, where it is then transported back to the cell body and can become latent.

### Clinical Symptoms

Most infections are **asymptomatic.** Initial symptoms may include vesicular ulcerating lesions of the genitals and perianal area. Like HSV-1, HSV-2 can also cause **herpetic whitlow** (Figure 4-79). HSV-2 may become latent in the **lumbosacral** ganglia and can be reactivated under conditions of stress, resulting in recurring genital lesions. **Neonatal HSV** can occur via transplacental transmission (TORCH) or during delivery. Infection may be local (mouth, eyes, skin), may affect multiple organs and cause congenital defects, or result in spontaneous abortion. HSV-2 can also cause **neonatal encephalitis.** Diagnosis of cutaneous lesions can be made by PCR or DFA test, by demonstration of multinucleate giant cells on a **Tzanck** smear (Figure 4-82), or by visualization of intranuclear inclusion bodies on skin **biopsy.**

### Treatment

Acyclovir to decrease the duration of active infection or prevent recurrence (not curative). **Cesarean section** is indicated for mothers with active lesions in the birth canal or prodromal symptoms (fever, pruritus, paresthesias).

## Varicella-Zoster Virus (VZV, Chickenpox, Zoster, Shingles)

### Characteristics

Highly contagious. More commonly occurs in the winter and early spring, with the highest prevalence rate in children aged 4–10 years (uncommon in preschoolers).

### Pathogenesis

Transmitted by respiratory secretions or contact with active lesions. Like HSV, VZV also causes local infection and can invade sensory nerve endings, where it is then transported back to the cell body and can become latent.

### Clinical Symptoms

- In **children,** VZV typically causes a mild, flulike illness with characteristic skin lesions (**varicella** or **chickenpox).**
- Often described as "**dew drops on a rose petal,**" these lesions appear initially as discrete papules on a macular erythematous base (Figure 4-83). The papules then vesiculate, become pustules, and eventually rupture and release additional virus particles before crusting over. However, children can remain infectious through respiratory contact for up to 10 days after crusting occurs.
- Lesions tend to spread distally from the trunk and are characteristically **asynchronous** (ie, multiple lesions observed at different stages of evolution).
- Infection is usually self-limited and resolves after a few weeks. In **adults,** primary infection can be much more severe and lead to **pneumonia** and **encephalitis.**
- **Reactivation** of latent VZV (**herpes zoster** or **shingles**) can also occur under conditions of stress.
- Zoster is often characterized by extremely **painful** vesicular lesions in a **unilateral dermatomal** distribution (due to reactivation of latent VZV in a single sensory nerve). It can also manifest in the ophthalmic division of the trigeminal nerve (herpes zoster ophthalmicus) and as a facial neuropathy (Ramsay Hunt syndrome). In **immunocompromised** patients, both primary and reactivated VZV infections are much more severe. Post-herpetic neuralgia after reactivation of latent VZV can last for months.

- Diagnosis of cutaneous lesions can be made by DFA test, demonstration of multinucleate giant cells on a **Tzanck** smear, or by the presence of intranuclear inclusion bodies on skin **biopsy.**

### Treatment

Usually supportive. In severe cases, acyclovir can be given. In immunocompromised patients, anti-VZV Ig (VZIG) can be given intravenously. **Reye syndrome** has often been associated with the use of aspirin to treat chickenpox in children. There are two **VZV vaccines**—one for children to prevent chickenpox and one for adults to prevent shingles. Long-term efficacy has not been proven with regard to decreasing zoster incidence, but its use in the pediatric population is widely accepted.

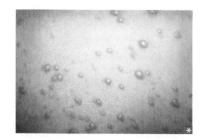

**FIGURE 4-83. Varicella-zoster virus (VZV) lesions.** VZV lesions are characterized by multiple papules and vesicles on an erythematous base.

### Epstein-Barr Virus (EBV, Infectious Mononucleosis)

### Characteristics

Symptomatic infections typically affect teenagers and young adults.

### Pathogenesis

Transmitted by saliva and respiratory secretions. EBV binds to CD21 on B cells. Selective transformation causes B cells to proliferate abnormally. The host's response to these infected B cells results in the clinical presentation.

### Clinical Symptoms

EBV can cause **infectious mononucleosis (kissing disease),** which presents with **flulike** symptoms, profound **fatigue,** painful **pharyngitis, lymphadenopathy** (characteristically occurring in the posterior cervical nodes), and **hepatosplenomegaly.** Peak incidence is at 15–20 years of age, consistent with the term *kissing disease* to describe disease transmission through the saliva. Patients are at risk for splenic rupture and should avoid contact sports. Infection is usually self-limited. In immunocompromised patients, sustained B-cell proliferation may result in mutations that predispose to future neoplasms **(Burkitt lymphoma** [Figure 4-84] and **nasopharyngeal cancers).**

### Diagnosis

- Presence of **atypical T lymphocytes** in the blood (cytotoxic T cells responding to the infection, not the proliferating B cells).
- Monospot test detects **heterophile antibodies** in the blood.
- Heterophile antibodies are produced during an active EBV infection and are able to agglutinate sheep RBCs. Both finding atypical lymphocytes and the heterophile antibody test are insensitive for acute EBV infection. IgM antibody to the EBV VCA antigen is useful in the acute phase; VCA IgG and EBNA antibodies arise after the acute phase of illness.

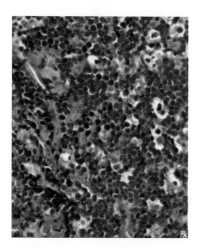

**FIGURE 4-84. Burkitt lymphoma.** Lymph node biopsy reveals numerous lymphoma cells with "starry sky" pattern.

### Treatment

Supportive.

### Cytomegalovirus (CMV)

### Characteristics

Common. Also can cause neonatal infection (one of the **TORCH** infections).

### Pathogenesis

Transmitted by close contact, body fluids, organ **transplantation,** and through the placenta. Infects many cell types.

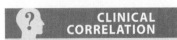
## Clinical Symptoms

Most infections are **asymptomatic** and become **latent.**

- Primary infections in **adults** can be similar to infectious mononucleosis, but do not result in the production of heterophile antibodies (**heterophile-** or **Monospot-negative mononucleosis**).
- In **newborns,** primary infection results in **cytomegalic inclusion disease.** Symptoms include microcephaly, hepatosplenomegaly, and CNS deficits.
- In **immunocompromised** patients, latent CMV can reactivate and cause severe infections such as retinitis, pneumonia, and esophagitis.
- Most common opportunistic viral colitis in HIV-positive patients.
- Diagnosis can be made with a tissue biopsy, based on the visualization of large cells with characteristic purple intranuclear inclusion bodies surrounded by a halo (**owl's eye inclusion bodies,** Figure 4-85). High EBV plasma viral load is associated with end-organ EBV disease and is often followed in transplant patients.

## Treatment

Ganciclovir (not acyclovir) and foscarnet (in the rare case of a ganciclovir-resistant virus).

## Human Herpesviruses 6 and 7 (HHV-6, HHV-7, Roseola)

### Characteristics

Affects infants or bone marrow transplant recipients (encephalitis). Route of transmission currently unknown.

### Pathogenesis

Infects B and T cells.

### Clinical Symptoms

Roseola (Figure 4-86) is characterized by a high fever for several days that can cause seizures, followed by the sudden appearance of a diffuse macular rash on the trunk.

### Treatment

Foscarnet for HHV-6 encephalitis. Roseola goes away on its own and is treated supportively.

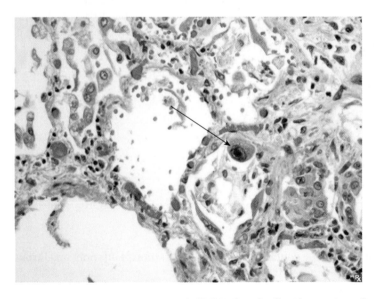

**FIGURE 4-85.** **Cytomegalovirus infection.** A CMV-infected cell with prominent "owl's eye" inclusion (*arrow*) is seen lining an alveolar space in an immunosuppressed patient with pneumonia.

Human Herpesvirus 8 (HHV-8, KSHV or Kaposi Sarcoma–Associated Herpesvirus)

### Characteristics

Affects patients with **HIV**, especially men. Transmitted via sexual contact.

### Pathogenesis

HHV-8 interacts with HIV to produce angioproliferative lesions.

### Clinical Symptoms

Kaposi sarcoma (KS) lesions can affect any organ, but are often seen as raised violaceous skin nodules containing extravasated RBCs (Figure 4-87).

### Treatment

Antiretroviral drugs can be effective by treating underlying HIV disease.

## Hepadnaviruses

### Hepatitis B Virus, HBV

### Characteristics

HBV has a complicated life cycle. After infecting host cells, the partial dsDNA genome is completed by viral DNA polymerase, thus becoming a fully double-stranded genome. Viral genes are then transcribed into mRNA. Viral mRNA is used both to make viral proteins **and** to regenerate the partially dsDNA viral genome through the action of a **viral RT.** Replicated genomic DNA and viral proteins are then repackaged into virion particles.

### Pathogenesis

Transmitted through blood (**transfusions**), sexual contact, and transplacentally (one of the **TOR<u>C</u>H** infections). Initial viremia leads to hepatocyte infection. A number of markers are used to track clinical course:

- **HBsAg** indicates either acute disease or a chronic carrier state.
- **Anti-HBsAg antibodies** indicate immunity to HBV, which can occur either through immunization or recovery from prior infection.
- **Hepatitis B core antigen (HBcAg)** and **anti-HBcAg antibodies.** Anti-HBcAg antibodies are positive during the equivalence zone or **window period** when HBsAg and anti-HBsAg are roughly equal in quantity, complex with each other, and thereby evade serologic detection. Thus, a positive HBcAb is often a helpful indicator of infection when the serologic profile is otherwise normal-appearing. One can also ascertain whether disease is recent (IgM HBcAb) or chronic (IgG). A positive HBcAb is the most reliable single marker of HBV infection.
- **Hepatitis B infectivity "e" antigen (HBeAg)** is an important indicator of active viral replication and both prognosis and transmissibility.

Conversely, the presence of **anti-HBeAg antibodies** indicates low transmissibility and better prognosis. **HBV PCR** is also used to measure viral load and monitor response.

Thus, depending on the serologic pattern observed, one can reliably interpret a patient's infectious status (Table 4-28). Laboratory tests are also helpful in differentiating viral from other causes of hepatitis. As a rule of thumb, alanine aminotransferase (ALT) is greater than aspartate aminotransferase (AST) in viral hepatitis (ALT > AST), but the reverse is true for alcoholic hepatitis (AST > ALT).

### Clinical Symptoms

Infection may be acute or chronic, depending on the host response. Infected hepatocytes can be killed by cytotoxic T cells; therefore, a robust immune response may result in a severe but acute course that ultimately clears the infection. A weaker immune response

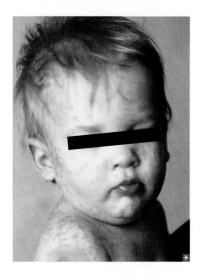

**FIGURE 4-86.** **Roseola.** Exanthem subitum (ie, "sudden rash"), otherwise known as sixth disease, or roseola, is typically caused by human herpesvirus 6 (HHV-6) infection and characterized by high fever followed by a blanching macular rash that appears one day after defervescence. Rash typically starts on neck and trunk and can spread to the face and extremities.

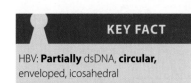

**KEY FACT**

HBV: **Partially** dsDNA, **circular,** enveloped, icosahedral

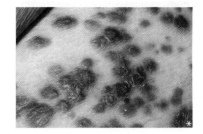

**FIGURE 4-87.** **Kaposi sarcoma of the skin.**

**TABLE 4-28.** **Serologic Patterns and Interpretation of HBV Infection**

|  | HBsAg | ANTI-HBS | HBeAg | ANTI-HBE | ANTI-HBc |
|---|---|---|---|---|---|
| Acute HBV | ✓ |  | ✓ |  | IgM |
| Window |  |  |  | ✓ | IgM |
| Chronic HBV (high infectivity) | ✓ |  | ✓ |  | IgG |
| Chronic HBV (low infectivity) | ✓ |  |  | ✓ | IgG |
| Recovery |  | ✓ |  | ✓ | IgG |
| Immunized |  | ✓ |  |  |  |

Reproduced with permission from Le T, et al. *First Aid for the USMLE Step 1 2016.* New York, NY: McGraw-Hill Education; 2016: 157.

results in a milder course, but the infection may not be cleared. Liver enzyme levels are elevated in both cases. Acute infection is characterized by **jaundice** and **fever** (Figure 4-88). Chronic infection may result in an asymptomatic **carrier** state. However, if a chronic inflammatory response is present, the host may develop **cirrhosis** or **hepatocellular carcinoma** (or both). A neonatal HBV infection presents as a high viral load with slightly elevated liver enzymes and carries a high risk of chronic infection.

### Treatment

Interferon alpha (INF-α), adefovir, tenofovir, lamivudine. There is also a recombinant HBV **vaccine** that contains HBsAg. Passive immunization with anti-HBsAg Ig is used in some cases (needlesticks and immediately after delivery of infants from infected mothers).

### Adenoviruses

#### Characteristics

One of the **most common causes of the common cold**; also causes nonpurulent conjunctivitis, pneumonia, gastroenteritis, and hemorrhagic cystitis (in children).

**MNEMONIC**

The common cold is **PRIMA**rily caused by:

**P**aramyxoviruses
**R**hinoviruses
**I**nfluenza viruses
**M**yxoviruses
**A**denoviruses

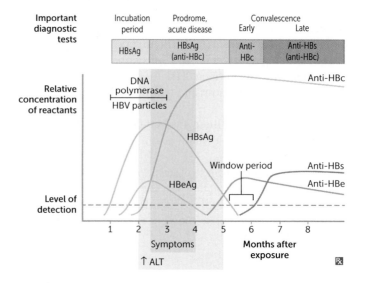

**FIGURE 4-88.** **Typical clinical and laboratory features of acute hepatitis B virus (HBV) infection.** ALT, alanine aminotransferase; HBc, hepatitis B core; HBeAg, hepatitis B infectivity "e" antigen; HBsAg, hepatitis B surface antigen.

### Pathogenesis

Transmitted via aerosolized droplets, contact, or fecal-oral route.

### Clinical Symptoms

There are over 40 serotypes, each of which has different manifestations, including rhinitis, pharyngitis, atypical pneumonia, conjunctivitis, hematuria, dysuria, and gastroenteritis with nonbloody diarrhea. Diagnosis can be confirmed by serology or viral cultures.

### Treatment

None.

## Parvoviruses

### Parvovirus B19

### Characteristics

This is the **smallest** clinically important virus, with a size of 20–25 nm. It is also one of the **five** most common pediatric viral exanthems (diseases that cause a **rash**).

### Pathogenesis

Transmitted via aerosolized droplets that inoculate the nasal cavity; infects erythroid progenitor cells.

### Clinical Symptoms

Immune complex deposition results in a lacy red rash (also called erythema infectiosum, fifth disease, or slapped-cheek fever) and arthralgias (Figure 4-89). Patients with hemolytic anemias such as thalassemia or sickle cell anemia may develop a **transient aplastic crisis.** Immunocompromised individuals may develop a **severe chronic anemia.** Infants may develop **hydrops fetalis** and severe anemia. Diagnosis can be confirmed with serology and complete blood count.

### Treatment

Supportive care with blood transfusions as needed. Immunocompromised patients may require IV immunoglobulins.

## Papillomaviruses

### Human Papillomavirus

### Characteristics

Human papillomavirus (HPV) infects squamous epithelial cells.

### Pathogenesis

Transmitted by close contact.

### Clinical Symptoms

Varies depending on the strain.

- HPV 6 and 11 cause benign warts, including anogenital and laryngeal warts (Figure 4-90).
- **HPV serotypes 16, 18, 31, 33, and 45 are associated with cervical cancer.**
- These strains produce two proteins that inactivate known tumor suppressor genes: **E6 inhibits *p*53; E7 inhibits *Rb*.**
- Diagnosis can be made by PCR, Papanicolaou (Pap) smear, and/or biopsy.

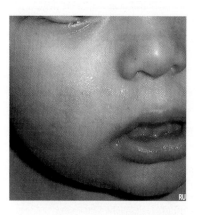

**FIGURE 4-89.** **Characteristic lacy red rash of parvovirus B19 infection, or fifth disease.**

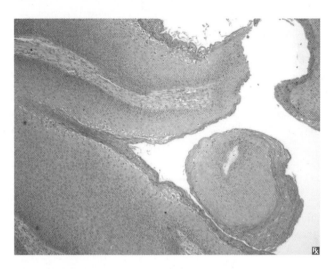

FIGURE 4-90. **Condyloma due to human papillomavirus (HPV).** Large warty projections of thickened epidermis with scale; note that infected cells have prominent haloes and are visible in the most superficial layers.

### Treatment

Most warts regress spontaneously after 1 or 2 years. Warts can also be ablated or surgically removed. With respect to cervical abnormalities, low-grade squamous intraepithelial lesions often regress and are monitored by regular Pap smears; higher-grade lesions are evaluated with a biopsy. Cervical cancer is managed according to stage (surgery or radiation, or both).

### Prevention

Vaccination (bivalent, for types 16,18; quadrivalent, for types 6, 11, 16, 18; or newest 9-valent, for types 6, 11, 16, 18, 31, 33, 45, 52, and 58), and barrier contraception.

## Polyomaviruses

BK and JC viruses

### Characteristics

Both BK and JC viruses are common in the general population; most people are asymptomatic carriers by the age of 18.

### Pathogenesis

Only cause clinical disease in immunocompromised individuals (eg, those with AIDS, chemotherapy, immunosuppressants).

### Clinical Symptoms

Reactivation of latent **JC virus** in immunocompromised individuals results in progressive multifocal leukoencephalopathy (**PML**). PML is a demyelinating, rapidly progressive, fatal disease that affects oligodendrocytes (ie, CNS) and is characterized by deficits in speech, coordination, and memory. Diagnosis is largely clinical, but can be confirmed by imaging (Figure 4-91) and PCR of the CSF. PML has also been linked to use of the monoclonal antibody natalizumab in multiple sclerosis, currently a "black box" warning. **BK virus** causes kidney disease and can be found in patients with solid organ (kidney) and bone marrow transplants.

### Treatment

Only treatment available is improving immune function, by reducing or stopping immunosuppressive drugs, or treating the underlying HIV/AIDS.

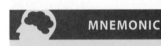

**ANSWER**

The patient's diagnosis is likely either EBV or CMV infection or possibly acute HIV. A Monospot test should be performed: positive indicates EBV infection; negative is inconclusive but points to a CMV or HIV infection. While CMV infections can be treated with ganciclovir or foscarnet, it is rarely necessary. Acute HIV infections can be diagnosed with 4th- and 5th-generation antigen-antibody tests or HIV RNA testing; treatment of HIV is discussed elsewhere.

**MNEMONIC**

**JC** virus affects the **C**erebrum.
B**K** virus affects the **K**idneys.

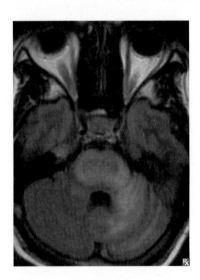

FIGURE 4-91. **Progressive multifocal leukoencephalopathy (PML).** MRI fluid-attenuated inversion recovery (FLAIR) image showing hyperintensities in the pons and left middle cerebellar peduncle.

## Poxvirus Family

Poxviruses are the **largest human viruses.** They are also the only viruses that **make their own envelope** and the only DNA viruses that replicate in the **cytoplasm.** Infected cells often have characteristic **cytoplasmic inclusion bodies** (in contrast to nuclear inclusion bodies in herpesvirus infections).

### Smallpox (Variola)

#### Pathogenesis

Transmitted as aerosolized droplets.

#### Clinical Symptoms

**Smallpox (variola)** is characterized by constitutional symptoms and a disseminated rash that is initially maculopapular, then forms vesicles, and later pustules (Figure 4-92). The rash begins on the face and extremities and spreads to the trunk (centripetal). Systemic illness results in a 10–30% mortality rate during the second week of symptoms.

#### Treatment

Supportive. The smallpox vaccine successfully eradicated smallpox infections in 1977. The vaccine contained an attenuated virus similar to smallpox **(vaccinia)** that served as the antigen. While there are only two known repositories of the virus worldwide (United States and Russia), there is concern that smallpox could be utilized as a bioterrorism agent in the future, given that populations are no longer widely vaccinated against the virus.

### Molluscum Contagiosum

#### Pathogenesis

Transmitted by physical contact.

#### Clinical Symptoms

Most often seen in children and immunocompromised patients and characterized by benign **umbilicated** papules on the skin that are small and flesh-colored (Figure 4-93). Infection is usually self-limited.

#### Treatment

None.

---

### POSITIVE (SINGLE)-STRANDED RNA VIRUSES—SS (+) RNA

#### General Characteristics

**All positive, single-stranded RNA viruses have an icosahedral capsid** with the exception of coronavirus, which has a helical capsid. RNA can either be enveloped or naked (exits host cells through budding or lysis, respectively; Table 4-29). Another helpful generalization that can be made is that **all positive single-stranded RNA viruses replicate in the cytoplasm** with the exception of HIV, which replicates in the nucleus (carries its own RNA-dependent DNA polymerase—RT).

### Hepevirus

#### Hepatitis E (Enteric Hepatitis)

##### Characteristics

Unique 30-nm hepatitis virus. It does not appear to cause chronic infection and is serologically distinct from hepatitis A virus (HAV). It is uncommon in the US, but endemic to Africa, southern Asia, and other parts of the world.

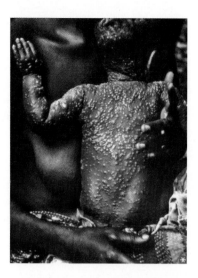

**FIGURE 4-92.** **Smallpox.** Multiple pustules can be seen on the back of this child. Note that all lesions are at the same stage of development.

**KEY FACT**

Poxviruses: dsDNA, linear, enveloped
- Large, complex viruses with a brick shape
- Includes smallpox (variola) and molluscum contagiosum

**MNEMONIC**

For the positive-sense RNA viruses, remember to **Cal/Pico** and **Fl**o **To Co**me **R**ight **A**way:

**Cal**iciviridae
**Pico**rnaviridae
**Fl**aviviridae
**To**gaviridae
**Co**ronavirus
**R**etro **A**stroviridae

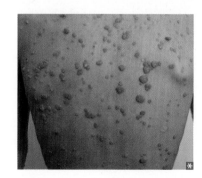

**FIGURE 4-93.** **Molluscum contagiosum.** Multiple translucent flesh-colored nodules of varying sizes with central umbilication.

**TABLE 4-29.**   **Positive-Stranded RNA Viruses**

| FAMILY | STRUCTURE | DISEASE | ROUTE OF TRANSMISSION | IMPORTANT FACTS |
|---|---|---|---|---|
| **Hepeviridae** | | | | |
| Hepatitis E (HEV) | Naked, icosahedral, nonsegmented, linear | Enteric hepatitis. | Fecal-oral. | Self-limiting disease (except in pregnant women, for whom there is a high mortality rate). |
| **Caliciviridae** | | | | |
| Norwalk and norovirus (Norwalk agent) | Naked, icosahedral, nonsegmented, linear | Epidemic adult gastroenteritis. | Fecal-oral. | Vomiting more frequent than diarrhea. |
| Sapovirus | Naked, icosahedral, nonsegmented, linear | Epidemic outbreaks of gastroenteritis. | Fecal-oral. | Associated with pediatric gastroenteritis. |
| **Picornaviridae** | | | | |
| Polioviruses | Naked, icosahedral | Abortive poliomyelitis, paralytic poliomyelitis (1%), aseptic meningitis. | Fecal-oral. | Immunization: natural infection confers lifelong immunity. |
| Echoviruses | Naked, icosahedral, nonsegmented, linear | Can cause mild or febrile illnesses, rashes, and aseptic meningitis. | Infection by viral invasion of nasopharyngeal mucosa. | High incidence during summer-fall. |
| Enteroviruses | Naked, icosahedral, nonsegmented, linear | Common cause of mild or febrile illness, aseptic meningitis. Enterovirus 70 can cause conjunctivitis. | Fecal-oral. | High incidence during summer-fall. |
| Rhinoviruses | Naked, icosahedral, nonsegmented, linear | Number 1 cause of common cold; > 100 serologic types. | Often spread by self-inoculation nose/throat; inactivated at low pH, so does not colonize the gut like other picornaviridae. | Clinical diagnosis from symptoms. |
| Hepatitis A (HAV) | Naked, icosahedral, nonsegmented, linear | Acute viral hepatitis. Not a chronic disease; no carriers. | Fecal-oral. | Anti-HAV IgG indicates person had a previous infection. |
| Coxsackieviruses | Naked, icosahedral, nonsegmented, linear | Group A viruses can cause herpangina, hand-foot-mouth disease, and pharyngitis. Group B viruses can cause myocarditis, aseptic meningitis, and pleurodynia. | Infection by viral invasion of nasopharyngeal mucosa. | High incidence during summer-fall. |

*(continues)*

**TABLE 4-29. Positive-Stranded RNA Viruses (continued)**

| FAMILY | STRUCTURE | DISEASE | ROUTE OF TRANSMISSION | IMPORTANT FACTS |
|---|---|---|---|---|
| **Flaviviridae** | | | | |
| Hepatitis C (HCV) | Enveloped, icosahedral | Acute, usually subclinical hepatitis; ~80% chronic. | Primarily parenteral (common cause of post-transfusion hepatitis and hepatitis among IV drug abusers); sexual (less common). | Associated with hepatocellular carcinoma; cirrhosis. |
| Saint Louis encephalitis virus | Enveloped, icosahedral | | *Culex* mosquito. | Most common encephalitis in elderly in the US. |
| West Nile virus | Enveloped, icosahedral | Fever, nausea, vomiting, and rash. | *Culex* mosquito. | Peaks in summer. |
| Japanese encephalitis virus | Enveloped, icosahedral | Mild febrile illness, acute meningoencephalitis. | *Culex* mosquito. | Reservoirs in pigs and birds. |
| Yellow fever virus | Enveloped, icosahedral | Chills, fever, black vomit, headaches. | *Aedes* mosquito. | With liver involvement, patients have jaundice with Councilman bodies (acidophilic inclusions). |
| Dengue virus | Enveloped, icosahedral | Mild fever, headache, bone aches, hemorrhagic shock syndrome (Southeast Asian variant). | *Aedes* mosquito. | Biggest arbovirus problem. |
| **Togaviridae** | | | | |
| Rubella (German measles, 3-day measles) | Enveloped, icosahedral, linear | Maculopapular rash, fever, conjunctivitis, sore throat. | Respiratory droplets. | Congenital rubella syndrome prevented if mother is vaccinated. |
| Western/Eastern/ Venezuelan equine encephalitis virus | Enveloped, icosahedral, linear | Flulike illness, encephalitis. | Mosquito vector. | |
| **Coronaviridae** | | | | |
| Coronaviruses | Enveloped, helical, nonsegmented | Second leading cause of common cold. Implicated in infant gastroenteritis. | Aerosols and respiratory droplets. | The only positive sense ssRNA virus with a helical capsid. |
| **Astroviridae** | | | | |
| Astroviruses | Naked, icosahedral, linear | Endemic gastroenteritis in neonates and young children. | Fecal-oral. | Outbreaks similar to rotavirus; peaks in winter in temperate climates and during rainy season in tropical climates. |

*(continues)*

**TABLE 4-29.    Positive-Stranded RNA Viruses** *(continued)*

| FAMILY | STRUCTURE | DISEASE | ROUTE OF TRANSMISSION | IMPORTANT FACTS |
|---|---|---|---|---|
| **Retroviridae** | | | | |
| Human immunodeficiency virus (HIV) | Enveloped, icosahedral, linear; diploid ss(+) RNA RNA-dependent DNA polymerase | Primary infection: mononucleosis-like syndrome. As disease progresses, virus infects and kills more CD4+ T cells; without these cells both humoral and cell-mediated arms of the immune system are weakened (CDC criteria). | Vertical, perinatal via breast milk, sex, blood transfusions, and needles. | Common opportunistic infections. At risk for thrush when CD4+ T cells < 400. At risk for *Pneumocystis jirovecii* pneumonia when CD4+ T cells < 200. At < 100 CD4+ T cells, risk of CMV, *Mycobacterium avium* complex, and toxoplasmosis. |
| Human T-cell lymphotrophic virus type I (HTLV-1) | Enveloped, icosahedral, linear | Causes adult T-cell leukemia and tropical spastic paraparesis (TSP). | Vertical, perinatal via breast milk, sex, blood transfusions, and needles. | TSP/HTLV-1–associated myelopathy: demyelination of the spinal cord pyramidal tract. Rapid onset. |

CDC, Centers for Disease Control and Prevention.

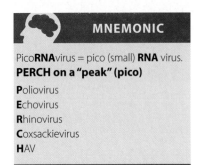

**MNEMONIC**

Pico**RNA**virus = pico (small) **RNA** virus.
**PERCH on a "peak" (pico)**

**P**oliovirus
**E**chovirus
**R**hinovirus
**C**oxsackievirus
**H**AV

### Pathogenesis

Like HAV, transmitted via the fecal-oral route and can cause water-borne outbreaks (water contamination with fecal material).

### Clinical Symptoms

It resembles HAV in its incubation, course, and severity; typically causes mild hepatitis in healthy individuals. It is self-limited but can cause **fulminant hepatitis in pregnant women.**

### Treatment

Supportive; no benefit from administering IFN-α. **Vaccine is in development.**

### Picornavirus Family

#### Polioviruses

Abortive poliomyelitis, paralytic poliomyelitis, postpolio syndrome.

#### Characteristics

Very small picornavirus (20–30 nm), which usually causes a subclinical syndrome. It is important, however, because it can also cause paralysis, which is completely preventable.

#### Pathogenesis

The portal of entry is the mouth, and viral replication occurs in the gut. Active virus is excreted in the feces for several weeks.

#### Clinical Symptoms

- Most common outcome is **abortive poliomyelitis,** which is a mild febrile syndrome.
- **Paralytic poliomyelitis** occurs in 1% of all cases. Paralysis results from viral damage to **anterior horn motor neurons.**

- Many years after resolution, some patients can develop **postpolio syndrome,** which causes further muscle atrophy.
- Also causes **aseptic meningitis.** (Other picornaviruses, notably echoviruses and coxsackieviruses, commonly cause this condition.)
- Diagnosis can be confirmed by serology, virus isolation or RT-PCR (reverse transcriptase-polymerase chain reaction), and DNA hybridization.

### Treatment

Supportive care.

- Prevention: Two types of vaccines are available—killed (**Salk; inactivated poliomyelitis vaccine [IPV]**) and live attenuated (**Sabin; oral polio vaccine [OPV]**) vaccinations.
- The IPV is given to immunocompromised patients.
- OPV contains three serotypes of poliovirus. This vaccine has also been known to cause **vaccine-associated paralytic poliomyelitis (VAPP)** as a result of reversion to wild-type virus.

### Hepatitis A (HAV)

Enteric, short incubation acute viral hepatitis.

### Characteristics

Positive sense, single-stranded 27-nm RNA virus associated with poor sanitation. Common childhood infection in developing countries.

### Pathogenesis

Similar to hepatitis E (HEV), acquired by the **fecal-oral route.**

- Incubation is between 2 and 6 weeks, with shedding of virus occurring during late incubation period and the prodrome.
- The virus is shed in stool and thus can be contracted through exposure to contaminated water, food, and shellfish.
- The highest prevalence is in densely populated areas and developing countries.

### Clinical Symptoms

Often asymptomatic and anicteric; experienced as flulike illness. Often manifests with jaundice and GI disturbances (watery diarrhea is most common). Fulminant hepatitis and carrier states are rare. The infection is usually self-limited and is **not** associated with chronic hepatitis or hepatocellular carcinoma. Diagnosis can be confirmed with tests for HAV antibody.

### Treatment

- Supportive care. Prevention involves hand washing.
- **Vaccine:** HAV vaccine is given to all patients with chronic liver disease (especially hepatitis C), travelers to high-risk countries, those with high-risk behavior, and those from high-risk communities. Anti-HAV antibody is 90% effective if given within 2 weeks of exposure.

### Coxsackieviruses

Herpangina, hand-foot-and-mouth disease, aseptic meningitis.

### Characteristics

This small, 20- to 30-nm, virus is the most common cause of aseptic meningitis (far more than all bacterial forms), followed by echovirus and mumps virus. It is highly contagious and manifests with rash.

**KEY FACT**

Young children receive four doses of Salk (IPV) vaccine. Sabin (OPV) is no longer available in the United States.

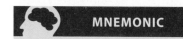

**MNEMONIC**

The Vowels Hit Your Bowels: Hepatitis A and E → Fecal-Oral Route

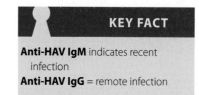

**KEY FACT**

**Anti-HAV IgM** indicates recent infection
**Anti-HAV IgG** = remote infection

**KEY FACT**

Coxsackievirus: ssRNA, linear, naked, icosahedral.

### Pathogenesis

Fecal-oral transmission.

### Clinical Symptoms

- **Group A** coxsackievirus is responsible for **herpangina** (Figure 4-94) and hand-foot-and-mouth disease.
- **Group B** coxsackievirus is responsible for cardiomyopathy (acute myocarditis and pericarditis), aseptic meningitis, and pleurodynia.

### Treatment

Supportive care.

## Flaviviruses

### Hepatitis C (HCV, Infectious Hepatitis)

### Characteristics

The HCV genome is a 10-kb positive-sense RNA genome, with a 42-nm capsid. It is a major cause of non-A, non-B (NANB) hepatitis worldwide.

### Pathogenicity

Mainly acquired through IV drug use or blood products. It can also be transmitted perinatally or sexually.

### Clinical Symptoms

Presentation is similar to that of hepatitis B, but less severe. Persistent infections may progress to chronic active hepatitis, cirrhosis, and hepatocellular carcinoma. Serodiagnostic test detects the antibodies to HCV, which indicate acute or chronic infection. RT-PCR and DNA assays are also used to determine the viral load.

### Treatment

Supportive care and an emerging panel of targeted therapies used for different HCV genotypes.

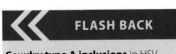

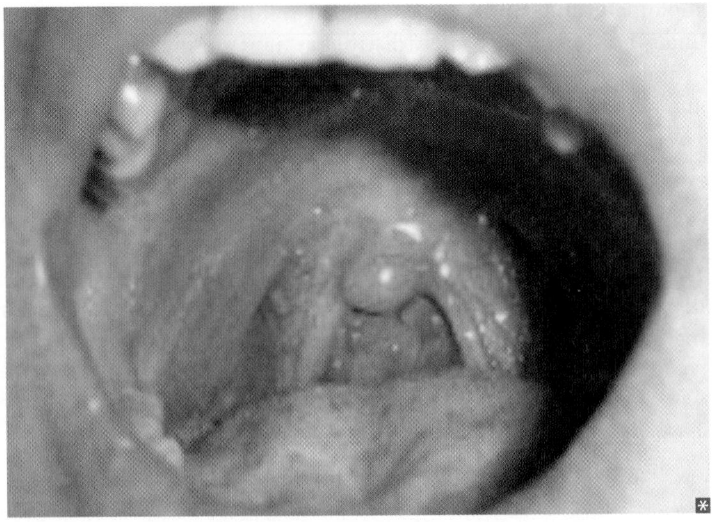

**FLASH BACK**

**Cowdry type A inclusions** in HSV lesions help to differentiate between HSV lesions and herpangina.

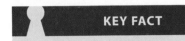

**KEY FACT**

Most hepatitis C viral infections develop into chronic hepatitis.

**FIGURE 4-94.    Infectious enanthem: herpangina.** Multiple, small vesicles and erosions with erythematous halos on the soft palate.

## Togaviruses

### Rubella (German Measles)

#### Characteristics

This togavirus can persist in humans for years with no detectable signs or symptoms. Rubella virus readily crosses the placenta and is highly teratogenic, causing deafness, blindness, and/or heart or brain defects in fetuses of mothers infected in the first trimester.

#### Pathogenesis

Spreads primarily through aerosolized particles. The mucosa of the upper respiratory tract is the portal of viral entry and initial site of virus replication.

#### Clinical Symptoms

Clinically apparent rubella is characterized by a truncal maculopapular rash, occipital and postauricular lymphadenopathy, low-grade fever, conjunctivitis, sore throat, and arthralgias.

#### Treatment

Supportive care.

#### Prevention

Live vaccine is available and confers long-term immunity to rubella. However, **the vaccine is not given to pregnant women.**

## Retroviruses

### Human Immunodeficiency Virus (HIV)

#### Characteristics

The genome consists of two identical subunits of single-stranded RNA (**diploid linear**), surrounded by a conical truncated capsid (Figure 4-95). These components are surrounded by a plasma membrane of host-cell origin, formed when the capsid buds from the host cell.

**KEY FACT**

Retroviruses, including HIV, are the **only** diploid viruses of clinical relevance to humans.

**KEY FACT**

**Structural genes:**
- *Gag*—group-specific antigen; encodes p24; p6, p7, and p9; p17.
- *Pol*—encodes RT; integrase; protease.
- *Env*—encodes gp120; gp41.

**Regulatory genes:**
- *Tat*—encodes transactivator proteins.
- *Rev*—encodes regulatory virion proteins.
- *Nef*—encodes negative factor.

**KEY FACT**

Major **risk factors** for contracting HIV:
- Unprotected sexual intercourse.
- Sharing contaminated needles.
- Birth from an infected mother.
- In underdeveloped countries, blood products and transfusions still pose major risk factors.

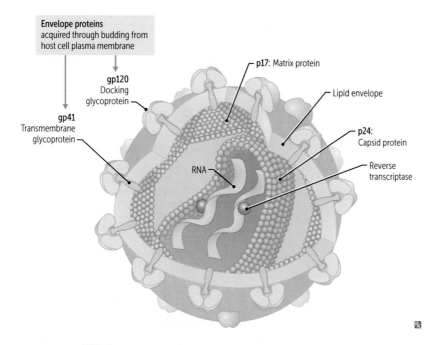

Envelope proteins acquired through budding from host cell plasma membrane

gp120 Docking glycoprotein

gp41 Transmembrane glycoprotein

p17: Matrix protein

Lipid envelope

p24: Capsid protein

Reverse transcriptase

RNA

**QUESTION**

A patient with a history of abdominal pain and swelling is examined and found to have yellowing of his sclerae and skin. Serology is as follows:

| | |
|---|---|
| Anti-HAV IgG | Positive |
| Anti-HAV IgM | Negative |
| Anti-HbcAg IgM | Positive |
| Anti-HBsAg | Positive |
| Anti-HBeAg | Positive |

What is the best interpretation of these test results?

**FIGURE 4-95.   HIV virus.**

- (ss) RNA: Bound to the nucleocapsid proteins and enzymes, such as **RT, integrase,** and **protease.**
- The main **matrix protein (p17)** surrounds the capsid (**p24–capsid protein**) and maintains the integrity of the virion particle.
- The **envelope** includes glycoproteins **gp120** and **gp41.**

The HIV genome is very complex and includes several major genes coding for **structural proteins** (expressed in all retroviruses), and several **regulatory genes,** unique to HIV.

### Pathogenesis

Transmission of HIV may occur secondary to sexual contact (semen, vaginal secretions), blood transfusions, IV drug use, and contact with other infected bodily fluids (plasma, CSF). HIV can also be transmitted through the placenta (intrauterine transmission), perinatally, and through breast milk.

HIV primarily infects macrophages and CD4+ T cells. Macrophages are thought to play a key role in primary HIV-1 infection. Infection of and replication in monocytes/macrophages results in the spread of HIV to other tissues.

- Viral entry to **CD4+ T cells** and macrophages is **initiated** through **interaction** of the envelope glycoproteins (**gp120**) with **CD4** molecules of target cells.
- Fusion with target cells is further facilitated through their own chemokine receptors (**CCR5** or **CXCR4**). CXCR4 is located on T cells, and CCR5 is located on macrophages.
- HIV invades CD4+ T cells, impairing both the humoral and cell-mediated arms of the immune system (Figure 4-96).

### Clinical Symptoms

The hallmarks of initial infection with HIV are an abrupt drop in the CD4+ T-cell count and rapid viral replication (increased **viral load**). Typical course of an HIV-infected individual is as follows (Figure 4-97):

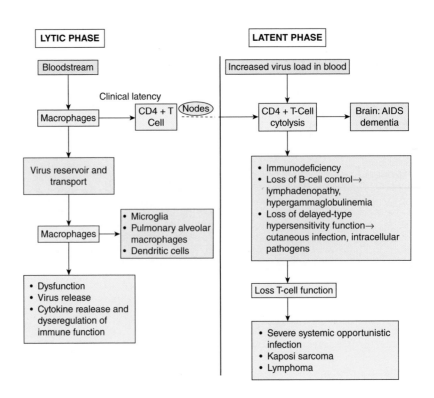

**FIGURE 4-96.    HIV/AIDS cycle and evasion.**

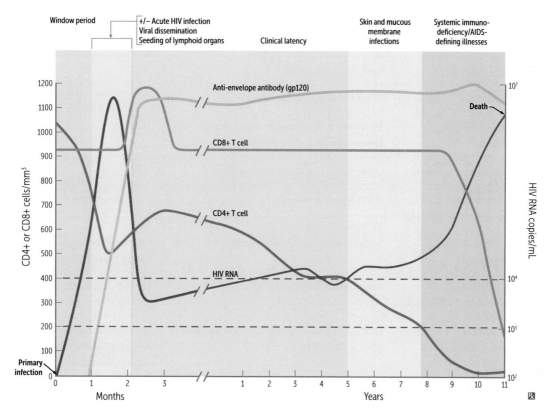

**FIGURE 4-97.** **Typical course of an HIV-infected individual.**

- **Primary infection; acute HIV syndrome (Centers for Disease Control and Prevention [CDC] category A):** Patients may experience mononucleosis-like syndrome, which usually occurs 4–8 weeks after initial infection. Major symptoms include, but are not limited to, **fever, generalized lymphadenopathy, headache, myalgia,** and **pharyngitis.**
- **Clinical latency stage:** CD4+ T-cell count rebounds, and most symptoms of the acute infection subside. However, lymphadenopathy can be present throughout the entire course of an HIV infection. During the latent phase, virus replicates in lymph nodes.
- **Disease progression and later stages (AIDS):** Dictated by the number of viable CD4+ T cells. As they decline over time, patients have an increased risk of acquiring common and not so common infections (**CDC categories B and C**). These conditions are summarized in Table 4-30.

### Diagnosis

- Tests for initial screening (sensitive, high false-positive rate, RULE OUT test): detects antibodies to viral antigens **p24, p17, gp120,** and **gp41.**
- HIV-1/2 discriminatory antibody test is used as a confirmatory test, positive patients are then referred to care and HIV viral load and genotype testing.
- **HIV RNA-PCR:** For monitoring effects of drug therapy on viral load. Also used to screen for HIV infection in newborns of HIV-positive mothers.
- **CD4+ T-cell count:** Used to assess treatment progress. AIDS diagnosis with ≤ 200 CD4+ cells/mm³ (normal: 500–1500). Considered HIV-positive if AIDS-defining condition is present or CD4/CD8 ratio < 1.5.

### Treatment

Patients are usually placed on highly active antiretroviral therapy (**HAART**).

- HAART includes at least two RT inhibitors combined with a protease inhibitor.
- Pregnant women are prescribed combination antiretroviral therapy, which has been shown to prevent perinatal transmission of the virus.

**CLINICAL CORRELATION**

HIV-positive patients are said to be at risk for developing **candidiasis** (thrush) and **TB** once their **CD4+** T-cell count drops **below 400.** These are AIDS-defining conditions.

**KEY FACT**

Antigen p24 is detectable shortly after initial infection, so it is often used as an early sign of HIV infection.

**KEY FACT**

Definitive diagnosis of HIV infection can be made only when there are antibodies to at least two viral antigens, as confirmed by Western blot analysis.

**TABLE 4-30.** **Commonly Encountered HIV-Associated Infections**

| | MANIFESTATION | KEY POINT | CAUSATIVE AGENT |
|---|---|---|---|
| Neoplasm | Hairy leukoplakia A | Often on lateral tongue | EBV |
| | Non-Hodgkin lymphoma | Often on oropharynx (Waldeyer ring) | |
| | Primary B-cell CNS lymphoma | More likely to have multiple lesions than in immunocompetent population | EBV |
| | Squamous cell carcinoma | Often in anus (gay male) or cervix (female) | HPV |
| Skin/mucosa | Thrush; fluffy white, "cottage-cheese" lesions B | Often on buccal mucosa | *Candida albicans* |
| | Superficial vascular proliferation | Biopsy reveals neutrophilic inflammation | *Bartonella henselae*—causes bacillary angiomatosis |
| | Superficial, neoplastic proliferation of vasculature | Biopsy reveals lymphocytic inflammation | HHV-8—causes Kaposi sarcoma |
| Systemic | Low-grade fevers, cough, hepatosplenomegaly | Oval yeast cells within macrophages; seen when CD4+ < 100 cells/mm$^3$ | *Histoplasma capsulatum*—causes only pulmonary symptoms in immunocompetent hosts |
| | Fever, diarrhea, abdominal pain, hepatosplenomegaly, lymphadenopathy | Seen when CD4+ < 50 cells/mm$^3$ | Disseminated *Mycobacterium avium-intracellulare* |
| GI | Chronic, watery diarrhea | Acid-fast cysts seen in stool; seen when CD4+ < 200 cells/mm$^3$ | *Cryptosporidium* or *Cystoisospora* |
| | Chronic ulcers or esophagitis | *Candida* esophagitis seen when CD4+ < 100 cells/mm$^3$ | HSV (also causes bronchitis/pneumonitis) |
| CNS | Meningitis | India ink stain reveals narrow-based budding | *Cryptococcus neoformans*—may also cause encephalitis |
| | Progressive multifocal leukoencephalopathy C | Due to reactivation of a latent virus; results in demyelination | JC virus (Polyomavirus) |
| | HIV encephalitis/AIDS dementia complex | Virus gains CNS access via infected macrophages | Occurs late in course of HIV infection; microglial nodules with multinucleated giant cells |
| | Abscesses | Many ring-enhancing lesions on imaging. Seen when CD4+ < 100 cells/mm$^3$ | *Toxoplasma gondii* |
| | Retinitis D | Cottonwool spots on funduscopic exam or blindness; seen when CD4+ < 50 cells/mm$^3$ | Cytomegalovirus |

*(continues)*

**TABLE 4-30.**  **Commonly Encountered HIV-Associated Infections** *(continued)*

| | MANIFESTATION | KEY POINT | CAUSATIVE AGENT |
|---|---|---|---|
| Respiratory | Interstitial pneumonia | Biopsy reveals cells with intranuclear and cytoplasmic inclusion bodies | |
| | Invasive aspergillosis | Pleuritic pain, hemoptysis, infiltrates on imaging | *Aspergillus fumigatus* |
| | Pneumonia E | Seen when CD4+ < 200 cells/mm³ | *Pneumocystis jirovecii* |

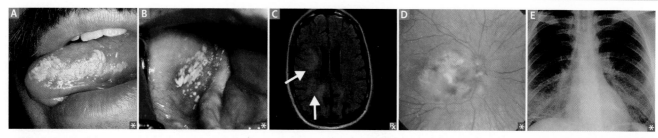

CD, cluster of differentiation; CNS, central nervous system; EBV, Epstein-Barr virus; HHV, human herpesvirus; HPV, human papillomavirus; HSV, herpes simplex virus.

## Prognosis

There is no cure for AIDS, but patients who are treated with combination antiretroviral therapy have a predicted lifespan approaching that of HIV-negative persons.

## NEGATIVE (SINGLE)-STRANDED RNA VIRUSES—SS (−) RNA

### General Characteristics

Negative, single-stranded RNA viruses have the largest variety in structure (Table 4-31). All are enveloped and replicate in the host cell cytoplasm with the exception of orthomyxoviruses and retroviruses, which replicate in the nucleus. The capsid shape varies from icosahedral to helical. There are also linear, circular, segmented, and nonsegmented genomes among the negative single-stranded RNA viruses.

## Paramyxoviridae

### General Characteristics

Large, enveloped, single-stranded, negative sense RNA, nonsegmented.

Paramyxoviruses are a major cause of upper and lower respiratory tract (URT and LRT) disease, as well as systemic illness. Paramyxoviruses causing LRT disease include parainfluenza and respiratory syncytial virus (RSV). Measles and mumps cause systemic disease. Paramyxoviruses are the most important cause of respiratory infection in children < 5 years old. Typical virus organization is depicted in Figure 4-98.

**Membrane fusion** and hemolysin activities are carried out by **F,** fusion glycoprotein. It exists as inactive **F0,** which is cleaved to the active **F1** form by cellular proteases. The fusion (F) glycoprotein is also responsible for large syncytia formation in cells infected with paramyxoviruses by causing respiratory epithelial cells to fuse.

## Parainfluenza

### Characteristics

Parainfluenza virus (PIV) primarily affects children 3–8 years old, although it may also affect adults. Viral infection may manifest in the upper or lower respiratory tract.

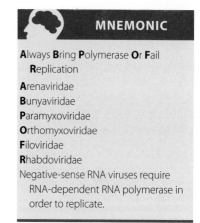

**MNEMONIC**

**A**lways **B**ring **P**olymerase **O**r **F**ail
   **R**eplication
**A**renaviridae
**B**unyaviridae
**P**aramyxoviridae
**O**rthomyxoviridae
**F**iloviridae
**R**habdoviridae
Negative-sense RNA viruses require RNA-dependent RNA polymerase in order to replicate.

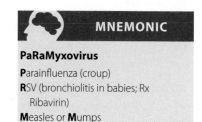

**MNEMONIC**

**PaRaMyxovirus**
**P**arainfluenza (croup)
**R**SV (bronchiolitis in babies; Rx Ribavirin)
**M**easles or **M**umps

**TABLE 4-31.**    **Negative-Stranded RNA Viruses**

| FAMILY | STRUCTURE | DISEASE | ROUTE OF TRANSMISSION | IMPORTANT FACTS |
|---|---|---|---|---|
| **Paramyxoviridae** | | | | |
| Parainfluenza | Enveloped, helical, linear | Croup, bronchiolitis, pneumonia | Droplets | Self-limiting disease |
| Measles | Enveloped, helical, linear | Cough, coryza, conjunctivitis, rash | Aerosol/airborne | Symptoms due to immune response |
| Mumps | Enveloped, helical, linear | Aseptic meningitis, meningoencephalitis, parotitis, unilateral nerve deafness, orchitis | Droplets | Infection confers lifelong immunity |
| Respiratory syncytial virus | Enveloped, helical, linear | Bronchiolitis, pneumonia | Droplets | Can be deadly to infants |
| **Rhabdoviridae** | | | | |
| Rabies | Enveloped, bullet/helical, linear | Fever, nausea, hydrophobia, delirium, paralysis, and coma | Animal bite | Evidence of infection, including symptoms and the detection of antibody; does not occur until too late for intervention |
| **Filoviridae** | | | | |
| Ebola/Marburg viruses | Enveloped, helical, linear | Viral hemorrhagic fevers, flulike symptoms, death in ~70% | Contact with body fluids; droplets | Most deadly hemorrhagic fevers |
| **Orthomyxoviridae** | | | | |
| Influenza | Enveloped, helical, segmented (eight segments) | Fever, arthralgias, malaise | Droplets | Undergoes antigenic shift and antigenic drift |
| **Deltaviridae** | | | | |
| HDV "delta agent" | Enveloped, helical, circular | Can coinfect or superinfect with HBV to worsen its prognosis. Chronic disease (carriers) | Same as HBV | Defective virus that requires HBsAg as its envelope |
| **Bunyaviridae** | | | | |
| Hantavirus | Enveloped, helical, linear → circular, segments | Hantavirus renal disease (HVRD), HV cardiopulmonary syndrome (HVCPS) | Inhaled rodent urine/feces | Treat with ribavirin |
| Rift Valley fever virus | Enveloped, helical, linear → circular, segments | Acute febrile illness (saddle-back fever), myalgias, low back pain, headache, anorexia, retroorbital pain | Tick-borne | Most common in sub-Saharan Africa, or in military personnel on tours of duty there |
| La Crosse virus | Enveloped, helical, linear → circular, segments | Viral encephalitis | Mosquito vector | Most important cause of insect encephalitis in the Midwest |
| California encephalitis | Enveloped, helical, linear → circular, segments | Viral encephalitis | Mosquito vector | |
| Crimean-Congo hemorrhagic fever | Enveloped, helical, linear → circular, segments | Hemorrhagic viral encephalitis | Mosquito vector | |

*(continues)*

**TABLE 4-31.    Negative-Stranded RNA Viruses (continued)**

| FAMILY | STRUCTURE | DISEASE | ROUTE OF TRANSMISSION | IMPORTANT FACTS |
|---|---|---|---|---|
| **Arenaviridae** | Ambisense | | | |
| Lymphocytic choriomeningitis virus (LCMV) | Enveloped, helical, circular, segmented | Aseptic meningitis or encephalitis; asymptomatic to mild febrile illness most common | Rat | No human–human transmission except mother to fetus and transplant recipients |
| Lassa fever | Enveloped, helical, circular, segmented | Hemorrhagic fever, multisystem involvement, often including encephalitis and facial swelling | Rat | High death rates in pregnant women in 3rd trimester and fetuses (~95% fetal mortality rate). *Complications*: Most common is deafness in ~1/3 of cases |

Although paramyxovirus infections tend to be minor and relatively short-lived, elderly and immunocompromised patients are at greater risk of serious complications.

### Pathogenesis

The virus is airborne and invades the mucosa of the URT. From there, it may travel to lower segments.

### Clinical Symptoms

Clinical manifestations include:

- **Common cold:** Acute URT infection typically lasting 7–10 days.
  - **Symptoms** include runny nose, nasal congestion, sneezing, sore throat, cough, and headache. Fever may or may not be present.

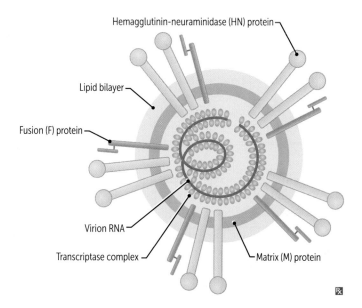

**FIGURE 4-98.    Schematic diagram of a paramyxovirus showing major components.** The lipid bilayer is shown as the light blue concentric circle; underlying the lipid bilayer is the viral matrix protein (dark blue concentric circle). Inserted through the viral membrane are the hemagglutinin-neuraminidase (HN) attachment glycoprotein and the fusion (F) glycoprotein. Inside the virus is the negative-strand virion RNA, with associated transcriptase complexes, leading to RNA-dependent RNA transcriptase activity.

- **Croup:** Affects the larynx, trachea, and bronchi (laryngotracheobronchitis). Mild cold usually persists for several days before the barking "seal-like" cough becomes evident.
  - **Symptoms** include fever, hoarse barking cough, laryngeal obstruction, and inspiratory stridor.
- **Bronchiolitis:** Begins as a mild URT infection that, over a period of 2–3 days, can develop into increasing respiratory distress with wheezing and a **tight, wheezy cough.** The peak incidence of bronchiolitis is during the first year of life; it dramatically declines until it virtually disappears by school age.
  - **Signs and symptoms** include fever, expiratory wheezing, tachypnea, retractions, crackles, and air trapping.
- **Pneumonia** is usually a complication in high-risk patients, including very young children, the elderly, and the immunocompromised.
  - **Signs and symptoms** include fever, crackles, and evidence of pulmonary consolidation.

In addition, **PIVs routinely cause** otitis media, pharyngitis, conjunctivitis, and coryza, occurring separately or in combination with an LRT infection.

### Treatment

Treatment is mainly supportive, with antivirals and antibiotics as needed. No vaccine is currently available.

- **Ribavirin** aerosol or systemic therapy has been used to treat PIV infections in children and adults who are severely immunocompromised. Broader use at this time is of uncertain clinical benefit.
- **Antibiotics** are used only when secondary bacterial infections (eg, otitis, sinusitis) develop.
- **Corticosteroids** and **nebulizers** are used to treat respiratory symptoms and to help reduce the inflammation and airway edema of croup.

### Respiratory Syncytial Virus

#### Characteristics

Respiratory syncytial virus (RSV) is an acute viral infection with short incubation period and recovery occurring within 7–12 days. RSV is the most important cause of LRT disease in young children. Almost all children have been infected with RSV by the age of 2.

#### Pathogenesis

The virus is transmitted via droplets, invades the mucosa of the URT, and replicates only within respiratory epithelium. RSV does not have HN or NA attachment proteins.

#### Clinical Symptoms

In most infants, the virus causes symptoms resembling those of the **common cold.** In infants born prematurely or those with chronic disease, RSV can cause a severe or even life-threatening disease.

- **Signs and symptoms** include low-grade fever, cough, tachypnea, cyanosis, retractions, wheezing, and crackles.
- Most common **complications** are ear infections. Less common, but serious complications include pneumonia (0.5–1%) and respiratory failure (2%).

#### Treatment

Mostly supportive with airway management (most important). **Ribavirin** is a nucleoside analog and is the only antiviral approved for use. However, it is not used routinely. Its main use is in high-risk infants prone to developing complications.

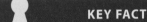

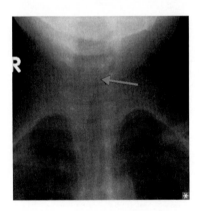

**FIGURE 4-99.** **Steeple sign.** X-ray of the neck showing steeple sign, narrowing of the trachea (arrow).

- **Prevention: Palivizumab (Synagis),** monoclonal antibody is indicated for the **prevention** of serious LRT disease caused by RSV in pediatric patients and prematurely born infants (at < 32 weeks' gestation).
- **No vaccine is available.** Strict hygiene and contact precautions with diseased individuals are imperative.

### Measles (Rubeola)

#### Characteristics

Measles is a highly infectious **childhood febrile exanthem** that has a long incubation period of approximately 2 weeks, followed by a classic viral prodrome and virus-specific immune response. Complete recovery ensues 7–10 days after onset of measles rash. The clearance of virus coincides approximately with fading of the rash. A differential diagnosis of rubeola with other common "red rashes of childhood" can be found in Table 4-32.

**Q    QUESTION**

A 6-year-old boy has a runny nose and sore throat, and has just developed a "seal-like," barking cough. What are some respiratory sequelae of the virus likely responsible?

**TABLE 4-32.    "Lots of Spots": Red Rashes of Childhood**

| CONDITION | DESCRIPTION |
|---|---|
| Rubella (German measles, 3-day measles) | A Rubivirus; rash begins at head and moves down; postauricular tenderness **A** |
| Rubeola (measles) | A paramyxovirus; beginning at head and moving down **B**; rash preceded by cough, coryza, conjunctivitis, and blue-white (Koplik) spots on buccal mucosa |
| Varicella (chickenpox) | A herpesvirus (VZV); rash begins at chest, spreads to face and extremities with lesions of different age **C** |
| Roseola (exanthem subitum, sixth disease) | A herpesvirus (HHV-6/HHV-7); macular truncal rash appearing suddenly after defervescence of high fever **D**; usually affects infants and young children |
| Erythema infectiosum (fifth disease) | A parvovirus (B19); "slapped cheek" rash on face that later appears over body in reticular, "lace-like" pattern **E** |
| *Streptococcus pyogenes* (scarlet fever) | Erythematous, sandpaper-like rash with fever and sore throat **F** |
| Variola (smallpox) | A poxvirus, thankfully eradicated, but potential bioterrorism threat **G** |
| Hand-foot-mouth disease | A coxsackievirus (type A); rash on palms and soles, ulcers in oral mucosa **H** |
| Molluscum contagiosum | Flesh-colored papule with central umbilication **I** |

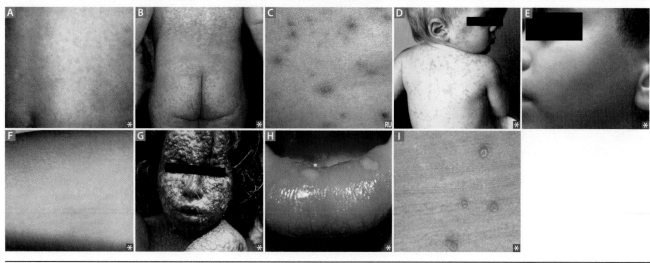

### Pathogenesis

The virus is airborne (transmitted by aerosolized particles), infects the respiratory tract, and replicates locally in the respiratory epithelium before spreading to regional lymphatic tissue and the rest of the body.

### Clinical Symptoms

Clinical picture develops in relation to previously described pathogenic characteristics.

- **Classic viral prodrome** occurs following the incubation period. It is commonly referred to as the **3 C's: Cough, Coryza, and Conjunctivitis** with photophobia.
  - Pathognomonic **Koplik spots** typically arise on the buccal, gingival, and labial mucosae within 2–3 days of initial symptoms. The Koplik spots are 1- to 2-mm blue-gray macules on an erythematous base (Figure 100).
  - **Giant-cell pneumonia,** characterized by **Warthin-Finkeldey cells** (multinucleated giant cells with eosinophilic nuclear and cytoplasmic inclusion bodies) found in the lungs and sputum. Rare condition found only in the immunosuppressed.
  - Additional **prodromal symptoms** may include fever, malaise, myalgias, photophobia, and periorbital edema.
- **Virus-specific immune response** is characterized by the appearance of the **rash.** Measles rash is a maculopapular erythematous rash.
  - Rash typically begins at the hairline and spreads caudally over the next 3 days as the prodromal symptoms resolve.
  - Lasts 4–6 days and then fades from the head downward. Lesion density is greatest above the shoulders, where macular lesions may coalesce.
  - Desquamation may be present but is generally not severe.
- **Complete recovery** from measles generally occurs within 7–10 days from onset of the rash.

### Treatment

Mainly supportive care; IV hydration, antipyretics. Secondary infections such as pneumonia and otitis media should be treated with antibiotics. Vitamin A may reduce mortality in select measles patients, notably in those who are vitamin deficient.

- **Postexposure prophylaxis** with immune globulin may be given within 6 days of exposure to high-risk patients such as immunocompromised children and pregnant women.

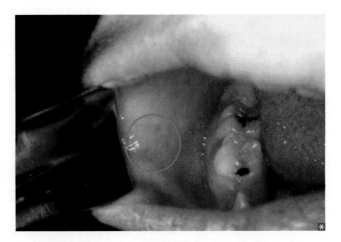

**FIGURE 4-100.    Koplik spots.** The spots manifest as white or bluish lesions with an erythematous halo on the buccal mucosa. They usually occur in the first 2 days of measles symptoms and may briefly overlap the measles exanthem. The presence of the erythematous halo differentiates Koplik spots from Fordyce spots (ectopic sebaceous glands), which occur in the mouths of healthy individuals.

- **Prevention:** There is one serotype worldwide; all cases are clinically apparent. The **MMR vaccine (3-in-1)** protects against measles, mumps, and rubella and consists of live attenuated virus. Infection produces lifelong immunity. Maternal antibody can protect newborns.
- **Complications:**
  - **Common:** Respiratory complications in up to 15% of cases.
  - **Uncommon and severe:** Postinfectious encephalomyelitis, subacute sclerosing panencephalopathy (SSPE), and bacterial superinfection due to immunosuppression.

## Mumps

### Characteristics

A systemic infection usually affecting unvaccinated children between the ages 2 and 12 but can occur in other age groups. Mumps usually spreads from person to person by saliva droplets or by direct contact with contaminated articles.

### Pathogenesis

The URT is the point of initial entry via the inhalation of respiratory droplets containing virus. The virus then spreads to draining lymph nodes and replicates in lymphocytes, after which it disseminates hematogenously to the salivary glands, as well as other glands.

- Long incubation period (an average of 16–18 days).
- No clinical indication of infection in approximately one-third of infected individuals; however, they can still transmit the disease.
- The period of communicability (transmissibility) is usually from 9 days before onset of parotid edema to 1–2 days after onset of swelling and occasionally lasts as long as 7 days after swelling.

### Clinical Symptoms

- **Parotid gland:** After initial presentation of fever, headache, and otitis, the parotid gland enlarges and rapidly progresses to maximum size in 1–3 days, displacing the lobe of the ear, resulting in increased pain and tenderness (Figure 101). Symptoms rapidly subside after swelling reaches its peak. The parotid gland gradually decreases in size in 3–7 days.
- **Epididymo-orchitis** is the second most common manifestation of adult mumps. Symptoms include:
  - Acute onset of fever, chills, nausea, vomiting, and lower abdominal pain following parotitis.
  - After the acute syndrome, the testes begin to swell rapidly. As the fever decreases, the pain and edema subside. A loss of turgor (typically unilateral) demonstrates atrophy. Impaired fertility is uncommon, but is a greater risk when the infection occurs after puberty.

### Treatment

Supportive.

### Prevention

There is only one serotype worldwide. Infection confers lifelong immunity. (Both humoral and cell-mediated immune response are induced.) Infants are protected for approximately 6 months by maternal antibodies. The MMR vaccine is used as described previously.

### Complications

Mumps infection can invade the epithelial cells of multiple organs, including the testes, ovaries, pancreas, meninges, thyroid, bladder, and kidneys.

**KEY FACT**

The MMR vaccine is the only live-attenuated vaccine that should be administered to HIV-positive patients without evidence of severe immunosuppression.

**KEY FACT**

Parotid glands are commonly, but not always, affected by mumps.

**KEY FACT**

Postpubertal males who develop mumps have a 15–20% risk of developing orchitis.

**CLINICAL CORRELATION**

In an adolescent with swollen parotid glands and no viral symptoms, suspect purging.

**MNEMONIC**

**POM: P**arotitis, **O**rchitis, **M**eningitis

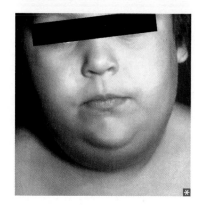
**FIGURE 4-101. Mumps.** Swollen neck and parotid glands.

- **Meningoencephalitis** is the most common complication in children and results from a primary infection of the neurons or postinfection encephalitis with demyelination.
- **Aseptic meningitis** is usually indistinguishable from other causes. The mumps virus can be isolated in the CSF.
- **Unilateral deafness,** permanent or transient, is uncommon. However, mumps is the leading cause of deafness worldwide.
- **Pancreatitis** is a severe but fortunately rare manifestation.
  - **Elevated amylase** is seen, regardless of the presence of pancreatitis.
  - **Lipase** is a more specific indicator of pancreatic involvement and should be tested if this complication is suspected.

### Orthomyxoviridae (Influenza A, B, and C Viruses)

#### General Characteristics

Large, enveloped, single-stranded, negative sense RNA virus, segmented. Unlike most RNA viruses, influenza **replicates** in the host cell's **nucleus.** (Recall that Orthomyxoviridae and Retroviridae are the only two RNA viruses to do this.) However, it acquires its envelope from the host cell membrane through budding. It has several important structural proteins (Table 4-33). Notably, HA promotes viral entry, whereas NA promotes progeny virion release, and the M2 membrane protein promotes viral uncoating. These three proteins are especially relevant because they serve as targets for anti-influenza drugs.

There are three known serotypes of influenza viruses: A, B, and C.

- Types A and B exhibit continual antigenic changes; type C does not.
- Influenza A has human and zoonotic hosts (aquatic birds, chickens, ducks, pigs, horses, and seals), whereas B and C types have human hosts only. Type A viruses are the most virulent and cause the most disease among humans.

#### Pathogenesis

Influenza causes protracted illness with a short incubation period (1–4 days) and exhibits both respiratory and systemic symptoms. It spreads by respiratory droplets or contact with contaminated surfaces and hands. It colonizes the respiratory epithelium and replicates locally. There is no viremia; systemic symptoms are ascribed to IFN and cytokines produced by the host. Antigenic variants of influenza virus are caused by **antigenic shift** and **antigenic drift.**

#### Clinical Symptoms

Major cause of local infections of respiratory tract with constitutional symptoms.

**KEY FACT**

Each year, hundreds of centers around the world keep track of which flu strains are predominant. This information is used to decide which strains should be targeted in the yearly vaccine.

**KEY FACT**

Swine flu and bird flu are serotype A, as they have both human and nonhuman hosts. They are able to undergo antigenic shifts.

**FLASH BACK**

**Antigenic drift:** Gradual change in antigenicity due to point mutations that affect major antigenic sites on the glycoprotein.
**Antigenic shift:** Abrupt change due to genetic reassortment with an unrelated strain.
**S**udden **S**hift (pandemic) is more deadly than gra**D**ual **D**rift (epidemic).

**TABLE 4-33.  Selected Structural and Functional Proteins of Influenza Viruses**

| ENCODED PROTEIN | FUNCTION |
| --- | --- |
| **HA** (hemagglutinin) | - Mediator of viral attachment to host cells<br>- Binds to sialic acid<br>- Fusion activity at acidic pH<br>- Host range determinant<br>- Vaccine/drug target; 95% of outer spikes |
| **NA** (neuraminidase) | - Cleaves sialic acid from HA–host cell complex; promotes virus release from cells<br>- Vaccine/drug target (zanamivir/oseltamivir); 5% of outer spikes |
| **M2** (membrane protein) | - Essential for virus uncoating, drug target (amantadine/rimantadine) |

- Uncomplicated influenza typically presents with cough, sore throat, runny or stuffy nose, fever, muscle aches and pains, headache, and fatigue.
- GI symptoms such as nausea, vomiting, and diarrhea also can occur but are more common in children than in adults.

### Treatment

- **Amantadine** (24–48 hours after onset of symptoms) and **rimantadine** target the M2 ion channel responsible for the alteration of pH required for viral uncoating and assembly. Both are specific for influenza A virus but are not prescribed owing to toxicity and high rates of resistance.
- **Zanamivir (Relenza)** and **oseltamivir phosphate (Tamiflu)** are neuraminidase inhibitors for **both** influenza **A and B,** and should be used within 24–48 hours of symptom onset for maximal effectiveness.

### Vaccine

Natural immunity toward a **single** influenza **strain** is long lasting and is provided by IgA of the respiratory tract. The single best way to prevent the flu is the flu vaccine. The flu vaccine is contraindicated for those with severe egg allergy, although in some cases it may still be safely given under the supervision of an allergist. There are two types of vaccines.

- Intramuscular **flu shot** is an inactivated vaccine. It contains three influenza strains (2As and 1B), and is approved for use in individuals older than 6 months of age, both healthy people and those with chronic medical conditions.
- The **nasal-spray** flu vaccine is a live, attenuated flu virus. It is approved for use in healthy people 5 years to 49 years of age who are not pregnant.

Antibodies develop within approximately 2 weeks following vaccination. Flu vaccines do not protect against flulike illnesses caused by noninfluenza viruses.

### Complications

Rare, affect specific populations.

- **Pneumonia:** Young children, immunocompromised patients, and elderly people in nursing homes are particularly susceptible. In some epidemics (depending on the viral strain), pregnant women are at high risk as well.
- Can be primary influenza, bacterial, or a combination of the two. Infection with *S aureus* is common post influenza and can be life-threatening.
- **Reye syndrome.**

## Rhabdoviridae (Rabies)

### Characteristics

Simple negative-sense enveloped single-stranded RNA virus. The key differentiating characteristic is its **bullet-shaped** capsid.

### Pathogenesis

The virus is secreted in the animal's saliva, and infection results from a bite of the rabid animal. More commonly acquired from bat, raccoon, and skunk bites than from dogs in the United States. Following local inoculation, the virus progresses to the peripheral nervous system and reaches the central nervous system by way of **retrograde axonal transport** after binding to nicotinic acetylcholine receptors. The incubation period may be 3 months or longer; hence, the rabies virus is considered a **slow virus.**

### Clinical Symptoms

The initial symptoms of rabies are fever, malaise, headache, pain or paresthesia at the bite site, GI symptoms, fatigue, and anorexia. After the initial "flulike" syndrome, the

**FLASH FORWARD**

Amantadine is also used in the treatment of Parkinson disease and to reduce drug-induced extrapyramidal effects. Its mechanism of action as an antiparkinsonian agent remains poorly understood, but it is thought to act as a partial dopamine agonist.

**MNEMONIC**

A man to dine takes off his coat: Amantadine blocks M2 membrane protein, which is essential for viral uncoating.

**FLASH FORWARD**

**Reye syndrome:** Hepatoencephalopathy resulting from the use of salicylates in children with URT infections, influenza A or B, or varicella.

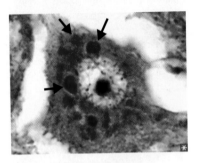

**FIGURE 4-102.    Negri body.** Characteristic cytoplasmic inclusions (arrows) in neurons infected by rabies virus.

patient develops **hydrophobia,** seizures, disorientation, and hallucinations. The final symptoms are paralysis, which may lead to respiratory failure and coma. Unfortunately, rabies cannot be diagnosed until it is too late to treat. **Negri bodies** in the cytoplasm of affected neurons are the hallmark diagnostic finding (Figure 102), but rabies diagnostic laboratories routinely perform DFA and PCR for definitive diagnosis. The only way to definitively diagnose rabies is with a brain biopsy.

### Treatment

**PEP** is used to prevent overt clinical illness in affected persons. The wound is cleaned and the patient is administered human rabies immunoglobulin and the rabies vaccination, which is a killed-virus vaccine.

## DOUBLE-STRANDED RNA VIRUSES

Double-stranded RNA viruses (ie, the Reoviruses) all lack an envelope and have an icosahedral capsid and segmented genome (Table 4-34). The segmented genome allows for switching of various segments among viruses within the same family. This is called **antigenic shift.**

### Rotavirus

#### Characteristics

This double-stranded segmented RNA virus is a common agent of diarrhea in children. Commonly found in the winter and in kindergartens/day care centers.

#### Pathogenesis

The virus is spread via the fecal-oral route and possibly the respiratory route. The mechanism is intestinal villous destruction and atrophy with decreased reabsorption of sodium and water, with consequent copious, osmotic diarrhea.

#### Clinical Symptoms

The major clinical findings are vomiting, diarrhea, fever, and dehydration. Because most patients have large quantities of virus in stool, the direct detection of viral antigen is the method of choice for diagnosis.

**TABLE 4-34.    Overview of Double-Stranded RNA Viruses**

| FAMILY | STRUCTURE | DISEASE | ROUTE OF TRANSMISSION | IMPORTANT FACTS |
|---|---|---|---|---|
| **Reoviridae** | | | | |
| Reovirus | Naked, icosahedral, segmented | Causes mild, self-limiting infections of the upper respiratory or GI tract | Droplet and fecal-oral | Very stable and have been detected in sewage and river water |
| Colorado tick fever virus | Naked, icosahedral, segmented | Causes serious hemorrhagic disease due to vascular endothelial infection. Symptoms of acute disease include fever and muscle/joint pain; can have subclinical cases | Transmitted by wood tick *Dermacentor andersoni* | Found in western and northwestern United States, as well as western Canada |
| Rotavirus | Naked, icosahedral, segmented | Diarrhea | Fecal-oral | Most common agent of infantile diarrhea worldwide, #1 cause of fatal diarrhea in children |

Treatment

Supportive care. The **pentavalent rotavirus (PRV) vaccine** is a pentavalent human–bovine reassortment and is currently recommended as a preventive measure for infants in the United States. The previous version, RotaShield, was removed from the market after being linked to **intussusception in children** (Figure 103).

## PRION DISEASES

Prion diseases are a related group of rare, fatal brain diseases that affect animals and humans. These diseases were previously thought to be viral in origin. The term prion is an abbreviation for proteinaceous infectious particle (PrP). Non-pathogenic PrP (PrPc) is composed of primarily alpha helices, whereas the pathologic variant (PrPsc) is composed of primarily β-pleated sheets. PrPsc induces normal proteins to misfold, further propagating itself.

Prion diseases are also known as **transmissible spongiform encephalopathies** (TSE) and include bovine spongiform encephalopathy (BSE, or mad cow disease) in cattle, Creutzfeldt-Jakob disease (CJD) in humans, and scrapie in sheep. TSEs can be sporadic, inherited, or acquired.

## Microbiology: Systems

## NORMAL FLORA

Although bacteria are commonly associated with infection, even healthy individuals harbor a variety of organisms, as described in Table 4-35. In fact, the average person's body contains 10 times more bacterial cells than human cells. This symbiosis begins when membrane rupture allows flora from the vagina and surrounding environment to migrate into the previously sterile fetus. Neonates delivered by cesarean section have no flora but are rapidly colonized after birth. *Normal flora* are permanently resident microorganisms found in all people, whereas *colonization* indicates a temporary or long-term presence of certain organisms not considered part of the normal flora.

**TABLE 4-35.** **Location of Dominant Normal Flora**

| LOCATION | MICROORGANISM |
| --- | --- |
| Skin | *Staphylococcus epidermidis, Propionibacterium acnes* |
| Nose | *S epidermidis, Corynebacterium* (benign species), may be colonized by *Staphylococcus aureus* |
| Oropharynx | Viridans group streptococci |
| Dental plaque | *Streptococcus mutans* |
| Colon | *Bacteroides fragilis* > *E coli* |
| Vagina | *Lactobacillus,* colonized by group B streptococcus and *Escherichia coli* |

Neonates delivered by C-section have no flora, but are rapidly colonized after birth. All neonates receive vitamin K to prevent intraventricular hemorrhage, as gut flora are responsible for normal vitamin K production.

**CLINICAL CORRELATION**

Intussusception is the telescoping of bowel into itself and classically presents with intermittent pain and bloody stools (Figure 4-103). The "target sign" on ultrasound is classic.

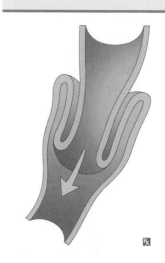

**FIGURE 4-103.** **Intussusception.** The telescoping of one segment of bowel into another.

**KEY FACT**

Vitamin K is essential for the production of clotting factors II, VII, IX, and X, as well as the anticoagulant proteins C and S.
Newborns receive vitamin K to prevent fatal hemorrhage.

**KEY FACT**

Glucocorticoids cause dose-dependent immunosuppression by blocking cytokine production and release, preventing leukocyte migration, impairing T-cell function, and inducing T-cell apoptosis.

**KEY FACT**

In a young adult with pharyngitis and tonsillar exudates, consider infectious mononucleosis caused by EBV. A positive monospot (heterophile antibody) test and atypical lymphocytes on blood smear are diagnostic. If the test is negative and the disease is prolonged, check for IgM and IgG against the viral capsid antigen (VCA) and IgG to nuclear antigen (EBNA).

**CLINICAL CORRELATION**

Group A strep commonly manifests itself with an erythematous throat, tonsillar exudates, and tender cervical lymphadenopathy. There is typically no cough.

**CLINICAL CORRELATION**

Children with epiglottitis often assume the "tripod position," or sitting upright with the neck extended to maximize airway patency. A lateral neck radiograph will show swelling of the epiglottis, dubbed the "thumbprint sign" (Figure 4-104).

## Beneficial Effects

By competing with pathogens, indigenous flora play an important role in **defense against infection.** Anaerobic bacteria in the intestines are a major source of **vitamin K,** help make **B vitamins,** and break down cellulose to aid digestion. The normal flora are essential for normal immune system development and probably have other significant functions still undiscovered.

## Role in Infection

Although usually harmless in their native environment, normal flora can cause infection if they migrate to otherwise sterile locations in the body or areas to which they are not indigenous. If the overall composition of the normal flora is altered, as by antibiotic use or immune deficiency, overgrowth of particular organisms can lead to disease. Chronic carriers harbor significant numbers of pathogenic organisms that can infect other persons.

- **UTIs** in sexually active women are often caused by intestinal *E coli* that spreads to the urinary bladder.
- **Endocarditis** can occur when viridans streptococci enter the bloodstream following dental procedures and lodge on susceptible heart valves.
- **Peritonitis** can occur when ruptured viscera from conditions such as appendicitis, diverticulitis, or a penetrating abdominal wound introduce mixed fecal bacteria into the peritoneal cavity.
- *C difficile* **(pseudomembranous) colitis** can develop when the composition of the normal flora of the GI tract is altered by **antibiotic therapy.** This leads to overgrowth of the opportunistic pathogen *C difficile,* whose toxin causes illness.
- **Candidiasis** is a fungal infection, commonly caused by *Candida albicans.* Vaginal candidiasis is common in women, and may or may not be secondary to antibiotic use. Oral candidiasis (thrush) may be an early sign of an immune deficiency, such as HIV/AIDS. Oral candidiasis may also be secondary to inhaled glucocorticoids, especially if the patient has not rinsed his/her mouth afterward.

### MICROBIAL DISEASES OF THE RESPIRATORY TRACT

## Upper Respiratory Infections

Infections of the upper respiratory tract (URIs) result from invasion of the oral and nasal cavities, sinuses, pharynx, and tonsils (Table 4-36). Middle respiratory tract infections involve the larynx, epiglottis, and trachea. Viruses are the most common cause of URIs. Bacteria may secondarily infect these tissues as a complication of a viral infection. Except for group A streptococcal pharyngitis, antibiotics are rarely indicated for URIs and should **not** be prescribed.

## Lower Respiratory Infections

Infections of the LRT involve the bronchi, bronchioles, alveoli, and extra-alveolar lung tissues. Bronchitis and bronchiolitis are, like URIs, more commonly caused by viruses than bacteria.

- **Laryngotracheal bronchitis (croup)** is most often caused by PIV. It classically manifests in a child who presents with a seal-like **barking cough.**
- **Pneumonia** is most often caused by bacteria and viruses, but fungi, mycobacteria, and parasites may also cause infection. Clues to the causative organism can be found in the patient's age (Table 4-37), where the infection was acquired (ie, community vs hospital), the patient's immune status, and other risk factors (Table 4-38).
- RSV

**TABLE 4-36.    Upper Respiratory Infections**

| SITE | COMMON ORGANISMS |
|------|------------------|
| Dental caries (cavities) | *Streptococcus mutans* |
| Periodontal (gum) disease | Anaerobic bacteria (*Bacteroides, Actinomyces, Prevotella*) |
| Rhinitis | Viruses (adenovirus, rhinovirus, coxsackie A, echovirus, influenza, RSV) |
| Acute sinusitis | *Streptococcus pneumoniae* or *Haemophilus influenzae* |
| Chronic sinusitis | More likely anaerobic organisms |
| Pharyngitis | Adenovirus, rhinovirus, coronavirus, influenza, Epstein-Barr virus, *Streptococcus pyogenes* ("strep throat") |
| Epiglottitis (Figure 4-104) | *Staphylococcus aureus* (*H influenzae* uncommon owing to vaccine) |

RSV, respiratory syncytial virus.

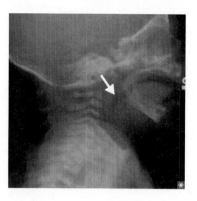

**FIGURE 4-104.    Thumbprint sign.** Radiographic thumbprint sign (arrow) of epiglottitis in a neonate.

## Community-Acquired Pneumonia

Causes of "**typical**" pneumonia include:

- *S pneumoniae*
- *H influenzae*
- *Moraxella catarrhalis*

Causes of "**atypical**" pneumonia include:

- *M pneumoniae* ("walking pneumonia")
- *Chlamydophila pneumoniae*
- *Legionella* (associated with contaminated aerosolized water, classically in air-conditioning systems)
- Viruses

**KEY FACT**

**Typical** community-acquired pneumonia is heralded by an abrupt onset of fever, chills or rigors, respiratory distress, and purulent or bloody sputum. Radiographs often demonstrate **lobar consolidation** (Figure 4-105) and the patient may have pleuritic chest pain.

**KEY FACT**

**Atypical** organisms cause diffuse interstitial disease, rather than lobar disease, and are characterized by the subacute onset of dry cough, malaise, myalgias, sore throat, fever, and headache. The chest film is usually either normal or shows diffuse rather than localized infiltrates.

**TABLE 4-37.    Causes of Pneumonia by Age Group**

| AGE GROUP | MOST LIKELY PATHOGEN | OTHER CAUSES |
|-----------|---------------------|--------------|
| Neonates (0–6 wk) | *Streptococcus agalactiae* (group B) | *E coli* <br> *Chlamydia trachomatis* |
| Children (6 wk–18 yr) | Viruses like respiratory syncytial virus (RSV), influenza, and parainfluenza | *Mycoplasma pneumoniae* <br> *Chlamydophila pneumoniae* <br> *Streptococcus pneumoniae* |
| Young adults (18–40 yr) | *M pneumoniae* <br> Viruses | *C pneumoniae* <br> *Streptococcus pneumoniae* |
| Older adults (40–65 yr) | *Streptococcus pneumoniae* <br> Viruses | *H influenzae* <br> *M pneumoniae* |
| Elderly (> 65 yr) | *Streptococcus pneumoniae* <br> Viruses | *H influenzae* <br> Gram-negative rods <br> *Moraxella catarrhalis* <br> *Mycobacterium tuberculosis* (reactivation) |

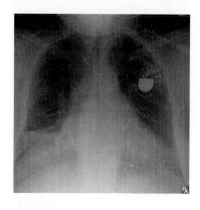

**FIGURE 4-105.    Pneumococcal pneumonia.** Well-defined infiltrate in the right middle lobe.

**TABLE 4-38.**    **Common Causes of Pneumonia in Special Groups**

| | |
|---|---|
| Alcoholic/IVDU | *Streptococcus pneumoniae, Klebsiella pneumoniae, Staphylococcus aureus* |
| Aspiration | Anaerobes (new right lower lobe infiltrate) |
| Atypical | Viruses, *Mycoplasma, Legionella, Chlamydophila pneumoniae* |
| Cystic fibrosis | *Pseudomonas, Staphylococcus aureus, Streptococcus pneumoniae, Burkholderia* |
| Immunocompromised | *Staphylococcus aureus,* enteric GNRs, fungi, viruses, PJP |
| Healthcare associated | *Staphylococcus aureus, Pseudomonas aeruginosa,* other GNRs |
| Postviral | *Staphylococcus aureus, Streptococcus pneumoniae, Haemophilus influenzae* |

GNRs, gram-negative rods; IVDU, IV drug user; PJP, *P jirovecii* pneumonia.

**KEY FACT**

Patients with epiglottitis require immediate intubation in the operating room in case there is a need for a surgical airway.

**Hospital-acquired (nosocomial) pneumonia** is most likely to be caused by *S aureus* as well as *P aeruginosa* and other gram-negative rods.

## MICROBIAL DISEASES OF THE CARDIOVASCULAR SYSTEM

### Infective Endocarditis

Infective endocarditis occurs when endothelial damage allows circulating microorganisms to colonize as a focal collection of platelets and fibrin on heart valves or other cardiac surfaces. Colonization leads to development of a **vegetation** and subsequent inflammatory, embolic, and immunologic complications. Clinical manifestations can include fever, heart murmur, and signs of systemic embolization such as painful indurated nodules on the fingers and toes (**Osler nodes**), painless erythematous macules on the palms and soles (**Janeway lesions**), red linear lesions in the nailbeds (**splinter hemorrhages**), retinal hemorrhages with clear centers (**Roth spots**) (Figure 4-106), and strokes. Septic emboli may localize to the distant sites and cause an abscess.

### Classification of Endocarditis

Endocarditis can be classified as **acute, subacute,** or **chronic,** depending on the virulence of the causative organism and the progression of the disease if no treatment is initiated (Table 4-39). The microbiology of native and prosthetic valve endocarditis is significantly different.

### Special Populations

**IV drug users** tend to get **right-sided** endocarditis, with vegetations on the **tricuspid** valve. Typical organisms in this population include *S aureus,* enteroccoci, gram-negative enteric bacilli, and *C albicans.*

**Prosthetic-valve** endocarditis is usually associated with gram-positive cocci such as *S aureus,* coagulase-negative staphylococci, and enterococci.

**HACEK** organisms are a group of gram-negative bacilli that are part of the normal oropharyngeal flora. They are slow-growing (mean and median time to detection of 3.4 and 3 days, respectively) and have a tendency to be involved in endocardial infections. These organisms cause infections in IV drug users who contaminate the needle or

**MNEMONIC**

**HACEK** (These organisms typically are culture negative.)

**H**aemophilus aphrophilus, H parainfluenzae, and H paraphrophilus
**A**ggregatibacter (formerly *Actinobacillus*) actinomycetemcomitans
**C**ardiobacterium hominis
**E**ikenella corrodens
**K**ingella kingae

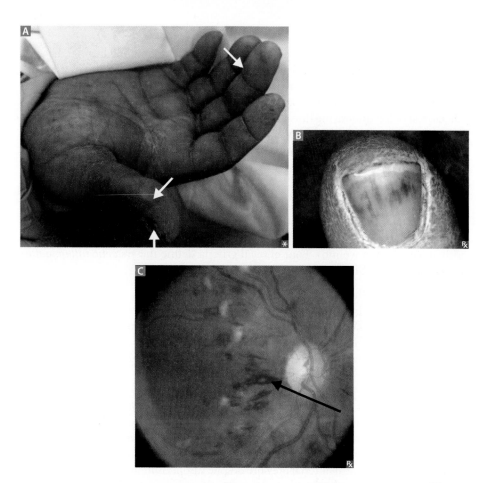

FIGURE 4-106. **Infective endocarditis.** A Janeway lesions; B splinter hemorrhage; C Roth spot.

injection site with saliva, as well as in patients with poor dental hygiene or preexisting valvular damage.

## MICROBIAL DISEASES OF THE BLOODSTREAM

### Bacteremia

Bacteremia is defined as the presence of viable bacteria in circulating blood. Transient bacteremia can occur during tooth brushing, menstruation, and other daily activities, but usually resolves quickly and asymptomatically secondary to leukocyte clearance of the bacteria.

**KEY FACT**

**Sepsis** is a life-threatening condition resulting from the immune response to bacteremia, characterized by fever, chills, and hypotension (shock).

TABLE 4-39. **Types of Endocarditis**

| TYPE OF ENDOCARDITIS | INCUBATION TIME | MOST COMMON CAUSE |
|---|---|---|
| Acute | Days to weeks | *Staphylococcus aureus;* β-hemolytic streptococci; gram-negative rods |
| Subacute | Weeks to months | Viridans streptococci; *Enterococcus*; occasionally fungi |
| Prosthetic valve | Varies | Coagulase-negative staphylococci and corynebacteria, in addition to the organisms associated with native-valve endocarditis |

### Key Sources of Bacteremia

Except in endocarditis and the transient daily bacteremias mentioned earlier, bacteremia is usually associated with a significant, localized infection elsewhere in the body. A common risk factor for bacteremia is an indwelling urinary catheter, which provides easy access for *E coli* to invade via the urinary tract. The microbiology of bacteremia reflects that of the underlying disease; bacteremia associated with pneumonia is caused by pneumonia pathogens (eg, *S pneumoniae*); bacteremia associated with abdominal trauma tends to be caused by colonic flora such as *E coli* and anaerobes. Bacteremia may also be due to infected hardware.

### Sepsis

Sepsis is defined as a systemic inflammatory state associated with either laboratory-confirmed bloodstream infection or an obvious source of contamination (eg, an obviously infected open wound). Four clinical criteria define the *systemic inflammatory response syndrome* (SIRS):

- Temperature, either > 38.5°C or < 35°C
- Heart rate, > 90 bpm
- Respiratory rate, either > 20 breaths per minute or measurement of the arterial $CO_2$ concentration < 32 mm Hg
- White blood cell count, > 12,000 cells/mm$^3$, < 4,000 cells/mm$^3$, or > 10% immature band forms

When two or more of these clinical criteria are present, the patient is said to have SIRS, which can result from noninfectious causes, and when SIRS is accompanied by infection, the patient has *sepsis*. This life-threatening condition can progress to severe sepsis (sepsis with acute organ failure), ***septic shock***, and refractory septic shock (septic shock with persistently low mean arterial pressure despite vasopressors and fluid resuscitation). The immediate goal in clinical management of sepsis is support of respiratory and cardiovascular function, followed by rapid administration of appropriate antimicrobial therapy.

Bacteremia in the setting of **gastrointestinal malignancy** may be due to *S bovis* and clostridia.

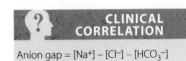

**KEY FACT**

Septic shock: Sepsis with hypotension despite adequate fluid resuscitation and pressors to maintain a mean arterial pressure > 65 mm Hg and a serum lactate > 2 mmol/L.

**CLINICAL CORRELATION**

Anion gap = [Na$^+$] – [Cl$^-$] – [HCO$_3^-$]

## MICROBIAL DISEASES OF THE GI TRACT

### Food-Poisoning Syndromes

Caused by eating food contaminated with bacterial toxins (Table 4-40) or live organisms (Table 4-41). Symptoms may include nausea, vomiting, abdominal cramps, diarrhea, fever, chills, weakness, and headache. Onset of symptoms varies with cause—from as few as 2–6 hours to 1 or 2 days after ingestion.

### Parasitic Causes of Diarrhea

**Amebiasis** is an infection caused by amoebae; *Entamoeba histolytica* is the primary pathogenic amoeba of humans. It is spread by cysts in fecally contaminated food and can lead to asymptomatic passage of cysts, nondysenteric infection characterized by watery diarrhea, or dysenteric infection characterized by **bloody diarrhea** and tenesmus, especially in malnourished or immunocompromised persons with "flask-shaped" lytic lesions elsewhere in the GI tract. This also causes right upper quadrant pain resulting from liver abscesses (typically in patients without diarrheal illness).

**TABLE 4-40.** Bacterial Sources of Food-Borne Illness

| ORGANISM | MECHANISM | DIARRHEA | ASSOCIATED FOODS | POINTS TO REMEMBER |
|---|---|---|---|---|
| *Bacillus cereus* | Preformed toxin | Nonbloody | Reheated rice and other starchy foods, undercooked meat or vegetables. | May cause emetic or diarrheal disease. Both *S aureus* and *B cereus* start and end relatively quickly. |
| *Campylobacter jejuni* | Bacterial infection | Bloody | Poultry, milk, contaminated water. | Most common invasive bacterial enterocolitis; produces crypt abscesses and ulcers resembling ulcerative colitis, causes explosive diarrhea with blood and/or mucus, may cause Guillain-Barré syndrome. Growth at 42°C (*Campylobacter* spp like the hot campfire). |
| *Clostridium botulinum* (adults) | Preformed toxin | Nonbloody | Inadequately preserved canned foods (bulging cans). | Neurotoxin binds synaptic vesicles in cholinergic nerves, blocks acetylcholine release, and causes paralysis and death. |
| *Clostridium botulinum* (infants) | Bacterial infection | Nonbloody | Honey. | Spores contaminate honey and germinate in infant's GI tract; neurotoxin blocks acetylcholine release and causes constipation and "floppy baby." |
| *Clostridium perfringens* | Preformed toxin | Nonbloody | Meat that is unrefrigerated or cooled too slowly. | Causes cramps and watery diarrhea lasting 24 hr. |
| *Listeria monocytogenes* | Bacterial infection | Nonbloody | Deli meats, unpasteurized milk and cheese. | Occurs sporadically, and rarely. Limited to pregnant and immunocompromised patients, though high mortality rate. |
| *Salmonella enteriditis* | Bacterial infection | Bloody (*Salmonella typhi* nonbloody) | Poultry, meat, fish, eggs. | Most common cause of noninvasive food poisoning in the United States; may cause watery or mucous diarrhea. Flagellar motility. Gallbladder is an important reservoir for organisms, thus cholecystectomy is indicated for asymptomatic carriers. Otherwise, not typically treated with antibiotics, as this may prolong the carrier state. |
| *Shigella dysenteriae* | Bacterial infection | Bloody | Raw vegetables. | Very small inoculum required to cause disease; often fecal-oral. |
| *Staphylococcus aureus* | Preformed toxin | Nonbloody | Potato salad, custard, mayonnaise, meats left at room temperature. | Severe vomiting and diarrhea appear 2–6 hr after ingestion. |
| *Vibrio cholera* | Preformed toxin | Nonbloody | Water, vegetables, seafood. | Rice-water diarrhea. Rehydration is critical. |
| *Vibrio parahaemolyticus, Vibrio vulnificus* | Bacterial infection | Nonbloody | Raw or undercooked seafood (usually oysters). | Causes vomiting and watery diarrhea that are self-limited. *V vulnificus* can also cause wound infections from contact with contaminated shellfish. |

See Table 4-42 for a more in-depth discussion of *E coli* infection.

Bloody diarrhea should always raise your suspicion of inflammatory bowel disease, *Salmonella, Shigella, Yersinia, E coli, Campylobacter,* and *Entamoeba*.

**TABLE 4-41.    Bacterial Causes of Non-Food-Borne Illness**

| ORGANISM | PATHOGENESIS | POINTS TO REMEMBER |
|---|---|---|
| Cholera (*Vibrio cholerae*) | Comma-shaped organism spread via fecal-oral route, usually through **contaminated water.** Cholera toxin activates **adenylate cyclase,** increases intracellular cAMP, and increases secretion of ions and water into the GI tract. | Secretory, "rice-water" diarrhea with a non-gap acidosis. May see dehydration, hypokalemia. Treatment includes oral rehydration therapy. Very rare in the United States. |
| *Shigella* | Spread through fecal-oral route. Invade colon, release shiga toxin, which inhibits the 60S ribosome and kills intestinal epithelial cells. | May see blood and pus in stool. A very small number of organisms may lead to widespread infection. Treatment: ciprofloxacin. |
| *Clostridium difficile* | Typically due to the death of normal intestinal flora secondary to antibiotic administration. The bacterium produces an enterotoxin and cytotoxin, leading to exudates (Figure 4-6). | Fever, cramping, severe diarrhea with or without blood. Creamy white/green **pseudomembranes** on colonoscopy. Diagnosis: Stool toxin assay. Treatment: PO/IV metronidazole or PO vancomycin. |
| *Yersinia enterocolitica* | May be spread via the fecal-oral route, ingestion of raw or contaminated pork, unpasteurized milk, contaminated water. | Bloody diarrhea, associated with outbreaks in daycare centers. May have right lower quadrant pain-- "pseudoappendicitis." |
| *Escherichia coli* | Normal bacteria acquires virulence factors. | See Table 4-42. |

**Giardiasis** is caused by the protozoan parasite *Giardia lamblia*, which is a single-celled parasite with a prominent ventral sucking disk and flagella (Figure 4-107). Patients may ingest cysts from **open water,** including clear-running mountain streams. Many patients remain asymptomatic; however, symptomatic disease can range from a self-limited acute diarrhea to severe chronic diarrhea. The diarrhea, when present, is typically greasy and light-colored. Treatment is with metronidazole.

**Cryptosporidiosis** is caused by protozoa of the genus *Cryptosporidium*, predominantly *C parvum* and *C hominis*. Ingestion of oocysts from fecally contaminated water results in infection of the brush border of the intestine, leading to a self-limited diarrheal illness in immunocompetent patients. In immunocompromised patients, however, the diarrhea is often severe and unrelenting. In HIV-infected patients HAART should be initiated to boost immunity. Treatment may include nitazoxanide.

**TABLE 4-42.    Types of *Escherichia coli* Causing Gastroenteritis**

| ORGANISM | VIRULENCE FACTOR | CLINICAL FEATURES |
|---|---|---|
| Enteropathogenic *E coli* [EPEC] | Bacteria adhere to intestinal epithelial cells and prevent fluid absorption. | Secretory diarrhea associated with epidemics in infants. |
| Enteroaggregative *E coli* [EAEC] | Aggregates of bacteria adhere to intestinal epithelial cells and prevent fluid absorption. | Secretory diarrhea—one cause of traveler's diarrhea. |
| Enterotoxigenic *E coli* [ETEC] | Heat-stable enterotoxin activates guanylate cyclase, inhibiting intestinal fluid uptake; heat-labile enterotoxin activates adenylate cyclase, stimulating hypersecretion of fluids (just like cholera toxin). | Secretory diarrhea (up to 20 L/day), most common cause of traveler's diarrhea. |
| Enterohemorrhagic *E coli* [EHEC] | Shiga-toxin positive, often type O157:H7. Has a very low $ID_{50}$ (10–100 organisms). Causes HUS in up to 10% of infected kids. Recognition of EHEC is critical, as antibiotic therapy causes **increased** morbidity and mortality. | Inflammatory diarrhea and dysentery and HUS. |
| Enteroinvasive *E coli* [EIEC] | Bacteria invade the epithelial cells lining the colon, then replicate and destroy the cells; also produces small amounts of Shiga-like toxin. | Inflammatory diarrhea. |

HUS, hemolytic-uremic syndrome; $ID_{50}$, median infective dose.

### Viral Causes of Diarrhea

Viral gastroenteritis is spread via the fecal-oral route. Viruses cause diarrhea by invading the intestinal epithelial cells and multiplying intracellularly. As they subvert host cell metabolism, fluid transport is disrupted, and cell destruction occurs, leading to decreased fluid reabsorption. The resulting nausea, vomiting, and watery diarrhea are usually self-limited but can lead to life-threatening dehydration in patients who are very young, malnourished, or immunocompromised.

- **Rotavirus** is the most common cause of diarrhea in children. Its incidence increases during the winter. Stool antigen testing may aid the diagnosis.
- **Norwalk virus** is a common cause of diarrheal outbreaks among adults and children, particularly on cruise ships, in nursing homes, and at camps.
- **Astrovirus** is an important cause of diarrhea in children younger than 1 year.
- **CMV** is an important cause of colitis, which produces chronic watery diarrhea in patients with HIV/AIDS and other profoundly immunosuppressed patients. Visualization of ulcers on colonoscopy may aid diagnosis.

## MICROBIAL DISEASES OF THE URINARY AND REPRODUCTIVE SYSTEMS

Infections commonly occur as a result of fecal contamination, sexual transmission, or as a complication of medical instrumentation (eg, catheterization).

### Urinary Tract Infections

Defined by the presence of bacteria in the urine (bacteriuria) in combination with symptoms such as dysuria, urgency, and frequency, as well as suprapubic pain and WBCs (but not WBC casts) in the urine. The urinary tract is normally sterile, but infection is frequently caused by ascension of bacteria such as *E coli* into the bladder via the urethra. Any cause of urinary stasis, such as a tumor, stone, enlarged prostate, neurogenic bladder, catheterization, diabetes, recent kidney surgery, or the presence of a foreign body can predispose to UTI. Common causative organisms are listed in Table 4-43.

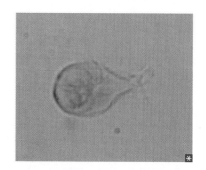

**FIGURE 4-107.** *Giardia lamblia* **trophozoites.** Wet mount stained with iodine.

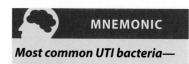

### MNEMONIC

**Most common UTI bacteria— SSEEK PP**

**S** marcescens
**S** taphylococcus saprophyticus
**E** coli
**E** cloacae
**K** pneumoniae
**P** aeruginosa
**P** mirabilis

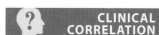

### CLINICAL CORRELATION

WBC casts are pathognomonic for pyelonephritis.

**TABLE 4-43.** **Bacteria Causing Urinary Tract Infections**

| SPECIES | FEATURES |
|---|---|
| *Escherichia coli* | Leading cause of UTI. Colonies show green metallic sheen on EMB agar |
| *Staphylococcus saprophyticus* | 2nd leading cause of UTI in sexually active women |
| *Klebsiella pneumoniae* | 3rd leading cause of UTI. Large mucoid capsule and viscous colonies |
| *Serratia marcescens* | Some strains produce a red pigment; often nosocomial and drug resistant |
| *Enterococcus* | Often nosocomial and drug resistant |
| *Proteus mirabilis* | Motility causes "swarming" on agar; produces urease; associated with struvite stones |
| *Pseudomonas aeruginosa* | Blue-green pigment and fruity odor; usually nosocomial and drug resistant |

EMB, eosin methylene blue.

Modified with permission from Le T, et al. *First Aid for the USMLE Step 1, 2017.* New York, NY: McGraw-Hill, 2017.

A urine sample should be obtained **midstream** after the initial urine in the urethra has been voided. Bacterial counts are highest in the first morning void as the bacteria have multiplied overnight and the sample is likely to be relatively concentrated. Classically, a value of $10^5$ colony-forming units (CFU) of *E coli* per milliliter is considered the cutoff to establish infection, but in samples collected by suprapubic aspirate CFUs as low as $10^2$ are associated with symptoms. In the typical well-collected, midstream urine sample, a useful rule of thumb is that a single isolate in a concentration of $10^4$–$10^5$ may be pathogenic; at a concentration $> 10^5$ it's probably pathogenic.

**Women,** especially sexually active young women, are at risk for developing UTIs because of the short length of the female urethra and the presence of fecal bacteria in female perineal flora. UTIs are 10 times more common in women than in men. Uncomplicated UTIs in the outpatient setting can be treated empirically with TMP-SMX, nitrofurantoin, or fluoroquinolones. Causative organisms include:

- Uropathogenic *E coli* (70–95%)
- *S saprophyticus* (10–15%)
- *K pneumoniae* and other gram-negative rods; occasionally yeasts.

**Hospitalized patients** are at increased risk for developing UTIs, typically secondary to the presence of Foley catheters. This is the most common hospital-acquired infection. *E coli* remains the most common causative organism, but other causative organisms, such as *Proteus, Klebsiella, Serratia, Pseudomonas, Enterobacter, Enterococcus,* and yeasts, are seen much more frequently than in outpatients. Urine culture should be performed in hospitalized patients to determine the specific bacteria causing the infection.

**Pregnancy** is frequently associated with asymptomatic bacteriuria from both pelvic compression by the fetus causing urinary stasis and high circulating levels of progesterone causing urinary tract dilation. Bacteriuria during pregnancy is a risk factor for pyelonephritis and also increases the risk for preterm labor and low birth weight. Because of these risks, bacteriuria in pregnant women is treated as if it were a true UTI, whereas otherwise bacteriuria without symptoms represents normal flora or colonization, and treatment is ineffective, or even harmful. Pregnant women should be screened for bacteriuria early in pregnancy and should always be treated, regardless of the presence of symptoms.

**Children with recurrent UTIs** should be evaluated for vesicoureteral reflux (VUR) and other congenital abnormalities. Frequent UTIs or other pelvic infections in children raise the concern for child abuse. UTIs in otherwise healthy men are also often associated with urinary tract pathology.

### Sexually Transmitted Infections

Sexually transmitted infections (STIs) are among the most common infectious diseases in the United States today. Because they share a common mechanism of transmission, it is not uncommon for a patient to present with more than one infection simultaneously. In many cases, individuals are asymptomatic while carrying (and transmitting) these infections. Women in particular are at risk for developing serious complications, such as pelvic inflammatory disease (PID), from even asymptomatic STIs. These infections are summarized in Table 4-44.

**Chlamydia** is the most commonly reported STI in the United States and is a leading cause of infertility in women. The causative organism, *C trachomatis,* is an obligate intracellular bacterium with 15 immunotypes. Immunotypes D–K cause genital tract infections and immunotypes L1–L3 cause genital ulcers (lymphogranuloma venereum). Most cases of chlamydia infection are **asymptomatic,** but the disease may cause dysuria and mucopurulent discharge from the urethra as well as subacute PID.

**TABLE 4-44. Sexually Transmitted Infections**

| DISEASE | ORGANISM | CLINICAL FEATURES | TREATMENT |
|---|---|---|---|
| Chlamydia | *Chlamydia trachomatis* (D–K) | Urethritis, cervicitis, conjunctivitis, pelvic inflammatory disease (PID), infertility, reactive arthritis (Reiter syndrome). | Doxycycline for 7 days or single-dose azithromycin. |
| Lymphogranuloma venereum | *C trachomatis* (L1–L3) | Ulcers, lymphadenopathy, rectal strictures. | Doxycycline for 21 days. |
| Gonorrhea | *Neisseria gonorrhoeae* | Urethritis, cervicitis, PID, prostatitis, epididymitis, arthritis, creamy purulent discharge. | Ceftriaxone (also treat for possible *Chlamydia*). |
| Primary syphilis (weeks) | *Treponema pallidum* | Painless chancre for several weeks. | Single dose of benzathine penicillin G IM. |
| Secondary syphilis (weeks to months) | *T pallidum* | Rash (affecting palms and soles), fever, lymphadenopathy, condylomata lata (weeks to months later). | Single dose of benzathine penicillin G IM. |
| Tertiary syphilis (years) | *T pallidum* | Gummas, aortitis. Meningitis, tabes dorsalis, general paresis, Argyll-Robertson pupils (years later). | Three doses of benzathine penicillin G IM. 10–14 days of aqueous crystalline penicillin G IV. |
| Genital herpes | Herpes simplex virus (usually HSV-2) | Painful penile, vulvar, or cervical ulcers; can cause systemic symptoms such as fever, headache, myalgia. | Acyclovir, famciclovir, or valacyclovir. Valacyclovir may be taken prophylactically depending on frequency of outbreaks. |
| AIDS | Human immunodeficiency virus (HIV) | Opportunistic infections, Kaposi sarcoma, lymphoma. | Highly active antiretroviral therapy (HAART). |
| Acute HIV | Human immunodeficiency virus (HIV) | Flulike symptoms, lymphadenopathy, diarrhea. | Highly active antiretroviral therapy (HAART). |
| Condylomata acuminata | Human papillomavirus (HPV), types 6 and 11 | Genital warts. | Cryotherapy or surgical excision. |
| Cervical cancer | Human papillomavirus (HPV), types 16, 18, 31, 33, and others | | Vaccine (prevention). Surgery, radiation, systemic therapy (depending on extent of disease). |
| Hepatitis B | Hepatitis B virus | Jaundice, liver failure. | Interferon-$\alpha$ (INF-$\alpha$), lamivudine, adefovir, or entecavir. |
| Chancroid | *Haemophilus ducreyi* | Painful genital ulcer, inguinal lymphadenopathy. | Azithromycin, ceftriaxone, or ciprofloxacin. |
| Granuloma inguinale (donovanosis) | *Klebsiella granulomatis* | Small papule or painless beefy red ulcer with rolled edges that bleed easily. | Doxycycline for 3–5 weeks until lesions resolve. |
| Bacterial vaginosis | *Gardnerella vaginalis*, anaerobes | Noninflammatory, clue cells, malodorous discharge (fishy smell); positive whiff test. | Metronidazole or clindamycin. |
| Trichomoniasis | *Trichomonas vaginalis* | Vaginitis, frothy vaginal discharge, "strawberry cervix." | Metronidazole (for patient and partners). |

IM, intramuscular.

**Gonorrhea** is a common STI characterized by acute **purulent urethral discharge** and painful or difficult urination. In contrast to chlamydia, gonorrheal PID is typically acute and associated with high fever. It is caused by *N gonorrhoeae*, aerobic gram-negative cocci that are characteristically coffee bean–shaped in pairs. Because coinfection with *C trachomatis* is common, patients diagnosed with gonorrhea should also be treated for chlamydia infection.

PID can be a serious complication of STIs in women. Chlamydia infection and gonorrhea are the most common primary causes, either alone or in combination. Organisms infecting the vagina and cervix ascend the female genital tract and cause disease in the uterus, fallopian tubes, and ovaries. The infection progresses to form scar tissue and adhesions. Sequelae can include **ectopic pregnancy, hydrosalpinx, tubo-ovarian abscess (TOA), infertility,** and **chronic pelvic pain.** Another complication is **Fitz-Hugh–Curtis syndrome** resulting from peritoneal spread of infection to the liver capsule with characteristic "violin string" adhesions of parietal peritoneum to liver. Serious PID is often polymicrobial in origin, when normal urogenital flora proliferate within the fallopian tubes and ovaries behind scarring and blockage associated with chlamydia or gonorrhea.

### Vaginal Infections

Vaginitis often manifests with symptoms such as itching, burning, irritation, and abnormal discharge. The three most common causes of vaginitis are bacterial vaginosis, candidiasis, and trichomoniasis, which together account for more than 90% of cases. Several diagnostic criteria used to differentiate these infections are listed in Table 4-45.

**Bacterial vaginosis** is the most common cause of vaginitis. It is caused by an overgrowth of organisms such as *G vaginalis, Mobiluncus, Mycoplasma hominis,* and *Peptostreptococcus.* It can manifest with a thin, white, adherent vaginal discharge, which releases a fishy odor when mixed with KOH (positive whiff test). Diagnosis is confirmed by saline wet mount showing epithelial cells covered in bacteria **(clue cells),** as seen in Figure 4-20.

**Candidiasis** is a fungal infection that can be associated with douching, antibiotic use, immunodeficiency, or idiopathic causes. Isolated frequent vaginal yeast infections should not necessarily be a cause for concern.

**Trichomoniasis** is an STI that produces a frothy vaginal discharge and a characteristic "strawberry cervix" due to punctate petechial hemorrhages dotting the cervix. This is a flagellated organism with "corkscrew" motility on wet prep. The protozoan can be isolated from up to 80% of male partners of infected women; therefore, both the patient and her partner(s) should be treated.

**TABLE 4-45.    Diagnostic Characteristics of Common Vaginal Infections**

|  | NORMAL | BACTERIAL VAGINOSIS | CANDIDIASIS | TRICHOMONIASIS |
|---|---|---|---|---|
| Complaints | None | Discharge, odor | Discharge, **itching** | Frothy discharge, itching, odor |
| Discharge | White, clear, flocculent | Thin, adherent, white-gray, homogeneous | White, curd-like | White to yellow-green, frothy |
| Amine odor | Absent | Present (fishy) | Absent | Variable |
| Microscopic | Lactobacilli | Clue cells, cocci | Budding yeast and pseudohyphae | Trichomonads |
| Vaginal pH | 3.8–4.2 | > 4.5 | < 4.5 | > 4.5 |

## Infections During Pregnancy

A number of infections can cause severe congenital problems if a patient contracts them during pregnancy. The acronym ToRCHHeS (toxoplasmosis, rubella, CMV, HIV, herpes, syphilis) identifies infectious diseases commonly screened for during pregnancy. Nonspecific findings common to many of these infections include hepatosplenomegaly, jaundice, thrombocytopenia, and growth retardation.

**Toxoplasmosis** is a parasitic disease contracted by eating undercooked meat or being exposed to aerosolized cat feces. It is usually asymptomatic or causes a mild flulike illness in healthy adults; however, when transmitted to the neonate, it can result in the classic "triad" of chorioretinitis, hydrocephalus, and intracranial calcification, often accompanied by mental retardation and/or or seizures.

All pregnant patients should be screened for **HIV.** Antiretroviral therapy with ZDV greatly reduces the likelihood that the virus will be transmitted to the fetus during pregnancy and delivery (from 25% to approximately 8%). HIV-positive women should be counseled not to breast feed their babies. The best way to prevent vertical transmission of HIV is through HAART.

**Rubella** is a viral infection typically transmitted via respiratory droplets that causes a mild rash and flulike illness in healthy adults. During the first trimester of pregnancy, however, it can lead to miscarriage, stillbirth, or serious birth defects. Congenital rubella syndrome includes the classic "triad" of **heart malformations** (most often patent ductus arteriosus or pulmonary hypoplasia), deafness, and cataracts. Other common manifestations include mental retardation and a "blueberry muffin" rash.

**CMV** infection can be transmitted during delivery or via breast milk. Usually asymptomatic or producing a heterophile-negative mononucleosis-like illness in adults; infected neonates may develop hearing loss, seizures, and mental retardation, and chorioretinitis.

**Herpes** is a common viral infection causing painful mucosal ulcers. A neonate typically becomes infected while passing through the birth canal during an active maternal outbreak. This leads to an often fatal neonatal encephalitis with widespread herpetic (vesicular) lesions of the skin and eye. Therefore, any mother with an active outbreak should undergo cesarean section.

**Syphilis** is an STI with a wide variety of clinical manifestations in adults. During pregnancy, treponemes can pass through the placenta to the fetus. Approximately 50% of these fetuses are aborted or stillborn. The remainder may present with the **Hutchinson triad** of notched teeth, eighth cranial nerve deafness, and interstitial keratitis. Infected infants may also present with other syphilitic stigmata such as a saddle nose, short maxilla, saber shins, and severe hydrops fetalis.

**Other** infections include parvovirus B19 (causes hydrops fetalis), group B streptococcus, and listeria (both are important causes of neonatal sepsis and meningitis).

## MICROBIAL DISEASES OF THE BONES, JOINTS, AND SKIN

### Osteomyelitis

#### Infection of the Bone

Osteomyelitis can occur as a result of trauma, postsurgical infection, hematogenous spread of bacteria into the bone (more common in children), invasion of the bone from a contiguous source of infection (more common in adults), or skin breakdown in the setting of vascular insufficiency. Direct spread from a soft tissue infection is most com-

**MNEMONIC**

**ToRCHHeS**

**To**xoplasma—Avoid domestic cats and cat litter during pregnancy.

**R**ubella—Screen for IgG immunity; vaccinate postpartum if nonimmune.

**C**MV—Amniocentesis for PCR if confirmed primary maternal infection.

**H**IV—Screen with ELISA test using an "opt-out" approach; treat with antiretroviral drugs to reduce transmission.

**He**rpes—Deliver by cesarean section if the mother has active lesions in the birth canal.

**S**yphilis—Screen with VDRL or RPR; confirm with FTA-Abs.

**MNEMONIC**

**Toxoplasmosis complications— CHIC**

**C**horioretinitis
**H**ydrocephalus
**I**ntracranial **C**alcifications

**QUESTION**

A woman with purulent vaginal discharge gets a swab taken for culture. There are no organisms, but many WBCs. What infection does she likely have?

**KEY FACT**

MRI is the best for detecting acute infection and detailing anatomic involvement (Figure 4-108 **A**). Radiographs are insensitive early on but may be used in chronic cases (Figure 4-108 **B**).

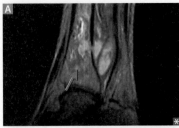
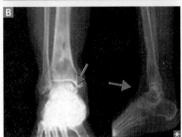

**FIGURE 4-108. Osteomyelitis.** Arrows point to areas of chronic inflammation.

mon in adults, whereas hematogenous spread is more common in children. Osteomyelitis is far more common in children. The most common cause of osteomyelitis overall is *S aureus* (*S pyogenes* is second), although certain populations may be predisposed to infection with other organisms (Table 4-46). Inflammatory markers CRP and ESR are typically elevated.

### Infectious Arthritis

Bacterial invasion of a joint. *S aureus* and *N gonorrhoeae* are the first and second most common causes, respectively, of infectious arthritis in adults. The disease typically affects a single large joint, producing pain, tenderness, warmth, and erythema. The synovial fluid is thick and cloudy with many white blood cells, although bacteria may not be evident on Gram stains or cultures.

Lyme disease is another significant cause of septic arthritis in endemic areas. The arthritis of Lyme may be mono- or polyarticular, and Gram stains and cultures are negative. Gonococcal arthritis may be a migratory polyarthritis.

### Cellulitis

Cellulitis is an acute, spreading infection of the skin extending into the deep dermis and subcutaneous tissues. Group A streptococci and *S aureus* are the most common causes.

**Erysipelas** involves the superficial dermis and dermal lymphatics. It most commonly manifests on the legs with lesions that are bright red, edematous, and indurated with a sharp, raised border. It is almost always caused by group A streptococci.

**Erythrasma** is a superficial infection caused by *Corynebacterium*. Scaly plaques are present between the toes, and erythematous plaques are found in the intertriginous areas. Diagnosis is confirmed with the Wood's lamp.

**TABLE 4-46. Osteomyelitis Risk Factors and Associated Infections**

| RISK FACTOR | ASSOCIATED INFECTION |
|---|---|
| Sexually active | *Neisseria gonorrhea* (rare, more likely to cause septic arthritis than osteomyelitis) |
| Sickle cell disease | *Salmonella* and *S aureus* |
| Prosthetic joint replacement | *S aureus* and *S epidermidis* |
| Vertebral involvement | *S aureus*, *M tuberculosis* (Pott disease) |
| Cat and dog bites | *Pasteurella multocida* (Do not primarily close the wound. Doing so prevents drainage and may lead to abscess formation in these wounds.) |
| IV drug abuse | *Pseudomonas, Candida, S aureus* |
| No information available | Assume *S aureus* (most common) |
| Skull base involvement | *Pseudomonas* (malignant otitis externa in diabetics), *Mucor* and *Rhizopus* species (invasive fungal sinusitis in diabetics and immunosuppressed patients) |

IV, intravenous.

### Erythema Chronicum Migrans; Lyme Disease

This characteristic target-shaped rash is indicative of **Lyme disease,** caused by the spirochete *B burgdorferi* and transmitted by *Ixodes* ticks in the United States. The rash may be accompanied by nonspecific constitutional symptoms in the first stage. Later manifestations include migratory arthralgias, meningitis, facial nerve palsy, AV nodal block, and arthritis. The diagnosis of Lyme disease at the ECM stage (prior to the development of antibody) is clinical, based on exposure history and the characteristic rash. The organism is difficult to culture and culturing is not routinely performed. For systemic syndromes consistent with Lyme disease, serology is the mainstay of diagnosis; IgM antibody appears within a month of infection, and IgG persists for many years. Despite a great deal of controversy in the popular literature, scientific evidence supports Lyme serology as a reliable diagnostic test, similar to other serodiagnostic methods. In addition, there is no evidence that prolonged antibiotic therapy, as given by some practitioners, provides benefit in chronic Lyme disease.

## MICROBIAL DISEASES OF THE EYE AND EAR

### Conjunctivitis

**Children and neonates** are particularly susceptible to conjunctivitis. Neonatal conjunctivitis can be classified according to its temporal presentation after birth:

- **Day 1:** Silver nitrate susceptibility.
- **Days 1–4:** *N gonorrhoeae.* Manifests with **hyperpurulent exudates.**
- **Days 3–10:** *C trachomatis.* Manifests with purulent exudates. Microscopic evaluation reveals **inclusion bodies** in cells. This infection may progress to blindness if left untreated.

### Postneonatal Period and Childhood

Purulent exudates suggest infection with *H influenzae* or *S pneumoniae.* Watery exudates and sore throat with recent swimming pool exposure suggest **a**denovirus ("pink eye").

- **Contact lens wearers** can develop conjunctivitis after leaving contacts in their eyes for long periods of time (*Pseudomonas*) or from using homemade saline (*Acanthamoeba*).
- **Conjunctivitis with vision loss** may be caused by *C trachomatis,* types A, B, and C. These immunotypes are uncommon in the United States, but chronic infection commonly causes corneal scarring and blindness in less developed countries.

### Otitis

**Otitis externa** is most commonly caused by *P aeruginosa* and *S aureus,* though many cases are polymicrobial. It causes severe tenderness and pain upon manipulation of the pinna. Swimmers and diabetics are at increased risk for this infection. Treatment is with antibiotic drops (typically an aminoglycoside or fluoroquinolone), with or without steroids.

**Otitis media** is an exceedingly common infection in children under the age of 6 years. It usually arises as a complication of a viral URT infection. Secretions and inflammation cause a relative obstruction of the eustachian tubes. As the mucosa of the middle ear absorbs air that cannot be replaced because of this obstruction, negative pressure is generated, and a serous effusion develops (Figure 4-109). This provides a fertile medium for bacterial growth. Common causal organisms include *S pneumoniae, H influenzae, Moraxella,* and viruses. Although otitis media with effusion is less prone to resolve with antibiotic therapy, AOM responds well to antibiotics, such as amoxicillin.

**CLINICAL CORRELATION**

It is imperative to distinguish conjunctivitis from preseptal (anterior to the septum) and orbital (posterior to the septum) cellulitis. Orbital cellulitis is a medical emergency and can be delineated by complaints of pain upon eye movement and visual symptoms.

**MNEMONIC**

*In chronologic order of presentation—*

**S**ome **N**eonates **C**an **H**ardly **S**ee **A**nything

**S**ilver nitrate susceptibility
***N*** *gonorrhoeae*
***C*** *trachomatis*
***H*** *influenzae*
***S*** *pneumoniae*
**A**denovirus

**CLINICAL CORRELATION**

Children older than 6 months should receive antibiotic therapy if they present with unilateral severe symptoms (otalgia 2 or more days, fever higher than 39°C). If nonsevere unilateral symptoms, may observe with appropriate follow-up. Bilateral acute otitis media (AOM) and AOM in children younger than 6 months should always be treated.

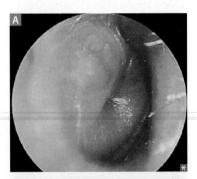
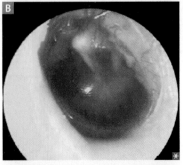
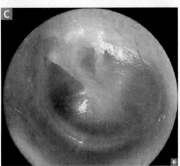

**FIGURE 4-109.    Three diagnostic categories of otitis media.** A Acute otitis media (AOM); B otitis media with effusion (OME); C and no effusion (NOE). AOM has a bulging, erythematous tympanic membrane, while OME has opacification of the tympanic membrane and possible air-fluid levels.

## MICROBIAL DISEASES OF THE NERVOUS SYSTEM

### Meningitis

Inflammation of the leptomeninges and underlying CSF. Symptoms include headache; fever; nuchal rigidity; and neurologic abnormalities including altered mental status, cranial nerve dysfunction, and seizures. As with pneumonia, the common causes of meningitis can be grouped according to the age of the patient (Table 4-47). The incidence of *H influenzae* type B meningitis, formerly the most common cause of meningitis in children, has declined significantly with the introduction of vaccine programs in the past 15–20 years. Bacterial, viral, and fungal causes of meningitis can be differentiated by characteristic patterns of the patient's CSF testing, as summarized in Table 4-48.

**HIV/AIDS** is associated with meningitis and other CNS manifestations caused by opportunistic pathogens such as *Cryptococcus*, *Toxoplasma*, CMV, and JC virus (progressive multifocal leukoencephalopathy).

### Brain Abscess

Suppurative infection of the brain parenchyma, usually ring-enhancing. Usually due to streptococci, staphylococci, and anaerobes (frequently polymicrobial). Toxoplasmosis and neurocysticercocis should be considered in the appropriate epidemiologic setting.

Brain abscesses may result from direct spread from a head/neck infection, direct inoculation (trauma), or hematogenous.

### Encephalitis

Usually due to HSV or arboviruses. Clinical manifestations usually include altered consciousness, headache, fever, and seizures. The presence of RBCs in the CSF without a history of trauma is pathognomonic for HSV encephalitis, although other infectious etiologies and subarachnoid hemorrhage must be considered. MRI may show temporal lobe abnormalities.

## NOSOCOMIAL INFECTIONS

Table 4-49 summarizes the pathogens commonly associated with various hospital-related risk factors.

**TABLE 4-47    Causes of Meningitis by Age Group**

| AGE GROUP | MOST COMMON PATHOGENS | OTHER CAUSES |
| --- | --- | --- |
| Newborn (0–6 mo) | Group B streptococci, *E coli* | *Listeria* |
| Children (6 mo–6 yr) | *Streptococcus pneumoniae* | *Neisseria meningitides* *Haemophilus influenzae* type B Enteroviruses |
| 6–60 yr | *N meningitidis* *S pneumoniae* | Enteroviruses Herpes simplex virus |
| Elderly (> 60 yr) | *S pneumoniae* | Gram-negative rods *Listeria* |

**TABLE 4-48. Cerebrospinal Spinal Fluid Findings in Meningitis**

| CAUSE | PRESSURE | CELL TYPE | PROTEIN | GLUCOSE |
|---|---|---|---|---|
| Bacterial | ↑ | ↑ PMNs | ↑ | ↓ |
| Fungal/TB | ↑ | ↑ Lymphocytes | ↑ | ↓ |
| Viral | Normal/↑ | ↑ Lymphocytes | Normal/↑ | Normal |

PMNs, polymorphonuclear leukocytes; TB, tuberculosis.

# Antimicrobials

## ANTIBACTERIAL DRUGS

Drugs may be characterized as either bactericidal or bacteriostatic, which is important for understanding the action of individual drugs as well as the synergistic or antagonistic effects of certain drug combinations. It is important to remember that exceptions exist where a drug that is usually bactericidal (or -static) may act in a different manner when used against certain bacteria or in certain organs. Figure 4-110 illustrates the sites of action of the drugs in the bacterial cell.

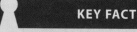

**KEY FACT**

Using two drugs that are both either bactericidal or bacteriostatic is often **synergistic** (eg, penicillin/aminoglycoside or TMP-SMX). Using a bacteriostatic drug with a bactericidal drug is often **antagonistic** (eg, penicillin/tetracycline).

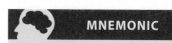

**MNEMONIC**

**Bacteriostatic:**

**ECSTaTiC**: **E**rythromycin, **C**lindamycin, **S**ulfamethoxazole, **T**rimethoprim, **T**etracyclines, **C**hloramphenicol

**Bactericidal:**

**V**ery **F**inely **P**roficient **A**t **C**ell **M**urder: **V**ancomycin, **F**luoroquinolones, **P**enicillin, **A**minoglycosides, **C**ephalosporins, **M**etronidazole

**TABLE 4-49. Healthcare Associated Infections**

| INFECTION | RISK FACTOR | PATHOGEN | SIGNS/SYMPTOMS |
|---|---|---|---|
| Aspiration pneumonia | Altered mental status | Polymicrobial, often gram-negative rods and anaerobes. | Purulent, malodorous sputum, new right lower/middle lobe infiltrate. |
| *Clostridium difficile* colitis | Antibiotic use (classically clindamycin, although many antibiotics are associated) | *Clostridium difficile.* | Watery diarrhea, leukocytosis, pseudomembranous colitis. |
| Infected wounds | Decubitus ulcers, recent surgery, drains | *Staphylococcus aureus*, gram-negative anaerobes. | Erythema, tenderness, purulence, induration from the wound site. |
| Catheter-associated bloodstream infections | IVs, catheters, and other lines | *S aureus, Staphylococcus epidermidis* (long term), *Enterobacter.* | Erythema, tenderness, purulence, induration from access site. |
| Ventilator-associated pneumonia | Mechanical ventilation, endotracheal intubation, recent surgery | *Pseudomonas, Acinetobacter, Klebsiella, S aureus.* | New infiltrate on chest x-ray, purulent sputum production. |
| Workplace-associated infections | Renal dialysis unit, needle stick injury | Hepatitis B virus, although HIV and HCV can be transmitted too. | Acute HIV infection: flulike symptoms, lymphadenopathy. Acute hepatitis may show fatigue, nausea, dark urine, abdominal discomfort, jaundice. |
| Urinary tract infection | Urinary catheterization | *Escherichia coli, Klebsiella, Proteus.* | Dysuria, leukocytosis, flank pain, lower abdominal discomfort, costovertebral angle tenderness. |
| Legionella pneumonia | Water | *Legionella.* | Pneumonia, GI symptoms, hyponatremia. |

GI, gastrointestinal; HCV, hepatitis C virus.

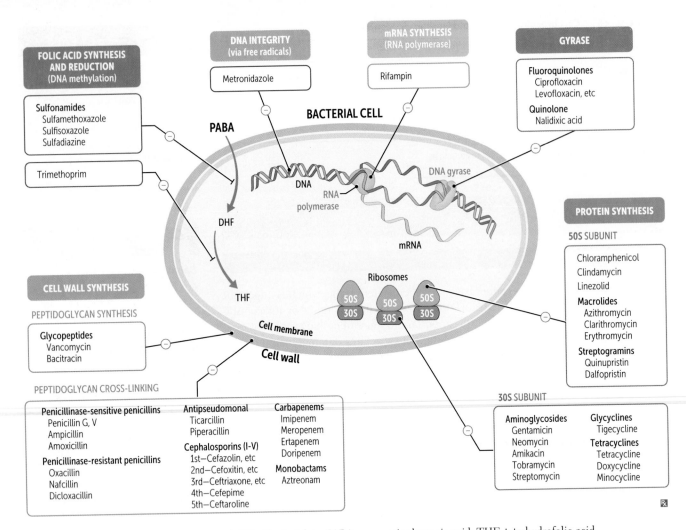

**FIGURE 4-110.** **Antimicrobial therapy.** DHF, dihydrofolate; PABA, para-aminobenzoic acid; THF, tetrahydrofolic acid.

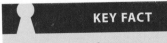

**KEY FACT**

Clavulanic acid, a β-lactam-like molecule, binds to and inactivates β-lactamase, conferring broader activity.

## Cell Wall Inhibitors

Bacterial cell walls contain peptidoglycans, which are repeating disaccharides with amino acid side chains. The side chains are cross-linked with one another via covalent bonds. Several antibiotics exert their effects through disruption of the bacterial cell wall. This may be accomplished by inhibiting peptidoglycan synthesis or cross-linking. Peptidoglycan cross-linking is inhibited by antibiotics, including the penicillins, cephalosporins, carbapenems, and monobactams, while peptidoglycan synthesis is inhibited by vancomycin and bacitracin.

Many inhibitors of peptidoglycan cross-linking fall into the category of β-lactam antibiotics (penicillins, cephalosporins, carbapenems, and monobactams), so named because of their ring (Figure 4-111). The β-lactam ring binds irreversibly to the bacterial transpeptidase enzyme, thereby disrupting peptidoglycan cross-linking. When this occurs, cell wall synthesis comes to a halt, and the bacterium dies.

Bacteria have evolved resistance mechanisms, which include:

- Inactivation of the β-lactam ring via β-lactamase
- Mutation of the binding site
- Decreased permeability or drug efflux

### Penicillin G, V

Penicillin G can be administered IV and intramuscularly (IM); Penicillin V can be administered orally (PO).

#### Mechanism

Irreversible inhibition of transpeptidase enzyme, activation of bacterial autolytic enzymes. Bactericidal.

#### Use

Mostly used for gram-positive organisms (*S pneumoniae*, *S pyogenes*, *Actinomyces*). Also used for gram-negative cocci (mainly *N meningitidis*) and spirochetes (namely *T pallidum*). Penicillinase sensitive.

#### Toxicity

Hypersensitivity reactions, hemolytic anemia.

#### Resistance

Penicillinase in bacteria (a type of β-lactamase) cleaves β-lactam ring.

### Amoxicillin, Ampicillin (Aminopenicillins)

#### Mechanism

Same as penicillin.

#### Use

Extended-spectrum penicillin. Amoxicillin has far greater oral availability than ampicillin.

Ampicillin is also first-line treatment for pregnant women and children younger than 8 years of age with Lyme disease, owing to the negative effects of doxycycline on bones.

#### Toxicity

Hypersensitivity reactions, rash, pseudomembranous colitis.

#### Resistance

Penicillinase.

### Cloxacillin, Dicloxacillin, Nafcillin, Oxacillin (Penicillinase-Resistant Penicillins)

#### Mechanism

Same as penicillin.

#### Use

*S aureus* (except MRSA, which is resistant owing to an altered transpeptidase/penicillin-binding protein target site). Dicloxacillin is available PO.

#### Toxicity

Hypersensitivity reactions, interstitial nephritis.

### Piperacillin, Ticarcillin (Antipseudomonal Penicillins)

#### Mechanism

Same as penicillin.

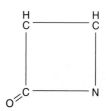

**FIGURE 4-111. β-lactam ring.** This chemical structure inhibits peptidoglycan cross-linking.

**KEY FACT**

β-lactams include:
- Penicillins
- Cephalosporins (all generations)
- Carbapenems
- Monobactams

**CLINICAL CORRELATION**

Some studies show that nearly 90% of patients who claim to have an allergy to penicillin do not in fact have one. Always be sure to ask patients with allergies what type of adverse reaction they have!

**MNEMONIC**

***Ampicillin/amoxicillin coverage—***

**HELPS S**laughter *Enterococcus*

**H** *influenzae*
**E** *coli*
**L** *Listeria*
**P** *mirabilis*
**S** *almonella*
**S** *higella*
**E** *nterococcus*

**MNEMONIC**

Am**O**xicillin is an **O**ral form of ampicillin.

### Use

Extended-spectrum penicillin is particularly effective against *Pseudomonas* and gram-negative rods. Typically combined with β-lactamase inhibitors (tazobactam, sulbactam, clavulanic acid).

### Toxicity

Hypersensitivity reactions.

### Resistance

Penicillinase.

## Cephalosporins (Generations I–IV)

### Mechanism

Same as penicillin.

### Use

First-generation (cefazolin, cephalexin): Gram-positive cocci. Frequently used for perioperative surgical wound prophylaxis.

Second-generation (cefoxitin, cefaclor, cefuroxime): Gram-positive cocci.

Third-generation (ceftriaxone, cefotaxime, ceftazidime): Serious gram-negative infections resistant to other β-lactams. Ceftriaxone is used for meningitis, gonorrhea, and disseminated Lyme disease. Ceftazidime is used for *Pseudomonas*.

Fourth-generation (cefepime): Gram-negative organisms, with enhanced activity against *Pseudomonas* and gram-positive organisms.

### Toxicity

Hypersensitivity (15% of those with penicillin allergies have cross-reactivity), autoimmune hemolytic anemia, disulfiram-like reaction, vitamin K deficiency.

### Resistance

Broad-spectrum β-lactamases and structural change in transpeptidases.

## Carbapenems (Imipenem, Meropenem, Ertapenem, Doripenem)

### Mechanism

Same as penicillin; β-lactamase resistant. Imipenem always is administered with cilastatin (decreases inactivation of drug in renal tubules).

### Use

Gram-positive cocci, gram-negative rods, anaerobes. Wide spectrum. Meropenem has lower risk of seizures and does not require cilastatin. Do **not** cover MRSA, VRE.

### Toxicity

Seizures, GI distress, skin rash.

## Monobactams (Aztreonam)

### Mechanism

Similar to penicillin.

### KEY FACT

Piperacillin + tazobactam = Zosyn
Ampicillin + sulbactam = Unasyn
Amoxicillin + clavulanic acid = Augmentin

### MNEMONIC

**Organisms covered by first-generation cephalosporins—PECK**

**P** mirabilis
**E** Coli
**K** lebsiella

### MNEMONIC

**Organisms covered by second-generation cephalosporins—HEN PECKS**

**H** influenzae
**E** nterobacter
**N** eisseria
**P** mirabilis
**E** Coli
**K** lebsiella
**S** marcescens

### Use

Gram-negative rods only! Synergistic with aminoglycosides. Used in penicillin-allergic patients and those with renal insufficiency who cannot tolerate aminoglycosides.

### Toxicity

No cross-hypersensitivity with penicillins. Occasional GI upset.

## Vancomycin

### Mechanism

Inhibits peptidoglycan synthesis by binding to D-ala D-ala portion of cell wall precursors. Bactericidal.

### Use

Gram-positive bugs only! For serious, multidrug-resistant organisms, including MRSA, coagulase-negative staph, certain species of *Enterococcus*, and *C difficile*.

### Toxicity

Nephrotoxicity, ototoxicity, thrombophlebitis. Also causes "red man syndrome," or diffuse flushing that can be prevented with pretreatment of antihistamines and slow infusion rate.

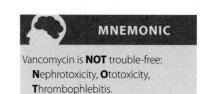

**MNEMONIC**

Vancomycin is **NOT** trouble-free: **N**ephrotoxicity, **O**totoxicity, **T**hrombophlebitis.

### Resistance

Not susceptible to β-lactamases. Bacteria change the binding site from D-ala D-ala to D-ala D-lac.

## PROTEIN SYNTHESIS INHIBITORS (FIGURE 4-112)

Drugs that target bacterial protein synthesis do so by targeting the ribosome, which is made of a 50S and a 30S subunit, which is distinct from the human 60S/40S ribosome.

## Aminoglycosides (Gentamicin, Neomycin, Amikacin, Tobramycin, Streptomycin)

### Mechanism

Bactericidal; irreversible inhibition of initiation complex through binding of the 30S subunit. Can cause misreading of mRNA. Also block translocation. Require $O_2$ for uptake; therefore, are ineffective against anaerobes.

### Use

Severe gram-negative rod infections. Synergistic with β-lactam antibiotics.

Neomycin for gut decontamination prior to bowel surgery.

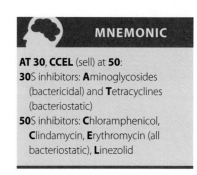

**MNEMONIC**

**AT 30**, **CCEL** (sell) at **50**:
**30**S inhibitors: **A**minoglycosides (bactericidal) and **T**etracyclines (bacteriostatic)
**50**S inhibitors: **C**hloramphenicol, **C**lindamycin, **E**rythromycin (all bacteriostatic), **L**inezolid

### Toxicity

Ototoxicity, nephrotoxicity, and neuromuscular blockade. Teratogenic.

### Resistance

Bacterial transferase enzymes inactivate the drug by acetylation, phosphorylation, or adenylation.

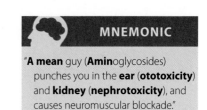

**MNEMONIC**

"**A mean** guy (**Amin**oglycosides) punches you in the **ear** (**ototoxicity**) and **kidney** (**nephrotoxicity**), and causes neuromuscular blockade."

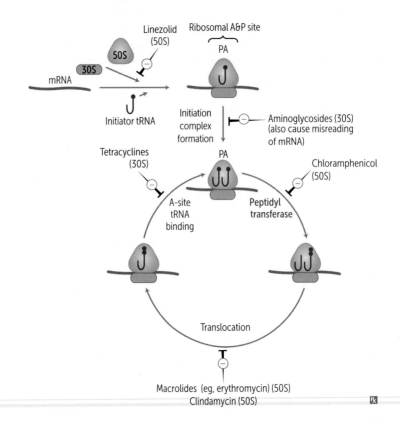

**FIGURE 4-112.** **Protein synthesis.** Depicted in the figure is normal protein synthesis, with the sites of action of antibiotics that work through this pathway. A&P, aminoacyl and peptidyl; mRNA, messenger ribonucleic acid; tRNA, transfer ribonucleic acid.

### Tetracyclines (Tetracycline, Doxycycline, Minocycline, Demeclocycline)

#### Mechanism

Bacteriostatic. Bind to 30S and prevent attachment of aminoacyl-tRNA. Tend to accumulate intracellularly.

#### Use

Excellent for

- Lyme disease
- *Mycoplasma*
- Intracellular organisms (*Rickettsia* and *Chlamydia*)

Also used for

- Acne
- Atypical pneumonia
- Syphilis (second-line therapy)

Have limited CNS penetration.

Doxycycline is fecally eliminated and can be used in patients with renal failure.

Patients should not take tetracyclines with milk ($Ca^{2+}$), antacids ($Ca^{2+}$ or $Mg^{2+}$), or iron-containing preparations, because divalent cations inhibit the drug's absorption in the gut.

Demeclocycline is used in syndrome of inappropriate antidiuretic hormone (SIADH), as it acts as a peripheral antagonist of the antidiuretic hormone (ADH) receptor.

### Toxicity

GI distress, discoloration of teeth and inhibition of bone growth in children, and photosensitivity. Contraindicated in pregnancy and young children.

### Resistance

Decreased uptake or increased efflux by plasmid-encoded transport pumps.

## Chloramphenicol

### Mechanism

Blocks peptidyl transferase at 50S ribosomal subunit. Bacteriostatic.

### Use

Meningitis (*H influenzae*, *N meningitidis*, *S pneumoniae*) and Rocky Mountain spotted fever (*Rickettsia rickettsii*).

Primarily used in developing countries because of low cost.

### Toxicity

Anemia (dose dependent), aplastic anemia (dose independent), gray baby syndrome (in premature infants, because they lack liver uridine diphosphate–glucuronyl transferase).

### Resistance

Plasmid-encoded acetyltransferase inactivates the drug.

## Clindamycin

### Mechanism

Blocks peptide transfer (translocation) at 50S ribosomal subunit. Bacteriostatic.

### Use

Anaerobic infections in aspiration pneumonia, lung abscesses, and oral infections (above the diaphragm). Also effective against invasive group A streptococcal infection.

### Toxicity

Pseudomembranous colitis (*C difficile* overgrowth), fever, diarrhea.

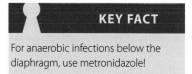

**KEY FACT**

For anaerobic infections below the diaphragm, use metronidazole!

## Linezolid

### Mechanism

Inhibits protein synthesis by binding to 50S subunit and preventing formation of the initiation complex.

### Use

Gram-positive species, including MRSA and VRE.

### Toxicity

Bone marrow suppression (especially thrombocytopenia), peripheral neuropathy, and serotonin syndrome.

### Resistance

Point mutation of ribosomal RNA.

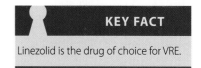

**KEY FACT**

Linezolid is the drug of choice for VRE.

## Macrolides (Azithromycin, Clarithromycin, Erythromycin)

### Mechanism

Inhibit protein synthesis by blocking translocation; bind to the 23S rRNA of the 50S ribosomal subunit. Bacteriostatic.

### Use

Atypical pneumonias.

Chlamydia.

Gram-positive cocci (streptococcal infections in patients allergic to penicillin).

Pertussis.

Prophylaxis against *M avium-intracellulare*.

Component of triple therapy against *H pylori*.

### Toxicity

Gastrointestinal motility issues, arrhythmia caused by prolonged QT interval, acute cholestatic hepatitis, rash, and eosinophilia.

Increases serum concentration of theophyllines, and oral anticoagulants. Clarithromycin and erythromycin inhibit cytochrome P450.

### Resistance

Methylation of 23S ribosomal ribonucleic acid (rRNA)-binding site prevents binding of drug.

## Streptogramins (Dalfopristin, Quinupristin)

### Mechanism

Bactericidal. Bind to the 50S ribosomal subunit and inhibit protein synthesis at two successive steps.

### Use

MRSA, VRE.

### Toxicity

Phlebitis, hyperbilirubinemia.

## FOLIC ACID SYNTHESIS INHIBITORS

These antibiotics work by inhibiting bacterial enzymes involved in the folic acid synthesis pathway (Figure 4-113).

### Trimethoprim

### Mechanism

Inhibits bacterial dihydrofolate reductase. Bacteriostatic.

### Use

Used in combination with sulfonamides (TMP-SMX), causing sequential block of folate synthesis.

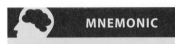

**MNEMONIC**

**MACRO**: GI **M**otility issues, **A**rrhythmia caused by prolonged QT interval, acute **C**holestatic hepatitis, **R**ash, e**O**sinophilia

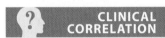

**CLINICAL CORRELATION**

Triple therapy for *H pylori* includes
- Amoxicillin (or metronidazole)
- Clarithromycin
- Proton pump inhibitor

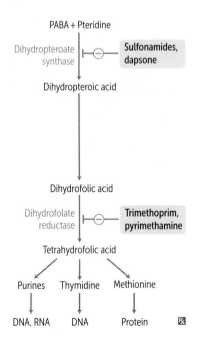

**FIGURE 4-113. Folic acid synthesis inhibitors**. Mechanism of action for sulfonamides, trimethoprim, and pyrimethamine. The words in green represent key enzymes inhibited by these antibiotics. PABA, para-aminobenzoic acid.

UTI.

Skin infections (staph, strep).

Bacterial diarrhea (*Shigella*, *Salmonella*).

*P jirovecii* pneumonia treatment and prophylaxis.

Toxoplasmosis prophylaxis.

### Toxicity

Megaloblastic anemia, leukopenia, granulocytopenia (may alleviate with supplemental folinic acid), severe skin reactions (particularly in HIV-infected patients).

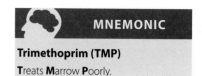

## Sulfonamides (Sulfamethoxazole [SMX], Sulfadiazine)

### Mechanism

Inhibit folate synthesis. *Para*-aminobenzoic acid (PABA) antimetabolites inhibit dihydropteroate synthase. Bacteriostatic (bactericidal when combined with trimethoprim).

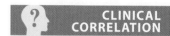

### Use

Gram-positives, gram-negatives, *Nocardia*, *Chlamydia*. Triple sulfas or SMX for simple UTI. See Trimethoprim.

### Toxicity

Hypersensitivity reactions, hemolysis if G6PD deficient, nephrotoxicity (tubulointerstitial nephritis), photosensitivity, and kernicterus in infants.

Displace other drugs from albumin (eg, warfarin).

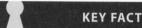

### Resistance

Altered bacterial dihydropteroate synthase, decreased uptake, or increased PABA synthesis.

## TOPOISOMERASE INHIBITORS

These antibiotics work by inhibiting prokaryotic topoisomerase II (DNA gyrase) and IV, which uncoil DNA to allow for efficient transcription.

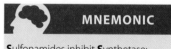

## Fluoroquinolones (Cipro-, Nor-, Levo-, O-, Moxifloxacin)

### Mechanism

Inhibit prokaryotic topoisomerases.

### Use

Gram-negative rods of urinary and GI tracts (including *Pseudomonas*), *Neisseria*, some gram-positive organisms.

### Toxicity

GI upset, superinfections, skin rashes, headache, dizziness.

Less commonly, can cause leg cramps and myalgias.

Contraindicated in pregnant women, nursing mothers, and children younger than 18 years owing to possible cartilage damage.

May cause tendonitis or tendon rupture in people older than 60 years and in patients taking prednisone.

### Resistance

Chromosome-encoded mutation in DNA gyrase, plasmid-mediated resistance, efflux pumps.

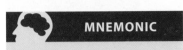

**MNEMONIC**

Fluoroquino**lones** hurt attachments to your **bones**.

## CELL MEMBRANE DISRUPTORS

These antibiotics insert into the bacterial cell membrane, where they aggregate, alter the membrane curvature, and allow rapid ion fluxes and ultimately depolarization and death of the bacterial cell.

### Daptomycin

#### Mechanism

Bacterial cell membrane disruptor.

#### Use

Only for resistant gram-positive cocci, notably MRSA and VRE. Also used for bacteremia and endocarditis.

Not used in pneumonia, as it is inactivated by surfactant.

#### Toxicity

Myopathy, rhabdomyolysis.

### Polymyxins

#### Mechanism

Membrane disruption. Bactericidal.

#### Use

Refractory gram-negative bugs only.

#### Toxicity

Nephrotoxicity (acute tubular necrosis), neurotoxicity.

#### Resistance

Altering cell membrane components.

## DNA DAMAGE INDUCERS VIA FREE RADICALS

These antibiotics form metabolites that function as free radicals, damaging bacterial DNA.

### Metronidazole

#### Mechanism

Free radical metabolites damage DNA.

### Use

See mnemonic.

### Toxicity

Disulfiram-like reaction (severe flushing, tachycardia, hypotension) with alcohol; headache, metallic taste.

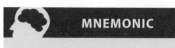
## ANTIMYCOBACTERIAL DRUGS

Important mycobacteria include *M tuberculosis*, MAI, and *M leprae* (Table 4-50; Figure 4-114).

### Rifamycins (Rifampin, Rifabutin)

#### Mechanism

Inhibit DNA-dependent RNA polymerase.

#### Use

*M tuberculosis*; delay resistance to dapsone when used for leprosy.

Used for meningococcal prophylaxis and chemoprophylaxis in contacts of children with *H influenzae* type B.

#### Toxicity

Minor hepatotoxicity and drug interactions (increase cytochrome P450), orange body fluids (nonhazardous side effect).

Rifabutin is favored over rifampin in patients with HIV infection, owing to less cytochrome P450 stimulation.

#### Resistance

Mutations reduce drug binding to RNA polymerase. Monotherapy rapidly leads to resistance.

### Isoniazid

#### Mechanism

Decreases mycolic acid synthesis.

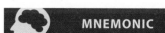
**TABLE 4-50.** **Mycobacterial Prophylaxis and Treatment**

| BACTERIUM | PROPHYLAXIS | TREATMENT |
|---|---|---|
| *M tuberculosis* | Isoniazid (INH) | **R**ifampin, **I**soniazid, **P**yrazinamide, Ethambutol (**RIPE** for treatment) |
| *M avium-intracellulare* | Azithromycin, rifabutin | More drug resistant than *M tuberculosis*<br>Azithromycin or clarithromycin + ethambutol<br>Can add rifabutin or ciprofloxacin |
| *M leprae* | N/A | Long-term treatment with dapsone and rifampin for tuberculoid form<br>Add clofazimine for lepromatous form |

**MYCOBACTERIAL CELL**

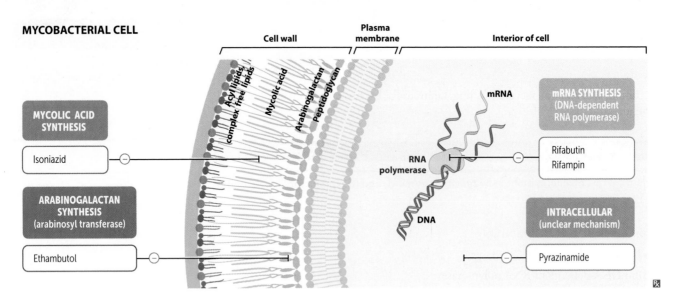

**FIGURE 4-114.** **Antimicrobials.** Schematic of mycobacterial cell with key components labeled, as well as sites of action of relevant antimicrobials.

**Use**

TB (prophylaxis when used alone).

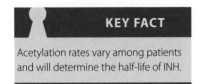

**Toxicity**

Neurotoxicity and hepatotoxicity. Vitamin $B_6$ can prevent neurotoxicity.

**Resistance**

Mutations in key proteins.

### Pyrazinamide

**Mechanism**

Uncertain.

**Use**

TB.

**Toxicity**

Hyperuricemia, hepatotoxicity.

### Ethambutol

**Mechanism**

Inhibits arabinosyltransferase.

**Use**

TB.

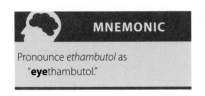

**Toxicity**

Optic neuropathy (red-green color blindness).

### Antimicrobial Prophylaxis

Table 4-51 describes clinical scenarios in which antimicrobial prophylaxis should be administered.

**TABLE 4-51.    Antimicrobial Prophylaxis**

| CLINICAL SCENARIO | MEDICATION |
|---|---|
| High risk for endocarditis and undergoing surgical or dental procedures | Amoxicillin |
| Exposure to gonorrhea | Ceftriaxone |
| History of recurrent urinary tract infections | Trimethoprim-sulfamethoxazole (TMP-SMX) |
| Exposure to meningococcal infection | Ceftriaxone, ciprofloxacin, rifampin |
| Pregnant woman carrying group B strep | Penicillin G |
| Prevention of gonococcal conjunctivitis in newborn | Erythromycin ointment |
| Prevention of postsurgical infection due to *S aureus* | Cefazolin |
| Prophylaxis of strep pharyngitis in child with prior rheumatic fever | Benzathine penicillin G or PO penicillin V |
| Exposure to syphilis | Benzathine penicillin G |

## ANTIFUNGAL THERAPIES

See Figure 4-115 for a description of antifungal drugs and their sites of action.

### Amphotericin B

Mechanism

Binds ergosterol, forms membrane pores leading to electrolyte leakage.

Use

Serious, systemic fungal infections. Can be used intrathecally for fungal meningitis.

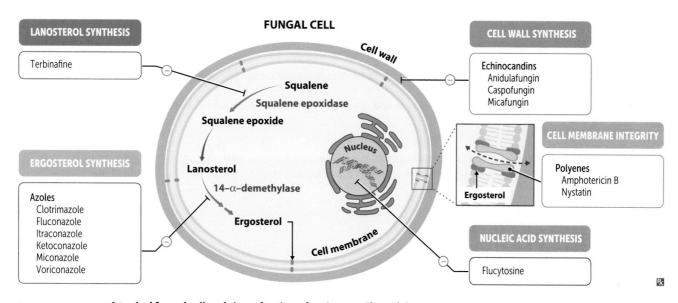

**FIGURE 4-115.    A typical fungal cell and sites of action of various antifungal drugs.**

### Toxicity

Fever/chills, nephrotoxicity, phlebitis ("amphoterrible"), arrhythmia, anemia. Hydration decreases nephrotoxicity, as do liposomal preparations.

## Nystatin

### Mechanism

Same as amphotericin B.

### Use

Used in a "swish and swallow" form for oral candidiasis, and topically for diaper rash/vaginal candidiasis.

## Flucytosine

### Mechanism

Inhibits DNA and RNA biosynthesis by conversion to 5-fluorouracil by cytosine deaminase.

### Use

Systemic fungal infections (primarily meningitis caused by *Cryptococcus*) in combination with amphotericin B.

### Toxicity

Bone marrow suppression.

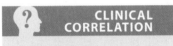

## Azoles (Clotrimazole, Fluconazole, Itraconazole, Ketoconazole, Miconazole, Voriconazole)

### Mechanism

Inhibit fungal sterol (ergosterol) synthesis by inhibiting the cytochrome P450 enzyme that converts lanosterol to ergosterol.

### Use

Local and less serious systemic mycoses.

Fluconazole for long-term suppression of cryptococcal meningitis in AIDS patients and candidal infections of all types.

Itraconazole for *Blastomyces*, *Coccidioides*, *Histoplasma*.

Clotrimazole and miconazole for topical fungal infections.

### Toxicity

Testosterone synthesis inhibition (gynecomastia, especially with ketoconazole), and liver dysfunction (inhibits cytochrome P450).

## Terbinafine

### Mechanism

Inhibits fungal squalene epoxidase.

### Use

Dermatophytoses (especially onychomycosis, fungal infection of the finger or toenail).

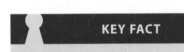

### Toxicity

GI upset, headaches, hepatotoxicity, taste disturbance (dysgeusia).

## Echinocandins (Caspofungin, Micafungin)

### Mechanism

Inhibit cell wall synthesis by inhibiting synthesis of β-glucan.

### Use

Invasive aspergillosis, candidiasis.

### Toxicity

GI upset, flushing (via histamine release).

## Griseofulvin

### Mechanism

Disrupts mitosis via microtubule dysfunction. Deposits in keratin-rich tissues, such as nails.

### Use

Oral treatment of superficial infections; inhibits growth of dermatophytes (tinea, ringworm).

### Toxicity

Teratogenic, carcinogenic, confusion, headaches, cytochrome P450 and warfarin metabolism.

## ANTIPARASITICS

Although the antiparasitics are a large and heterogeneous group of drugs, their spectrum of activity somewhat relates to the taxonomy of the parasites—that is, antinematode, antihelminth, antimalarial.

## Albendazole

### Mechanism

Inhibits parasite microtubule polymerization.

### Use

Cestode (tapeworm) infection, *T solium* neurocysticercosis, *Echinococcus* hydatid disease. May be used second-line in some nematode infections.

### Toxicity

Headache, liver function test (LFT) elevation, GI.

## Praziquantel

### Mechanism

Blocks voltage-gated calcium channels, increasing calcium influx, leading to severe spasms and paralysis of the worm's muscles.

**KEY FACT**

Corticosteroids must be given with albendazole in the treatment of cysticercosis, as the degenerating cysts elicit a strong immune response.

**Use**

Cestodes, trematodes (flukes): *T solium*, schistosomiasis, clonorchiasis, *P westermani*.

**Toxicity**

Cramps, diarrhea.

### Mebendazole/Pyrantel Pamoate

#### Mechanism

Mebendazole: Prevents glucose absorption, leading to loss of energy.

Pyrantel pamoate: Paralyzes the nematode.

#### Use

*E vermicularis* (pinworm), *T trichiura* (whipworm), *A lumbricoides* (giant roundworm), *A duodenale* (hookworm).

#### Toxicity

GI complaints.

### Thiabendazole

#### Mechanism

Blocks mitochondrial fumarate reductase.

#### Use

*Strongyloides*, trichinosis.

#### Toxicity

Hallucinations, diarrhea, nausea/vomiting, paresthesias.

### Ivermectin

#### Mechanism

Paralyzes and kills offspring of adult nematode.

#### Use

Filariasis and other nematode infections, sometimes in combination with thiabendazole. Onchocerciasis (river blindness).

#### Toxicity

Arthralgias, painful glands, tachycardia, and ocular irritation.

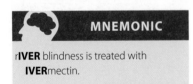

**MNEMONIC**

r**IVER** blindness is treated with **IVER**mectin.

### Diethylcarbamazepine

#### Mechanism

Effective against microfilarial diseases.

#### Use

Bancroft filariasis, loiasis, onchocerciasis (river blindness), and toxocariasis.

#### Toxicity

Swelling/itching of face, loss of vision, and arthralgias with long-term use.

## Chloroquine

### Mechanism

Generates toxic heme by-products that kill the parasite within infected RBCs.

### Use

Prophylaxis and treatment of malaria (not used in *P falciparum* owing to high resistance rates).

### Toxicity

Severe hemolysis in G6PD-deficient patients, blurred vision, and pruritis.

## Quinine

### Mechanism

Depresses oxygen uptake and intercalates into DNA.

### Use

Prophylaxis and treatment of malaria (especially severe infections).

### Toxicity

Cinchonism (tinnitus, deafness), proarrhythmic, hemolysis in G6PD-deficient patients; hypoglycemia.

## Mefloquine

### Mechanism

Unknown.

### Use

Prophylaxis and treatment of malaria and chloroquine-resistant malaria.

### Toxicity

Mood changes, suicidality, and unusual dreams.

## Atovaquone/Proguanil

### Mechanism

The two are synergistic.

### Use

Prophylaxis and treatment of malaria and chloroquine-resistant malaria. Especially useful in *P falciparum*.

### Toxicity

Fever, skin rash.

## Artemether

### Mechanism

Unknown.

### Use

Antimalarial.

**KEY FACT**

Malaria is resistant to chloroquine in many areas of the world; it is necessary to check local susceptibility before prescribing prophylaxis.

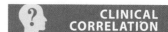

**CLINICAL CORRELATION**

The antimalarials (as well as sulfonamides, INH, aspirin, nitrofurantoin, and fava beans) are triggers for hemolysis in patients with G6PD deficiency.

**Toxicity**

Mild GI upset.

### Nifurtimox

**Mechanism**

Formation of free radicals.

**Use**

Chagas disease (*T cruzi*).

**Toxicity**

Hypersensitivity, GI, and neuropathy.

### Suramin/Melarsoprol

**Mechanism**

Depletes the organism of energy by inactivating pyruvate kinase (inhibits ATP production).

**Use**

African sleeping sickness (*T gambiense* and *T rhodanese*): Suramin when in blood, melarsoprol when in CSF.

**Toxicity**

Suramin: Urticaria, nausea and vomiting, and adrenal cortical damage.

Melarsoprol: Extremely toxic. Only used in extreme cases.

### Sodium Stibogluconate

**Mechanism**

Unknown.

**Use**

Leishmaniasis.

**Toxicity**

Phlebitis of injected veins, pancreatitis, cardiac conduction abnormalities, and GI disturbances.

### Pyrimethamine/Sulfadiazine

**Mechanism**

Often used in combination; pyrimethamine interrupts folate synthesis by inhibiting dihydrofolate reductase, while sulfadiazine inhibits dihydropteroate synthetase, thereby preventing DNA and RNA synthesis.

**Use**

Toxoplasmosis.

**Toxicity**

Folate deficiency (add leucovorin to prevent this).

## ANTI-MITE/LOUSE THERAPY

Permethrin (blocks sodium channels), malathion (acetylcholinesterase inhibitor), and lindane (blocks GABA channels) are used to treat scabies (*Sarcoptes scabiei*) and lice.

## ANTIVIRAL THERAPY

Different viruses have distinct life cycles, which can be exploited in the development of a host of antiviral drugs (Figure 4-116).

### Anti-Influenza

#### AMANTADINE, RIMANTADINE

Mechanism

Block viral penetration/uncoating; may buffer pH of endosome. Cause the release of dopamine from intact nerve terminals.

Use

Prophylaxis and treatment for influenza A; Parkinson disease.

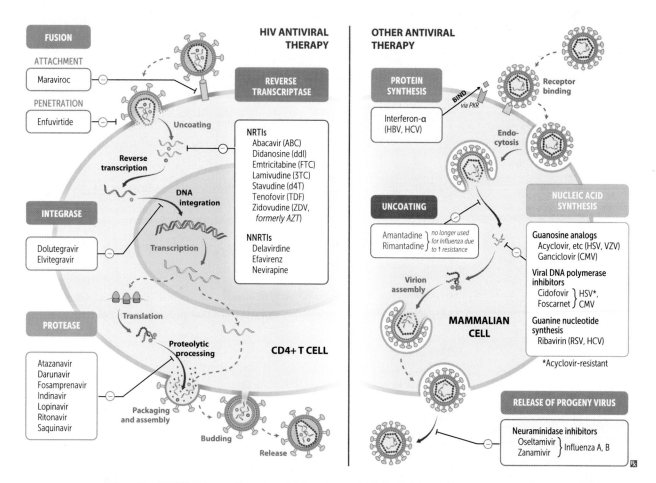

**FIGURE 4-116.    Life cycle of HIV (left) as well as that of other viruses (right), along with the mechanisms of action of several antivirals and the stages in which they work.** CMV, cytomegalovirus; HBV, hepatitis B virus; HCV, hepatitis C virus; HSV, herpes simplex virus; PKR, interferon-α–induced protein kinase; RSV, respiratory syncytial virus; VZV, varicella-zoster virus.

### Toxicity

Ataxia, dizziness, slurred speech, and hallucinations.

Rimantadine has fewer CNS side effects.

### Resistance

Mutation in the M2 protein (widespread, making this drug largely ineffective).

### OSELTAMIVIR, ZANAMIVIR

### Mechanism

Inhibit influenza neuraminidase, decreasing release of viral progeny.

### Use

Shorten duration of flu A/B symptoms by 1–2 days. Must be administered early in illness.

## Anti–Herpes Virus Medications

### ACYCLOVIR, FAMCICLOVIR, VALACYCLOVIR

### Mechanism

Guanosine analogs that are phosphorylated by HSV/VZV and thymidine kinase and not phosphorylated in uninfected cells. Inhibition of the viral DNA polymerase leads to chain termination.

### Use

HSV and VZV. Weak activity against EBV and no activity against CMV. Does not affect latent virus.

For herpes zoster, famciclovir is preferred.

### Toxicity

Crystalline nephropathy and renal failure if inadequate hydration.

### Resistance

Mutated viral thymidine kinase.

### GANCICLOVIR

### Mechanism

Guanosine analog, preferentially inhibits viral DNA polymerase via chain termination.

### Use

CMV, especially in immunocompromised patients. Valganciclovir, a prodrug of ganciclovir, has better oral bioavailability.

### Toxicity

Leukopenia, neutropenia, thrombocytopenia, renal toxicity. More toxic to host enzymes than acyclovir.

### Resistance

Mutated viral kinase.

**FLASH FORWARD**

Parkinson disease is due to degeneration of dopaminergic neurons found in the substantia nigra pars compacta. Therefore, amantadine may alleviate symptoms by increasing dopamine release from remaining neurons.

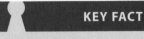

**KEY FACT**

Acyclovir, famciclovir, and valacyclovir do not work against CMV because the virus lacks thymidine kinase.

## FOSCARNET

### Mechanism

Viral DNA/RNA polymerase inhibitor and HIV RT inhibitor. Binds to pyrophosphate-binding site of enzyme. Does not require activation by viral kinase.

### Use

CMV retinitis in immunocompromised patients when ganciclovir fails; acyclovir-resistant HSV.

### Toxicity

Nephrotoxicity; electrolyte abnormalities (hypo- or hypercalcemia, hypo- or hyperphosphatemia, hypokalemia, hypomagnesemia) can lead to seizures.

### Resistance

Mutated DNA polymerase.

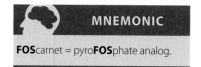

**MNEMONIC**

**FOS**carnet = pyro**FOS**phate analog.

## CIDOFOVIR

### Mechanism

Preferentially inhibits viral DNA polymerase. Does not require phosphorylation by viral kinase.

### Use

CMV retinitis in immunocompromised patients; acyclovir-resistant HSV. Long half-life.

### Toxicity

Nephrotoxicity (coadminister with probenecid and IV saline to decrease toxicity).

## HIV Therapy

HAART is now recommended at the time of HIV diagnosis.

HAART consists of three drugs to minimize the potential for resistance: two nucleoside RT inhibitors (NRTIs) plus either one non-NRTI (NNRTI), protease inhibitor, or integrase inhibitor. Many drugs come in combination pills, greatly reducing the potential for medication errors. Reviewing Figure 4-116, from the beginning of this section, on the HIV life cycle will deepen understanding of these drug classes.

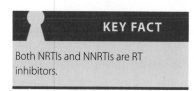

**KEY FACT**

Both NRTIs and NNRTIs are RT inhibitors.

## PROTEASE INHIBITORS (END IN -*NAVIR*): INDINAVIR, LOPINAVIR, RITONAVIR, SAQUINAVIR

### Mechanism

HIV protease (*pol* gene) cleaves the polypeptide products of HIV mRNA into their functional parts. Protease inhibitors, therefore, prevent viral maturation.

### Use

Ritonavir can boost other drug concentrations by inhibiting cytochrome P450.

### Toxicity

Hyperglycemia, nausea, diarrhea, lipodystrophy, thrombocytopenia (indinavir).

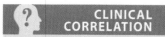

**CLINICAL CORRELATION**

Rifampin is a potent cyp450 inducer and decreases protease inhibitor concentrations. Therefore, these drugs should not be administered together.

## NUCLEOSIDE REVERSE TRANSCRIPTASE INHIBITORS (ABACAVIR, DIDANOSINE, EMTRICITABINE, LAMIVUDINE, STAVUDINE, TENOFOVIR, ZIDOVUDINE)

### Mechanism

Competitively inhibit nucleotide binding to RT, terminating the DNA chain, as it lacks a 3′OH group. Tenofovir is a nucleoTide; the rest are nucleosides.

Use

Zidovudine (ZDV, formerly AZT) is used for general prophylaxis and during pregnancy to reduce vertical transmission.

Toxicity

Bone marrow suppression (reversible with erythropoietin and granulocyte colony-stimulating factor), peripheral neuropathy, lactic acidosis, anemia (ZDV), pancreatitis (didanosine [ddI]), hypersensitivity (abacavir), and lactic acidosis.

### NON–NUCLEOSIDE REVERSE TRANSCRIPTASE INHIBITORS (NEVIRAPINE, EFAVIRENZ, DELAVIRDINE)

Mechanism

Bind to RT at a different site than the NRTIs. Phosphorylation not required.

Use

HAART.

Toxicity

Rash, hepatotoxicity.

Efavirenz: Vivid dreams, CNS symptoms.

Delavirdine and efavirenz are contraindicated in pregnancy.

### INTEGRASE INHIBITOR (RALTEGRAVIR)

Mechanism

Inhibits HIV integration into host cell genome by reversibly inhibiting HIV integrase.

Use

HAART.

Toxicity

Increased creatine kinase.

### FUSION INHIBITORS (ENFUVIRTIDE, MARAVIROC)

Mechanism

Enfuvirtide: Bind gp41, inhibiting viral entry.

Maraviroc: Bind CCR-5 on T cells/monocytes, inhibiting interaction with gp120.

Use

HAART.

Toxicity

Skin reaction at injection sites.

### Hepatitis C Therapy

The use of IFN/ribavirin is waning owing to IFN's adverse-effect profile and resultant low treatment compliance. With newer antivirals, HCV can be eliminated in the vast majority of patients. Combinations of drugs, such as sofosbuvir/ledipasvir, boceprevir/telaprevir, sofosbuvir/ribavirin, and ombitasvir/paritaprevir/ritonavir/dasabuvir, are currently on the market. The most important drugs in HCV treatment are sofosbuvir,

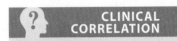

**CLINICAL CORRELATION**

The most effective method of reducing maternal-fetal HIV transmission is continuation of HAART.

which inhibits RNA-dependent RNA polymerase, and boceprevir, which binds to HCV protease. Combination therapy typically lasts 12 or 24 weeks, depending on whether the patient has cirrhosis or has been previously treated. HCV genotyping is incredibly important, as sustained virologic response varies with genotype.

## OTHER ANTIVIRAL DRUGS

IFNs are glycoproteins synthesized by virus-infected cells and exhibit a diverse range of antiviral and antitumor properties. IFN-α was previously used in HBV and HCV, as well as several solid and hematologic malignancies. IFN-β is used in multiple sclerosis, and IFN-γ is used in chronic granulomatous disease (CGD). IFNs have neutropenia, myopathy, and severe flulike symptoms as toxicities. They are falling out of use in favor of more effective therapies with more benign side-effect profiles.

**NOTES**

# Pathology

## NEOPLASIA

**Neoplasia** is an abnormal excessive and unregulated cell growth that typically arises from clonal proliferation of a single cell. These cells are unresponsive to normal cell regulation and continue to divide and grow beyond the normal needs of the organism. The word *neoplasia* is derived from the Greek *neo* (new) and *plasia* (growth). Before a tissue becomes neoplastic, other cellular changes are usually detected, as listed below.

### Definitions

- **Hyperplasia:** Increase in the **number** of cells (reversible adaptation). *Hyper-* = excessive.
- **Metaplasia:** Replacement of one adult cell type by another (can be reversible). Often secondary to irritation or environmental exposure (eg, squamous metaplasia in the trachea and bronchi of smokers). *Meta-* = transformation.
- **Dysplasia:** Abnormal growth with loss of cellular orientation, irregular cell shape and size compared with normal tissue maturation. Usually epithelial, can be premalignant. *Dys-* = abnormal.
- **Anaplasia:** Abnormal cells that show very little or no differentiation, appearing very primitive. *Ana-* = backward.

### Cell Types

Neoplasms usually consist of cells of **epithelial** or **mesenchymal** origin. Epithelial tissues are derived from either the embryological ectoderm or endoderm. Mesenchymal tissues derived from embryological mesoderm include blood cells, vessels, smooth muscle, skeletal muscle, bone, and fat. Tumors consisting of cells derived from all three germ layers are called **teratomas**.

### Nomenclature

- **Prefix:** The prefix used for a neoplasm depends on the tissue type, as seen in Table 5-1.
- **Suffix, benign:** The suffix *-oma* is generally used for benign neoplasms.
- **Suffix, malignant:** Malignant neoplasms of epithelial origin end in *-carcinoma*, whereas those of mesenchymal origin end in *-sarcoma*.
- **Exception:** Some malignant neoplasms end in *-oma* (eg, melanoma, mesothelioma, immature teratoma, lymphoma).

**TABLE 5-1. Tumor Nomenclature by Cell Type and Type of Neoplastic Process**

| CELL TYPE | BENIGN | MALIGNANT |
|-----------|--------|-----------|
| Epithelium | <ul><li>Adenoma</li><li>Squamous cell papilloma</li></ul> | <ul><li>Adenocarcinoma</li><li>Squamous cell papillary carcinoma</li></ul> |
| Blood cells | By convention, no blood cell neoplasms are considered benign | <ul><li>Leukemia</li><li>Lymphoma</li></ul> |
| Blood vessels | Hemangioma | Angiosarcoma |
| Smooth muscle | Leiomyoma | Leiomyosarcoma |
| Skeletal muscle | Rhabdomyoma | Rhabdomyosarcoma |
| Bone | Osteoma | Osteosarcoma |
| Fat | Lipoma | Liposarcoma |
| > 1 Cell type | Mature teratoma | Immature teratoma |

## Neoplastic Progression

Neoplastic cells accumulate genetic mutations that allow them to advance through successive steps in malignant progression, including invasion and metastasis, as outlined in Figure 5-1.

## Tumor Grade and Stage

### Grade

Classification system that describes the degree of cellular differentiation and mitotic activity of tumor cells based on histologic characteristics.

- Usually graded on a four-tier (I-IV: well-, moderately-, poorly- and undifferentiated) or two-tier (low- and high-grade) scale.
- Higher grade = more advanced tumor.

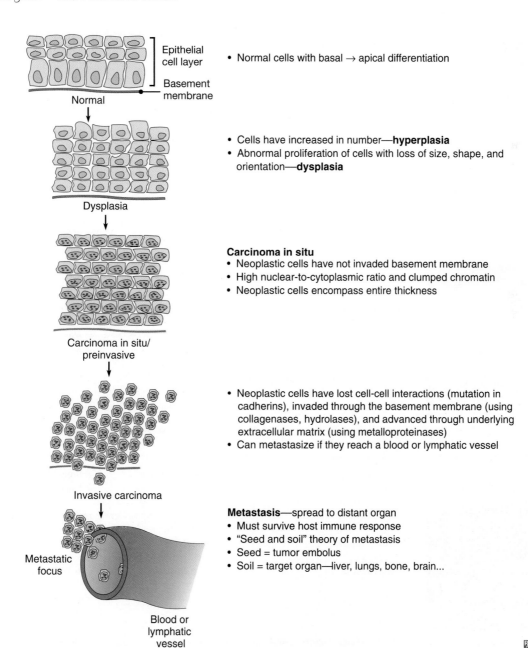

- Normal cells with basal → apical differentiation

- Cells have increased in number—**hyperplasia**
- Abnormal proliferation of cells with loss of size, shape, and orientation—**dysplasia**

**Carcinoma in situ**
- Neoplastic cells have not invaded basement membrane
- High nuclear-to-cytoplasmic ratio and clumped chromatin
- Neoplastic cells encompass entire thickness

- Neoplastic cells have lost cell-cell interactions (mutation in cadherins), invaded through the basement membrane (using collagenases, hydrolases), and advanced through underlying extracellular matrix (using metalloproteinases)
- Can metastasize if they reach a blood or lymphatic vessel

**Metastasis**—spread to distant organ
- Must survive host immune response
- "Seed and soil" theory of metastasis
- Seed = tumor embolus
- Soil = target organ—liver, lungs, bone, brain...

**FIGURE 5-1.   Neoplastic progression.**

## Stage

- Greater prognostic value than grade.
- Indicates the spread of tumor in a specific patient at a given point in time (ie, at the time of the staging procedure—usually a surgical operation).
- Based on the site and size of the primary tumor, spread to regional lymph nodes, and the presence or absence of metastases.
- A commonly used staging system is **TNM staging: T** for size of **T**umor, **N** for lymph **N**ode involvement, and **M** for **M**etastases.

## Characteristics of Neoplastic Cells

Benign and malignant neoplasms have features that distinguish them from each other, as seen in Table 5-2.

## Metastasis

Malignant neoplasms have the potential to metastasize to distant sites. Other than metastasis to regional lymph nodes, the lung, liver, brain, and bone are the most common sites.

## Metastasis to Liver

- Metastatic disease of the liver is much more common than primary liver neoplasms (Figure 5-2).
- Primary neoplasms that metastasize to the liver, in order of decreasing frequency:
  - Colon
  - Stomach
  - Pancreas
  - Breast
  - Lung

**TABLE 5-2.    Properties of Benign and Malignant Tumors**

| PROPERTY | BENIGN | MALIGNANT |
|---|---|---|
| Differentiation | Well-differentiated | Usually poorly differentiated |
| Mitotic figures | ▪ Few<br>▪ No atypical mitotic figures | ▪ Many<br>▪ Atypical mitotic figures |
| Nuclear-to-cytoplasm (N/C) ratio | Normal | Increased |
| Pleomorphism | Absent or minimal | Present |
| Hyperchromasia | Absent or minimal | Present |
| Circumscription and encapsulation | ▪ Well-circumscribed<br>▪ May be encapsulated | ▪ Poorly circumscribed<br>▪ Irregular<br>▪ Not encapsulated |
| Homogeneity | Homogeneous | May be heterogeneous |
| Rate of growth | Usually slow | Rapid |
| Metastatic potential | Does not metastasize | Can metastasize |
| Necrosis | No necrosis | May have necrosis/ hemorrhage |
| Physical examination findings | ▪ Mobile<br>▪ Well-defined | ▪ Fixed<br>▪ Irregular; poorly defined |

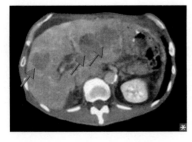

**FIGURE 5-2.    Liver metastases.** Axial CT scan showing liver metastases (arrows).

## Metastasis to Brain

- Approximately half of brain malignancies are due to metastatic disease from primary neoplasms located elsewhere (Figure 5-3).
- Primary neoplasms that metastasize to brain:
    - Lung
    - Breast
    - Skin (melanoma)
    - Kidney (renal cell carcinoma)
    - GI tract

## Metastasis to Bone

- Metastatic disease of bone is much more common than primary bone tumors, and has a predilection for the axial skeleton (Figure 5-4).
- The most common primary sites are breast and prostate.
- Primary neoplasms that metastasize to bone:
    - Lungs: mixed lesions
    - Kidney: lytic lesions
    - Thyroid: lytic lesions
    - Prostate: blastic lesions
    - Testes: lytic lesions
    - Breast: mixed lesions

## Direct (Local) Effects of Tumor Growth

- Destruction of normal surrounding architecture due to local tumor growth (**infiltration**).
    - **Nonhealing ulcers** from destruction of epithelial surfaces, such as those of the stomach, colon, mouth, or bronchus.
    - **Hemorrhage** or **infarction** due to erosion or compression of blood vessels.
    - **Pain** due to tumor involvement with sensory nerve endings. Most tumors are initially painless.
    - **Seizures and increased intracranial pressure** from space-occupying brain tumors.
    - **Perforation** of a visceral ulcer can lead to **peritonitis** (infection and inflammation of the peritoneum, the serous membrane that lines the abdominal cavity and the viscera) and **free air (air in the abdominal cavity)**.
    - **Bone involvement** can lead to pathologic fractures.
    - **Inflammation** of a serosal surface leads to **pleural effusion, pericardial effusion, and ascites**.

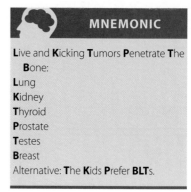

**MNEMONIC**

Lots of **B**ad **S**tuff **K**ills **G**lia:
**L**ung
**B**reast
**S**kin
**K**idney
**G**I tract

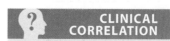

**MNEMONIC**

**L**ive and **K**icking **T**umors **P**enetrate **T**he **B**one:
**L**ung
**K**idney
**T**hyroid
**P**rostate
**T**estes
**B**reast
Alternative: **T**he **K**ids **P**refer **BLT**s.

**CLINICAL CORRELATION**

Lung cancer frequently presents as cough with hemoptysis due to tumor erosion of vasculature.

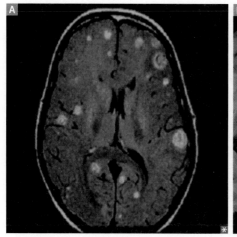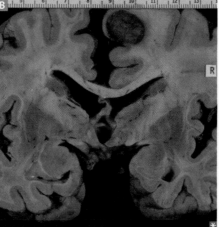

**FIGURE 5-3.    Brain metastases. A** MRI showing multiple intracranial metastases with surrounding edema. **B** Coronal view of cortical brain metastasis.

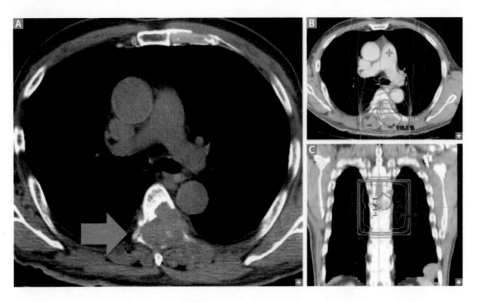

**FIGURE 5-4. Bone metastases.** **A** **B** Axial and **C** coronal CT scans showing metastases to a thoracic vertebral body.

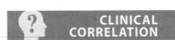
- Local neurologic deficits: Loss of sensory or motor function caused by nerve compression or destruction (eg, recurrent laryngeal nerve involvement by lung or thyroid cancer results in hoarseness).
- Pressure effects on normal organs (can also occur through infiltration, eg, pressure atrophy of glandular organs from a tumor growing nearby).
- **Obstruction:**
  - Obstructed bronchus → **pneumonia**
  - Obstructed biliary tree → **jaundice**
  - Obstructed intestines → **constipation, strangulation**
  - Obstructed venous or lymphatic drainage → **edema, superior vena cava syndrome**

### Paraneoplastic Effects

Various signaling molecules or immunogenic substances may be secreted by tumors without regulation, leading to systemic effects, as seen in Table 5-3.

### Carcinogenesis

Genetic damage can disturb the normal mechanisms that regulate cell proliferation and DNA repair. One genetic disruption often leaves cells vulnerable to others. Damage accumulating over time results in a process called **tumor progression.** Progression often leads to more aggressive tumor cells.

Cancer-related genes can be described under two separate categories:

### Proto-Oncogenes

- **Action:** Cause cells to grow and proliferate.
- **How they lead to cancer:** Mutations or translocations lead to **activation/overexpression** of these genes, causing uncontrolled cell proliferation. Associated diseases are listed in Table 5-4.
- **Required hits:** Cancerous growth can occur with a single gene mutation.

### Tumor Suppressor Genes/Antioncogenes

- **Action:** Regulate normal cell growth and differentiation by inhibiting cell cycle, mediating DNA repair, or initiating apoptosis when too much cell damage has occurred.

**KEY FACT**

The following can lead to cancer:
**Proto-oncogenes:** Turned ON
**Tumor suppressor genes:** Turned OFF

**TABLE 5-3.** **Paraneoplastic Effects of Tumors**

| HORMONE/MEDIATOR | EFFECT | NEOPLASM(S) |
|---|---|---|
| Adrenocorticotropic hormone (ACTH) or ACTH-like peptide | Cushing syndrome | Small-cell lung carcinoma, renal cell carcinoma |
| Antidiuretic hormone | SIADH | Small-cell lung carcinoma, intracranial neoplasms |
| Antibodies against pre-synaptic $Ca^{2+}$ channels at NMJ | Lambert-Eaton myasthenic syndrome | Small-cell lung carcinoma, thymoma |
| Erythropoietin | Polycythemia | Renal cell carcinoma, hemangioblastoma, hepatocellular carcinoma, leiomyoma, pheochromocytoma |
| Gonadotropin-releasing hormone, growth hormone | Acromegaly | Carcinoid tumors, small-cell lung carcinomas |
| Parathyroid hormone–related peptide | Hypercalcemia | Squamous cell lung carcinoma, renal cell carcinoma, breast carcinoma |
| TNF-α, IL-2 | Cachexia, fever, inflammation | Breast carcinoma, multiple myeloma, bone metastasis |

IL, interleukin; NMJ, neuromuscular junction; SIADH, syndrome of inappropriate antidiuretic hormone secretion; TNF, tumor necrosis factor.

- **How they lead to cancer:** Mutations or translocations **inactivate** these genes, leading to genetic instability or unchecked cell proliferation. See Table 5-5 for associated cancers, and Figure 5-5 for a commonly tested pathway to colon cancer.
- **Required hits:** Usually cause cancer only if both genes are inactivated; **"two-hit"** hypothesis.

**TABLE 5-4.** **Proto-Oncogenes and Their Associated Tumor**

| GENE | CHROMOSOME | GENE PRODUCT | ASSOCIATED TUMOR |
|---|---|---|---|
| BCR-ABL | 9,22 - Philadelphia chromosome | Tyrosine kinase | CML, ALL |
| BCL-2 | 18 | Antiapoptotic molecule (inhibits apoptosis) | Follicular and undifferentiated lymphomas |
| BRAF | 7 | Serine/threonine kinase | Melanoma, non-Hodgkin lymphoma |
| c-kit | 4 | Cytokine receptor | Gastrointestinal stromal tumor (GIST) |
| c-myc | 8 | Transcription factor | Burkitt lymphoma |
| HER2/neu (c-erbB2) | 17 | Tyrosine kinase | Breast, ovarian, and gastric carcinomas |
| L-myc | 1 | Transcription factor | Lung tumor |
| N-myc | 2 | Transcription factor | Neuroblastoma |
| RAS | — | GTPase | Colon cancer, lung cancer, pancreatic cancer |
| RET | 10 | Tyrosine kinase | Medullary thyroid cancer, MEN 2A and 2B |

ALL, acute lymphoblastic leukemia; CML, chronic myelogenous leukemia; GTP, guanosine triphosphate; MEN, multiple endocrine neoplasia.

**TABLE 5-5.** **Tumor Suppressor Genes and Associated Tumors**

| GENE | CHROMOSOME | ASSOCIATED TUMOR | ACTION |
|---|---|---|---|
| *APC* | 5q | Colorectal cancer | Inhibition of signal transduction |
| *BRCA1* and *BRCA2* | 17q, 13q | Breast and ovarian cancer | DNA repair |
| *DCC* | 18q | **C**olon cancer | Cell surface receptor |
| *DPC* | 18q | **P**ancreatic cancer | Cell surface receptor |
| *DPC4/SMAD4* | 18 | Pancreatic cancer | Nuclear transcription through TGF-β1. |
| *MEN1* | 11 | MEN 1 | Nuclear transcription |
| *NF1* | 17q | Neurofibromatosis type 1 | Inhibition of *ras* signal transduction |
| *NF2* | 22q | Neurofibromatosis type 2 | Signaling and cytoskeletal regulation |
| *p16* | 9**p** | Melanoma | Cell cycle control/DNA repair |
| *p53* | 17**p** | ■ Most human cancers<br>■ Li-Fraumeni syndrome | Regulation of the cell cycle and apoptosis after DNA damage |
| *PTEN* | 10 | Breast cancer, prostate cancer, endometrial cancer | PTEN dephosphorylates $PIP_3$ |
| *Rb* | 13q | ■ Retinoblastoma<br>■ Osteosarcoma | Regulation of the cell cycle |
| *TSC1, TSC2* | TSC1: 9, TSC2:16 | Tuberous sclerosis | TSC2 inhibits mTOR |
| *VHL* | 3 | von Hippel-Lindau disease, renal cell carcinoma | VHL inhibits hypoxia inducible factor 1a |
| *WT1/WT2* | 11q | Wilms tumor | Nuclear transcription |

MEN, multiple endocrine neoplasia; mTOR, mammalian target of rapamycin; PIP3, phosphoinositol 3,4,5-triphosphate; PTEN, phosphatase and tensin homolog; TSC2, tuberous sclerosis protein 2.

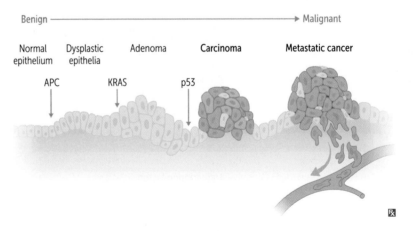

**FIGURE 5-5.** **Neoplastic progression and evolution of colon cancer from normal epithelia.** Acquired mutations allow colonic epithelial cells to progress through sequential steps to increasingly more advanced lesions from normal epithelium to adenomas and eventually invasive carcinoma (multistep carcinogenesis). APC, antigen-presenting cell.

## Carcinogenic Agents

Genetic damage can be inherited or can result from exposure to carcinogens such as chemicals, radiation, and/or viruses/microbes.

- **Chemicals:** Cancers associated with chemical exposure are listed in Table 5-6.
  - **Initiators** are chemicals that lead to irreversible damage to a cell's DNA.
  - **Promoters** do not affect the DNA, but promote cell growth and differentiation by other methods; their effects are usually reversible.
- **Radiation:** Penetrant high-energy waves can directly damage DNA.
  - **Ultraviolet (UV) rays** lead to squamous cell carcinoma, basal cell carcinoma, and melanoma in the skin.
  - **UVB rays** specifically lead to the formation of **pyrimidine dimers** in DNA. Usually, the nucleotide excision repair pathway repairs these dimers, but the damage can exceed the cell's ability to repair itself.
  - **Ionizing radiation** predominantly causes single- and double-stranded chromosome breaks. It is associated with a variety of cancers, including **leukemia** in those exposed to atomic blasts, **thyroid cancers** in those who have had previous head and neck radiation, and **osteosarcoma** in watch-dial workers who are exposed to radium.
- **Viruses and microbes:** Can cause cellular or direct DNA damage and thus predispose to cancer, as seen in Table 5-7.

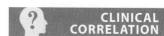

**CLINICAL CORRELATION**

In **xeroderma pigmentosum,** an autosomal recessive disease, the nucleotide excision repair pathway itself is dysfunctional. Those affected have a high incidence of skin cancer.

## Tumor Immunity

Affected cells often display tumor antigens that can stimulate the immune system. Tumor antigens may be specific (tumor-specific antigens [**TSAs**]) if expressed only in tumor cells or associated (tumor-associated antigens [**TAAs**]) if expressed in both normal and tumor cells. These antigens may also be used clinically to confirm the diagnosis, monitor for tumor recurrence, and monitor the response to therapy (Table 5-8). Because

**TABLE 5-6.** **Chemical Carcinogens**

| TOXIN | ASSOCIATED CANCER |
| --- | --- |
| Aflatoxins | Hepatocellular carcinoma |
| Alcohol | Hepatocellular carcinoma |
| Alkylating agents | Leukemia |
| Arsenic | Squamous cell carcinoma of the skin |
| Asbestos | Mesothelioma and bronchogenic carcinoma |
| Benzene | Acute leukemia |
| Carbon tetrachloride ($CCl_4$) | Centrilobular necrosis and fatty changes of the liver |
| Cigarette smoke | Carcinoma of the larynx and lung |
| Diethylstilbestrol (DES) | Clear cell adenocarcinoma of the vagina in offspring of mothers given the drug during pregnancy |
| Ionizing radiation | Papillary thyroid carcinoma |
| Naphthalene (aniline) dyes | Transitional cell carcinoma |
| Nitrosamines | Esophageal and gastric cancer |
| Radon | Lung cancer (2nd leading cause after cigarette smoke) |
| Vinyl chloride | Angiosarcoma of the liver |

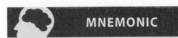

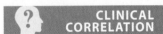

**TABLE 5-7.** **Viruses and Microbes, Associated Cancers, and Mechanisms**

| VIRUS/MICROBE | ASSOCIATED CANCER | MECHANISM |
|---|---|---|
| HPV 16,18 | Cervical, vulvar, penile, and anal carcinoma | HPV viruses produce E6 and E7 proteins. E7 inactivates *Rb*; E6 disables *p53* |
| HTLV-1 | Adult T-cell leukemia | The *tax* gene leads to a high rate of proliferation of T cells, which are subsequently vulnerable to mutations and translocations |
| HBV, HCV | Hepatocellular carcinoma | Causes chronic liver injury and regenerative hyperplasia, which can increase vulnerability to transformation |
| EBV | ▪ Burkitt lymphoma<br>▪ Nasopharyngeal carcinoma | Leads to proliferation of B cells; high rate of mutations and translocations |
| HHV-8 | ▪ Kaposi sarcoma<br>▪ B-cell lymphoma | Common in immunocompromised patients |
| *Helicobacter pylori* | Gastric adenocarcinoma, MALT lymphoma | Chronic inflammation |
| Liver fluke (*Clonorchis sinensis*) | Cholangiocarcinoma | Chronic inflammation |
| *Schistosoma haematobium* | Bladder cancer (squamous cell) | Chronic inflammation |

EBV, Epstein-Barr virus; HBV, hepatitis B virus; HCV, hepatitis C virus; HHV, human herpesvirus; HPV, human papillomavirus; HTLV, human T-lymphotropic virus; MALT, mucosa-associated lymphoid tissue.

these antigens are not expressed by normal tissues or are expressed at relatively low amounts, **cytotoxic T lymphocytes** and **natural killer cells** can recognize and destroy the neoplastic cells. The cancer cells can also escape the immune system through many mechanisms, including:

▪ Selection for cells that do not express TSAs, TAAs, human leukocyte antigen (HLA), or costimulatory receptors.
▪ Immunosuppression.

### Epidemiology

Cancer is the second leading cause of death in the United States (after heart disease). For this reason, it is important to understand the epidemiology of cancer.

**Common cancers** are listed below from most to least common:

▪ **Males:** Prostate, lung, and colorectal.
▪ **Females:** Breast, lung, and colorectal.

**Highest mortality rate** (from most to least common):

▪ **Males:** Lung, prostate.
▪ **Females:** Lung, breast.

**TABLE 5-8.** **Tumor Antigens and Associated Cancers**

| ANTIGEN | ASSOCIATED CANCER |
|---|---|
| Alkaline phosphatase | ▪ Metastases to bone |
| α-Fetoprotein | ▪ Hepatocellular carcinomas<br>▪ Nonseminomatous germ cell tumors of the testis (eg, yolk sac tumor) |
| β-hCG | ▪ Hydatidiform moles<br>▪ Choriocarcinomas<br>▪ Gestational trophoblastic tumors |
| Bombesin | ▪ Neuroblastoma<br>▪ Lung and gastric cancer |
| CA 15-3/CA 27-29 | Breast cancer |
| CA 19-9 | Pancreatic adenocarcinoma |
| CA-125 | Ovarian malignant epithelial tumors |
| Calcitonin | Medullary thyroid carcinoma |
| Carcinoembryonic antigen | ▪ Colorectal, pancreatic, gastric, and breast cancers<br>▪ Nonspecific; also used to monitor colorectal cancer recurrence after initial treatment/resection |
| Chromogranin | Neuroendocrine tumors/carcinoid |
| Prostate-specific antigen (PSA) | ▪ Prostatic carcinoma<br>▪ Can be elevated in benign prostatic hyperplasia and prostatitis<br>▪ Questionable risk/benefit for screening<br>▪ Used for monitoring recurrence and tumor load |
| S-100 | ▪ Melanoma<br>▪ Neural tumors<br>▪ Astrocytomas |
| Tartrate-resistant acid phosphatase | Hairy cell leukemia |

β-hCG, beta human chorionic gonadotropin.

**Note:** Lung cancer deaths are decreasing in males (due to smoking reduction), but increasing in females.

Other cancers are associated with particular diseases, as shown in Tables 5-9 and 5-10.

## CELL DEATH

There are two major forms of cell death: **apoptosis** and **necrosis.** Apoptosis occurs physiologically, but either type of cell death can occur in pathologic situations. Each type of cell death results in a distinct morphologic appearance.

### Apoptosis

Apoptosis is a form of programmed cell death that requires adenosine triphosphate (ATP) to perform a series of distinct and highly regulated steps. Intracellular enzymes

---

**KEY FACT**

**Apoptosis:** Programmed cell death, characterized by activation of cytosolic caspaces, leading to cellular breakdown in a structured fashion. The end result is fragmentation of cells into apoptotic bodies with intact plasma membrane, which do not generate a significant inflammatory response. The apoptotic bodies are then phagocytosed by macrophages.

**Necrosis:** Enzymatic degradation of a cell secondary to an exogenous injury. This leads to enlarged cell size (swelling, loss of plasma membrane integrity). The release of intracellular components leads to an inflammatory response.

**TABLE 5-9.**    **Diseases and Associated Neoplasms**

| CONDITION | NEOPLASM |
|---|---|
| Down syndrome | - Acute lymphoblastic leukemia<br>- Acute myelogenous leukemia |
| Albinism | - Melanoma<br>- Basal and squamous cancer of the skin |
| Chronic atrophic gastritis | Gastric adenocarcinoma |
| Pernicious anemia | |
| Postsurgical gastric remnants | |
| Tuberous sclerosis | - Giant cell astrocytomas<br>- Renal angiomyolipomas<br>- Cardiac rhabdomyomas<br>(Tumors may become malignant.) |
| Actinic keratosis | Squamous cell carcinoma of the skin |
| Barrett esophagus/chronic gastroesophageal reflux | Esophageal adenocarcinoma |
| Plummer-Vinson syndrome | Squamous cell carcinoma of the esophagus |
| Cirrhosis (alcoholic; hepatitis B or C) | Hepatocellular carcinoma |
| Ulcerative colitis | Colonic adenocarcinoma |
| Paget disease of bone | - Osteosarcoma |
| | - Fibrosarcoma |
| Immunodeficiency | Malignant lymphomas |
| AIDS | - Aggressive malignant lymphomas<br>  (non-Hodgkin)<br>- Kaposi sarcoma |
| Autoimmune disease (eg, Hashimoto thyroiditis, myasthenia gravis) | Benign and malignant thymomas |
| Acanthosis nigricans | Visceral malignancy (stomach, lung, breast, uterus) |
| Dysplastic nevus | Malignant melanoma |
| Dermato- and polymyositis | Associated with visceral malignancies, particularly genitourinary |
| Multiple seborrheic keratoses | Gastrointestinal, breast, lung, and lymphoid malignancies |
| Li-Fraumeni syndrome | *p53* mutation predisposes to various cancer types at a young age (eg, sarcoma, breast, leukemia, adrenal gland) |
| Radiation exposure | High risk of developing leukemia, sarcoma, papillary thyroid cancer, breast cancer |

**FLASH FORWARD**

Li-Fraumeni syndrome: a deficiency in *p53*. *p53* has many roles, including DNA repair, proliferation, apoptosis, and others. In Li-Fraumeni syndrome, the decreased apoptosis results in unregulated cell growth and tumorigenesis.

are activated to degrade DNA and proteins. The resulting apoptotic bodies can be cleared by phagocytosis. Because the cellular contents are not released, apoptosis does *not* result in an **inflammatory response** (Figure 5-6).

Causes

Apoptosis may be physiologic, usually induced by specific activation of death receptors or loss of growth factors:

**TABLE 5-10.** **Inherited Diseases Associated with Cancers**

| SYNDROME | INHERITANCE | ASSOCIATED CANCER | GENE (LOCATION) |
|---|---|---|---|
| Familial adenomatous polyposis coli | Autosomal dominant | Colon adenocarcinoma | *APC* (chromosome 5) |
| Multiple endocrine neoplasia (MEN) | Autosomal dominant | ■ 1: Carcinoma of the thyroid, parathyroid, adrenal cortex, pancreas, pituitary<br>■ 2A: Pheochromocytoma, medullary carcinoma of the thyroid<br>■ 2B: Pheochromocytoma, medullary carcinoma of the thyroid, mucocutaneous neuromas | *RET* (chromosome 10; only MEN 2A and MEN 2B) |
| Neurofibromatosis | Autosomal dominant | ■ Neurofibroma<br>■ Pheochromocytoma<br>■ Wilms tumor<br>■ Rhabdomyosarcoma<br>■ Leukemia | *NF1* (chromosome 17)<br>*NF2* (chromosome 22) |
| Von Hippel–Lindau syndrome | Autosomal dominant | ■ Hemangioblastoma<br>■ Adenomas<br>■ Renal cell carcinoma (frequently bilateral) | *VHL* (chromosome 3) |
| Xeroderma pigmentosa | Autosomal recessive (DNA repair) | ■ Melanoma<br>■ Squamous and basal cell carcinoma of the skin | *XPA* (chromosome 9) |
| Ataxia-telangiectasia | Autosomal recessive (DNA repair) | Lymphomas (sensitivity to ionizing radiation) | *ATM* (chromosome 11) |
| Bloom syndrome | Autosomal recessive (DNA repair) | Leukemia/lymphoma | *BLM* (chromosome 15) |
| Fanconi anemia | Autosomal recessive (DNA repair) | Myelodysplastic syndrome/leukemia (sensitivity to mitomycin C) | Many genes |
| Hereditary nonpolyposis colorectal cancer syndrome | Autosomal dominant | ■ Colon cancer<br>■ Breast cancer<br>■ Ovarian cancer | *MSH2* (chromosome 2)<br>*MLH1* (chromosome 3) |

- **Programmed tissue removal** during embryogenesis (eg, webbings between the digits).
- Tissue loss in an adult, usually hormone dependent.
- **Cell turnover,** as in intestinal epithelia.
- Death of a host cell after its function has been fulfilled (ie, the end of an immune response).
- Lymphocyte selection (eg, elimination of self-reactive lymphocytes during development).
- Death induced by cytotoxic T cells.

Apoptosis can also occur pathologically as a response to cellular damage, usually resulting from mild injuries. Common examples include:

- **DNA damage** from radiation or cytotoxic drugs.
- Certain viral infections (eg, hepatitis).
- Pathologic atrophy (eg, after duct obstruction due to a tumor).

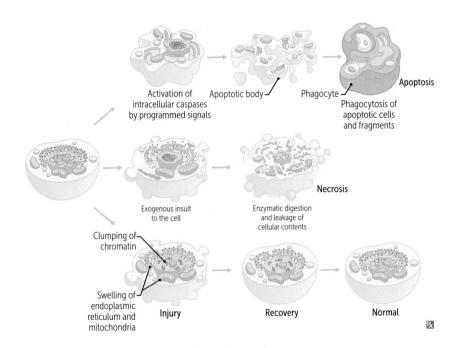

FIGURE 5-6.    **Comparison of apoptosis and necrosis.**

- Tumor cell regression or turnover.
- Accumulation of misfolded proteins (eg, in degenerative diseases).

### Morphology

The distinctive features of apoptotic cells allow for easy identification by electron microscopy. These include:

- Cell shrinkage with dense cytoplasm. **Pyknosis:** nuclear shrinkage and basophilia. **Karyorrhexis:** nuclear fragmentation.
- **Condensation of chromatin** at the periphery of the nuclear membrane.
- Membrane **cytoplasmic blebs** and cellular fragmentation into apoptotic bodies.
- **Phagocytosis** of apoptotic cells or bodies.

Typically, the plasma membrane remains intact and prevents the cellular contents (eg, lysosomal enzymes) from damaging adjacent tissue or stimulating an inflammatory response. On histologic section, apoptotic cells appear **strongly eosinophilic** with dense chromatin, and are generally found in small groups.

### Mechanisms of Apoptosis

Apoptosis occurs when signals activate **caspases,** which are a family of cysteine proteases. The activated caspases cleave the cellular cytoskeleton proteins and activate DNAses, which fragment the nuclear DNA into 50- to 300-kilobase pieces. This is seen as a **DNA ladder** when extracted DNA is run on gel electrophoresis. Apoptotic cells also flip **phosphatidylserine** from the inner to the outer layer of their plasma membrane, which targets the cell for clearance by macrophages.

Apoptosis can be induced by two separate pathways, as seen in Figure 5-7: Extrinsic (death receptor–initiated) or intrinsic (mitochondrial).

- The **extrinsic pathway** is activated when **death receptors,** such as the type 1 tumor necrosis factor receptor, or Fas, on the cell surface are stimulated. Cross-linking of these death receptors leads to signaling that activates caspase-8. This pathway of apoptosis is blocked by a protein called FLIP.
- The **intrinsic pathway** involves the release of proteins, including **cytochrome c,** from a leaky mitochondrion. These proteins activate caspase-9. Intrinsic apoptosis

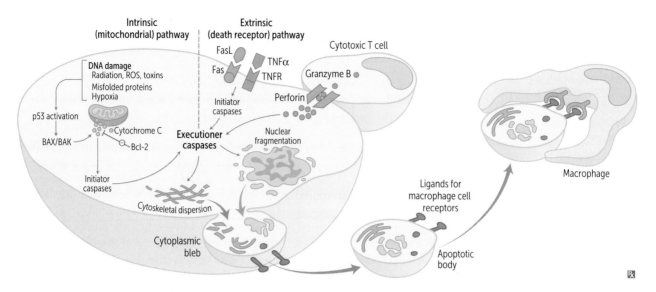

**FIGURE 5-7.** **Two major pathways of apoptosis.** Both the intrinsic (mitochondrion-based) and extrinsic (death receptor) signaling pathways are shown. Apaf, apoptotic proteinase-activating factor; BAX, Bcl-2 associated X protein; Bcl-2, B-cell lymphoma 2; FasL, Fas ligand.

is regulated by a balance between proapoptotic cellular molecules Bak, Bax, and Bim and antiapoptotic molecules Bcl-2 and Bcl-xL.

Both of these pathways converge on the same cascade of activated caspases. Each caspase exists as a zymogen, or inactive proenzyme, and is activated through cleavage by the previous caspase in the cascade. Caspases, including caspase-3 and caspase-6, function as "ultimate executioners" and promote protein cleavage and DNA breakdown within the cell.

## Necrosis

**Necrosis** is uncontrolled degradation of cells in living tissues following irreparable cellular damage. The plasma membrane is often disrupted, releasing cellular contents into the surrounding area, resulting in tissue damage and an inflammatory response. Debris are enzymatically digested and ultimately phagocytosed. If necrotic cells are not removed, they promote mineral deposition, leading to **dystrophic calcification.**

### Causes

Necrosis is generally considered to be due to irreversible exogenous injury that exceeds the body's ability to repair itself. There are several forms of cellular injury:

- **Ischemia/hypoxia** is the most common type of cell injury and results from reduced blood flow.
- **Ischemia/reperfusion injury** can occur when blood flow returns to ischemic tissue, causing free radical formation as a result of rapid oxygen influx and mitochondrial dysfunction.
- Chemical/toxic injury.

### Morphology

The appearance of damaged cells lies on a continuum between reversibly injured and necrotic cells. Several hallmarks are visible on histologic sections:

- Increased cytoplasmic eosinophilia.
- **Myelin figures** (whorled phospholipids) from damaged cell membranes.
- Nuclear breakdown occurs in a consecutive process:
  - Pyknosis: Increased nuclear basophilia and shrinkage.
  - Karyorrhexis: nuclear fragmentation.
  - Karyolysis: nuclear dissolution and disappearance of basophilia (DNA enzymatically degraded by endonucleases).

**CLINICAL CORRELATION**

In follicular lymphoma, a type of non-Hodgkin lymphoma, translocation of chromosomal arms of 14 and 18 results in uncontrolled Bcl-2 expression, which prevents apoptosis and leads to uncontrolled cell growth.

**KEY FACT**

Irreversible injuries occur when the cell cannot reverse the disturbances in mitochondrial and membrane function.

Types of Necrosis

There are several morphologically distinct patterns of cell necrosis, depending on the type of tissue injured and the mechanism of injury.

- **Coagulative necrosis** (Figure 5-8A) occurs most often from ischemic injury. Both structural proteins and enzymes become denatured and nonfunctional. As a result, there is no proteolysis of the dead cells, which retain their form/outline having lost their nuclei (anucleate ghost cells). Tissue architecture is similarly preserved (Figure 5-8). Coagulative necrosis results in two types of infarction: (1) pale (**white infarct**), which occurs with arterial occlusion in solid organs that have a single blood supply and dense tissue limiting diffusion of RBCs (eg, heart, spleen, kidney) and (2) hemorrhagic (**red infarct**), which occurs with venous occlusion (eg, testicular torsion), in loose spongy tissue (eg, the lungs), in organs with dual circulation (eg, lungs, intestines), or when blood flow is reestablished to a site previously infarcted due to arterial inclusion (eg, reperfusion after angioplasty or thrombolysis).
- Bacterial and some fungal infections cause **liquefactive** (Figure 5-8B). Neutrophils release lysosomal enzymes that digest the tissue, causing the loss of structure and cell outlines. Liquefactive necrosis is also observed following hypoxic injury to the central nervous system (CNS) for unknown reasons.
- **Caseous necrosis** (Figure 5-8C) is usually found in granulomas following infection with tuberculosis or systemic fungi. Macrophages wall off the infecting organism, causing granular debris. The appearance is often described as white and "cheesy." Cells are amorphous, and tissue architecture is completely degraded.
- **Fat necrosis** (Figure 5-8D) is not a strict morphologic pattern of necrosis, but refers to necrotic destruction of large areas of fat. Usually due to acute pancreatitis, in which activated pancreatic enzymes degrade adipocytes. Released fatty acids from adipocytes combine with calcium, resulting in **fat saponification.** Also occurs in breast trauma.
- **Fibrinoid necrosis** (Figure 5-8E) is a type of necrosis seen in the walls of blood vessels (usually arteries) from the deposition of immune complexes (in the setting of immunologic reactions) and resulting deposition of fibrin, damaging the vessel wall.
- **Gangrenous necrosis** (Figure 5-8F) is seen in the distal extremities after ischemia. It is categorized as either dry gangrene (coagulative necrosis) or wet gangrene (liquefactive necrosis due to superinfection).

Any form of necrosis can result in the release of cellular contents, with subsequent inflammation.

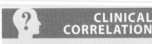

**CLINICAL CORRELATION**

Elevated enzymes in the blood can reveal the source of necrosis:
- Lipase: Enzyme released due to pancreatic cell necrosis
- Troponin: Enzyme released due to cardiac myocyte necrosis
- Creatine kinase: Enzyme released due to skeletal or myocardial necrosis

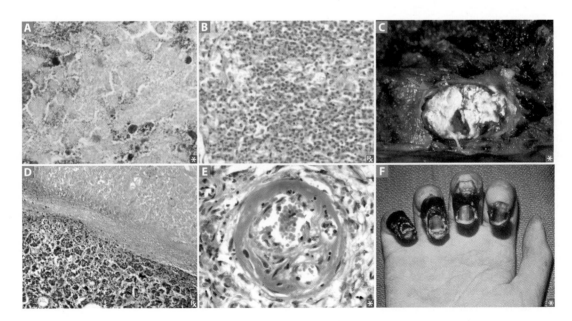

**FIGURE 5-8.** **Necrosis.** A Coagulative necrosis; B liquefactive necrosis; C caseous necrosis; D fat necrosis; E fibrinoid necrosis; F acral gangrene.

## Inflammation

Inflammation is the immune system's response to toxic agents or damaged tissues. This response can be divided into **vascular and cellular reactions,** involves the **secretion of mediators,** and is followed by attempted tissue repair.

### Vascular Reaction

Changes in the vasculature allow immune cells and mediators to migrate from the blood vessel to the site of injury. Changes occur in the following order:

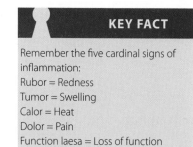

- Ultra-short neurogenic reflex of vasoconstriction lasting seconds.
- **Vasodilation** in the arterioles and capillary beds mainly due to the action of histamine and nitric oxide on vascular smooth muscle resulting in increased blood flow to the injured area (causing redness and heat).
- Histamine-mediated increased **permeability** of the vessel wall along with increased hydrostatic pressure from increased blood flow result in loss of protein-rich fluid into the extracellular tissues (causing swelling).
- Loss of fluid results in increased cellular concentrations in the blood, so flow is slowed, causing **stasis.**
- Stasis allows for increased leukocyte migration through the endothelium.

### Cellular Reaction

Leukocytes, particularly neutrophils and macrophages, are responsible for the removal of offending agents and damaged tissue. Chemotactic factors, such as **complement component 5a** (C5a), interleukin (IL)-8, leukotriene $B_4$ (LTB$_4$), kallikrein, and platelet-activating factor, recruit leukocytes to the site of injury. Leukocytes must travel from the blood vessel lumen to the interstitial tissue in a process called **extravasation** (Figure 5-9). This occurs in four steps:

- **Margination and rolling:** Leukocytes migrate to the vessel periphery and move along the endothelium. Endothelium expresses **selectins,** which bind with low affinity to **Sialyl-Lewis X glycoproteins** on leukocytes.
- **Adhesion:** Leukocytes bind firmly to endothelial cells. The endothelium expresses immunoglobulin **vascular cell adhesion molecule 1 (VCAM-1)** and intercellular **adhesion molecule 1 (ICAM-1),** which bind with high affinity to **integrins** on leukocytes.

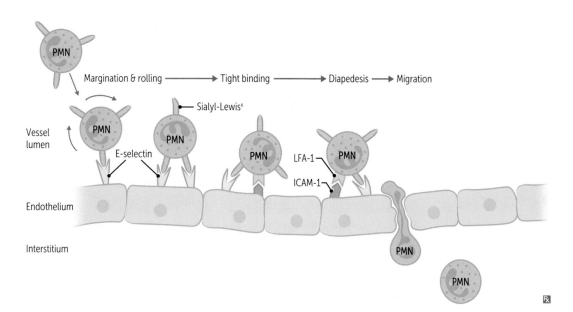

**FIGURE 5-9.** **Extravasation.** Extravasation occurs in four steps: margination and rolling, adhesion, transmigration or diapedesis, and migration to the site of injury.

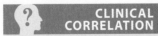
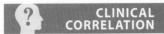

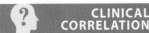
- **Transmigration (diapedesis):** Leukocytes travel through the vessel wall. **Platelet endothelial cell adhesion molecule (PECAM-1)** or **CD31** in the interendothelial space facilitates movement.
- **Migration** through the interstitium to the site of injury.

On arrival, leukocytes attempt to remove the microbe or other agent via **phagocytosis** and release substances such as lysosomal enzymes, reactive oxygen intermediates, and prostaglandins. These mediators can damage the endothelium and surrounding tissues. Many acute and chronic human diseases result from an excessive inflammatory response.

### Chemical Mediators of Inflammation

Mediators are produced in response to microbial products or host proteins activated by microbes or damaged tissues. These chemicals can be activated from precursors in plasma or may be newly produced by cells. Mediators are generally short-lived once they are activated, which helps limit the damage caused by inflammation. They fall into several categories (Table 5-11).

The roles of these mediators in inflammation are summarized in Table 5-12.

Laboratory findings associated with inflammation are summarized in Table 5-13.

**TABLE 5-11.** **Inflammatory Mediators**

| COMPOUND | SOURCE | FUNCTION |
|---|---|---|
| Histamine/serotonin | Stored preformed in mast cells, platelets, and enterochromaffin cells | ▪ Dilates arterioles<br>▪ Increases permeability of venules |
| Complement cascade (C3a, C5a) | Plasma | ▪ Functions in innate and adaptive immunity<br>▪ Increases vascular permeability |
| Coagulation system | Thrombin found in plasma | Promotes vascular permeability and leukocyte migration |
| Kinin system | Plasma | Release of bradykinin causes contraction of smooth muscle in lung and dilation of blood vessels |
| Prostaglandins/ leukotrienes | Many cells | Contributes to pain and fever during inflammation |
| Cytokines | Many cells | Systemic acute-phase responses (eg, fever, loss of appetite, neutrophilia) |
| Nitric oxide | Constitutively expressed or induced by cytokine activation | ▪ Potent vasodilator<br>▪ Reduces platelet aggregation<br>▪ Microbicidal |
| Lysosomal enzymes | Leukocytes | ▪ Microbicidal<br>▪ Destructive to endothelium and surrounding tissues |
| $O_2$-derived free radicals | Leukocytes (NADPH oxidative system) | ▪ Microbicidal<br>▪ Destructive to endothelium and surrounding tissues |

NADPH, reduced form of nicotinamide adenine dinucleotide phosphate.

**TABLE 5-12.**    **Functions of Chemical Mediators in the Cardinal Signs of Inflammation**

| SIGN | REACTION | MEDIATORS |
|------|----------|-----------|
| Redness (rubor) | Vasodilation | Histamine, prostaglandins, nitric oxide (NO) |
| Heat (calor) | Vasodilation, fever | Histamine, prostaglandins, NO, interleukin-1, tumor necrosis factor (TNF) |
| Swelling (tumor) | Increased vascular permeability | Histamine, serotonin, bradykinin, leukotrienes |
| Pain (dolor) | Release of mediators | Prostaglandins, bradykinin |
| Loss of function | Tissue damage | NO, lysosomal enzymes, $O_2$-derived free radicals |

## Acute Inflammation

Acute inflammation is a rapid vascular and cellular response to an agent causing tissue damage. Onset occurs in seconds to minutes, and the reaction lasts for several hours or days.

### Stimuli

Acute inflammatory responses can have multiple causes:

- Microbial infections or toxins.
- Tissue necrosis from any cause (eg, hypoxia).
- Physical (trauma, frostbite) or chemical damage.
- Foreign bodies.
- Hypersensitivity reactions.

### Major Cells Involved

Neutrophils are recruited to the site of injury and are responsible for clearing the area. Other cell types produce inflammatory mediators.

**TABLE 5-13.**    **Associated Lab Findings in Inflammation**

| LAB | FINDINGS | MECHANISM/SIGNIFICANCE |
|-----|----------|------------------------|
| WBC | Leukocytosis; left shift; toxic granulation | IL-1 and TNF mediate leukocytosis, resulting in presence of premature WBCs. |
| ESR | Elevated ESR | Inflammatory factors promote RBC rouleaux formation, resulting in prolongation of the rate of RBC settling in a vertical tube. |
| CRP | Elevated; an acute-phase reactant | Sensitive indicator of acute inflammation. May be used as a marker to monitor disease states and therapy. |
| Albumin | Decreased | Due to catabolic action of inflammation. The liver synthesizes acute-phase reactants from albumin breakdown. Prealbumin is not affected by inflammation and may be a better marker of protein nutritional state. |
| LFTs | Elevated | Liver enzymes such as AST and ALT may be elevated in inflammatory states secondary to cellular damage in the liver. |

ALT, alanine aminotransferase; AST, aspartate aminotransferase; CRP, C-reactive protein; ESR, erythrocyte sedimentation rate; IL, interleukin; LFTs, liver function tests; RBC, red blood cells; TNF, tumor necrosis factor; WBC, white blood cells.

## Outcomes

Acute inflammation has three possible outcomes:

- **Progression** to chronic inflammation.
- **Resolution,** resulting in clearance of the harmful stimulus and rebuilding of injured tissue. The tissue regains its normal function.
- **Fibrosis,** in which the damaged tissue is replaced with scar tissue. The tissue loses its function permanently.

## Chronic Inflammation

Inflammation, tissue destruction, and tissue repair proceed simultaneously for a longer duration.

### Causes of Chronic Inflammation

- **Persistent microbial and viral infection:** Characteristically caused by tuberculosis, syphilis, or particular viral, fungal, or parasitic infections. Organisms evoke a delayed-type hypersensitivity reaction from the host. Incomplete clearance of the organism leads to chronic inflammation.
- **Prolonged exposure to a toxic agent:** May be exogenous, as in silicosis due to long-term inhalation of silica, or endogenous, such as the reaction to plasma lipids in atherosclerosis.
- **Autoimmune diseases,** in which the inflammatory response to autoantigens results in tissue damage.

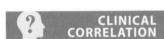

**CLINICAL CORRELATION**

The delayed-type hypersensitivity reaction in tuberculosis is the basis for the purified protein derivative (PPD) skin test, where macrophages are the principle cell in the indurated region.

### Major Cells Involved

Chronic inflammation is marked by infiltration of mononuclear cells and fibroblasts. Macrophages promote fibrosis and angiogenesis through their production of growth factors and cytokines but also cause tissue damage by releasing reactive oxygen species and proteases. Lymphocytes, plasma cells, eosinophils, and mast cells may also be involved.

### Morphologic Features

Generally, chronic inflammation is characterized by the presence of mononuclear cells, damaged tissue, and tissue repair. Repair is visible as fibrosis (formation of connective tissue) and angiogenesis (growth of new blood vessels).

**Granulomatous inflammation** is a distinctive type of chronic inflammation. Causes of granulomatous inflammation include: (1) **infectious** (eg, tuberculosis, histoplasmosis) and (2) **noninfectious** (eg, sarcoidosis, Crohn disease). Granulomatous inflammation is characterized by the formation of granulomas, focal sites of inflammation consisting of **central caseous necrosis** surrounded by macrophages, some of which form giant cells with multiple nuclei at the periphery (**Langhans-type giant cells**). The periphery of the granuloma is surrounded by lymphocytes and the occasional plasma cell. Granulomas can also have **noncaseous necrosis,** usually in response to foreign bodies or in sarcoidosis, as seen in Figure 5-10. In these cases, giant cells have nuclei scattered throughout the cell (foreign body–type giant cell).

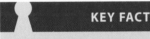

**KEY FACT**

Caseous necrosis indicates an infectious disease, prototypically tuberculosis. Noncaseous necrosis is found in sarcoidosis and Crohn disease.

### Outcomes

Chronic inflammation causes fibrosis, with resultant loss of function.

## HLA ASSOCIATIONS

Major histocompatibility complex (MHC) alleles associated with autoimmune diseases are primarily located within the classical MHC II loci. MHC II presents antigen to CD4+ T cells, which in turn activate B cells to produce antibody. Therefore, the binding specificities of these alleles are directly linked to the capacity of MHC II to bind self-antigen and initiate an autoimmune disease.

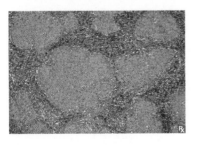

**FIGURE 5-10. Sarcoidosis.** Photomicrograph shows numerous tightly formed granulomas of a lymph node.

## HLA Genes

In humans there are four **HLA genes** known as *HLA-A*, *HLA-B*, *HLA-C*, and *HLA-D*. *HLA-A*, *HLA-B*, and *HLA-C* produce MHC class I molecules, which are expressed by almost all nucleated cells. They allow immune cells to monitor the cytoplasmic contents of each cell, especially during intracellular infections.

*HLA-D*, on the other hand, produces MHC class II molecules, which are only expressed by specialized cells (such as B cells, macrophages, dendritic cells, and other "antigen presenting cells") which display material acquired from extracellular spaces (eg, bacterial proteins). *HLA-D* is now recognized to contain three separate genes known as *HLA-DP*, *HLA-DQ*, and *HLA-DR*, with *HLA-DR* being the most extensively studied and related to certain human diseases.

## HLA Polymorphism and Disease Risk

Each HLA gene is highly **polymorphic,** which is to say that there are many variants or alleles in the human population. Each variant is given a different number, such as *HLA-B8*, *HLA-B27*, *HLA-DR2*, or *HLA-DR3*. (Note that a single individual can, at most, have two variants for any particular HLA gene, one from each of his or her parents.)

Because HLA molecules are in the business of presenting antigens, it is thought that they may be able to bind self-proteins and elicit autoimmunity. Some alleles predispose to certain autoimmune diseases, whereas others are associated with increased incidence and severity as summarized in Table 5-14.

**TABLE 5-14.   HLA-Associated Diseases**

| HLA TYPE | DISEASE ASSOCIATION |
|----------|---------------------|
| A3 | ▪ Hemochromatosis |
| B8 | ▪ Graves disease<br>▪ Celiac disease |
| B27 | ▪ Ankylosing spondylitis<br>▪ Reactive arthritis<br>▪ Reiter syndrome<br>▪ Acute anterior uveitis<br>▪ Psoriasis<br>▪ Inflammatory bowel disease |
| DR2 | ▪ Goodpasture syndrome<br>▪ Multiple sclerosis<br>▪ Narcolepsy<br>▪ SLE<br>▪ Hay fever<br>▪ *Protective* in type 1 diabetes mellitus (type 1 DM) |
| DR3 | ▪ Celiac disease<br>▪ Myasthenia gravis<br>▪ SLE<br>▪ Graves disease<br>▪ Type 1 DM<br>▪ Idiopathic Addison disease |
| DR4 | ▪ Rheumatoid arthritis<br>▪ Type 1 DM<br>▪ Pemphigus vulgaris |

**TABLE 5-14.** **HLA-Associated Diseases** *(continued)*

| HLA TYPE | DISEASE ASSOCIATION |
|----------|---------------------|
| DR5 | ▪ Hashimoto thyroiditis<br>▪ Pernicious anemia |
| DR7 | ▪ Steroid-responsive nephrotic syndrome |
| DR11 | ▪ Hashimoto thyroiditis<br>▪ Celiac disease |
| DQ2/DQ8 | ▪ Celiac disease |
| Dw3 | ▪ Sjögren syndrome |
| Dw4 | ▪ Rheumatoid arthritis |

SLE, systemic lupus erythematosus.

# CHAPTER 6

# General Pharmacology

# Pharmacokinetics and Pharmacodynamics

The general topic of pharmacology can be divided into two main subtopics: **pharmacokinetics** and **pharmacodynamics.**

**Pharmacokinetics** describes the metabolism and movement of drugs into, out of, and within the body. In other words, pharmacokinetics details how the body processes the drugs that enter it.

**Pharmacodynamics** describes a drug's mechanism of action and its physiologic effects—in other words, what the drug does and how it does it.

Both pharmacokinetics and pharmacodynamics depends on the drug's route of **administration.** Possible routes of administration are as follows:

- Transdermal (across the skin)
- Across a mucous membrane
    - Sublingual
    - Rectal
    - Vaginal
- Enteral (oral)
- Parenteral (by injection)
    - Subcutaneous
    - Intramuscular
    - Intravenous (IV)/intra-arterial
- Intrathecal (into the subarachnoid space)

## PHARMACOKINETICS

A drug's pharmacokinetics relates to its **a**bsorption, **d**istribution, **m**etabolism, and excretion.

### Absorption

A particular drug's absorption depends on its specific chemical properties and its route of administration. The fraction of the administered drug that reaches the systemic circulation unchanged is its **bioavailability (F).** By definition, IV administration results in a bioavailability of 100%. Oral administration typically results in a bioavailability lower than 100% due to incomplete absorption and first-pass metabolism (Figure 6-1).

### Distribution

Once a drug reaches the systemic circulation, it has access to nearly every target organ in the body, with the exception of the **brain** and the **testes.** These regions are relatively protected from the general systemic circulation by physiologic barriers. The drug then can be distributed from the bloodstream into various body compartments. Specific distribution depends on the drug's individual characteristics, such as molecular size, charge, and protein interactions. The unique nature of a particular drug's distribution can be understood in terms of its **volume of distribution** ($V_d$), which is a theoretical calculation of the fluid volume that would be needed to contain the total amount of absorbed drug at the concentration of drug found in the plasma at steady state.

$$V_d = \frac{\text{amount of drug in the body (mg)}}{\text{plasma drug concentration (mg/L)}}$$

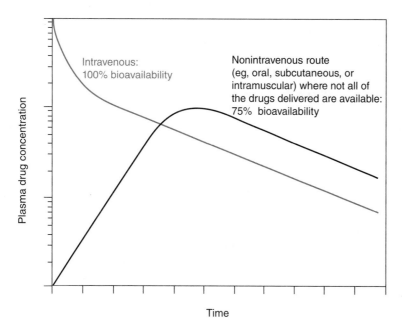

Intravenous:
100% bioavailability

Nonintravenous route
(eg, oral, subcutaneous, or
intramuscular) where not all of
the drugs delivered are available:
75% bioavailability

*Plasma drug concentration* (y-axis)

*Time* (x-axis)

**FIGURE 6-1.    Bioavailability.** Note that because medication administered intravenously has a 100% bioavailability, its plasma drug concentration starts high and then declines as it undergoes metabolism. This is in contrast to nonintravenous route of administration where the plasma drug concentration takes time to build up as the medication is being absorbed.

Drugs that are **small** and **lipophilic** tend to sequester into tissue and fat. As such, they have a **high** $V_d$ because their plasma drug concentration at steady state is very low. In other words, tissues serve as a "sink" and bind much of the protein such that there is very little distributed in the plasma. Therefore, to achieve the low plasma concentration (mg/mL) despite having such a large amount of drug in the body (mg), one would have to contain that large amount of drug in a large theoretical fluid volume (as though diluting the drug).

On the other hand, drugs that are **large, charged,** and **bound to plasma proteins** tend to sequester in the blood. In this case, the amount of drug in the body is mostly contained in the plasma. Therefore, the $V_d$ will be approximately equivalent to the volume of blood (relatively **low**). Of note, a single drug can be distributed in more than one compartment.

Table 6-1 describes the general features of drugs with low, medium, and high $V_d$.

> **KEY FACT**
>
> **Plasma drug concentration** is the **amount** of drug in plasma, regardless of whether the drug is protein bound or free in the plasma.

> **KEY FACT**
>
> The most abundant plasma protein is **albumin.** Although measurements of plasma drug levels include both free and protein-bound levels, protein-bound drugs are inactive.

**TABLE 6-1.    Volume of Distribution for Different Drug Types**

| $V_d$ | COMPARTMENT | DRUG TYPES |
|---|---|---|
| Low | Blood | Large/charged molecules; plasma protein bound |
| Medium | Extracellular fluid | Small hydrophilic molecules |
| High | All tissues including fat | Small lipophilic molecules, especially if bound to tissue protein |

Reproduced with permission from Le T, et al. *First Aid for the USMLE Step 1 2016.* New York, NY: McGraw-Hill Education; 2016: 237.

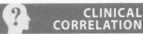

**CLINICAL CORRELATION**

Geriatric patients lose phase I first.

**FLASH FORWARD**

In addition to being metabolized by the cytochrome P450 system, many drugs also either induce or inhibit the system. This in turn affects the metabolism of other drugs and forms the basis for many clinically important drug-drug interactions. This is discussed further in Table 6-2.

**MNEMONIC**

Geriatric patients have **GAS**—

**G**lucuronidation
**A**cetylation
**S**ulfation

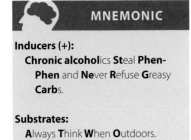

**MNEMONIC**

**Inducers (+):**
   **Chronic alcohol**ics **S**teal **Phen-Phen** and **Ne**ver **R**efuse **G**reasy **Carb**s.

**Substrates:**
   **A**lways **T**hink **W**hen **O**utdoors.

**Inhibitors (−):**
   **AAA RACKS IN GQ M**agazine.

## Metabolism

All orally ingested drugs are first metabolized by the liver before entering the systemic circulation; this is called **first-pass metabolism.** The path taken by oral medications is gastrointestinal (GI) system → portal circulation → liver → hepatic vein → inferior vena cava → heart → systemic circulation → target organs.

Parenterally administered drugs directly enter systemic circulation and bypass first-pass metabolism.

Metabolism occurs in two phases: phase I and phase II. Both of these phases occur in the liver, which is the primary site of drug biotransformation and metabolism.

### Phase I Reaction

Phase I reactions depend on the **cytochrome P450 system,** which is a superfamily of enzymes found mainly in the smooth endoplasmic reticulum of hepatocytes. These enzymes catalyze the metabolism of both endogenous compounds and exogenous drugs and toxins. Generally, phase I metabolism produces slightly polar, **water-soluble** metabolites, which are still **active.** This occurs via **reduction, oxidation,** or **hydrolysis,** which adds or unmasks a polar moiety in the drug.

### Phase II Reaction

Phase II reactions add more soluble moieties to the drug to make it more polar (and thus **more water soluble**) and often **inactive,** such that it can be renally excreted. This occurs via **conjugation** through either **gluroconidation, acetylation,** or **sulfation.** Although drugs are usually detoxified after phase II, in some cases, the metabolites are more toxic than the parent compound. Acetaminophen is one such example.

### Excretion

Just as drugs can enter the body via several different routes, they can also be excreted by the body in several ways.

The rate of drug elimination depends on whether the drug undergoes **zero-order elimination** or **first-order elimination** (Figure 6-2).

**TABLE 6-2.** Cytochrome P450 Interactors [Selected Inducers (+), Substrates, and Inhibitors (−)]

| INDUCERS (+) | SUBSTRATES | INHIBITORS (−) |
|---|---|---|
| Chronic alcohol use | Antiepileptics | Acute alcohol abuse |
| St. John's wort | Theophylline | Ritonavir |
| Phenytoin | Warfarin | Amiodarone |
| Phenobarbital (barbiturates) | Oral contraceptives (OCPs) | Cimetidine |
| Nevirapine | | Ketoconazole |
| Rifampin | | Sulfonamides |
| Griseofulvin | | Isoniazid (INH) |
| Carbamazepine | | Grapefruit |
| Cigarette smoke | | Quinidine |
| Omeprazole | | Macrolides (except azithromycin) |
| Doxorubicin | | Fluoxetine |
| Nefazodone | | Verapamil |
| Valproic acid | | Disulfiram |
| Zileuton | | Metronidazole |
| | | Ciprofloxacin |
| | | Gemfibrozil |

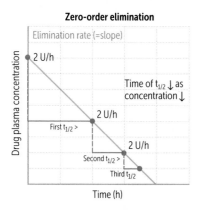
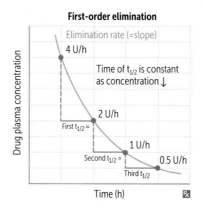

**FIGURE 6-2.** **Drug elimination rates.** In zero-order elimination, the elimination rate is fixed (2 U/hr), resulting in a linear decrease in drug concentration over time. In first-order elimination, the elimination rate is proportional to the drug concentration, resulting in an exponential decrease in drug concentration over time.

In **zero-order elimination,** the rate of elimination is **constant,** regardless of plasma concentration. In other words, a constant **amount** of drug is eliminated per unit time. In this scenario, the plasma concentration decreases **linearly** with time. This type of elimination is also called **capacity-limited** elimination. **P**henytoin, **e**thanol, and **a**spirin (at high concentrations) are eliminated in this manner.

In **first-order elimination,** the rate of elimination is directly **proportional** to the drug concentration. In other words, a constant **fraction** of drug is eliminated per unit time. In this scenario, the plasma concentration decreases **exponentially** with time. This type of elimination is also called **flow-dependent** elimination. Most drugs are eliminated in this manner.

### Half-Life (T$_{1/2}$)

One property of first-order elimination is half-life (T$_{1/2}$), which is the time required to change the amount of drug in the body by one-half during elimination (or constant infusion) (Table 6-3).

$$T_{1/2} = \frac{0.693 \times V_d}{clearance}$$

A drug infused at a constant rate takes 4–5 half-lives to reach steady state. It takes 3.3 half-lives to reach 90% of the steady-state level (Table 6-4).

### Clearance

Clearance (Cl) is the volume of plasma cleared of a drug per unit time. The clearance may be impaired with defects in cardiac, hepatic, or renal function.

$$Cl = \frac{\text{rate of elimination of the drug}}{\text{plasma drug concentration}} = V_d \times K_e \text{ (elimination constant)}$$

### Renal Excretion

The primary site of drug excretion are the kidneys. Drugs or drug metabolites excreted via this route are **hydrophillic** (water soluble). Renal excretion is affected by several factors:

- Glomerular filtration rate (GFR): Determines how quickly the drug can be filtered.
- Serum protein-binding affinity: Determines how much drug can be filtered, as serum-bound proteins cannot be filtered due to to size exclusion.
- Urine pH: Determines the maximum concentration that can be excreted into the urine based on solubility.

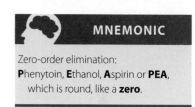

**MNEMONIC**

Zero-order elimination:
**P**henytoin, **E**thanol, **A**spirin or **PEA**, which is round, like a **zero**.

**KEY FACT**

T$_{1/2}$ = 0.7 × V$_d$/Cl, where V$_d$ is volume of distribution and Cl is clearance.

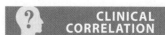

**CLINICAL CORRELATION**

Patients with impaired renal function (eg, diabetes patients, elderly) are susceptible to drug overdose due to impaired renal excretion.

**TABLE 6-3.    Percentage of Drug Remaining After Serial Half-lives**

| Number of half-lives | 1 | 2 | 3 | 4 |
|---|---|---|---|---|
| % remaining | 50% | 25% | 12.5% | 6.25% |

Ionized species are trapped in the urine and quickly cleared, whereas neutral forms can be reabsorbed in the renal tubules.

Drugs that are **weak acids** are trapped in basic environments. As such, alkalinizing the urine with bicarbonate can increase clearance:

$$RCOOH \text{ (lipid soluble, weak acid)} \leftrightarrow RCOO^- + H^+ \text{ (water-soluble in basic environment)}$$

Drugs that are **weak bases** are trapped in acidic environments. As such, acidifying the urine with ammonium chloride can increase clearance:

$$RNH_2 + H^+ \text{ (lipid soluble, weak base)} \leftrightarrow RNH_3^+ \text{ (water-soluble in acidic environment)}$$

### Biliary Excretion

The liver is also a site of drug elimination via biliary excretion of lipophilic drugs. Lipophilic drugs are solubilized in the bile, delivered into the small intestine, and ultimately excreted in feces. However, these drugs can be absorbed by the gut into the enterohepatic circulation and re-enter the systemic circulation.

### Dosage Calculations

In the hospital, drugs are often administered in either loading or maintenance doses. The purpose of the **loading dose** is to achieve a desired drug plasma concentration rapidly when the clinical situation is urgent (eg, therapeutic levels of antiarrhythmic drug must quickly be reached during a potentially fatal arrhythmia event). **Maintenance doses,** on the other hand, are used once a drug has reached steady state, in order to offset the rate of clearance and maintain drug levels within the therapeutic window.

### Loading Dose

- **Loading dose** $= C_P \times V_d/F$, where $C_P$ = target plasma concentration, $V_d$ = volume of distribution, and $F$ = bioavailability.
- In urgent situations or when administering drugs with long half-lives, a large loading dose may be used to rapidly reach therapeutic plasma levels.

### Maintenance Dose

- **Maintenance dose** $= \dfrac{C_p \times Cl \times \tau}{F}$

  where $C_p$ = target plasma concentration, $V_d$ = volume of distribution, $F$ = bioavailability, and $\tau$ = dosage interval (time between doses). $\tau$ can be excluded if the drug is administered continuously.

**TABLE 6-4.    Percentage of Steady State as a Function of Half-life**

| Number of half-lives | 1 | 2 | 3 | 3.3 | 4 |
|---|---|---|---|---|---|
| Concentration (%) | 50 | 75 | 87.5 | 90 | 93.75 |

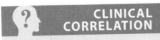

**CLINICAL CORRELATION**

Weak acid drugs: Phenobarbital, methotrexate, aspirin.
Weak base drugs: Amphetamines.
Weak acid drug overdose: Treat with bicarbonate.
Weak base drug overdose: Treat with ammonium chloride.

- To maintain a therapeutic concentration, the maintenance dose must be given to ensure that input = output.
- Patients with impaired hepatic or renal function often receive the same loading dose but a reduced maintenance dose.
- Time to steady state depends primarily on half-life and is independent of dose and dosing frequency.

## PHARMACODYNAMICS

A drug's **pharmacodynamics** relates to its receptor interactions, efficacy, potency, and toxicity.

### Receptor Interactions

Drugs can be broadly classified as agonists or antagonists depending on their action at a target site or receptor. A single drug can have multiple actions; it may act as an agonist at one type of receptor and an antagonist at another.

### Agonists

Agonists bind to a receptor and stabilize it in an active conformation.

- **Full agonists:** Produce a maximum response after binding to the receptor.
- **Partial agonists:** Produce a less-than-maximum response after binding to the receptor.
- When both full agonists and partial agonists are present in a system, the overall response may be less than the response to full agonists. Depending on the binding affinity, partial agonist molecules may preferentially bind to receptors and prevent full agonists from binding to the same receptors and exerting a maximum response. Thus, partial agonists may also be called **partial antagonists** or **mixed agonist-antagonists.**

### Antagonists

Antagonists inhibit the action of an agonist, but have no effect in the absence of the agonist. They are broadly categorized as receptor antagonists or nonreceptor antagonists (Figure 6-3).

- **Nonreceptor antagonists:** Do not bind to receptors but inhibit the ability of the agonist to initiate its action.
- **Receptor antagonists:** Bind to either the active site or an allosteric site.

The active site is where agonists bind to produce a response. **Allosteric sites** are sites other than the active site that are involved in receptor activation. In both cases, binding of the antagonist prevents agonists from activating the receptor; an active site antagonist prevents agonist binding, whereas an allosteric site antagonist prevents receptor activation without preventing agonist binding.

#### Nonreceptor Antagonists

- Inhibit agonists directly or affect the downstream pathway of the agonist.
- Divided into **chemical antagonists** or **physiologic antagonists.**
  - Chemical antagonists inactivate the agonist directly. Examples are antibodies and protamine, which bind heparin directly to inactivate heparin.
  - Physiologic antagonists mediate a response opposite that of the agonist receptor. An example is atropine, which is a type of muscarinic adrenergic antagonist that produces mydriasis.

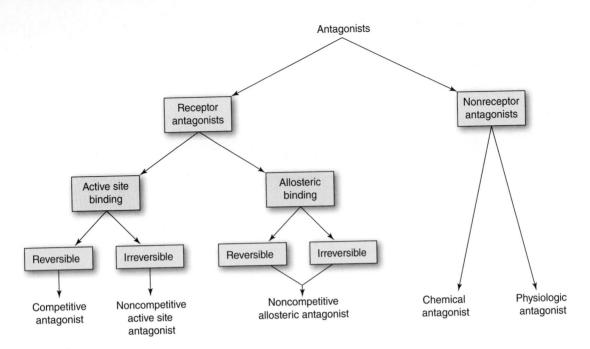

**FIGURE 6-3.** **Antagonist categories.**

### Competitive Antagonists

- Compete with agonists for the same active site and bind reversibly.
- By occupying the active site, the competitive antagonist blocks agonists from binding and activating the receptor.
- Antagonist effects can be overcome by flooding the system with another molecule (ie, an agonist) that binds to the same site, thereby outnumbering and outcompeting the competitive antagonist.

### Noncompetitive Antagonists

- Bind to an allosteric site on the receptor.
- Exert effect by changing the conformation of the receptor such that agonists cannot activate the receptor, even if they can bind to the active site.
- Effect cannot be overcome by flooding the system with an agonist molecule.

### Irreversible Antagonists

- Bind irreversibly to either the active site or to an allosteric site on the receptor.
- Bind to the site with very high affinity; their antagonist effects cannot be overcome either by saturating the system with an agonist molecule or by washing the antagonist out of the system.

### Enzyme Kinetics

Drug-receptor interactions can be considered substrate-enzyme interactions. As such, principles of **enzyme kinetics** are central to the understanding of drug-receptor interactions.

**Michaelis-Menton kinetics:** Michaelis-Menton kinetics (Figure 6-4A) is a model for enzyme kinetics, where [S] = concentration of a substrate is plotted against the **V** = velocity of the reaction. $K_m$ represents the concentration of the substrate at one-half the maximum velocity of the reaction and is inversely related to the affinity of the enzyme for its substrate. Maximum volume ($V_{max}$) is directly proportional to the enzyme concentration.

The linear transformation of Figure 6-4A results in the **Lineweaver-Burk plot** (Figure 6-4B).

In it, the y-intercept represents the inverse of the **maximum reaction velocity**. The x-intercept represents the negative inverse of the $K_m$.

The Lineweaver-Burk plot is a great tool for understanding **receptor inhibition** (Figure 6-4C). Note that competitive inhibitors bring the $K_m$ of the receptor closer to zero because they reduce the drug's affinity for the receptor. However, the y-intercept is unchanged because competitive inhibitors can be overcome by increasing the drug concentration. On the other hand, noncompetitive inhibitors have a reduced $V_{max}$ (higher y-intercept) because they effectively reduce the number of receptors available to bind drug. However, the $K_m$ is unchanged because the drug's affinity for the receptor is unchanged.

The preceding information is summarized in Table 6-5.

## Dose Response

Dose-response curves represent the elicited response as a function of drug dose (Figures 6-5 and 6-6).

## Affinity

- A measure of how tightly a drug binds to a receptor.
- Inversely related to $K_d$, the dissociation constant for the drug-receptor complex.

## Potency

- The amount of drug needed for a given effect.
- Measured by the half-maximal effective concentration ($EC_{50}$).
- The higher the **potency** of a drug, the lower the concentration needed to produce an effect (the lower the $EC_{50}$).
- Note that drug potency has **no relationship to drug efficacy.**
- Drug X is more potent than drug Y because a lower concentration is required for a given effect.

## Efficacy

- Measured by the **maximal response** that can be achieved by the drug.
- Drug efficacy is represented by the $V_{max}$.
- Partial agonists have **less** efficacy than full antagonists.
- Two drugs are equally efficacious if they can achieve the same **maximal response** (regardless of the drug dose needed for that response).
- Note that efficacy has no **relationship to potency.**

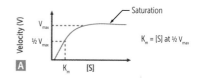
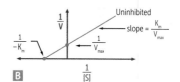
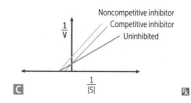

**FIGURE 6-4.** **Enzyme kinetics.** A Michaelis-Menton kinetics, B Lineweaver-Burk plot, and C receptor inhibition.

**TABLE 6-5.** **Properties of Drug-Receptor Interactions in the Presence of Antagonists**

| ANTAGONIST TYPE | EFFECT ON POTENCY ($K_M$) | EFFECT ON EFFICACY ($V_{MAX}$) | REVERSIBILITY |
|---|---|---|---|
| Competitive antagonist (reversible) | Decreased ($\uparrow K_m$; Figure 6-7A) | No change | Reversible with $\uparrow$ agonist |
| Noncompetitive antagonist | No change | Decreased ($\downarrow V_{max}$; Figure 6-7B) | Cannot be reversed |
| Partial agonist (mixed agonist-antagonist) | Decreased or no change ($\uparrow K_m$ or no change) | Decreased or no change ($\downarrow V_{max}$ or no change; Figure 6-7C) | Reversibility depends on relative binding affinity and concentrations |

$K_m$, Michaelis-Menten constant; $V_{max}$, maximum velocity.

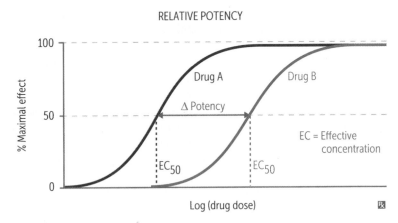

**FIGURE 6-5.** **The effect of increased potency on a drug's EC$_{50}$.** Drug A is more potent than Drug B, because Drug A produces 50% of its maximal effect at a **lower** drug concentration than Drug B.

Figure 6-7 shows the dose-response curve of an agonist alone and when an agonist is combined with a competitive antagonist (A), a noncompetitive antagonist or an irreversible competitive agonist (B), and a partial agonist (C), respectively. The x-axis is a log scale of agonist dose, and the y-axis is the percent response at each dose of agonist.

### Spare Receptors

- Not all receptors have to be occupied for maximal response.
- In the presence of spare receptors, maximal response occurs at a lower agonist dose than that required for receptor saturation.
- Less than 50% of receptors need to be bound to achieve half-maximal response, such that potency $< K_d$.

### Therapeutic Index

- Important clinical tool for measuring the dose-related toxicity of a drug, and a measure of overall drug safety.
- **TD$_{50}$** — toxic drug dose at which 50% of patients experience **adverse effects.**
- **ED$_{50}$** — effective drug dose at which 50% of patients experience **desired therapeutic effects.**
- **Therapeutic index (TI)** — ratio of TD$_{50}$ to the ED$_{50}$ (Figure 6-8).
- **High TI** drugs — those that achieve therapeutic doses well before causing toxicity and are relatively safe.

**CLINICAL CORRELATION**

Fewer spare nicotinic acetylcholine (nACh) receptors occur in the eyelid muscles than elsewhere in the body. Therefore, in **myasthenia gravis,** a reduction in the number of nACh receptors initially manifests clinically as **eyelid droop.**

**CLINICAL CORRELATION**

**Drugs with low TI:**
- Digoxin
- Lithium
- Theophylline
- Warfarin

**MNEMONIC**

**TITE:**
**T**herapeutic **I**ndex = **T**D$_{50}$/**E**D$_{50}$

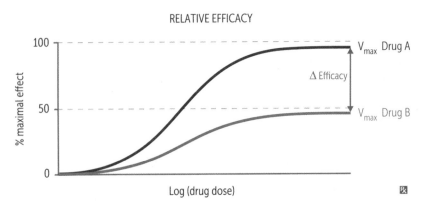

**FIGURE 6-6.** **The effect of increased efficacy on a drug's maximal effect.** Drug A is more efficacious than Drug B, because Drug A has a higher V$_{max}$ than Drug B.

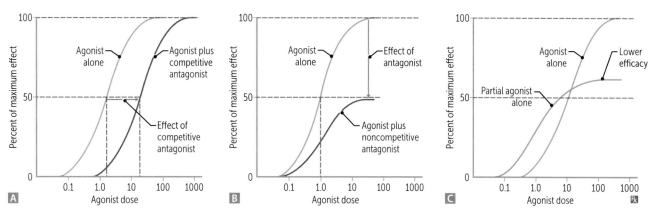

**FIGURE 6-7.** **The effect of antagonist on receptor binding properties.** **A** Competitive antagonists decrease an agonist's potency (or increase its $K_m$). **B** Noncompetitive antagonists decrease a drug's efficacy (or decrease its $V_{max}$). **C** Partial agonists may decrease an agonist's potency or efficacy, but this depends on the partial agonist's receptor affinity and concentration relative to the agonist.

- Drugs with a **low or narrow TI** have a smaller dosing margin that separates desired effects from toxicity.
- **Therapeutic window** is a measure of clinical drug effectiveness for a patient.

Therefore, drugs with a low TI must be used precisely and serum levels should be monitored closely.

## Toxicology

Table 6-6 lists in alphabetical order the most common toxic drugs, nondrug toxins, and their antidotes. For adverse reactions associated with drugs, see Table 6-8 in the next section.

### CARBON MONOXIDE

**Mechanism**

Binds to hemoglobin with much higher affinity (240×) than $O_2$, thereby inhibiting $O_2$ transport.

**Effects**

Headache, confusion, seizures, death.

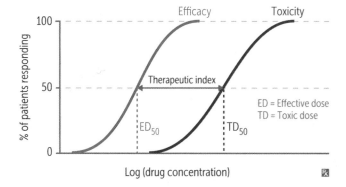

**FIGURE 6-8.** **Therapeutic index.**

**TABLE 6-6.    Common Toxic Drugs, Nondrug Toxins, and Antidotes**

| DRUG OR TOXIN | ANTIDOTE (MECHANISM, IF KNOWN) |
|---|---|
| Acetaminophen | *N*-acetylcysteine (replenishes glutathione) |
| Amphetamines | Ammonium chloride (acidifies urine) |
| Anticholinergics | Physostigmine salicylate (inhibits anticholinesterase) |
| Anticholinesterases, organophosphates | Atropine (competitively binds to muscarinic acetylcholine receptor) followed by pralidoxime (replenishes active acetylcholinesterase) |
| Aspirin | Sodium bicarbonate (alkalinization of blood and urine), dialysis, activated charcoal (absorbs aspirin) |
| Benzodiazepines | Flumazenil (competitively inhibits benzodiazepine receptor site on GABA receptors) |
| β-blockers | Glucagon, calcium gluconate, dextrose-insulin therapy (treats hypoglycemia) |
| Carbon monoxide | 100% $O_2$, hyperbaric $O_2$ (increase oxygen binding to hemoglobin) |
| Cyanide | Amyl nitrite, sodium thiosulfate, hydroxocobalamin (see text for discussion) |
| Digitalis/digoxin | Anti-digoxin Fab antibodies (promotes dissociation of digoxin from Na/K ATPase) |
| Ethylene glycol (antifreeze), methanol | Fomepizole (competitive inhibition of alcohol dehydrogenase), ethanol (competes for alcohol dehydrogenase [substrate inhibition]) |
| Heparin | Protamine sulfate (sequesters heparin) |
| Isoniazid (INH) | Pyridoxine (vitamin $B_6$) (sequesters INH) |
| **Meth**emoglobinemia (drugs causing) | **Meth**ylene blue (promotes reduction of methemoglobin) |
| Opioids | Naloxone (opioid receptor antagonist) |
| Quinidine | Hypertonic sodium bicarbonate, lidocaine, magnesium sulfate |
| Strychnine | Benzodiazepines (reduce muscle activity) |
| Theophylline | β-blockers (prevent cardiac arrhythmia), benzodiazepines (prevent seizures) |
| Tissue plasminogen activator (tPA), streptokinase, urokinase | Aminocaproic acid (sequesters plasminogen) |
| Tricyclic antidepressants (TCAs) | Sodium bicarbonate (to treat hypotension or cardiac arrhythmia), benzodiazepines (to control agitation) |
| Warfarin | Vitamin K: delayed effect (replenishes vitamin K stores needed for synthesis of clotting factors), fresh-frozen plasma; immediate dose effect (replenishes clotting factors) |

ATPase, adenosine triphosphatase; GABA, γ-aminobutyric acid.

Antidote

100% $O_2$, hyperbaric $O_2$.

### CYANIDE

Mechanism

Reacts with iron in cytochrome oxidase in mitochondria (see Figure 2-45 in the Biochemistry chapter), thereby inhibiting electron transport and adenosine triphosphate (ATP) formation.

## Effects

Tachycardia followed by bradycardia, hypotension, lactic acidosis, seizures, coma, and rapid death. $O_2$ utilization is diminished at the tissue level, and so venous $O_2$ concentration is elevated. Clinically, this manifests as brighter red venous blood than normal.

## Antidote

Amyl nitrite and sodium nitrite prevent and reverse binding of cyanide to cytochrome oxidase. Nitrites oxidize hemoglobin ($Fe^{2+}$) to methemoglobin ($Fe^{3+}$). Cyanide then binds to the oxidized iron in methemoglobin instead of the iron in cytochrome oxidase. Sodium thiosulfate donates a sulfur group to cyanide, producing thiocyanate, which detoxifies cyanide and accelerates its excretion. Hydroxocobalamin chelates cyanide, forming cyanocobalamin, which accelerates its excretion and prevents it from binding to cytochrome oxidase.

## ETHANOL

### Mechanism

Poorly understood. May exert effects at γ-aminobutyric acid (GABA) receptors or by modifying ion channels in biologic membranes. Figure 6-9 illustrates the metabolism of ethanol.

### Effects

Euphoria, disinhibition, sedation, respiratory depression, pancreatitis, hepatitis, Wernicke-Korsakoff syndrome, gynecomastia, testicular atrophy, fetal alcohol syndrome.

### Antidote

Benzodiazepines are used for acute withdrawal. Thiamine is used for prevention of Wernicke-Korsakoff syndrome. Disulfiram is used to treat chronic alcoholism.

## METHANOL

### Mechanism

Metabolized by alcohol dehydrogenase to formaldehyde, which is metabolized by formaldehyde dehydrogenase to formic acid (Figure 6-10). Formic acid accumulation causes retinal and optic nerve toxicity.

**QUESTION**

A patient with congestive heart failure (CHF) presents with **nausea, vomiting, abdominal pain,** and **scotomas.** He complains that "most objects look yellow." ECG shows atrial **tachycardia with a slow ventricular response.** He has been on digoxin, and his dose of **furosemide** was just increased for worsening edema and shortness of breath. What is causing the patient's symptoms?

**CLINICAL CORRELATION**

Although patients with CO poisoning have less $O_2$ bound to hemoglobin, standard pulse oximetry methods will report a **normal functional $O_2$ saturation ($SpO_2$)** despite a truly **low oxygen saturation.** This is because standard methods **cannot** discriminate between oxyhemoglobin and carboxyhemoglobin.

Therefore, patients with CO poisoning will present with **normal $PaO_2$** and **normal $SpO_2$** but will have pathognomonic **cherry-red blood.**

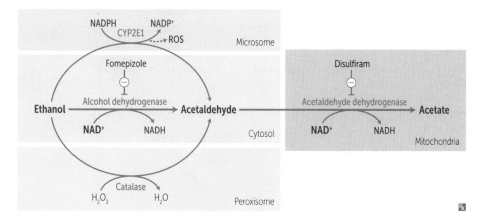

**FIGURE 6-9.    Ethanol metabolism.** Note that disulfiram prevents acetaldehyde dehydrogenase from converting acetaldehyde into acetate. This causes acetaldehyde to accumulate, which produces "hangover"-like symptoms. CYP2E1, cytochrome P450 2E1; NAD+, oxidized nicotinamide adenine dinucleotide; NADH, reduced nicotinamide adenine dinucleotide; ROS, reactive oxygen species.

**ANSWER**

Furosemide given for fluid overload also causes urinary K+ wasting, leading to hypokalemia, which precipitates digoxin toxicity. This patient exhibits all of the neurologic, gastrointestinal, and cardiac features classically associated with **digoxin toxicity.**

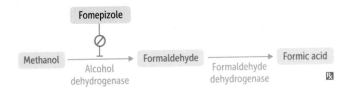

**FIGURE 6-10.    Methanol metabolism.** Note that fomepizole prevents the metabolism of methanol, which ultimately prevents the formation of toxic formic acid.

### Effects

Blindness, metabolic acidosis, and death.

### Antidote

Ethanol acts as a competitive substrate for alcohol dehydrogenase; fomepizole inhibits alcohol dehydrogenase.

**FLASH BACK**

Recall that lead blocks heme synthesis in two ways:
- Inhibiting δ-aminolevulinic acid dehydratase.
- Inhibiting ferrochelatase.

### HEAVY METALS

Exposure to heavy metals can lead to significant morbidity and mortality. Some heavy metals are necessary for biological function in small amounts (ie, iron), but can lead to toxicity in high amounts, whereas others are toxic even in small doses. The precise mechanism of toxicity, clinical manifestations, and antidote for several heavy metals are described in Table 6-7.

**TABLE 6-7.    Heavy Metals**

| HEAVY METAL | MECHANISM OF TOXICITY | CLINICAL MANIFESTATIONS | ANTIDOTE |
|---|---|---|---|
| Arsenic | *Trivalent arsenic (+3):* Binds to sulfhydryl groups on proteins and interferes with multiple enzymatic processes<br>*Pentavalent arsenic (+5):* May uncouple oxidative phosphorylation | *Early:* Garlic breath, bloody diarrhea<br>*Late:* Hair loss, neuropathy, hyperpigmentation, lung cancer | Dimercaprol, dimercaptosuccinic acid, D-penicillamine |
| Cadmium | Complexes with metallothionein | Metallic taste, GI corrosive, renal, bone (osteoporosis and fractures), and pulmonary disease | Supportive therapy (chelators have uncertain efficacy in patients) |
| Gold | Unknown | Pruritus, dermatitis, stomatitis, proteinuria; rarely, hepatotoxicity and pulmonary disease | Dimercaprol |
| Iron | Direct GI corrosive, forms reactive oxidative species, disrupts oxidative phosphorylation | 5 overlapping phases (time post ingestion):<br>1. GI corrosive (30 mins–6 hr)<br>2. Latent/stable phase (6–24 hr)<br>3. Shock and metabolic acidosis (6–72 hr)<br>4. Hepatotoxicity/hepatic necrosis (12–96 hr)<br>5. Bowel obstruction, bloody diarrhea, coma, leukocytosis, hyperglycemia (2–8 wk) | De**fer**oxamine, de**fer**asirox |

*(continues)*

**TABLE 6-7.    Heavy Metals** *(continued)*

| HEAVY METAL | MECHANISM OF TOXICITY | CLINICAL MANIFESTATIONS | ANTIDOTE |
|---|---|---|---|
| Lead | Inhibits heme synthesis | Anemia, abdominal pain, **lead lines** (see Figure 3-116 in Biochemistry chapter), motor neuropathy, encephalopathy | EDTA, dimercaprol, dimercaptosuccinic acid, D-penicillamine |
| Mercury | Inhibits multiple enzyme processes | Pneumonitis, nephrotoxicity, gum inflammation, intention tremor, psychiatric symptoms | D-penicillamine, dimercaptosuccinic acid, dimercaprol |
| Copper | Accumulates in tissue, impairing physiologic function | Acute: GI manifestations, including pain, vomiting, and diarrhea<br>Chronic: hepatotoxicity, encephalopathy, cardiac and renal failure | D-penicillamine |

EDTA, ethylenediaminetetraacetic acid.

## STRYCHNINE

### Mechanism

Competitive antagonist of the glycine receptor in central nervous system (CNS), leading to loss of normal inhibitory tone and subsequent **over-excitation.**

### Effects

Seizure with contraction of all voluntary muscles, resulting in full extension of limbs and vertebrae (opisthotonos).

### Antidote

Benzodiazepines and neuromuscular blockade.

## COMMON DRUG SIDE EFFECTS

Table 6-8 presents some commonly tested drug adverse effects and causative agents by organ system. This list is not comprehensive. Please refer to each organ system in the text for more details.

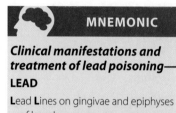

**MNEMONIC**

***Clinical manifestations and treatment of lead poisoning—*** **LEAD**

**L**ead **L**ines on gingivae and epiphyses of long bones

**E**ncephalopathy and **E**rythrocyte basophilic stippling

**A**bdominal pain and microcytic **A**nemia

**D**rops—wrist and foot drop from neuropathy; **D**imercaprol, **D**imercaptosuccinic acid and E**D**TA

**TABLE 6-8.    Common Drug Reactions**

| SYSTEM | ADVERSE REACTION | DRUG | MNEMONIC |
|---|---|---|---|
| **Neurologic** | Cinchonism | Quinidine, quinine, aspirin | |
| | Parkinsonism | Haloperidol, chlorpromazine, reserpine, MPTP | |
| | Tardive dyskinesia | Antipsychotics (long-term use), metoclopramide | |
| | Extrapyramidal side effects | Chlorpromazine, thioridazine, haloperidol | |
| | Seizures | Imipenem, antipsychotics, tricyclic antidepressants, buprenorphine, bupropion, lithium | |
| | Peripheral neuropathy | Vinca alkaloids | |
| **Cardiovascular** | Dilated cardiomyopathy | Doxorubicin, daunorubicin | |
| | Torsades de pointes | Class III (sotalol), class IA (quinidine) antiarrhythmics, macrolide antibiotics, antipsychotics, tricyclic antidepressants | |

*(continues)*

**TABLE 6-8.    Common Drug Reactions** *(continued)*

| SYSTEM | ADVERSE REACTION | DRUG | MNEMONIC |
|---|---|---|---|
| **Cardiovascular** *(continued)* | Coronary vasospasm | Cocaine, sumatriptan, ergot alkaloids | |
| **Pulmonary** | Pulmonary fibrosis | **B**leomycin, **A**miodarone **B**usulfan, **M**ethotrexate | **B**reathing **A**ir **B**adly from **M**edications. |
| | Dry cough | ACE inhibitors | |
| **Gastrointestinal** | Hepatitis | **H**alothane, **Is**oniazid | **H**epatit**Is.** |
| | Focal to massive hepatic necrosis | **H**alothane, **A**manita mushroom, **V**alproic acid, **Ac**etaminophen | Liver "**HAVAc.**" |
| | Pseudomembranous colitis | Broad-spectrum antibiotics (eg, clindamycin, ampicillin, cephalosporins) | |
| | Gingival hyperplasia | Phenytoin, verapamil, nifedipine (calcium channel blockers), cyclosporine | |
| **Renal** | Lactic acidosis | Metformin, nucleoside reverse-transcriptase inhibitors | |
| | Tubulointerstitial nephritis | Sulfonamides, furosemide, methicillin, rifampin, NSAIDs (except aspirin) | |
| | Diabetes insipidus | Lithium, demeclocycline | |
| | Fanconi syndrome | Expired tetracyclines, heavy metals | |
| **Heme** | Hemolysis in G6PD-deficient individuals | **S**ulfonamides, **I**soniazid **P**rimaquine, **P**yrimethamine, **I**buprofen, **N**itrofurantoin, **A**spirin, **D**apsone, **C**hloramphenicol | **SIPPIN' A D**iet **C**oke. |
| | Thrombosis | Oral contraceptives: estrogens, progestins | |
| | Agranulocytosis | **D**apsone, **C**lozapine, **C**arbamazepine, **C**olchicine, **M**ethimazole, **P**ropylthiouracil, **P**rocainamide | **D**rugs **CCC**rush **M**yeloblasts and **P**romyelocytes **P**lenty. |
| | Aplastic anemia | **C**arbamazepine, **M**ethimazole, **S**ulfonamides, **N**SAIDs, **B**enzene, **C**hloramphenicol, **P**ropylthiouracil, Gold salts | **C**an't **M**ake or **S**ynthesize **N**ew **B**lood **C**ells **P**roperly. |
| **Endocrine** | Adrenocortical insufficiency | Glucocorticoid withdrawal | |
| | Hot flashes | Tamoxifen, clomiphene | |
| | Gynecomastia | **S**pironolactone, **D**igitalis, **C**imetidine, **E**strogen, Chronic **A**lcohol abuse, **K**etoconazole | **S**ome **D**rugs **C**reate **E**xtremely **A**wesome **K**nockers. |
| | Hyperprolactinemia | Tricyclic antidepressants, methyldopa, reserpine, phenothiazines | |
| | SIADH | **C**yclophosphamide, **C**arbamazepine, **C**hlorpromazine, **A**CE inhibitors, **S**SRIs, vincristine | **C**an't **C**oncentrate **S**erum **S**odium. |
| | Hypothyroidism | Lithium, amiodarone, sulfonamides | |

*(continues)*

**TABLE 6-8.** **Common Drug Reactions** *(continued)*

| SYSTEM | ADVERSE REACTION | DRUG | MNEMONIC |
|---|---|---|---|
| **Dermatologic** | **Photo**sensitivity | **S**ulfonamides, **A**miodarone, **T**etracyclines, 5-**FU** | **SAT F**or a **photo.** |
| | Cutaneous flushing | **V**ancomycin (red man syndrome), **A**denosine, **N**iacin, **C**alcium channel blockers | **VANC.** |
| | Stevens-Johnson syndrome | Anti**epileptic** drugs (ethosuximide, carbamazepine, lamotrigine, phenytoin, phenobarbital), **all**opurinol, **Sulfa drugs, penicillin** | **Steven Johnson** has **epileptic A**llergy to **Sulfa drugs** and **Penicillin.** |
| | Gray baby syndrome | Chloramphenicol | |
| **Musculoskeletal** | Tendonitis, tendon rupture, and cartilage damage | Fluoroquinolones | |
| | Osteoporosis | Corticosteroids, heparin | |
| **Multiple** | Ototoxicity and nephrotoxicity | Aminoglycosides, loop diuretics, cisplatin | |
| | Neurotoxicity and nephrotoxicity | **Poly**myxi**Ns** | Toxic to **Poly**, **Ns** (neuro, nephrotoxic). |
| **Systemic** | Anaphylaxis | Penicillin and many others | |
| | SLE-like syndrome | **S**ulfa-drugs, **H**ydralazine, **I**soniazid, **P**rocainamide, **P**henytoin, **P**enicillamine, **E**tanercept, minocycline, methyldopa, chlorpromazine | Having lupus is **SHIP-PE.** |
| | Disulfiram-like reaction | Some **C**ephalosporins, **P**rocarbazine, **S**ulfonylureas, **Metro**nidazole | **C**an't **P**ound **S**hots on the **Metro.** |
| | Atropine-like side effects | Tricyclic antidepressants | |

ACE, angiotensin-converting enzyme; 5-FU, 5-fluorouracil; G6PD, glucose-6-phosphate dehydrogenase; MPTP, 1-methyl-4-phenyl-1, 2, 3, 6-tetrahydropyridine; NSAIDs, nonsteroidal anti-inflammatory drugs; SIADH, syndrome of inappropriate antidiuretic hormone secretion; SLE, systemic lupus erythematosus; SSRI, selective serotonin reuptake inhibitor.

**NOTES**

# Public Health Sciences

## Epidemiology

Increasingly, emphasis has been placed on the concept of evidence-based medicine. Every year, more questions about the techniques used to conduct research and interpret basic tests appear in Step 1. An understanding of the methodology and interpretation of research studies and the significance of diagnostic test results is very helpful.

Common types of questions include:

- Given a description of the population studied and the methods used, what type of study is this?
- Given a description of the study population and the goals of the research, what type of study is most appropriate?
- Perform common calculations and understand the mathematical definitions and significance of terms such as *false-positive* and *false-negative*.

**KEY FACT**

Epidemiologic questions are easy points, but only if students know the definitions and understand the basic calculations.

### STUDY METHODS

Studies can be divided into two types: observational and experimental. **Observational studies** look at events that happen with little or no manipulation by the researcher. **Experimental studies** often require the researcher to assemble subjects, design a study protocol, and perform some type of intervention.

### Observational Studies

#### Case Study or Case Series

These studies are written descriptions of a patient or particular problem, generally used to document a unique manifestation of a disease, a previously unrecognized association or risk factor, the first incidence of a new disease, or some clinical presentation that might be of interest to other physicians. A case series is simply a collection of case studies, typically consecutive, that document a similar patient presentation or disease manifestation.

**Example:** Case studies documented rare opportunistic infections in apparently healthy young patients and were some of the earliest documentations of HIV/AIDS before the disease was recognized.

#### Cross-Sectional Study

A cross-sectional study collects data at a particular point in time from a group of people to assess the frequency of disease and related risk factors. It answers basic questions, such as, "In a given population, how many people have a disease?" or "How many people have risk factors in population X?"

**Example:** In the 1980s, some physicians noticed that hemophiliacs had a high incidence of AIDS. To determine what proportion of hemophiliacs had HIV/AIDS in 1988, a cross-sectional study, or survey, could be performed in this population.

#### Case-Control Study

A case-control study retrospectively compares a group of people who already have a disease or condition with a group that does not to determine disease risk factors. Once a group with the condition is identified (the case), it is matched with a demographically similar group without the condition (the control). The two groups are then compared for differences that may provide insight into possible causes or risk factors, as illustrated in Figure 7-1.

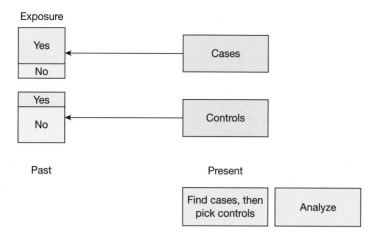

FIGURE 7-1. **Case-control study.**

**Example:** To determine why some hemophiliacs contracted HIV/AIDS in the 1980s when many others did not, a case-control study was performed. In this study a group of HIV-positive hemophiliacs was matched by age, sex, race, and location with a control group of hemophiliacs who did not have the disease. When the data were analyzed for differences between the two groups, it was found that the HIV-positive hemophiliacs were far more likely to have received more blood transfusions than the controls.

## Cohort Study

A cohort study examines a large group and watches it evolve over time. It includes people with different exposures and follows all of these people to see which ones will develop the disease. At the outset, the participants do not usually have the condition or disease being studied. It is expected that some individuals in the study will develop the condition or complication being studied (Figure 7-2).

A cohort can be retrospective or prospective. A prospective cohort is identified in the present and followed into the future for analysis. A retrospective cohort is identified in the past, observed over time, and followed up to the present for analysis.

**Example:** To determine the risk of HIV transmission in IV drug users, identify a cohort of HIV-negative IV drug users and follow them for 10 years.

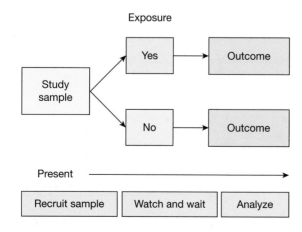

FIGURE 7-2. **Cohort study.**

**KEY FACT**

In a case-control study, the cases already have a condition or illness, and controls are chosen retrospectively. In a prospective cohort study, participants do not yet have the condition or illness at the outset, and are grouped based on status of exposure to the risk factor of interest, and observed over time to see if the condition develops.

**KEY FACT**

The Framingham Heart Study is a very well-known cohort study that has followed the residents of Framingham, Massachusetts, for decades. More than 1000 papers on cardiac health have come out of this study.

**QUESTION**

A researcher wants to determine whether glioblastoma, which has a prevalence of 1 in 100,000, is associated with cell phone use. What study design is best suited to answer this question?

### Studies of Heritability and Environment

Two observational studies that measure heritability and the influence of environmental factors are twin concordance studies and adoption studies. In a **twin concordance study,** monozygotic and dizygotic twins are compared. If a factor is highly heritable, it is expected to appear more frequently in both twins if they are monozygotic due to their near-identical genes. In an **adoption study,** siblings, or matched controls, are observed as they are raised in different households. Different outcomes between these groups may then be attributable to their different environments.

### Experimental Studies

### Clinical Trial

A clinical trial is a direct test of a drug, technique, or other intervention. Subjects are divided into at least two groups: one group acting as a control receives either a placebo or the current standard-of-care treatment; the other group is given the intervention being studied (Figure 7-3). Often, such trials are double-blind, meaning that neither the subjects nor the experimenters know who is receiving the actual treatment and who is receiving the placebo. Clinical drug trials comprise four stages (Table 7-1).

**Example:** To test a new HIV drug, similar HIV-positive subjects are recruited and divided randomly into treatment and placebo groups. Experimenters and participants are blinded so they do not know who is receiving the actual drug versus the placebo. At the end of the experiment, the group assignment is revealed to allow for comparison of the outcomes.

### Crossover Study

Participants are randomized into one of two treatment groups, with the control group often given a placebo. The experiment is performed once, after which there is a time delay for the effects of the treatment to wear off. Then, each participant is switched to the other arm of the study (ie, crossed over) to receive the other treatment. Thus, each participant receives both treatments at different times and can act as his or her own control (see Figure 7-4).

**Example:** A drug that may temporarily raise CD4 T-cell counts in HIV-positive individuals is being tested. Half of the subjects are assigned to a treatment group and the other half to a placebo group; then effects are measured. Because the effect is not permanent, one could repeat the experiment with switched groups. One can compare each subject's response to the drug and the placebo.

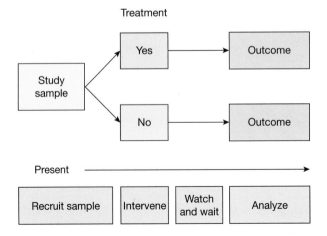

FIGURE 7-3. **Clinical trial.**

**TABLE 7-1.    Phases of Clinical Drug Trials**

| DRUG TRIAL | TYPICAL STUDY SAMPLE | PURPOSE |
|---|---|---|
| Phase I | Small number of healthy volunteers | "Is it safe?" Assesses safety, toxicity, pharmacokinetics, and pharmacodynamics |
| Phase II | Small number of patients with disease of interest | "Does it work?" Assesses treatment efficacy, optimal dosing, and adverse effects |
| Phase III | Large number of patients randomly assigned either to the treatment under investigation or to the best available treatment (or placebo) | "Is it as good or better?" Compares the new treatment to the current standard of care |
| Phase IV | Postmarketing surveillance of patients after treatment is approved | "Can it stay?" Detects rare or long-term adverse effects. Can result in treatment being withdrawn from market |

Reproduced with permission from Le T, et al. *First Aid for the USMLE Step 1 2017*. New York, NY: McGraw-Hill Education, 2017.

## Meta-Analysis

A meta-analysis combines the data from many preexisting studies on the same topic to produce what is essentially one big study. It is not necessary to understand the statistical techniques for the USMLE.

**Example:** Many studies have assessed the effectiveness of treatments to prevent immunosuppression in HIV. However, no one study is large enough to state unequivocally that the treatment is truly effective. By combining the results of multiple studies, more definitive conclusions are possible.

Any time studies are combined, think meta-analysis. A meta-analysis is only as good as the studies it combines. Even when the studies are based on good data, it is hard to accurately combine studies because the methodology of each must be controlled.

All studies described earlier are compared in Table 7-2.

> **KEY FACT**
>
> Case-control vs cohort studies:
> - Cohort: Starts with the exposure and looks for the outcome
> - Case-control: Starts with the outcome and looks for the possible exposure

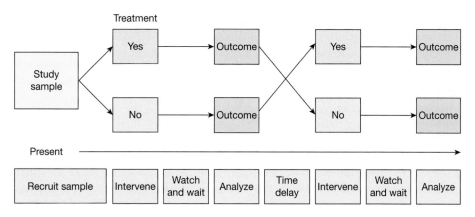

**FIGURE 7-4.    Crossover study.**

**TABLE 7-2.** **Comparison of Study Types**

| OBSERVATIONAL STUDIES | |
| --- | --- |
| **Case Studies/Case Series** | **Cross-Sectional Studies** |
| ▪ Easy | ▪ Fairly easy |
| ▪ Purely descriptive | ▪ Purely descriptive |
| ▪ Do not address causality | ▪ Do not address causality |
| ▪ Do not provide prevalence statistics or other epidemiologic data | ▪ Do provide prevalence statistics or other epidemiologic data |
| **Case-Control Studies** | **Cohort Studies** |
| ▪ Retrospective | ▪ Prospective or retrospective |
| ▪ Can be quick | ▪ Can take a long time |
| ▪ Do not provide prevalence statistics or other epidemiologic data | ▪ Do provide prevalence statistics or other epidemiologic data |
| ▪ Good for rare diseases | ▪ Not good for rare diseases |
| EXPERIMENTAL STUDIES | |
| **Clinical Trials** | **Crossover Studies** |
| ▪ Good if intervention is permanent | ▪ Good if intervention is temporary |
| ▪ Prone to bias | ▪ Prone to bias and unanticipated permanent effects |
| ▪ Gold standard if randomized and blinded | |

## BIAS

In statistics, bias refers to any part of the study that **may inadvertently favor one outcome or result over another.** Bias is often unintentional, but has the potential to invalidate conclusions. It is possible to detect certain forms of bias by analyzing the study in question.

### Types of Bias

### Confounding Bias

A confounding bias can occur when a hidden or unknown variable is closely related to both the independent and dependent variables under study. If the researcher does not appreciate the relationship, the incorrect variable may be thought to cause the disease or the condition being studied.

**Example:** A scientist notes that certain people stand outside every day during their breaks at work. He also notices that these same people often develop lung cancer. He collects data and finds that the more time one spends standing outside during work breaks, the more likely one is to develop lung cancer. He concludes that being outside causes lung cancer. In reality, the people who stand outside a lot develop lung cancer because they smoke.

### Sampling Bias

Sampling bias occurs when the sample of people chosen for the study (or one group within the study) is not representative of the pool from which they were chosen.

**Example:** To test a new treatment for diabetes, 1000 men over the age of 65 are enrolled in a study. The drug appears to be effective in controlling symptoms. However, when marketed to the general population, the results are less favorable because the original study excluded younger patients or women, who respond poorly to the medication.

### Recall Bias

When people are asked to recall information retrospectively, their responses are often influenced by knowledge gained after the fact, such as whether they received a placebo or a real drug.

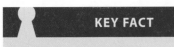

**KEY FACT**

**Bias:** Deviation from the truth.
**Validity:** Accuracy of results.
**Reliability:** Consistency among repeated trials.

**Example:** In a case-control study investigating a link between cell phone use and brain cancer, patients who develop cancer (the cases) may be more likely to recall their cell phone use.

### Selection Bias

When the investigators or clinicians choose how to group participants for the purposes of the study, a selection bias results. In this situation, the distribution of subjects within the groups is often not random.

**Example:** Investigators or the patient's treating clinician are given the choice of whether subjects with cancer receive the standard chemotherapy treatment or an experimental treatment. The investigators or clinicians disproportionately choose the experimental treatment for subjects with advanced cancer because they know that the standard treatment is ineffective for late-stage cancer. Those receiving the experimental treatment might do worse on average, due not to the inherent ineffectiveness of the drug, but to the disproportionate number of very sick patients who receive this treatment.

### Late-Look Bias

The results in studies with a late-look bias are recorded at the wrong time, skewing the outcomes.

**Example:** Persons with a certain stage of colon cancer have, on average, 5 months to live. Half are given an experimental treatment, and they are found to have lived an average of 3 months. The investigators conclude that the treatment actually shortens life expectancy by 2 months. However, they overlooked the fact that treatment itself took 3 months. In this situation, the treated group actually lived 1 month longer!

### Reducing Bias

Two common ways to reduce bias include **blinding** and **randomization.**

### Blinding

In blinded studies, participants or the investigators may not be told which intervention is being given. In a single-blind study, either the participants or the researchers performing the test are not told the intervention. In a double-blind study, neither party is aware who is receiving which intervention. Blinding **prevents recall bias.**

**Example:** Use of a **placebo** is the classic way to blind participants in a study. A placebo is an inactive treatment that looks, tastes, and feels identical to the actual drug; thus, participants do not know which treatment they are receiving.

### Randomization

Participants are grouped randomly into study groups. Randomization **prevents selection bias** because neither subjects nor study conductors participate in the decision of whether subjects receive the experimental treatment.

**Example:** After a pool of subjects for a study is chosen, the subjects are placed in the intervention group or the placebo group, based on some random method such as a coin toss. Potential differences between subjects that may skew results are more likely to be randomly distributed into both groups.

### Prevalence, Incidence, and Duration

**Prevalence** is how many people in a sample group have a condition **at a certain point in time.** Often written as a ratio, such as "1 in 4 persons over the age of 40 has high cholesterol."

**KEY FACT**

Randomized, double-blind clinical trials are the gold standard for robust studies.

**KEY FACT**

For diseases of very short duration, incidence = prevalence.

**Incidence** is how many people will **newly acquire** a condition in a given period, such as "1 in 50 per year."

**Duration** is how long a given condition lasts, on average.

These three terms are related by the formula:

$$\text{Prevalence} = \text{Incidence} \times \text{Duration}$$

**Example:** In a given population, 1 in 100 persons acquires a new plantar wart each year (incidence). On average, the wart will last two years (duration). Survey this population in any given year, and roughly 2 in 100 persons will have a plantar wart (Incidence × Duration = Prevalence).

### Sensitivity, Specificity, and Predictive Value

When a patient is given a test to determine the presence of a condition, the test most often yields one of two results: positive or negative. However, no test is 100% accurate. Thus, there are four possibilities:

- **True-positive (TP)** is a positive test result in a person who has the condition.
- **False-positive (FP)** is a positive test result in a person who does not have the condition.
- **True-negative (TN)** is a negative test result in a person who does not have the condition.
- **False-negative (FN)** is a negative test result in a person who does have the condition.

**True-positives** and **false-negatives** actually have the condition being tested for. **True-negatives** and **false-positives** do not have the condition (Figure 7-5). False-positive rate = 1 – Specificity.

These four outcomes for any test are used to calculate **sensitivity, specificity,** and **predictive values.**

Sensitivity and specificity describe the accuracy of a diagnostic test (Figure 7-6).

**Sensitivity** is a measure of how often a given test will detect the presence of disease *in those who have the disease.* In other words, it is a measure of how reliable the test is in identifying the disease. It is the percentage of positive test results (TP) among a population with the tested condition (TP + FN). It measures the percentage of those who have the condition that test positive in the test.

**Specificity** is a measure of how often a given test will detect the absence of a disease **in those who do not have the disease** (that is, true-negatives). It is a measure of how well the test identifies disease-free individuals. It is the percentage of negative test results

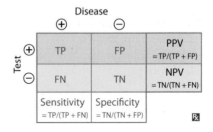

**FIGURE 7-5.** **Positive and negative test results.** FN, false negative; FP, false positive; TN, true negative; TP, true positive; NPV, negative predictive value; PPV, positive predictive value.

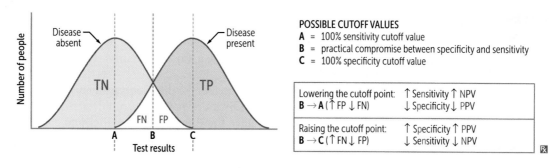

**FIGURE 7-6.    Relationship between sensitivity and specificity.** FN, false negative; FP, false positive; TN, true negative; TP, true positive; NPV, negative predictive value; PPV, positive predictive value.

(TN) among a population without the tested condition (TN + FP). It measures the percentage of those who do not have the condition that test negative in the test.

**Predictive value describes the likelihood that a patient has (or does not have) the disease in question, based on the results of the diagnostic test.**

**Positive predictive value** is the likelihood that a positive test result truly means that a patient has a given condition, that is, the number of correct positive tests (TP) out of the total number of positive tests (TP + FP).

**Negative predictive value** is the likelihood that a negative test result truly means that a patient does not have a given condition, that is, the number of correct negative tests (TN) out of the total number of negative tests (TN + FN).

The interrelationships between these values are depicted in Figure 7-7.

> **KEY FACT**
>
> Positive predictive value = TP / (TP + FP)
>
> Negative predictive value = TN / (TN + FN)

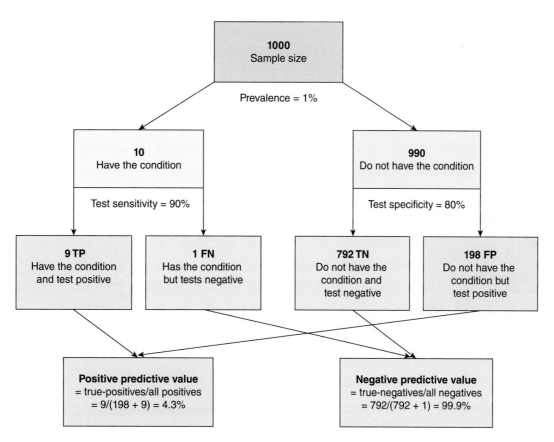

**FIGURE 7-7.    Integrating prevalence, sensitivity, specificity, and predictive values.** FN, false negative; FP, false positive; TN, true negative; TP, true positive.

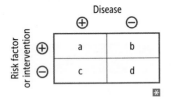

FIGURE 7-8. **Outcomes matrix after exposure to a risk factor or intervention.**

Steps to solve the common board questions related to sensitivity and specificity:

- Pick an easy number to use for the sample patient population (any number works).
- Use prevalence to calculate how many in the sample do and do not actually have the disease.
- For those who do have the disease, use the test's sensitivity to determine how many would test positive (true-positives) and how many would test negative (false-negatives).
- For those who do not have the disease, use specificity to calculate how many will test negative for the disease (true-negatives) and how many will test positive (false-positives).
- Calculate the positive predictive value by dividing the true-positives by all positive test results. Calculate the negative predictive value by dividing the true-negatives by all negative results.

### Odds Ratio and Relative Risk

**Odds ratios** and **relative risk** express how much more likely something is to occur if a certain condition is met, such as a patient being exposed to an illness or receiving a particular treatment. These are calculated based on known outcomes, as in the example in Figure 7-8.

### Absolute Risk

Relative risks and odds ratios are calculated from a chart similar to Figure 7-8 using **absolute risk,** which is the likelihood of an outcome over time without comparison to another group. That is, it is the probability of something occurring. The risk is not compared to any other risks.

$$\text{Absolute Risk (of dying if exposed)} = A / (A + B)$$
$$\text{Absolute Risk (of dying if not exposed)} = C / (C + D)$$

### Attributable Risk

Absolute risk (if not exposed) demonstrates that some subjects will have the outcome being studied, even when the condition is not met. To calculate how much risk is actually due to the condition being studied, use **attributable risk.**

$$\text{Attributable Risk} = \text{Absolute Risk (if exposed)} - \text{Absolute Risk (if not exposed)} = \frac{a}{a + b} - \frac{c}{c + d}$$

### Relative Risk

Relative risk is the comparison of risks between two different conditions or groups of people. For example, the relative risk of developing lung cancer for nonsmokers as compared to that for smokers is different.

$$\text{Relative risk} = \frac{a/(a + b)}{c/(c + d)}$$

Relative risk is the measurement of probability of something happening in condition 1 relative to condition 2. In the example shown in Figure 7-8, there is a 2.4 times greater chance of dying after being exposed to the pathogen versus not being exposed.

### Odds Ratio

Relative risk and odds ratio are two distinct statistical concepts. Odds ratio is the probability of an event happening divided by the probability of an event not happening in a particular condition. Odds ratio is the odds of condition 1 divided by the odds of condition 2.

In our example, if people are exposed to a particular pathogen, the odds of dying are 20/5 = 4. The odds of dying without exposure are 10/20 = 0.5.

Thus, the odds of dying if one is exposed to the pathogen compared to not having been exposed are 8 times higher (4/0.5 = 8).

$$\text{Odds Ratio} = (A\,/\,B)\,/\,(C\,/\,D)$$

Studies that **create a sample population based on outcome,** such as case-control studies, must **use odds ratios.**

Studies that create a **sample population based on exposure or treatment,** such as a controlled trial or cohort study, can **use relative risk.**

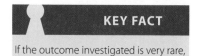

**KEY FACT**

If the outcome investigated is very rare, odds ratio ~ relative risk.

### Precision, Accuracy, and Error

**Precision, accuracy,** and **error** describe the quality of measurements, such as those produced by a laboratory test.

- **Precision** (reliability) is the reproducibility of a measurement.
- **Accuracy** (validity) is how close a measurement is to the true value.
- **Systematic errors** are errors that **occur the same way every time** a measurement is taken. As a result, the measurements are wrong in the same way each time and thus are not accurate, but are precise.
- **Random error** is unavoidable error that is **different each time a measurement is taken.** This reduces precision. It also reduces accuracy if the amount of error is large.

These differences are shown in Figure 7-9.

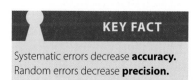

**KEY FACT**

Systematic errors decrease **accuracy.**
Random errors decrease **precision.**

## Statistics

### MEASURES OF CENTRAL TENDENCY AND STATISTICAL DISTRIBUTION

The term **distribution** describes the **frequency** of observations in a population or data set as plotted on a graph.

Distribution of a set of observations is defined by the measures of central tendency:

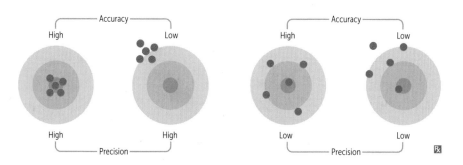

FIGURE 7-9. **Relationship of error to precision and accuracy.**

- **Mean (arithmetic mean** or **average)** is the most common measure of central tendency. It represents the ratio between the sum of all individual observations ($\Sigma X$) over the number of observations (***n***):

$$\text{Mean} = \Sigma X / n$$

The mean, however, may not be an appropriate measure of central tendency for skewed distributions or in data sets that contain outliers.

- **Median (middle observation)** represents the **50th percentile of a distribution,** or the point at which half of the observations are smaller and half are larger. The median is often a more appropriate measure of central tendency for skewed distributions or in situations with large outliers.

- **Mode** represents the most frequent value in a distribution and is commonly used for a large number of observations to identify the value that occurs most frequently.

All three are used for continuous data (ie, data that can be expressed along a numerical continuum, such as weight); the median may also be used for ordinal categorical data (eg, grades of cancer, asthma severity grades, etc).

A **frequency curve** may be produced from the data set (Figure 7-10).

Terms that describe the curves created include:

- **Gaussian:** Also known as a "normal," or "bell-shaped," curve. It indicates **symmetrical distribution** of the observations.
  - The mean, median, and mode are identical.
- **Bimodal:** The curve produces two "peaks" due to two separate areas of increased frequency of data in the population or data set. These curves may indicate **symmetrical** or **asymmetrical distribution** of observations.
- **Positive skew:** Asymmetrical curve with the tail to the right of the peak. Outliers are located at larger values.
  - **Mean > median > mode**
- **Negative skew:** Asymmetrical curve with the tail to the left of the peak. Outliers are located at smaller values.
  - **Mean < median < mode**

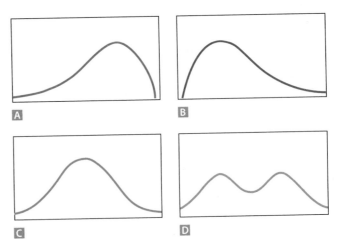

**FIGURE 7-10.**  **Shapes of common distributions of observations.** A Negatively skewed; B positively skewed; C Gaussian; D bimodal.

## STATISTICAL HYPOTHESIS

A statistical hypothesis is a formal statement regarding the expected outcome of an experiment. There are two major types of hypotheses, differentiated by how the statement is framed:

- **Null hypothesis ($H_0$):** A statement that there is **no difference**, or association **between two or more variables.** In medicine, this normally relates to disease and risk factors. $H_0$ is tested for possible rejection under the assumption that the hypothesis is true.
- **Alternative hypothesis ($H_1$):** A statement that **there is an association between two or more variables,** and contrary to the null hypothesis, the observations are the result of a real effect (Figure 7-11).

### Type I Error ($\alpha$)

Type I error results when one states or determines that there **is** an effect or difference when in reality one does not exist. Stated another way, the **alternative** hypothesis is accepted when in actuality the **null** hypothesis is correct. Type I error is also known as a **"false-positive."**

- The probability of making a Type I error is known as the level of significance, denoted as the Greek letter $\alpha$.
- The normal accepted $\alpha$ is usually $< 0.05$, which means that there is a less than 5% chance of making a type I error, or that the data will show something that **is not really true.**

### Type II Error ($\beta$)

Type II error results when one states or determines that there **is not** an effect or difference when in reality one does exist. In other words, the **null** hypothesis fails to be rejected when in actuality the **alternative** hypothesis is correct (Figure 7-11). Type II error is also known as **"false-negative."**

### Power

Power is the probability of rejecting the null hypothesis when it is in fact false. The power is affected by sample size and the variability or spread of the observations. The power is calculated as $1 -$ probability of a Type II error ($\beta$).

$$\text{Power} = 1 - \beta$$

## STANDARD DEVIATION VERSUS ERROR

**Standard deviation** is a statistical measurement used to describe the spread of the data around the mean within a statistical distribution (Figure 7-12). It is used to describe the spread of values within a particular distribution.

All forms of measurement have some inherent error. For this reason, the **standard error of the mean** (SEM) is used to estimate the amount of variability that exists between the sample mean and the true population mean of which the sample mean is an estimate.

$$\text{SEM} = \sigma / \sqrt{n}$$
$$\sigma = \text{standard deviation}$$
$$n = \text{sample size}$$

**CLINICAL CORRELATION**

An example of a **null hypothesis** is, "There is no difference in average blood pressure between those with low and high sodium intake."

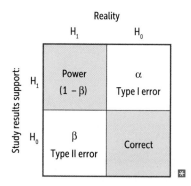

**FIGURE 7-11. Summary of possible results of any hypothesis test.**

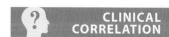

**CLINICAL CORRELATION**

An example of an **alternative hypothesis ($H_1$)** is, "Increased sodium intake leads to increased blood pressure."

**MNEMONIC**

**Type I ($\alpha$) and type II ($\beta$) errors:**

$\alpha$ = You s$\alpha$w a difference that did not exist.

$\beta$ = You were $\beta$lind to a difference that did exist.

**KEY FACT**

**SEM $< \sigma$ and SEM decreases** as $n$ **increases.**

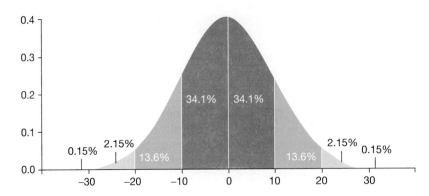

**FIGURE 7-12.** **Standard deviation.** Dark red is less than one standard deviation from the mean. For the normal distribution, this accounts for about 68% of the set (dark red), while two standard deviations from the mean (medium and dark red) account for about 95%, and three standard deviations (light, medium, and dark red) account for about 99.7%.

## Confidence Intervals

A confidence interval (CI) is a range, with upper and lower values, in which a specified probability of the means of the repeated samples would be expected to fall. The confidence interval sets boundaries within which the true population mean falls.

The CI can be determined by using the SEM.

For a 95% CI, that is the interval within which 95% of the sample means lie it can be calculated as:

$$CI = mean \pm 1.96 \, (SEM)$$

- If the CI for the difference between two means includes zero, the null hypothesis is **not rejected** (ie, there is **no difference** between the two group means).
- If the CI for the difference does not contain zero, the null hypothesis is **rejected** (ie, there is a **difference** between the two group means).

**Example:** Imagine a study in which 50 people in a town have their blood pressure measured (independent samples from a population). Their blood pressure should be reported as a range, which is best expressed as a CI. A 95% CI for blood pressure tells readers that there is a 95% chance that the true mean blood pressure of the population will lie within this interval.

## *t*-TEST, ANOVA, AND CHI-SQUARE ($\chi^2$) TEST

### *t*-Test

The *t*-test is used to determine the difference between the mean values of two groups of observations. This test is based on the *t* distribution, which involves **degrees of freedom (df)**.

- For **groups with a large df** value, the *t* distribution is indistinguishable from the normal distribution.
- As the **df decreases,** the *t* distribution becomes increasingly spread out.
- The *t* distribution for a given df value can be graphed, and the corresponding *p* value can be looked up in a table for that distribution.

### ANOVA

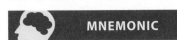
ANOVA is used to determine the statistical difference between the means of three or more groups of observations.

### Chi-Square ($\chi^2$) Test

Chi-square test is used to determine the statistical difference among two or more percentages or proportions of categorical outcomes (not mean values). It is a categorical test used to determine the probability that the observed distribution of data is due to chance (sampling error).

## CORRELATION COEFFICIENT

The **correlation coefficient ($r$)** is a numerical value that always falls between **–1 and 1**. It indicates the strength and direction of a linear relationship (correlation) between two or more different and independent variables. Values approaching 1 indicate a strong correlation between the variables. A value of 0 indicates no correlation, and values approaching –1 indicate an inverse relationship.

The **coefficient of determination ($R^2$)** is the proportion of **variability** (or **sum of squares**) in a data set that is accounted for by a statistical model, using regression analysis. It helps to determine whether a linear relationship exists between the response variable and the "regressors."

If $R^2 = 1$, the regression line perfectly fits the data.

**CLINICAL CORRELATION**

An example of the **chi-square test** is a clinical trial comparing a 28-day survival rate of subjects in a treatment group versus those in a control group. The percentage of survivors versus controls can be compared using this test.

# Public Health

## FORMS OF DISEASE PREVENTION

Public health officials try to limit the spread of disease through primary, secondary, or tertiary prevention.

### Primary Disease Prevention

**Primary disease prevention stops the disease before it starts.** For example, vaccination is used to build immunologic resistance and thus limit the infectivity and spread of a disease. Examples are human papillomavirus (HPV) vaccination for the prevention of cervical cancer. Another example is advertising to lower the smoking rate. If a person does not begin smoking, the risk of developing cancer, and other smoking-related diseases, drops dramatically.

**MNEMONIC**

**PST:**

**P**revent (**P**rimary)
**S**creen (**S**econdary)
**T**reat (**T**ertiary)

### Secondary Disease Prevention

**Secondary disease prevention seeks to detect disease early in its course before it becomes clinically apparent to reduce the associated morbidity and mortality.** Examples of secondary disease prevention include cervical cancer screening through Papanicolaou (Pap) smears, which detect cellular atypia that may progress to cancer; colonoscopy for the detection of colon cancers; and mammogram screening for the detection of breast cancers. Early detection can reduce the morbidity and mortality of the disease and also prevent epidemics.

Disease screening tests usually are very **sensitive** in order to capture as many true positives as possible, but may result in a significant number of false positives.

### Tertiary Disease Prevention

**Tertiary disease prevention aims to reduce the disability or morbidity resulting from disease.** Examples include exogenous insulin for diabetes and surgical treatment of cancers. Tertiary disease prevention aims to treat the disease through available medical or surgical management.

## REPORTING AND MONITORING DISEASE

### Reportable Diseases

By requiring clinicians to report certain infectious diseases, public health officials can monitor, track, and try to control the spread of contagious diseases. **Reportable infectious diseases** are shown in Table 7-3, and leading causes of death are reported in Table 7-4.

### Medical Surveillance

The effort to continuously monitor and detect the occurrence of health-related events is known as medical surveillance. Through **medical surveillance,** it is possible to determine the **incidence** of disease (the rate of new disease in a given period), the number of deaths resulting from the disease (**case fatality**), the **mortality rate** (combination of incidence rate and case fatality), **rate ratios** (a ratio of the incidence rates of two different groups, resulting in a comparison of the rate of disease occurrence), and **mortality patterns.** Figures 7-13, 7-14, and 7-15 show examples of incidence rates, mortality rates or patterns, and rate ratios, respectively.

**T A B L E  7 - 3 .**   **Reportable Diseases**

| DISEASE | CAUSATIVE AGENT | COMMUNICABILITY |
|---|---|---|
| Acquired immune deficiency syndrome (AIDS) | HIV | Spread by sexual contact, parenteral exposure, perinatal exposure where there is contact with blood or blood products |
| Chickenpox | Varicella zoster virus (VZV) | Spread by inhalation of vesicles or close contact |
| Gonorrhea | Gram-negative diplococcus *Neisseria gonorrhoeae* | Sexual contact |
| Hepatitis A | Hepatitis A virus (HAV) | Fecal-oral transmission |
| Hepatitis B | Hepatitis B virus (HBV) | Sexual contact, parenteral and perinatal exposure |
| Hepatitis C | Hepatitis C virus (HCV) | More likely parenteral, less likely sexual contact, perinatal exposure |
| Measles (rubeola) | Paramyxovirus | Inhalation of respiratory droplets |
| Mumps | Paramyxovirus | Inhalation of respiratory droplets, perinatal exposure |
| Rubella (German measles) | Togavirus | Inhalation of respiratory droplets |
| Salmonella | Gram-negative bacilli *Salmonella typhi* | Contaminated food or water |
| Shigella | Gram-negative bacilli *Shigella dysenteriae* | Contaminated food |
| Syphilis | Spirochete *Treponema pallidum* | Sexual contact, perinatal exposure |
| Tuberculosis | *Mycobacterium tuberculosis* | Droplet transmission |

**TABLE 7-4.    Leading Causes of Death in the United States by Age**

| AGE GROUP | LEADING CAUSE OF DEATH |
|---|---|
| Infants | ▪ Congenital anomalies<br>▪ Short gestation/low birth weight<br>▪ Sudden infant death syndrome |
| Age 1–14 | ▪ Unintentional injuries<br>▪ Cancer<br>▪ Congenital anomalies<br>▪ Homicide<br>▪ Heart disease |
| Age 15–34 | ▪ Injuries (especially motor vehicle accidents)<br>▪ Suicide<br>▪ Homicide |
| Age 35-44 | ▪ Injuries<br>▪ Cancer<br>▪ Heart disease |
| Age 45–64 | ▪ Cancer<br>▪ Heart disease<br>▪ Unintentional injuries |
| Age 65+ | ▪ Heart disease<br>▪ Cancer<br>▪ Chronic respiratory disease<br>▪ Stroke |

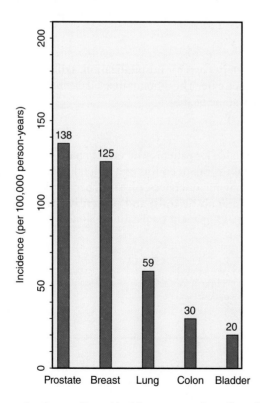

**FIGURE 7-13.    Example of age-adjusted incidences rates.** Age-adjusted incidence rates of the leading cancers in men and women in the United States from 2008–2012. (Data from Howlader N, Noone AM, Krapcho M, et al. (eds). *SEER Cancer Statistics Review, 1975–2012*, National Cancer Institute. Bethesda, MD, http://seer.cancer.gov/csr/1975_2012/, based on November 2014 SEER data submission, posted to the SEER website, April 2015.)

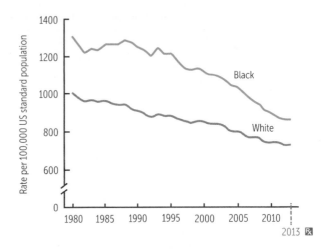

**FIGURE 7-14.** **Example of age-adjusted total mortality rates.** Age-adjusted total mortality rates by calendar year and race in the United States, 1980–2013. (Data from National Center for Health Statistics: National Vital Statistics Report, 2013.)

## GOVERNMENT FINANCING OF MEDICAL INSURANCE

Medical costs can be paid several ways: out-of-pocket payments, individual private insurance, employment-based private insurance, or government financing. The two major types of government financing are Medicare and Medicaid.

### Medicare and Medicaid

Medicare is a government-sponsored program financed through Social Security, federal taxes, and monthly premiums that provides financial coverage for hospital and physician services for persons 65 years and older. It consists of **Medicare Part A** and **Medicare Part B.**

### Medicare Part A

This portion covers **certain costs for hospitalization, skilled nursing facilities, home health care, and hospice care.** The amount that Medicare Part A will reimburse varies with the length of stay at the facility.

### Medicare Part B

Medicare Part B is available for patients who elect to pay a separate monthly premium. The rest of the program is financed through federal taxes. Medicare Part B covers **medical expenses for physician services; physical, occupational, and speech therapy; medical equipment; diagnostic tests; and preventive care** (eg, Pap smears, mammograms, vaccinations). Outpatient medications, along with eye, hearing, and dental services, are **not** covered.

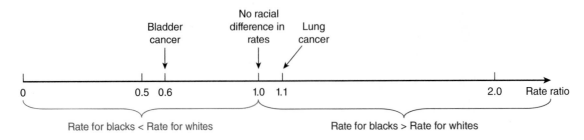

**FIGURE 7-15.** **Example of incidence rate ratio.** Schematic representation of black-to-white incidence rate ratio for cancers of the lung and bladder in the United States, 2008–2012. (Data from Howlader N, Noone AM, Krapcho M, et al. (eds). *SEER Cancer Statistics Review, 1975–2012,* National Cancer Institute. Bethesda, MD, http://seer.cancer.gov/csr/1975_2012/, based on November 2014 SEER data submission, posted to the SEER website, April 2015.)

### Medicare Part D

Medicare Part D, which went into effect in 2006, is administered by private insurance companies to cover prescription drugs. It is only available to those who are eligible for Medicare Part A or B. To receive the benefit, a person must enroll in one of the many available prescription plans offered by the numerous private insurance companies and pay a separate monthly premium.

### Medicare Part C

Medicare Advantage (Medicare Part C) is a private insurance option for Medicare-eligible persons. These plans are administered by private companies and are approved by Medicare. They must offer at least the same services as are covered by Parts A and B, and they typically offer additional benefits such as vision, dental, and/or prescription coverage.

### Medicaid

Medicaid is a state-sponsored program, although the federal government contributes 50–80% of the funds (more money comes from the federal government in poorer states, as measured by per capita income). Medicaid provides **coverage for a number of services,** including **hospital fees, physician services, laboratory services, radiographs, prenatal care, preventive care, nursing home care, and home health services.** Requirements that need to be met to qualify for Medicaid vary from state to state. However, typically, low-income families with children, individuals (disabled, blind, or elderly) who receive cash assistance under the Supplemental Security Income (SSI) program, and pregnant women whose family income is ≤ 133% of the deferral poverty level are eligible.

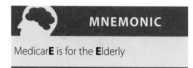

**MNEMONIC**

Medicar**E** is for the **E**lderly

## Patient Safety and Quality Improvement

Ensuring patient safety while delivering health care extends beyond simply making the right diagnosis and providing appropriate treatment. Steps must be taken to identify sources of error that can lead to missed diagnoses and/or inappropriate treatments. Patients may be exposed to potential harm before, during, and after a medical encounter; and quality improvement efforts are structured ways to analyze and minimize such harm. The cost of medical errors in the US is enormous, and part of that cost is due to preventable hospital readmissions. A report from the Medicare Payment Advisory Commission in 2005 estimated that up to $12 billion a year is spent on preventable readmissions. As a result, the Centers for Medicare & Medicaid Services (CMS) has started a Hospital Readmissions Reduction Program (HRRP) to attempt to limit excess readmissions. One of the program's measures includes penalties for readmissions involving acute myocardial infarction, heart failure, or pneumonia. See Table 7-5 for common reasons for readmissions based on different insurer types.

### PATIENT SAFETY

Medical errors are defined as actions (or lack of action) during planning or execution of care that lead to or could lead to an unintended result. Although some medical errors are not preventable, many are. Errors can be further subdivided into **active** and **latent errors.**

- **Active error** occurs at the level of a **frontline operator.** For example, a physician orders the wrong medication for a patient.
- **Latent error** occurs more indirectly and is commonly **systems-based.** For example, an electronic health system interface offers multiple drugs with similar names without clear differentiation. In this case there is no direct harm to a patient, but rather a potential harm in the future should the incorrect drug be prescribed by a physician due to a missed selection.

 **QUESTION**

An intern who is covering the entire floor of patients at night is called to see a patient who is in a double room. For privacy reasons related to the Health Insurance Portability and Accountability Act (HIPAA), patient names are not displayed at the room entrances. After the intern evaluates the patient, a note is entered and orders are placed. A short time later, the nurse discovers that the patient's roommate was erroneously examined instead. What factors (patient, physician, and/or system) were involved and what types of error (active and/or latent) occurred?

**TABLE 7-5. Five Hospitalized Conditions with the Most Frequent Readmissions***

| MEDICARE PATIENTS | MEDICAID PATIENTS | PRIVATE INSURANCE PATIENTS | UNINSURED PATIENTS |
|---|---|---|---|
| Congestive heart failure | Mood disorders | Maintenance chemotherapy; radiotherapy | Mood disorders |
| Septicemia | Schizophrenia and other psychotic disorders | Mood disorders | Alcohol-related disorders |
| Pneumonia | Diabetes mellitus with complications | Complications of surgical procedures or medical care | Diabetes mellitus with complications |
| COPD and bronchiectasis | Other complications of pregnancy | Complication of device; implant or graft | Pancreatic disorders (not diabetes) |
| Cardiac dysrhythmias | Alcohol-related disorders | Septicemia | Skin and subcutaneous tissue infections |

COPD, chronic obstructive pulmonary disease.

*Readmission for any reason within 30 days of index hospitalization.

There are multiple factors involved in medical errors, including those that arise from the patient, the physician, and the healthcare system.

- Patient factors include health literacy, cultural factors, socioeconomic status, and health compliance.
- Physician factors include deficits in knowledge, errors in judgment, fatigue or other impairment, and biases associated with decision-making processes.
- Systemic factors include the design and availability of hospital equipment, processes involved in ordering and administering medications, and the culture of a hospital team.

All of these factors are potential sources of error, and they can manifest in different ways. There are errors associated with **transition of care** when communication breaks down between clinicians changing shifts, or while admitting or discharging a patient. Medication errors are unfortunately common and can often be traced back to patient factors (eg, the patient misunderstood the medication instructions), physician factors (eg, mathematical error in dosing or faatigue and inattention when writing prescriptions), or systemic factors (eg, different doses or formulations of medication being labeled similarly and being stored next to each other).

The following strategies and systems can be used to analyze and reduce medical errors:

- **Root cause analysis** occurs after an error has taken place and uses records and participant interviews to identify the underlying problems that led to an error. The goal is to prevent a recurrence of that kind of error in the future.
- **Failure mode and effects analysis** is performed before a process is implemented with the goal of preventing errors. It seeks to identify the different ways a new process might fail, along with its probability of occurrence, effect, and method to preempt error.
- Medical errors can be reduced through the use of validated approaches designed to improve patient safety. A **safety culture** can be implemented to empower everyone involved in patient care to speak up when they feel that a patient is at risk for a medical error. When the hierarchy is flattened in settings where patients are at risk, healthcare workers are less afraid to report potential risks.
- Another systems approach is **human factors engineering,** in which the system prevents certain types of error by modulating human behavior. An example of this is creating different kinds of connections on different types of tubing, so that, for example, a feeding tube cannot physically be connected to an IV line.

A key analogy for how errors occur is the **"Swiss cheese model"** of failure (Figure 7-16). The entire system can be thought of as a stack of individual slices of Swiss cheese, each

**ANSWER**

This scenario involves active physician error, likely due to provider fatigue and the information overload of covering multiple new patients overnight. It also involves latent systems-based errors, in that patients are roomed together without clear differentiation of which patient is in which bed.

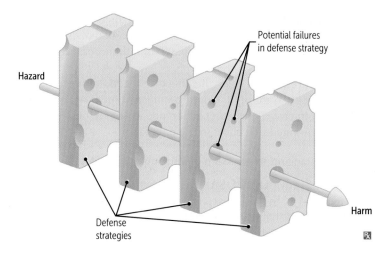

**FIGURE 7-16.    Swiss cheese model of error.**

with their own holes that represent ways latent or active errors can occur. When stacked together, the holes often do not overlap and so active errors made at one stage in the system can be blocked by safeguards and redundancies at other levels in the system. When the holes line up, however, errors can propagate through several layers of defenses and result in patient harm.

## QUALITY IMPROVEMENT

Health care is a complex system, and as a result there is potential for wide variability and unpredictability of outcomes. Quality improvement is the systematic analysis of a system's performance aimed at improving outcomes. Various quality metrics can be measured and displayed on run and control charts. In its most basic form, a **run chart** is a simple plot of a variable through time to report its values over time. A chart of a patient's blood pressure can be presented as a run chart (Figure 7-17). A **control chart** adds additional information by overlaying the desired characteristics of that measure, such as including lines demarcating the cutoffs for hypo- and hypertension. Categories of quality metrics include:

- **Outcome measures,** which measure the direct impact on patients. An example is a patient's HbA1c over time, or the average HbA1c of a population.

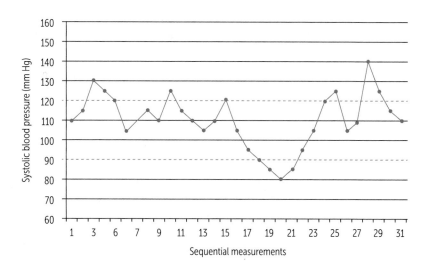

**FIGURE 7-17.    Control chart of blood pressure over time.**

**CLINICAL CORRELATION**

Run and control charts are frequently used in the hospital to identify subtle trends in patient lab values. A patient's weight and hemoglobin A1c may rise gradually and imperceptibly for months or years if each measurement is seen in isolation, but when graphed the trends become clearer and physicians can intervene sooner.

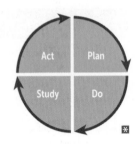

**FIGURE 7-18.** **PDSA cycle.**

■ **Process measures,** which seek to track the performance of a system according to planned parameters. An example would be the proportion of diabetics in a population whose HbA1c was measured in the past 6 months according to recommended guidelines.

■ **Balancing measures,** which track the effects that certain new processes have on different measures. An example would be measurement of hypoglycemia rates among diabetics to ensure that strict adherence to HbA1c outcome measures was not having an unwanted side effect in the population.

There are several paradigms to approach quality improvement in overlapping ways.

■ The **Plan, Do, Study, Act (PDSA) cycle** is first used to plan or develop a new process (Figure 7-18). In the Do step the plan is implemented and is followed by a Study of the results. Finally, in the Act step, as a result of the study, new actions to be implemented are determined, and the cycle begins anew.

The goal of all quality improvement efforts is to ensure high quality health care. Delivery of health care in this setting is as follows:

■ High-value: Costs are minimized and diagnostic tests are not overutilized.
■ Equitable: Access to the health care system is uniform.
■ Patient-centered: Focus is on patient autonomy.
■ Timely: Care is delivered as early as possible to avoid complications caused by delays.

## Ethics

### AUTONOMY

Patient autonomy is the right of patients to actively participate in and make final medical decisions that affect their health. Autonomy and justice are the most deeply seated principles in bioethics (and in the US legal system) regarding medical decision making. Autonomy means that people have **the right to choose** (accept or refuse) treatment.

**Example:** A police officer does not have the right to search an individual's home without a warrant. Similarly, a doctor does not have the right to perform a lung biopsy without the patient's consent.

■ **Patients** have **the right to accept or refuse treatments** that the physician may recommend because the patient "owns" his or her body and therefore has the right to make his or her own choices regarding health care.

■ **Physicians** have an **obligation to respect patients' autonomy,** and they must honor patient preferences for care.

**A patient's autonomy** can be **breached** under the following circumstances:

■ The patient is infected with a highly infectious and dangerous disease (eg, TB).
■ The patient has greatly impaired decision-making capacity (eg, a delusion impairing understanding of the decision).
■ The patient's autonomy is legally waived by the US government (eg, epidemics).

**Justice Cardozo** established the legal medical autonomy standard in the 1914 case of *Schloendoff vs Society of New York Hospital* (105 N.E. 92). The case involved a patient who consented to an examination of a fibroid tumor under ether, but explicitly denied consent for surgery. The surgeons performed the operation during the ether examination without her consent or knowledge.

**Justice Cardozo stated,** "Every human being of adult years and sound mind has a right to determine what shall be done with his own body; and a surgeon who performs an operation without his patient's consent, commits an assault, for which he is liable in damages."

**This is true except** in cases of emergency, when the patient is unconscious, and situations in which it is necessary to take action before consent can be obtained (life-threatening events).

## BENEFICENCE

Beneficence is **"the principle of doing good."** Physicians have a special ethical responsibility to act in the patient's best interest. This is known as a **fiduciary** relationship.

**Patient autonomy may conflict with beneficence.** If the patient makes an informed decision, then ultimately the patient has the right to decide what is in his or her best interest.

The practice of doing whatever the physician feels is best for the patient without consideration of the patient's wishes is called **paternalism.** This old form of medical practice is no longer acceptable in most circumstances.

**Case 3:** An intern is riding the subway home after a long shift at the hospital. She witnesses one of her fellow passengers falling onto the floor because of a cardiac arrest.

Although the exhausted intern is now off duty, she is **morally obligated** to help the unfortunate passenger **within the limits of her expertise and the established guidelines of care.** This obligation to act is often referred to as the **duty to rescue.**

> **KEY FACT**
>
> **Four general obligations for beneficence:**
> 1. One ought not to inflict evil or harm (what is bad).
> 2. One ought to prevent evil or harm.
> 3. One ought to remove evil or harm.
> 4. One ought to promote or do good.

## NONMALEFICENCE

The principle **"first do no harm"** is derived from *primum non nocere* in the Hippocratic oath. Nonetheless, if the benefits of an intervention outweigh the risks, ethically, the physician must act, as when there is an emergency.

Key issues that can be addressed by this principle include:

- Killing versus letting die.
- Intending versus foreseeing harmful outcomes.
- Withholding versus withdrawing life-sustaining treatment.
- Extraordinary versus ordinary circumstances.

Many of these issues center on the terminally ill and the seriously ill and injured.

> **KEY FACT**
>
> From the Hippocratic oath: "I will use treatment to help the sick according to my ability and judgment, but I will never use it to injure or wrong them."

## JUSTICE

The principle of justice in medical ethics relates to a fair distribution of resources in society. It is generally agreed that all persons should qualify for equal treatment, but limited resources (eg, organ donation or disaster events) constrain our ability to deliver equal resources to all. The principle of justice attempts to provide a framework for addressing the allocation of care in these resource-limited settings as well as in society as a whole.

## INFORMED CONSENT

Informed consent implies that the patient must have been fully informed of all options (benefits and risks) by the physician. This principle is ethically rooted in the concept of respect for the patient's autonomy.

Informed consent requires all of the following:

- **Disclosure** of relevant information, including the risks and benefits of treatment, as well as the consequences of no treatment.
- **Understanding** of the patient about the risks, benefits, and alternatives (including no treatment).
- **Capacity** of the patient to assess the risks and benefits and see how they align with the patient's own goals of care.
- **Voluntary** choice, free of coercion.

The idea is for the patient and physician to engage in a conversation in which negotiation and conflict resolution are welcomed to enhance patient autonomy.

**Key facts to remember about informed consent:**

- Consent is implied in the case of an emergency.
- Consent is necessary for **each** specific procedure.
- The health care worker performing the procedure **should** be the one to obtain consent.
- Beneficence does **not** obviate the need for consent.
- Consent received via the telephone **is** legitimate, but must be documented and usually requires witnesses.
- Pregnant women **can** refuse therapy for a fetus. (Once the child is born, life-saving therapy cannot be refused.)
- Decisions made by patients at a time when they were competent **continue** to be valid, even when they have lost the capacity to consent (ie, loss of consciousness).
- A health care proxy, living will, or medical power of attorney is the best method of obtaining consent (beforehand) from someone who has **lost** capacity.
- Informed consent must come from a parent/legal guardian (in the case of a minor), third-party court-appointed individual, or "substituted judgment" (an individual who ideally knows the patient well and can make decisions based on what he or she believes the patient would want). This prior preference may not be known for a **continuously** incompetent person (eg, a patient with severe Down syndrome). Then, the risks and benefits predominate.

**INFORMED ASSENT**

**Informed assent** consists of a **child's agreement** to medical procedures in the situation that he or she is not legally authorized or does not have the capacity to give consent competently (eg, participation in clinical trials, terminal illness).

In line with the World Health Organization (WHO) Research Ethics Review Committee, the following recommendations must be honored:

- Before seeking consent and assent to involve children in research, it must be demonstrated that comparable research cannot be done with adults to the same effect and scientific effect.
- Researchers must obtain consent from a parent or guardian on an informed consent form (ICF) for all children.
- Children should be provided with detailed information and a description of the research to be conducted, geared to the child's age, and should have their questions and concerns addressed. They have the right to express their agreement or lack of agreement to participate.
- Researchers should consider asking for assent from children older than 7 years, while accepting assent from all children older than 12 years.
- Children express their agreement to participate on an informed assent form (IAF) written in age-appropriate language. This form is **in addition to,** and **does not replace,** parental consent on an ICF.
- **Assent that is denied by a child should be taken very seriously.**

## DECISION-MAKING CAPACITY

A question of decision-making **capacity** arises when there is a conflict of ethical principles between autonomy and beneficence. Health care professionals are often faced with the difficult task of determining if a patient has or does not have the capacity to make decisions.

The components of capacity include "**CRAM**":

- The patient **Communicates** a stable choice.
- The patient understands the **Relevant** information.
- The patient can **Appreciate** the situation and the consequences of the choice.
- The patient can **Manipulate** the information.

**Example:** A patient who is refusing psychiatric hospitalization often needs a psychiatric evaluation to determine whether he or she has the capacity to make medical decisions. This may be the case even when a patient is involuntarily hospitalized because of a suicide attempt, for instance, or because of other circumstances in which he or she presents a danger to self or others.

## LEGAL COMPETENCE

The components of legal competence generally include:

- The patient has the capacity to understand the material information and the ability to state a preference.
- He or she can reason through a logical decision and make a judgment about the information in light of his or her values.
- The patient intends a certain outcome.
- The patient is able to freely communicate his or her wish to caregivers or investigators.

**KEY FACT**

Competency is different from capacity. Competency is a legal determination.

Although some ethical principles consider that individuals can fall anywhere on a spectrum, **competence is an "all or nothing" concept.** The patient is either competent or not. Thus, the legal process for determining that a patient is indeed **incompetent** is often painstaking.

## ADVANCE DIRECTIVES

**Advance directives** are written while a person is competent and are used to direct future health care decisions. Thus, patients can maintain autonomy even when they lack legal competence.

### Types of Written Advance Directives

There are two types of written advance directives:

- A **living will** is a statement of exactly which procedures are acceptable or unacceptable, and under what circumstances. It describes the types of treatments the patient wishes to receive or not receive if he or she becomes incapacitated and cannot communicate about treatment decisions.
- **Medical power of attorney** grants a specific surrogate person the authority to perform certain actions on behalf of the person who signs the document. The surrogate acts as the health care proxy on behalf of the person. The health care proxy retains the power unless it is revoked by the patient. It is more flexible than a living will.

### Oral Versus Written Advance Directives

**Oral advance directives** are taken from an incompetent patient's previous oral statements. These should be written in the patient's chart whenever possible.

**Example:** A woman is hospitalized after a motor vehicle collision and is placed on a ventilator before her family arrives. Upon arrival, the family recalls the patient's desire never to be placed on a ventilator because of her experience with her mother's death after a prolonged period on a ventilator. This recollection acts as an **oral advance directive.**

Unfortunately, people can often misinterpret an incapacitated person's previous statements. Thus, the following criteria add more validity to oral statements:

- The patient is informed.
- The directive is specific.
- The patient makes a choice.
- The decision is repeated over time.

**Written advance directives** are preferred because they provide stronger evidence of the patient's wishes.

Potential problems with advance directives:

- Relatively few persons have them.
- Designated decision makers may be unavailable, incompetent, or have a conflict of interest (eg, inheritance).
- Some people change their treatment preferences, but do not change the legal document.
- They leave no legal basis for health care providers to overturn instructions that turn out not to be in the patient's best medical interest, although the patient could not have reasonably anticipated this circumstance while competent.

## CONFIDENTIALITY

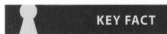

**KEY FACT**

The *Tarasoff* case: This classic case took place in California in 1976. This case highlighted the limits of confidentiality and established that clinicians are allowed to breach confidentiality if someone else is in danger.

**KEY FACT**

The suicidal or homicidal patient may be held against his or her will.

Confidentiality in the medical setting refers to keeping secret any personal information a patient discloses to his or her physician. Clinicians must respect the patient's privacy and autonomy, thus building a doctor-patient relationship based on trust. Patients may specify any information that they would like the physician to share with their family; anything that is not so specified should be kept confidential.

Certain **exceptions exist to the rule of confidentiality.** Such exceptions center around the risk of harm to the patient or others:

- The patient indicates suicidal or homicidal intent.
- Child abuse and elder abuse require mandatory reporting.
- Infectious diseases: The physician must report certain infectious diseases that pose significant public health risks (Table 7-3). In some cases, individuals at risk must be notified (eg, sexual partners of someone newly diagnosed with HIV), an action referred to as "**contact tracing.**"
- Impaired drivers, either due to substance abuse or neurologic conditions.

**Case 4:** A 47-year-old woman is diagnosed with metastatic breast cancer and is told she will probably not survive more than one year. She does not wish for her family to know about her disease or prognosis. The physician feels certain that the patient and her family will benefit by knowing the truth so that the family can support the patient and so they can make the most of their last months together.

**What should the physician do?**

The physician **may certainly urge** the patient to consider informing her family, but the **physician should not break her confidence.**

## MALPRACTICE

Medical malpractice is a civil suit that is taken out by patients or their family members against a physician or other health professional due to some form of **negligence,** malfeasance, or nonfeasance (inaction that allows or results in harm to a person) by the physician or a direct subordinate that has caused some type of harm to the patient. Causes can be a direct act or an omission by the medical team that results in a deviation from the standard accepted practice and results in a negative consequence.

Four conditions must be met for the plaintiff (patient or family member) to prove that malpractice has occurred, which together are known as **the four D's of malpractice.**

1. **Duty:** The physician is responsible for the medical care of the person harmed.
2. **Dereliction:** The physician deviated from the standard of medical care for the patient.
3. **Damage:** Because of a dereliction of one's duty to the patient, a direct harm occurs.
4. **Direct:** There is a direct link between the dereliction and the damage that was caused.

Without the fulfillment of these four criteria, malpractice cannot be proven in a court of law, and the physician is **not legally liable** for the damages that the patient has received.

It must be remembered that accidents that can cause harm frequently occur. Not all of these accidents result in malpractice suits; however, for a case to be made, all four conditions must have occurred.

> **KEY FACT**
>
> For malpractice to occur, the doctor must be responsible for the patient harmed and there must be proof of a deviation from standard practice that directly caused harm.

# Life Cycle

## DEVELOPMENT

### Apgar Score

- Each letter in the name Apgar stands for a sign assessed in newborns, as summarized in Table 7-6.
- The Apgar examination is fast, easy to perform, and helpful for determining whether medical intervention, including resuscitation, is needed. However, it is not particularly accurate as a prognostic indicator.

### Scoring

The Apgar score is determined at 1 and 5 minutes after birth. Reassessment may be performed after 5 minutes, and thereafter, if the Apgar score is abnormal.

**TABLE 7-6.  Apgar Signs and Scoring Criteria**

| SIGN | 0 POINTS | 1 POINT | 2 POINTS |
| --- | --- | --- | --- |
| **A**ppearance (skin color) | Cyanotic appearance throughout (pale, bluish-gray appearance) | Normal color except for cyanotic extremities | Normal color |
| **P**ulse | Absent | < 100 | ≥ 100 |
| **G**rimace (reflex irritability/response to stimulation) | No response | Grimace | Grimace and cough, pull away and/or sneeze |
| **A**ctivity (muscle tone) | None | Some | Active movement |
| **R**espiration | None | Weak, irregular | Strong, regular |

- Each of the five signs is scored as 0, 1, or 2; the Apgar score is the sum of the five scores.
- 7–10: Normal.
- 4–6: Some resuscitation may be needed.
- 0–3: Immediate resuscitation is necessary.

## LOW BIRTH WEIGHT

Low birth weight (LBW) is defined as birth weight below 2500 g and is caused by premature birth or intrauterine growth restriction (IUGR). LBW infants are at increased risk for the following complications:

- **Sepsis:** With possible negative sequelae of septic shock and disseminated intravascular coagulation (DIC).
- **Infant respiratory distress syndrome (hyaline membrane disease):** The infant's lungs produce inadequate surfactant, a protein normally secreted by type II pneumocytes in mature lungs. Surfactant (short for "surface active agent") facilitates inflation of alveoli and helps prevent alveolar collapse.
- **Necrotizing enterocolitis:** This is the most common neonatal gastrointestinal emergency; its cause remains uncertain, but is thought to be multifactorial. It is characterized by tissue necrosis in the gastrointestinal tract, and if supportive care (bowel rest and fluid replenishment) fails, surgical resection of necrotic bowel may be required.
- **Intraventricular hemorrhage:** Spontaneous bleeding into the ventricular system of the brain. This may result in long-term complications including cerebral palsy and delayed development.
- **Persistent pulmonary hypertension of the newborn (persistent fetal circulation):** Increased pressure in the pulmonary vasculature causes shunting of deoxygenated blood into the systemic circulation, resulting in hypoxemia.

## REFLEXES OF THE NEWBORN

Infants exhibit characteristic reflexes at birth that fade and then vanish at certain points in development. These reflexes are:

- **Moro:** Infant spreads then unspreads the arms when startled. Generally disappears around three to six months; persists in certain conditions, such as cerebral palsy.
- **Babinski:** Toes fan upward upon plantar stimulation. Generally disappears around 12–14 months; persists in certain neurologic conditions.
- **Palmar:** Infant grasps objects that come in contact with the palm. Generally disappears around 2–3 months.
- **Rooting:** Nipple seeking. Generally disappears around 3–4 months.

## DEVELOPMENTAL MILESTONES

Developmental milestones are skill sets (described in Table 7-7) acquired by children at certain ages and are useful for determining whether a child is progressing at the expected rate. Variation among healthy children can be considerable.

## INFANT DEPRIVATION

**History:** In the 1950s, psychologist Harry F. Harlow demonstrated that rhesus monkeys deprived of affection and physical contact developed abnormally. Later studies have suggested the existence of a similar phenomenon in humans: Long-term infant deprivation results in multiple long-term sequelae.

**FLASH FORWARD**

Infants born at 37–42 weeks' gestation are designated **term** infants; those born before 37 weeks' gestation are considered **premature**. A **LBW** infant need not be premature; he or she may have experienced IUGR or inappropriately low growth for gestational age.

**MNEMONIC**

**My Baby's Primary Reflexes:**

**M**oro
**B**abinski
**P**almar
**R**ooting

**KEY FACT**

In general, motor development proceeds cephalocaudally head to toe, from medial to lateral and from proximal to distal. Ulnar precedes radial, grasp precedes release, and pronation precedes supination.

**TABLE 7-7.** **Early Developmental Milestones**

| AGE | MOTOR | SOCIAL | VERBAL/COGNITIVE |
|---|---|---|---|
| INFANT | **P**ARENTS | **S**TART | **O**BSERVING |
| 0–12 mo | **P**rimitive reflexes disappear—Moro (by 6 mo), rooting (by 4 mo), palmar (by 6 mo), Babinski (by 12 mo)<br>**P**osture—lifts head up prone (by 1 mo), rolls and sits (by 6 mo), crawls (by 8 mo), stands (by 10 mo), walks (by 12–18 mo)<br>**P**icks—passes toys hand to hand (by 6 mo), **P**incer grasp (by 10 mo)<br>**P**oints to objects (by 12 mo) | **S**ocial smile (by 2 mo)<br>**S**tranger anxiety (by 6 mo)<br>**S**eparation anxiety (by 9 mo) | **O**rients—first to voice (by 4 mo), then to name and gestures (by 9 mo)<br>**O**bject permanence (by 9 mo)<br>**O**ratory—says "mama" and "dada" (by 10 mo) |
| TODDLER | **C**HILD | **R**EARING | **W**ORKING |
| 12–36 mo | **C**ruises, takes first steps (by 12 mo)<br>**C**limbs stairs (by 18 mo)<br>**C**ubes stacked—number = age (yr) × 3<br>**C**ultured—feeds self with fork and spoon (by 20 mo)<br>**K**icks ball (by 24 mo) | **R**ecreation—parallel play (by 24–36 mo)<br>**R**approchement—moves away from and returns to mother (by 24 mo)<br>**R**ealization—core gender identity formed (by 36 mo) | **W**ords—**200** words by age 2 (**2 zeros**), 2-word sentences |
| PRESCHOOL | **D**ON'T | **F**ORGET, THEY'RE STILL | **L**EARNING |
| 3–5 yr | **D**rive—tricycle (3 wheels at 3 yr)<br>**D**rawings—copies line or circle, stick figure (by 4 yr)<br>**D**exterity—hops on one foot (by 4 yr), uses buttons or zippers, grooms self (by 5 yr) | **F**reedom—comfortably spends part of day away from mother (by 3 yr)<br>**F**riends—cooperative play, has imaginary friends (by 4 yr) | **L**anguage—**1000** words by age 3 (**3 zeros**), uses complete sentences and prepositions (by 4 yr)<br>**L**egends—can tell detailed stories (by 4 yr) |

Reproduced with permission from Le T, et al. *First Aid for the USMLE Step 1 2017*. New York, NY: McGraw-Hill Education, 2017.

**Major effects of long-term infant deprivation:**

- **Illness:** Increased vulnerability to physical ailments.
- **Floppy:** Decreased muscle tone.
- **Wordless:** Language deficiencies.
- **Mistrust:** Difficulty in forming emotional bonds, sense of abandonment.
- **Thin:** Weight loss, failure to thrive.
- **Withdrawn:** Deficient socialization skills.
- **Anaclitic depression:** Relating to one person's physical and emotional dependence on another person (eg, infant's dependence on mother).

The term **anaclitic depression** refers to the deteriorated psychologic and physical health of infants who are separated from their caregivers and placed in cold, unstimulating institutional environments. Deprivation for > 6 months can lead to irreversible changes, such as withdrawn state, unresponsiveness, failure to thrive, and in severe cases, death.

## CHILD ABUSE

Abuse of children by caregivers can be physical, emotional, or sexual; physical and sexual abuse are covered in Table 7-8. The most common form of child maltreatment is **neglect,** which is the failure to provide a child with adequate food, shelter, supervision, education, and/or affection.

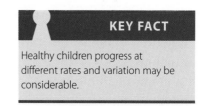

**KEY FACT**

Healthy children progress at different rates and variation may be considerable.

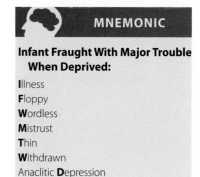

**MNEMONIC**

**Infant Fraught With Major Trouble When Deprived:**

**I**llness
**F**loppy
**W**ordless
**M**istrust
**T**hin
**W**ithdrawn
Anaclitic **D**epression

**TABLE 7-8.**    **Characteristics of Child Abuse**

|  | PHYSICAL ABUSE | SEXUAL ABUSE |
|---|---|---|
| EVIDENCE | Fractures (eg, ribs, long bone spiral, multiple in different stages of healing), bruises (eg, trunk, ear, neck; in pattern of implement), burns (eg, cigarette, buttocks/thighs), subdural hematomas, retinal hemorrhages. During exam, children often avoid eye contact | Genital, anal, or oral trauma; STIs; UTIs |
| ABUSER | Usually biologic mother | Known to victim, usually male |
| EPIDEMIOLOGY | 40% of deaths in children < 1 year old | Peak incidence 9–12 years old |

Reproduced with permission from Le T, et al. *First Aid for the USMLE Step 1 2017*. New York, NY: McGraw-Hill Education, 2017.

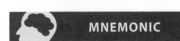

**MNEMONIC**

**Six S's of Aging**

**S**ex (slower erection, vaginal shortening)
**S**leep (decreased sleep)
**S**lowing (cognitive)
**S**ickness (increased susceptibility to chronic and infectious disease)
**S**uicide
p**S**ychiatric problems (depression)

## NORMAL CHANGES OF AGING

As adults move into late adulthood, certain patterns of physiologic and psychologic change are notable.

- Sexual changes (male): Slower erection and ejaculation; longer refractory periods.
- Sexual changes (female): Vaginal shortening, thinning, and dryness.
- Sleep pattern changes: Decreased rapid eye movement (REM) and slow-wave sleep, and increased time to increased sleep latency (time to sleep onset). The sleep period, or time from sleep onset to morning awakening, does not decrease. However, true sleep time does decrease due to increased awakening during the night.
- Certain medical conditions become more common: heart disease, some cancers, arthritis, hypertension, cataracts.
- Psychiatric problems, such as depression, are more common.
- Higher suicide rate.
- Thinking becomes less theoretical and more concrete.

## NORMAL GRIEF

Elisabeth Kübler-Ross defined the stages of grief in her landmark book, *On Death and Dying*. (Victims of physical or psychologic trauma [eg, rape] and various forms of personal loss may also experience these stages.) Although this order is typical, some individuals experience these stages in a different sequence. More than one stage may be present at a given time, and not all individuals experience all five stages.

- **Denial:** The reality of the loss is denied initially in an attempt to avoid emotional distress. One might understand the situation intellectually without experiencing the full emotional and psychologic impact.
- **Anger:** Anger and resentfulness are experienced and possibly expressed toward the departed, family and friends, or caregivers. It is important for physicians to see the anger as normal and to not personalize it.
- **Bargaining:** The bereaved may try, in essence, to "make a deal," on the assumption that circumstances might improve if he or she alters his or her behavior or attitudes. In this stage, patients and family members may try excessively to be "good."
- **Despair** or **depression:** The loss is now acknowledged, with a passive, sad emotional response.
- **Acceptance:** One integrates the experience into his or her world and copes successfully.

# Psychology

## INTELLIGENCE QUOTIENT (IQ)

Intelligence testing originated in the early 20th century for the purpose of identifying intellectually disabled children who would benefit from enrollment in special education programs.

IQ is:

- Correlated with genetic factors.
- More highly correlated with educational achievement and socioeconomic status.
- Generally stable throughout life.

In addition to IQ tests, assessment of one's actual living skills is sometimes performed and is required for the diagnosis of intellectual disability. This refers to one's abilities in such areas as self-care, self-direction, social functioning, and communication. The Vineland Adaptive Behavioral Scale, which is based on information provided by a close observer, such as a parent or teacher, is one such test.

Interpretation of IQ tests:

- Most IQ tests measure an individual as compared to a group mean, usually set at 100 with a standard deviation of 15.
- Intellectual disability is defined as an IQ less than 70.
- Intellectual disability is subdivided into four degrees of severity, as described in Table 7-9.

## ERIK ERIKSON'S PSYCHOSOCIAL DEVELOPMENT THEORY

Erikson's theory outlines eight stages through which a normal individual proceeds, as shown in Table 7-10. Each stage consists of a **basic crisis** that must be successfully overcome to proceed to the next stage. Although the stages correspond approximately to certain chronologic phases of life, the rate of progression varies among individuals.

**FLASH FORWARD**

Mental degeneration can be assessed by administering an IQ test and comparing the result with that expected for the patient's educational level and occupational achievement. Pathology may be harder to detect in individuals with a high baseline IQ because their scores may appear normal despite a decline from their previous levels.

**KEY FACT**

The average IQ is 100 with a standard deviation (SD) of 15. Intellectual disability is 2 or more SDs below the mean, or an IQ of 70.

**TABLE 7-9.  Degrees of Intellectual Disability and Corresponding IQ Ranges**

| DEGREE OF INTELLECTUAL DISABILITY | IQ RANGE |
| --- | --- |
| Mild | 55–69 |
| Moderate | 40–55 |
| Severe | 25–40 |
| Profound | < 25 |

**TABLE 7-10.    Erikson's Stages of Psychosocial Development**

| STAGE | BASIC CRISIS |
| --- | --- |
| Infancy (birth–1 year) | Trust versus mistrust |
| Early childhood (1–3 years) | Autonomy versus shame and self-doubt |
| Play age (3–5 years) | Initiative versus guilt |
| School age (6–11 years) | Industry versus inferiority |
| Adolescence (11–21 years) | Identity versus role confusion |
| Young adulthood (21–40 years) | Intimacy versus isolation |
| Adulthood (40–65 years) | Generativity versus stagnation |
| Late adulthood (over 65 years) | Integrity versus despair |

## CONDITIONING

Conditioning is the alteration of behavior by consequences.

### Classical Conditioning

Classical conditioning was first described by the Russian physiologist Ivan Pavlov. In his experiments with dogs, an unconditioned stimulus (UCS) of food elicited a characteristic unconditioned response (UCR) of salivation. Pavlov then introduced a new neutral conditioned stimulus (CS). In this case, a bell that was rung right before the food (UCS) was presented. Eventually the ringing bell (CS) alone elicits the salivation, which is now a conditioned response (CR). For the CS to effectively elicit a CR, it must precede the UCS during the training phase.

**Example:** A young child naturally cries (UCR) in response to sharp pain (UCS). If the child is brought to a physician's office for a vaccination, sees the syringe (CS), and immediately experiences sharp pain from the needle, the child will associate the needle with the pain and cry (CR) in response to the mere sight of the needle (CS), even before the vaccination is given.

### Operant Conditioning

Operant conditioning was first described by B. F. Skinner, who observed that the likelihood of voluntary behavior is increased by subsequent **reinforcement** or decreased by subsequent **punishment**. Reinforcement can be positive or negative.

- **Positive reinforcement:** A reward follows the desired behavior (eg, food appears after a button is pressed).
- **Negative reinforcement:** An unpleasant experience is removed (eg, a loud continuous noise stops after a button is pressed).
- **Positive punishment:** An unpleasant experience occurs after a behavior (eg, an electric shock is administered after a button is pressed).
- **Negative punishment:** A pleasant experience is removed after a behavior (eg, food is taken away after a button is pressed).

Beware of confusion between punishment and negative reinforcement. Any reinforcement, either positive or negative, encourages the reinforced behavior.

**Extinction** is the process by which a previously reinforced behavior is no longer reinforced, leading to its elimination. For example, in classical conditioning, visits to the doctor who no longer gives shots will lead to decreased association of the needle with pain. In operant conditioning, a rat that no longer receives food when pressing a bar will stop associating this behavior with food and stop responding. In other words, conditioned behavior can be unlearned as well as learned.

### Reinforcement Schedules

The two main categories of reinforcement schedules are **ratio** and **interval**. In the ratio schedule, reinforcement occurs based on behavioral events, regardless of time intervals. In the interval schedule, reinforcement occurs based on time intervals, regardless of the frequency of behavioral events. In either category, reinforcement can be **fixed** or **variable.**

- **Fixed-ratio** schedule: Reinforcement occurs after a set number of behaviors. Example: Salesman bonus for every tenth car sold.
- **Variable-ratio** schedule: Reinforcement occurs after a varying number of behaviors. Example: Casino slot machines.
- **Fixed-interval** schedule: Reinforcement occurs after a set time interval (and a response on the part of the organism). Example: Timed pet feeders.

**KEY FACT**

All reinforcement of behavior increases the probability of such behavior in the future, and all punishment decreases the probability of such behavior.

**KEY FACT**

Reinforcement is most effective when presented in such a way that the individual can clearly perceive the connection between the behavior and the reinforcement. Thus, effective reinforcement generally occurs shortly following the behavior.

**KEY FACT**

Classical conditioning causes a previously neutral stimulus to produce a characteristic (and preexisting) response. Operant conditioning uses effective reinforcement and punishment to alter voluntary behavior.

**KEY FACT**

Intermittent/variable reinforcement is more resistant to extinction than is continuous reinforcement.

- **Variable-interval** schedule: Reinforcement occurs at varied times. Example: Pop quizzes.

## EGO DEFENSE MECHANISMS

Anna Freud, Sigmund Freud's daughter and a renowned psychoanalyst in her own right, believed strongly in the importance of unconscious drives in determining behavior, but she also emphasized the importance of the ego, or executive decision making, in the functioning of the person. One aspect thereof is the **ego defense mechanism.** These mechanisms are automatic, unconscious, and act in response to psychologic stress or threat. Some are mature (Table 7-11); others are immature (Table 7-12).

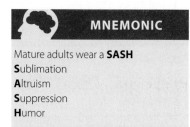

**MNEMONIC**

Mature adults wear a **SASH**
**S**ublimation
**A**ltruism
**S**uppression
**H**umor

**TABLE 7-11. Mature Defense Mechanisms**

| DEFENSE MECHANISM | DEFINITION | EXAMPLE |
| --- | --- | --- |
| Altruism | Generosity and personal sacrifice to bring pleasure to others and for internal satisfaction | Mafia boss making a large donation to charity |
| Humor | Appreciation of the amusing aspects of an anxiety-inducing setting | Nervous medical student joking about the boards |
| Sublimation | Redirecting unacceptable impulses into more acceptable actions | Aggressive tendencies redirected toward competitive sports |
| Suppression | Voluntarily keeping a thought away from consciousness | Refusing to think about a big game until it is time to play |

**TABLE 7-12.** **Immature Defense Mechanisms**

| DEFENSE MECHANISM | DEFINITION | EXAMPLE |
|---|---|---|
| Acting out | Unacceptable thoughts and feelings are expressed through actions | Temper tantrums |
| Denial | Pretending, believing, and/or acting as though an undesirable reality is nonexistent | Common response in patients newly diagnosed with cancer or AIDS |
| Displacement | Feelings one wishes to avoid are directed at a neutral party | Man arguing with his wife after being reprimanded by his boss |
| Dissociation | Avoidance of stress by a temporary drastic change in personality, memory, consciousness, or motor behavior | In extreme cases, dissociative identity disorder can result in which the individual develops multiple identities |
| Fixation | Partially remaining at an age-inappropriate level of development | Functional adult nibbling on her nails |
| Identification | Learning behavior from a model | Abused child identifying with an abuser |
| Intellectualization | Focusing on the intellectual aspects of a situation to avoid unacceptable emotions | Doing vigorous research on one's terminal disease to distract oneself from distress |
| Isolation | Separation of feelings from ideas and events | Attending a loved one's funeral without emotion |
| Passive aggression | Expressing negativity and performing below what is expected as an indirect show of opposition | Disgruntled employee is repeatedly late to work |
| Projection | Attributing an unacceptable impulse to an outside source rather than to oneself | Man who wants another woman thinking that his wife is cheating on him |
| Rationalization | Creating a logical argument to avoid blaming oneself | A woman who is passed over for a desirable promotion saying that her current position is better |
| Reaction formation | Unconsciously behaving in a manner opposite to how one truly feels in order to avoid anxiety | A patient with libidinous thoughts enters a monastery |
| Regression | Reverting to an earlier stage of development to avoid handling an unpleasant situation according to one's current developmental stage | Previously toilet-trained child wetting the bed |
| Repression | Keeping anxiety-provoking thoughts and feelings from consciousness | Involuntary or unconscious burying of memories of child abuse |
| Splitting | Perceiving people as either all good or all bad | Patient saying that all nurses are cold, but all doctors are friendly |

# Image Acknowledgments

In this edition, in collaboration with MedIQ Learning, LLC, and a variety of other partners, we are pleased to include the following clinical images and diagrams for the benefit of integrative student learning.

**Rx** Portions of this book identified with the symbol **Rx** are copyright © USMLE-Rx.com (MedIQ Learning, LLC).

**RU** Portions of this book identified with the symbol **RU** are copyright © Dr. Richard Usatine and are provided under license through MedIQ Learning, LLC.

**✳** Portions of this book identified with the symbol **✳** are listed below by Figure number.

This symbol ⊚ refers to material that is available in the public domain.

This symbol ⊚ refers to the Creative Commons Attribution license, full text at http://creativecommons.org/licenses/by/3.0/legalcode.

This symbol ⊚ refers to the Creative Commons Attribution-Share Alike license, full text at: http://creativecommons.org/licenses/by-sa/4.0/legalcode.

## Anatomy and Histology

**Figure 1-9**    **Peripheral blood smear with neutrophilia.** This image is a derivative work, adapted from the following source, available under ⊚: Mare TA, et al. The diagnostic and prognostic significance of monitoring blood levels of immature neutrophils in patients with systemic inflammation. *Crit Care.* 2015;19(1):57. doi:10.1186/s13054-015-0778-z.

**Figure 1-10**    **Electron microscopy of neutrophils: Image A.** Highly activated neutrophils with apoptotic neutrophils and cell debris. This image is a derivative work, adapted from the following source, available under ⊚: Rydell-Törmänen K, Uller L, Erjefält JS. Neutrophil cannibalism—a back up when the macrophage clearance system is insufficient. *Resp Res.* 2006;7(1):143. doi:10.1186/1465-9921-7-143. The image may have been modified by cropping, labeling, and/or captions. All rights to this adaptation by MedIQ Learning, LLC are reserved.

**Figure 1-11**    **Eosinophil microscopy: Image A.** Mature eosinophil with bright red granules. This image is a derivative work, adapted from the following source, available under ⊚: Rosenberg HF. Eosinophil-Derived Neurotoxin (EDN/RNase 2) and the Mouse Eosinophil-Associated RNases (mEars): Expanding Roles in Promoting Host Defense. *Int J Mol Sci.* 2015;16(7):15442-15455.

**Figure 1-11**    **Eosinophil microscopy: Image B.** Electron microscopy of eosinophils with bilobed nuclei and specific granules in the shape of a football with a crystalline core made from major basic protein. This image is a derivative work, adapted from the following source, available under ⊚: Rosenberg HF. Eosinophil-Derived Neurotoxin (EDN/RNase 2) and the Mouse Eosinophil-Associated RNases (mEars): Expanding Roles in Promoting Host Defense. *Int J Mol Sci.* 2015;16(7):15442-15455.

**Figure 1-12**    **Basophil microscopy: Image A.** Electron micrograph of a normal intact mast cell with homogenous electron-dense granules. This image is a derivative work, adapted from the following source, available under ⊚: Friesen CA, Neilan N, Daniel JF, et al. Mast cell activation and clinical outcome in pediatric cholelithiasis and biliary dyskinesia. *BMC Res Notes.* 2011;4:322. doi:10.1186/1756-0500-4-322.

**Figure 1-12**    **Basophil microscopy: Image B.** Basophil. Courtesy of Dr. Kristine Krafts.

**Figure 1-13**    **Macrophage microscopy: Image A.** Active macrophage. This image is a derivative work, adapted from the following source, available under ⊚: Mercer RR, Scabilloni JF, Hubbs AF, et al. Extrapulmonary transport of MWCNT following inhalation exposure. *Part Fibre Toxicol.* 2013;10:38. doi:10.1186/1743-8977-10-38. The image may have been modified by cropping, labeling, and/or captions. All rights to this adaptation by MedIQ Learning, LLC are reserved.

**Figure 1-13**    **Macrophage microscopy: Image B.** Multinucleated giant cell. Le T, et al. *First Aid for the USMLE Step 1.* New York, NY: McGraw-Hill, 2010.

**Figure 1-14**    **Light microscopy of a lymphocyte from a blood smear.** Courtesy of Dr. Kristine Krafts.

**Figure 1-18**    **Inguinal area.** Le T, et al. *First Aid for the USMLE Step 1.* New York, NY: McGraw-Hill Education, 2017.

**Figure 1-22**    **Histology of Peyer patches in small intestine.** This image is a derivative work, adapted from the following source, available under ⊚: Carvalho LJ, et al. Germinal center architecture disturbance during Plasmodium berghei ANKA infection in CBA mice. *Malar J.* 2007;6:59. doi:10.1186/1475-2875-6-59. The image may have been modified by cropping, labeling, and/or captions. All rights to this adaptation by MedIQ Learning, LLC are reserved.

**Figure 1-23**    **Diagram of the functional units of the spleen and histologic section of splenic sinusoid: Image B.** Histologic section of the splenic sinusoid showing vascular channels through the red pulp and T cells in the PALS. This image is a derivative work, adapted from the following source, available under ⊚: Heinrichs S, Conover LF, Bueso-Ramos CE, et al. MYBL2 is a sub-haploinsufficient tumor suppressor gene in myeloid malignancy. *eLife* 2013;2:e00825. doi 10.7554/eLife.00825. The image may have been modified by cropping, labeling, and/or captions. All rights to this adaptation by MedIQ Learning, LLC are reserved.

**Figure 1-26**  **Histology of the Purkinje cell of the cerebellum, demonstrating characteristic extensive dendritic branching.** This image is a derivative work, adapted from the following source, available under ⓒⓞ: Reeber SL, Otis TS, Sillitoe RV. New roles for the cerebellum in health and disease. *Front Syst Neurosci.* 2013;7:83. doi:10.3389/fnsys.2013.00083. The image may have been modified by cropping, labeling, and/or captions. All rights to this adaptation by MedIQ Learning, LLC are reserved.

**Figure 1-27**  **Electron micrograph of myelinated axons in the optic nerve.** This image is a derivative work, adapted from the following source, available under ⓒⓞ: Frühbeis C, Fröhlich D, Kuo WP, et al. Extracellular vesicles as mediators of neuron-glia communication. *Front Cell Neurosci.* 2013;7:182. doi:10.3389/fncel.2013.00182. The image may have been modified by cropping, labeling, and/or captions. All rights to this adaptation by MedIQ Learning, LLC are reserved.

**Figure 1-31**  **Erb palsy.** Claw hand. Winged scapula. Le T, et al. *First Aid for the USMLE Step 1.* New York, NY: McGraw-Hill Education, 2017.

**Figure 1-38**  **Lung alveolus.** Le T, et al. *First Aid for the USMLE Step 1.* New York, NY: McGraw-Hill Education, 2015.

**Figure 1-39**  **Gas exchange barrier.** Le T, et al. *First Aid for the USMLE Step 1.* New York, NY: McGraw-Hill, 2011.

**Figure 1-40**  **Lungs and bronchi: Image A.** Right bronchus is more vertical and wider in diameter than the left bronchus. Le T, et al. *First Aid for the USMLE Step 1.* New York, NY: McGraw-Hill Education, 2017.

## Biochemistry

**Figure 2-3**  **Base structures of pyrimidines and purines.** Le T, et al. *First Aid for the USMLE Step 1.* New York, NY: McGraw-Hill Education, 2017.

**Figure 2-25**  **Xeroderma pigmentosum.** This image is a derivative work, adapted from the following source, available under ⓒⓞ: Halpern J, Hopping B, Brostoff JM. Photosensitivity, corneal scarring and developmental delay: Xeroderma Pigmentosum in a tropical country. *Cases Journal.* 2008;1:254. doi:10.1186/1757-1626-1-254. The image may have been modified by cropping, labeling, and/or captions. All rights to this adaptation by MedIQ Learning, LLC are reserved.

**Figure 2-37**  **Osteogenesis imperfecta.** This image is a derivative work, adapted from the following source, available under ⓒⓞ: van Dijk HA, Fred H. Images of memorable cases: 40, 41, & 42. OpenStax CNX. Dec 3, 2008. Available at: *http://cnx.org/contents/_on798ZB@3/Images-of-Memorable-Cases-Case.*

**Figure 2-38**  **Menkes disease.** This image is a derivative work, adapted from the following source, available under ⓒⓞ: Datta AK, Ghosh T, Nayak K, Ghosh M. Menkes kinky hair disease: A case report. *Cases J.* 2008;1:158. doi:10.1186/1757-1626-1-158. The image may have been modified by cropping, labeling, and/or captions. All rights to this adaptation by MedIQ Learning, LLC are reserved.

**Figure 2-39**  **Reticular fibers (silver stain).** This image is a derivative work, adapted from the following source, available under ⓒⓞ: Seidensticker M, et al. Quantitative in vivo assessment of radiation injury of the liver using Gd-EOB-DTPA enhanced MRI: tolerance dose of small liver volumes. *Radiat Oncol.* 2011;6:40. doi:10.1186/1748-717X-6-40. The image may have been modified by cropping, labeling, and/or captions. All rights to this adaptation by MedIQ Learning, LLC are reserved.

**Figure 2-62**  **Alanine synthesis.** Modified with permission from Le T, et al. *First Aid for the USMLE Step 1.* New York, NY: McGraw-Hill, 2010.

**Figure 2-71**  **Amino acid derivatives.** Le T, et al. *First Aid for the USMLE Step 1.* New York, NY: McGraw-Hill Education, 2017.

**Figure 2-74**  **Amino acid carbon skeleton recycling.** Le T, et al. *First Aid for the USMLE Step 1.* New York, NY: McGraw-Hill, 2010.

**Figure 2-76**  **Pellagra.** This image is a derivative work, adapted from the following source, available under ⓒⓞ: van Dijk HA, Fred H. Images of memorable cases: case 2. Connexions Web site. Dec 4, 2008. Available at: *http://cnx.org/contents/3d3dcb2e-8e98-496f-91c2-fe94e93428a1@3@3/.* The image may have been modified by cropping, labeling, and/or captions. All rights to this adaptation by MedIQ Learning, LLC are reserved.

**Figure 2-78**  **Hypersegmented neutrophil.** This image is a derivative work, adapted from the following source, available under ⓒⓞ: De Tommasi AS, Otranto D, Furlanello T, et al. Evaluation of blood and bone marrow in selected canine vector-borne diseases. *Parasit Vectors.* 2014;7:534. doi:10.1186/s13071-014-0534-2. The image may have been modified by cropping, labeling, and/or captions. All rights to this adaptation by MedIQ Learning, LLC are reserved.

**Figure 2-79**  **Ecchymosis secondary to vitamin C deficiency.** This image is a derivative work, adapted from the following source, available under ⓒⓞ: Alqanatish JT, et al. Childhood scurvy: an unusual cause of refusal to walk in a child. *Pediatr Rheumatol Online J.* 2015;13:23. doi:10.1186/s12969-015-0020-1. The image may have been modified by cropping, labeling, and/or captions. All rights to this adaptation by MedIQ Learning, LLC are reserved.

**Figure 2-84**  **Warfarin prevents conversion of vitamin K epoxide to vitamin K.** Le T, et al. *First Aid for the USMLE Step 1.* New York, NY: McGraw-Hill Education, 2017.

**Figure 2-91**  **Structure of proinsulin and insulin.** Modified with permission from Le T, et al. *First Aid for the USMLE Step 1.* New York, NY: McGraw-Hill Education, 2017.

**Figure 2-100**  **Xanthoma of elbow.** This image is a derivative work, adapted from the following source, available under ⓒⓞ: Reproduced with permission from Kardaş F, Cetin A, Solmaz M, et al. Successful treatment of homozygous familial hypercholesterolemia using cascade filtration plasmapheresis. *Turk J Haematol.* 2012;29(4):334-41. doi: 10.5152/tjh.2011.20.

**Figure 2-101** **Multiple tendon xanthoma.** This image is a derivative work, adapted from the following source, available under [cc]: Kumar AA, Shantha GPS, Srinivasan Y, et al. Acute myocardial infarction in an 18-year-old South Indian girl with familial hypercholesterolemia: a case report. *Cases J.* 2008;1:71. doi:10.1186/1757-1626-1-71.

**Figure 2-102** **Acanthocyte ("spur cell").** Courtesy of Dr. Kristine Krafts.

**Figure 2-111** **Hemoglobin.** Le T, et al. *First Aid for the USMLE Step 1.* New York, NY: McGraw-Hill Education, 2017.

**Figure 2-114** **Lead lines on the metaphysis of long bone.** Reproduced, with permission, from Dr. Frank Gaillard and *www.radiopaedia.org.*

**Figure 2-116** **Hemoglobin binding curve.** Le T, et al. *First Aid for the USMLE Step 1.* New York, NY: McGraw-Hill Education, 2017.

**Figure 2-117** **Carboxyhemoglobin binding curve.** Le T, et al. *First Aid for the USMLE Step 1.* New York, NY: McGraw-Hill Education, 2017.

**Figure 2-127** **Example of SDS-PAGE.** This image is a derivative work, adapted from the following source, available under [cc]: Chacko AD, et al. Voltage dependent anion channel-1 regulates death receptor mediated apoptosis by enabling cleavage of caspase-8. *BMC Cancer.* 2010;10:380. doi:10.1186/1471-2407-10-380.

**Figure 2-129** **ELISA.** Le T, et al. *First Aid for the USMLE Step 1.* New York, NY: McGraw-Hill Education, 2015.

**Figure 2-131** **Hardy-Weinburg formula.** Le T, et al. *First Aid for the USMLE Step 1.* New York, NY: McGraw-Hill Education, 2017.

**Table 2-31** **Sphingolipidoses: Image A.** Fabry disease. This image is a derivative work, adapted from the following source, available under [cc]: Burlina AP, Sims KB, Politei JM, et al. Early diagnosis of peripheral nervous system involvement in Fabry disease and treatment of neuropathic pain: the report of an expert panel. *BMC Neurol.* 2011;11:61. doi 10.1186/1471-2377-11-61. The image may have been modified by cropping, labeling, and/or captions. All rights to this adaptation by MedIQ Learning, LLC are reserved.

**Table 2-31** **Sphingolipidoses: Image B.** Gaucher disease. This image is a derivative work, adapted from the following source, available under [cc]: Sokołowska B, Skomra D, Czartoryska B, Tomczaket W, et al. Gaucher disease diagnosed after bone marrow trephine biopsy—a report of two cases. *Folia Histochem Cytobiol.* 2011;49:352-356. doi 10.5603/FHC.2011.0048. The image may have been modified by cropping, labeling, and/or captions. All rights to this adaptation by MedIQ Learning, LLC are reserved.

**Table 2-31** **Sphingolipidoses: Image C.** Niemann-Pick disease. This image is a derivative work, adapted from the following source, available under [cc]: Prieto-Potín I, Roman-Blas J, Martínez-Calatrava M, Gómez R, et al. Hypercholesterolemia boosts joint destruction in chronic arthritis. An experimental model aggravated by foam macrophage infiltration. *Arthritis Res Ther.* 2013;15(4):R81. doi:10.1186/ar4261. The image may have been modified by cropping, labeling, and/or captions. All rights to this adaptation by MedIQ Learning, LLC are reserved.

**Table 2-31** **Sphingolipidoses: Image D.** Tay-Sachs disease. This image is a derivative work, adapted from the following source, available under [cc]: Courtesy of Dr. Jonathan Trobe.

**Table 2-34** **Summary of diseases of hemoglobin synthesis: Image A.** Microcytic anemia with basophilic stippling. This image is a derivative work, adapted from the following source, available under [cc]: van Dijk HA, Fred HL. Images of memorable cases: case 81. Connexions Web site. Dec 3, 2008. Available at: *http://cnx.org/contents/3196bf3e-1e1e-4c4d-a1ac-d4fc9ab65443@4@4.*

## Immunology

**Figure 3-2** **The spleen: Image B.** Normal spleen showing red pulp and white pulp. This image is a derivative work, adapted from the following source, available under [cc]: Heinrichs S, Conover LF, Bueso-Ramos CE, et al. MYBL2 is a sub-haploinsufficient tumor suppressor gene in myeloid malignancy. *eLife.* 2013;2:e00825. doi 10.7554/eLife.00825. The image may have been modified by cropping, labeling, and/or captions. All rights to this adaptation by MedIQ Learning, LLC are reserved.

**Figure 3-4** **Peyer patches.** This image is a derivative work, adapted from the following source, available under [cc]: Song Y, Liang C, Wang W, et al. Immunotoxicological Evaluation of Corn Genetically Modified with Bacillus thuringiensis Cry1Ah Gene by a 30-Day Feeding Study in BALB/c Mice. Fuchs S, ed. *PLoS ONE.* 2014;9(2):e78566. doi:10.1371/journal.pone.0078566. The image may have been modified by cropping, labeling, and/or captions. All rights to this adaptation by MedIQ Learning, LLC are reserved.

**Figure 3-6** **Macrophage.** [cc] Courtesy of the US Department of Health and Human Services and Dr. Francis W. Chandler. The image may have been modified by cropping, labeling, and/or captions. All rights to this adaptation by MedIQ Learning, LLC are reserved.

**Figure 3-7** **Dendritic cells.** This image is a derivative work, adapted from the following source, available under [cc]: Courtesy of Dr. Ed Uthman.

**Figure 3-8** **The complement system.** Le T, et al. *First Aid for the USMLE Step 1.* New York, NY: McGraw-Hill Education, 2017.

**Figure 3-24**    **Granulocytes in Chédiak-Higashi syndrome.** This image is a derivative work, adapted from the following source, available under ⊚🄯: Bharti S, Bhatia P, Bansal D, et al. The accelerated phase of Chediak-Higashi syndrome: the importance of hematological evaluation. *Turk J Haematol*. 2013;30:85-87. doi: 10.4274/tjh.2012.0027. The image may have been modified by cropping, labeling, and/or captions. All rights to this adaptation by MedIQ Learning, LLC are reserved.

**Figure 3-25**    **Malar rash.** Le T, et al. *First Aid for the USMLE Step 1*. New York, NY: McGraw-Hill Education, 2015.

**Figure 3-27**    **Systemic sclerosis.** This image is a derivative work, adapted from the following source, available under ⊚🄯: Russo RA, Katsicas MM. Clinical characteristics of children with Juvenile Systemic Sclerosis: follow-up of 23 patients in a single tertiary center. *Pediatr Rheumatol Online J*. 2007;5:6. doi:10.1186/1546-0096-5-6. The image may have been modified by cropping, labeling, and/or captions. All rights to this adaptation by MedIQ Learning, LLC are reserved.

**Figure 3-28**    **Telangiectasias on the lips.** This image is a derivative work, adapted from the following source, available under ⊚🄯: Fred HL, van Dijk HA. Images of memorable cases: cases 115 & 116. Connexions Web site. Dec 4, 2008. Available at: *http://cnx.org/contents/444f9696-2955-4c70-998c-18f0ac4f4fba@3*.

**Figure 3-29**    **Sjögren syndrome.** ⊚🄯 Courtesy of the US Department of Health and Human Services.

**Figure 3-30**    **Sarcoidosis: Image A.** Noncaseating granulomas. Le T, et al. *First Aid for the USMLE Step 1*. New York, NY: McGraw-Hill Education, 2017.

**Figure 3-30**    **Sarcoidosis: Image B.** Chest x-ray showing bilateral adenopathy and coarse reticular opacities. This image is a derivative work, adapted from the following source, available under ⊚🄯: Lønborg J, Ward M, Gill A, et al. Utility of cardiac magnetic resonance in assessing right-sided heart failure in Sarcoidosis. *BMC Med Imaging*. 2013;13:2. doi 10.1186/1471-2342-13-2. The image may have been modified by cropping, labeling, and/or captions. All rights to this adaptation by MedIQ Learning, LLC are reserved.

**Figure 3-30**    **Sarcoidosis: Image C.** CT showing hilar and mediastinal adenopathy. This image is a derivative work, adapted from the following source, available under ⊚🄯: Lønborg J, Ward M, Gill A, et al. Utility of cardiac magnetic resonance in assessing right-sided heart failure in Sarcoidosis. *BMC Med Imaging*. 2013;13:2. doi 10.1186/1471-2342-13-2. The image may have been modified by cropping, labeling, and/or captions. All rights to this adaptation by MedIQ Learning, LLC are reserved.

## Microbiology

**Figure 4-5**    **Alpha-hemolysis and beta-hemolysis on blood agar.** ⊚🄯 Courtesy of the US Department of Health and Human Services and Dr. Richard R. Facklam.

**Figure 4-7**    **Photomicrograph of *Streptococcus pyogenes* in long chains.** ⊚🄯 Courtesy of the US Department of Health and Human Services.

**Figure 4-8**    **Impetigo.** ⊚🄯 Courtesy of the US Department of Health and Human Services and Dr. Herman Miranda and A. Chambers.

**Figure 4-10**    **Staphylococcal scalded skin syndrome.** This image is a derivative work, adapted from the following source, available under ⊚🄯: Duijsters CE, Halbertsma FJ, Kornelisse RF, et al. Recurring staphylococcal scalded skin syndrome in a very low birth weight infant: a case report. *J Med Case Rep*. 2009;3:7313. doi:10.4076/1752-1947-3-7313.

**Figure 4-11**    **Infective endocarditis.** ⊚🄯 Courtesy of the US Department of Health and Human Services and Dr. Edwin P. Ewing, Jr.

**Figure 4-12**    **Pseudomembranous colitis.** This image is a derivative work, adapted from the following source, available under ⊚🄯: Kircher S, Wössner R, Müller-Hermelink H-K, Völker H-U. Lethal pneumatosis coli in a 12-month-old child caused by acute intestinal gas gangrene after prolonged artificial nutrition: a case report. *J Med Case Rep*. 2008;2:238. doi:10.1186/1752-1947-2-238. The image may have been modified by cropping, labeling, and/or captions. All rights to this adaptation by MedIQ Learning, LLC are reserved.

**Figure 4-13**    **Cutaneous anthrax on a forearm.** ⊚🄯 Courtesy of the US Department of Health and Human Services and Archil Navdarashvili. The image may have been modified by cropping, labeling, and/or captions. All rights to this adaptation by MedIQ Learning, LLC are reserved.

**Figure 4-14**    ***Corynebacterium diphtheriae.*** ⊚🄯 Courtesy of the US Department of Health and Human Services and Graham Heid. The image may have been modified by cropping, labeling, and/or captions. All rights to this adaptation by MedIQ Learning, LLC are reserved.

**Figure 4-16**    ***Neisseria gonorrhoeae.*** ⊚🄯 Courtesy of the US Department of Health and Human Services and Bill Schwartz. The image may have been modified by cropping, labeling, and/or captions. All rights to this adaptation by MedIQ Learning, LLC are reserved.

**Figure 4-17**    **Purpura fulminans.** This image is a derivative work, adapted from the following source, available under ⊚🄯: Hon K-L, So K-W, Wong W, et al. Spot diagnosis: An ominous rash in a newborn. *Ital J Pediatr*. 2009;35:10. doi:10.1186/1824-7288-35-10.

**Figure 4-18**    **Urethral discharge secondary to gonorrhea.** ⊚🄯 Courtesy of the US Department of Health and Human Services and Susan Lindsley.

**Figure 4-19**    **Infection from *Haemophilus ducreyi.*** ⊚🄯 Courtesy of the US Department of Health and Human Services and Dr. Pirozzi. The image may have been modified by cropping, labeling, and/or captions. All rights to this adaptation by MedIQ Learning, LLC are reserved.

**Figure 4-21**    **Rose spots of typhoid fever.** ⊚🄯 Courtesy of the US Department of Health and Human Services, Armed Forces Institute of Pathology, and Charles N. Farmer. The image may have been modified by cropping, labeling, and/or captions. All rights to this adaptation by MedIQ Learning, LLC are reserved.

**Figure 4-22** *Vibrio cholerae.* Courtesy of the US Department of Health and Human Services.

**Figure 4-23** **Bubonic plague.** Courtesy of the US Department of Health and Human Services. The image may have been modified by cropping, labeling, and/or captions. All rights to this adaptation by MedIQ Learning, LLC are reserved.

**Figure 4-24** **Caseating granuloma from lung parenchyma infected with *Mycoplasma tuberculosis.*** Le T, et al. *First Aid for the USMLE Step 1.* New York, NY: McGraw-Hill Education, 2017.

**Figure 4-25** **An anteroposterior x-ray of advanced bilateral pulmonary tuberculosis.** Courtesy of the US Department of Health and Human Services.

**Figure 4-27** **Lepromatous leprosy.** This image is a derivative work, adapted from the following source, available under : Fu X, Liu H, Zhang F. Borderline Lepromatous Leprosy with Type 1 (Reversal) Reactions in a Chinese Man. *Am J Trop Med Hyg.* 2015;93(2):207-209. doi:10.4269/ajtmh.14-0491. The image may have been modified by cropping, labeling, and/or captions. All rights to this adaptation by MedIQ Learning, LLC are reserved.

**Figure 4-28** **Chancre of primary syphilis.** Courtesy of the US Department of Health and Human Services and Susan Lindsley. The image may have been modified by cropping, labeling, and/or captions. All rights to this adaptation by MedIQ Learning, LLC are reserved.

**Figure 4-29** **Gumma of nose due to a long-standing tertiary syphilitic *Treponema pallidum* infection.** Courtesy of the US Department of Health and Human Services and J. Pledger.

**Figure 4-30** **Pathognomonic erythematous rash (erythema chronicum migrans).** Courtesy of the US Department of Health and Human Services and James Gathany.

**Figure 4-31** **Scanning electron micrograph of *Leptospira interrogans.*** Courtesy of the US Department of Health and Human Services, Rob Weyant, and Janice Haney Carr.

**Figure 4-33** **Histoplasma morphologies: Image A.** Tissue form. Courtesy of the US Department of Health and Libero Ajello.

**Figure 4-33** **Histoplasma morphologies: Image B.** Intracellular form. Courtesy of the US Department of Health and Dr. D.T. McClenan.

**Figure 4-34** **Blastomyces morphology.** Courtesy of the US Department of Health and Human Services.

**Figure 4-35** **Coccidioides morphologies: Image A.** Courtesy of the US Department of Health and Dr. Hardin.

**Figure 4-35** **Coccidioides morphologies: Image B.** Courtesy of the US Department of Health and Human Services and Dr. Lucille K. Georg.

**Figure 4-36** **Paracoccidioides—"pilot's wheel."** Courtesy of the US Department of Health and Human Services and Dr. Lucille K. Georg.

**Figure 4-37** **Dermatophytes: Image A.** Macroconidia budding from multiseptate conidiophores. Courtesy of the US Department of Health and Human Services and Dr. Libero.

**Figure 4-37** **Dermatophytes: Image B.** Spindle-shaped macroconidia of *Microsporum.* Courtesy of the US Department of Health and Human Services and Dr. Lucille K. Georg.

**Figure 4-38** **Tineas: Image A.** Tinea capitis. Courtesy of the US Department of Health and Human Services and Dr. Lucille K. Georg.

**Figure 4-38** **Tineas: Image B.** Tinea corporis. Courtesy of the US Department of Health and Human Services and Dr. Lucille K. Georg.

**Figure 4-39** **Hypopigmented, patchy rash of tinea versicolor.** Courtesy of the US Department of Health and Human Services and Dr. Lucille K. Georg.

**Figure 4-40** *Malassezia furfur.* Courtesy of the US Department of Health and Human Services and Dr. Lucille K. Georg.

**Figure 4-41** ***Candida* morphology.** Courtesy of the US Department of Health and Human Services and Dr. Stuart Brown.

**Figure 4-42** ***Candida.*** "Germ tube" morphology. Courtesy of the US Department of Health and Human Services, Mercy Hospital, and Dr. Brian Harrington.

**Figure 4-43** ***Cryptococcus* morphology.** Courtesy of the US Department of Health and Human Services and Dr. Leanor Haley.

**Figure 4-45** **Classic clinical presentation of *Pneumocystis jirovecii* pneumonia.** Courtesy of the US Department of Health and Human Services and Dr. Jonathan W.M. Gold.

**Figure 4-46** ***Aspergillus* morphology: Image B.** Conidial head with spores. Courtesy of the US Department of Health and Human Services and Dr. Lucille K. Georg.

**Figure 4-48** ***Sporothrix schenckii* morphologies and clinical presentation: Image A.** Branching conidiophores and numerous conidia of the mold form. Courtesy of the US Department of Health and Human Services and Dr. Libero Ajello.

**Figure 4-48** ***Sporothrix schenckii* morphologies and clinical presentation: Image B.** Cigar-shaped budding yeast. Courtesy of the US Department of Health and Human Services and Dr. Lucille K. Georg.

**Figure 4-49** ***Giardia lamblia* cyst.** Courtesy of the US Department of Health and Human Services.

**Figure 4-50** ***Entamoeba histolytica.*** This image is a derivative work, adapted from the following source, available under : Hung C-C, et al. Increased Risk for Entamoeba histolytica Infection and Invasive Amebiasis in HIV Seropositive Men Who Have Sex with Men in Taiwan. Bhattacharya A, ed. *PLoS Negl Trop Dis.* 2008;2(2):e175. doi:10.1371/journal.pntd.0000175.

**Figure 4-101** **Mumps.** Courtesy of the US Department of Health and Human Services.

**Figure 4-102** **Negri body.** Courtesy of the US Department of Health and Human Services and Dr. Daniel P. Perl. The image may have been modified by cropping, labeling, and/or captions. All rights to this adaptation by MedIQ Learning, LLC are reserved.

**Figure 4-104** **Thumbprint sign.** This image is a derivative work, adapted from the following source, available under : Noble J, Devor R, Rogalski FJ, et al. Aphonia and epiglottitis in neonate with concomitant MRSA skin infection. *Respirol Case Rep.* 2014;2(3):116-119. doi:10.1002/rcr2.66. The image may have been modified by cropping, labeling, and/or captions. All rights to this adaptation by MedIQ Learning, LLC are reserved.

**Figure 4-106** **Infective endocarditis: Image A.** Janeway lesions. This image is a derivative work, adapted from the following source, available under : Ji Y, Kujtan L, Kershner D. Acute endocarditis in intravenous drug users: a case report and literature review. *J Community Hosp Intern Med Perspect.* 2012;2(1):10.3402/jchimp.v2i1.11513. doi:10.3402/jchimp.v2i1.11513. The image may have been modified by cropping, labeling, and/or captions. All rights to this adaptation by MedIQ Learning, LLC are reserved.

**Figure 4-107** **Giardia lamblia trophozoites.** Courtesy of the US Department of Health and Human Services.

**Figure 4-108** **Osteomyelitis: Images A and B.** This image is a derivative work, adapted from the following source, available under : Pandey V, Rao SP, Rao S, et al. *Burkholderia pseudomallei* musculoskeletal infections (melioidosis) in India. *Indian J Orthop* 2010;44:216-220. doi 10.4103/0019-5413.61829. The image may have been modified by cropping, labeling, and/or captions. All rights to this adaptation by MedIQ Learning, LLC are reserved.

**Figure 4-109** **Three diagnostic categories of otitis media: Image A.** Acute otitis media. This image is a derivative work, adapted from the following source, available under : Kuruvilla A, Shaikh N, Hoberman A, Kovačević J. Automated Diagnosis of Otitis Media: Vocabulary and Grammar. *Int J Biomed Imaging.* 2013;2013:327515.

**Figure 4-109** **Three diagnostic categories of otitis media: Image B.** Otitis media with effusion. This image is a derivative work, adapted from the following source, available under : Kuruvilla A, Shaikh N, Hoberman A, Kovačević J. Automated Diagnosis of Otitis Media: Vocabulary and Grammar. *Int J Biomed Imaging.* 2013;2013:327515.

**Figure 4-109** **Three diagnostic categories of otitis media: Image C.** No effusion. This image is a derivative work, adapted from the following source, available under : Kuruvilla A, Shaikh N, Hoberman A, Kovačević J. Automated Diagnosis of Otitis Media: Vocabulary and Grammar. *Int J Biomed Imaging.* 2013;2013:327515.

**Table 4-30** **Commonly Encountered HIV-Associated Infections: Image A.** Hairy leukoplakia. Courtesy of the US Department of Health and Human Services, Dr. J.S. Greenspan, and Dr. Sol Silverman, Jr.

**Table 4-30** **Commonly Encountered HIV-Associated Infections: Image B.** *Candida albicans.* Courtesy of the US Department of Health and Human Services and Dr. Sol Silverman.

**Table 4-30** **Commonly Encountered HIV-Associated Infections: Image C.** Progressive multifocal leukoencephalopathy. Courtesy of Dr. Vanja Douglas.

**Table 4-30** **Commonly Encountered HIV-Associated Infections: Image D.** CMV retinitis. Courtesy of the US Department of Health and Human Services.

**Table 4-30** **Commonly Encountered HIV-Associated Infections: Image E.** *Pneumocystis jirovecii.* Courtesy of the US Department of Health and Human Services and Dr. Jonathan W.M. Gold. The image may have been modified by cropping, labeling, and/or captions. All rights to this adaptation by MedIQ Learning, LLC are reserved.

**Table 4-32** **"Lots of Spots": Red Rashes of Childhood: Image A.** Rubella. Courtesy of the US Department of Health and Human Services.

**Table 4-32** **"Lots of Spots": Red Rashes of Childhood: Image B.** Rubeola (measles). Courtesy of the US Department of Health and Human Services.

**Table 4-32** **"Lots of Spots": Red Rashes of Childhood: Image D.** Roseola. Courtesy of the US Department of Health and Human Services.

**Table 4-32** **"Lots of Spots": Red Rashes of Childhood: Image E.** Erythema infectiosum. Courtesy of the US Department of Health and Human Services and Dr. Philip S. Brachman.

**Table 4-32** **"Lots of Spots": Red Rashes of Childhood: Image F.** *Streptococcus pyogenes* (scarlet fever). Courtesy of the US Department of Health and Human Services.

**Table 4-32** **"Lots of Spots": Red Rashes of Childhood: Image G.** Smallpox. Courtesy of the US Department of Health and Human Services and James Hicks. The image may have been modified by cropping, labeling, and/or captions. All rights to this adaptation by MedIQ Learning, LLC are reserved.

**Table 4-32** **"Lots of Spots": Red Rashes of Childhood: Image H.** Hand, foot and mouth disease. This image is a derivative work, adapted from the following source, available under : Rao PK, Veena K, Jagadishchandra H, Bhat SS, Shetty SR. Hand, Foot and Mouth Disease: Changing Indian Scenario. *Int J Clin Pediatr Dent.* 2012;5(3):220-222. doi:10.5005/jp-journals-10005-1171. The image may have been modified by cropping, labeling, and/or captions. All rights to this adaptation by MedIQ Learning, LLC are reserved.

**Table 4-32** **"Lots of Spots": Red Rashes of Childhood: Image I.** Molluscum bumps. Courtesy of the US Department of Health and Human Services and Dr. L. Sperling, MD.

## Pathology

**Figure 5-2**   **Liver metastases.** This image is a derivative work, adapted from the following source, available under [cc]: Takeyama H, Sawai H, Wakasugi T, et al. Successful paclitaxel-based chemotherapy for an alpha-fetoprotein-producing gastric cancer patient with multiple liver metastases. *World J Surg Oncol.* 2007;5:79. doi:10.1186/1477-7819-5-79. The image may have been modified by cropping, labeling, and/ or captions. All rights to this adaptation by MedIQ Learning, LLC are reserved.

**Figure 5-3**   **Brain metastases: Image A.** MRI showing multiple intracranial metastases with surrounding edema. This image is a derivative work, adapted from the following source, available under [cc]: Alsidawi S, Malek E, Driscoll JJ. MicroRNAs in Brain Metastases: Potential Role as Diagnostics and Therapeutics. *Int J Mol Sci.* 2014;15(6):10508-10526. doi:10.3390/ijms150610508. The image may have been modified by cropping, labeling, and/or captions. All rights to this adaptation by MedIQ Learning, LLC are reserved.

**Figure 5-3**   **Brain metastases: Image B.** Coronal view of cortical brain metastasis. [cc] Courtesy of the US Department of Health and Human Services and Armed Forces Institute of Pathology. The image may have been modified by cropping, labeling, and/or captions. All rights to this adaptation by MedIQ Learning, LLC are reserved.

**Figure 5-4**   **Bone metastases.** This image is a derivative work, adapted from the following source, available under [cc]: Yuasa T, Kitsukawa S, Sukegawa G, et al. Early onset recall pneumonitis during targeted therapy with sunitinib. *BMC Cancer.* 2013;13:3. doi:10.1186/1471-2407-13-3. The image may have been modified by cropping, labeling, and/or captions. All rights to this adaptation by MedIQ Learning, LLC are reserved.

**Figure 5-8**   **Necrosis: Image A.** Coagulative necrosis. [cc] Courtesy of the US Department of Health and Human Services and Dr. Steven Rosenberg. The image may have been modified by cropping, labeling, and/or captions. All rights to this adaptation by MedIQ Learning, LLC are reserved.

**Figure 5-8**   **Necrosis: Image B.** Liquefactive necrosis. Courtesy of Dr. Robert W. Novak.

**Figure 5-8**   **Necrosis: Image C.** Caseous necrosis. This image is a derivative work, adapted from the following source, available under [cc]. Courtesy of Dr. Yale Rosen. The image may have been modified by cropping, labeling, and/or captions. MedIQ Learning, LLC makes this image available under [cc].

**Figure 5-8**   **Necrosis: Image E.** Fibrinoid necrosis. This image is a derivative work, adapted from the following source, available under [cc]. Courtesy of Dr. Yale Rosen. The image may have been modified by cropping, labeling, and/or captions. MedIQ Learning, LLC makes this image available under [cc].

**Figure 5-8**   **Necrosis: Image F.** Acral gangrene. [cc] Courtesy of the US Department of Health and Human Services and William Archibald. The image may have been modified by cropping, labeling, and/or captions. All rights to this adaptation by MedIQ Learning, LLC are reserved.

## Public Health Sciences

**Figure 7-8**   **Outcomes matrix after exposure to a risk factor or intervention.** Le T, et al. *First Aid for the USMLE Step 1.* New York, NY: McGraw-Hill Education, 2017.

**Figure 7-11**   **Summary of possible results of any hypothesis test.** Le T, et al. *First Aid for the USMLE Step 1.* New York, NY: McGraw-Hill Education, 2017.

**Figure 7-18**   **PDSA cycle.** Le T, et al. *First Aid for the USMLE Step 1.* New York, NY: McGraw-Hill Education, 2017.

# Index

**NOTES**

**NOTES**

**NOTES**

**NOTES**

## NOTES

**NOTES**

**NOTES**

**NOTES**

**NOTES**

# About the Senior Editors

### Tao Le, MD, MHS

Tao developed a passion for medical education as a medical student. He currently edits more than 15 titles in the *First Aid* series. In addition, he is Founder and Chief Education Officer of USMLE-Rx for exam preparation and ScholarRx for undergraduate medical education. As a medical student, he was editor-in-chief of the University of California, San Francisco (UCSF) *Synapse,* a university newspaper with a weekly circulation of 9000. Tao earned his medical degree from UCSF in 1996 and completed his residency training in internal medicine at Yale University and fellowship training at Johns Hopkins University. Tao subsequently went on to cofound Medsn, a medical education technology venture, and served as its chief medical officer. He is currently chief of adult allergy and immunology at the University of Louisville.

### William L. Hwang, MD, PhD

William is currently a resident physician-scientist in the Harvard Radiation Oncology Program. He previously completed an Internal Medicine internship at Massachusetts General Hospital. In 2015, William graduated summa cum laude from the Harvard/MIT MD-PhD program and was awarded the Seidman Prize for Best Senior Thesis. He earned his PhD in Biophysics in the laboratory of Xiaowei Zhuang, elucidating the mechanism and regulation of chromatin remodeling using a combination of single-molecule biophysics and molecular biology approaches. Prior to that, William completed his undergraduate studies at Duke University with degrees in Biomedical Engineering, Electrical and Computer Engineering, and Physics on an Angier B Duke Scholarship. He then made the hop across the pond to complete a Masters in Chemistry at the University of Oxford as a Rhodes Scholar. Outside of the clinic/lab, he is passionate about educational outreach and directs a nonprofit educational organization, United InnoWorks Academy, which develops innovative STEM programs for underserved youth. In his free time, he enjoys traveling with his wife, Katie, and playing volleyball.

# About the Editors

### Luke R.G. Pike, MD, DPhil

Luke is a resident physician at the Harvard Radiation Oncology Program in Boston, Massachusetts. He grew up in Newfoundland, Canada, where he was awarded an honors degree in biochemistry and chemistry at Memorial University. He went on to earn a DPhil in medical oncology at Oxford University on a Rhodes Scholarship. His research focused on the molecular mechanisms by which cancer cells survive the hypoxic tumor microenvironment and ways in which those might be exploited in cancer therapy. He obtained a medical degree at Yale, followed by an internship in internal medicine at Massachusetts General Hospital, before beginning advanced training in radiation oncology. He is a competitive power lifter and has previously won the Canadian national championship and competed at the world championships in France and India. In his spare time, he enjoys adventure motorcycling and has done 3000+ mile trips in Europe/Scandinavia, South Africa, Namibia, and New Zealand.

### M. Scott Moore, DO

Scott's passions in medicine are clinical pathology, osteopathy, and education. After earning an AAS degree in clinical laboratory sciences and a BA in German from Weber State University, a DO from Midwestern University's Arizona College of Osteopathic Medicine, and completing a pathology internship at the University of Arizona, he was hired as a clinical research fellow at Affiliated Dermatology in Scottsdale. He and his wife have been married since college and they just welcomed twins to their family. In his free time he is an avid runner, guitarist, his wife's sous-chef, and plays his fair share of peek-a-boo.

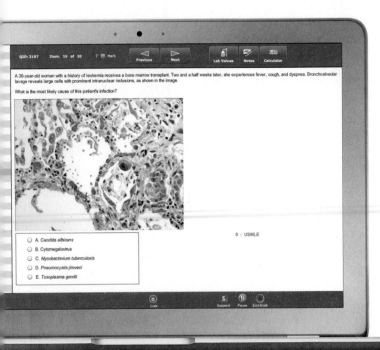
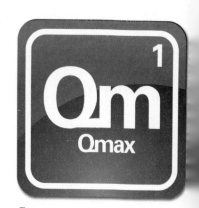